Clinical Nutrition

Edited on behalf of the Nutrition Society by

Michael J Gibney, Marinos Elia,
Olle Ljungqvist and Julie Dows~

Blackwell
Science

NS

© 2005 The Nutrition Society

Published by Blackwell Science,
a Blackwell Publishing company

Editorial offices:
Blackwell Science Ltd, 9600 Garsington Road, Oxford OX4 2DQ, UK
  Tel: +44 (0) 1865 776868
Blackwell Publishing Professional, 2121 State Avenue, Ames, Iowa 50014-8300, USA
  Tel: +1 515 292 0140
Blackwell Science Asia Pty, 550 Swanston Street, Carlton, Victoria 3053, Australia
  Tel: +61 (0)3 8359 1011

First published 2005

Library of Congress Cataloging-in-Publication Data
is available

ISBN-10: 0-632-05626-6
ISBN-13: 978-0-632-05626-2

A catalogue record for this title is available from the British Library

Set in Minion
by Sparks, Oxford – www.sparks.co.uk
Printed and bound in India
by Replika Press Pvt Ltd, Kundli

The publisher's policy is to use permanent paper from mills that operate a sustainable forestry policy, and which has been manufactured from pulp processed using acid-free and elementary chlorine-free practices. Furthermore, the publisher ensures that the text paper and cover board used have met acceptable environmental accreditation standards.

For further information on Blackwell Publishing, visit our website:
www.blackwellpublishing.com

The Human Nutrition Textbook Series

The International Scientific Committee

Editor-in-Chief
Professor Michael J Gibney
Trinity College, Dublin, Ireland

Assistant Editor
Julie Dowsett
Trinity College, Dublin, Ireland

Professor Lenore Arab
University of North Carolina, USA

Professor Yvon Carpentier
Université Libre de Bruxelles, Belgium

Professor Marinos Elia
University of Southampton, UK

Professor Frans J Kok
Wageningen University, Netherlands

Professor Olle Ljungqvist
Ersta Hospital, Karolinska Institute, Sweden

Professor Ian Macdonald
University of Nottingham, UK

Professor Barrie Margetts
University of Southampton, UK

Professor Kerin O'Dea
Menzies School of Health Research, Darwin, Australia

Dr Helen Roche
Trinity College, Dublin, Ireland

Professor Hester H Vorster
Potchefstroon, South Africa

Textbook Editors

Introduction to Human Nutrition
Editor-in-Chief
Professor Michael J Gibney
Trinity College, Dublin, Ireland

Professor Hester H Vorster
Potchefstroon, South Africa

Professor Frans J Kok
Wageningen University, Netherlands

Nutrition and Metabolism
Editor-in-Chief
Professor Michael J Gibney
Trinity College, Dublin, Ireland

Professor Ian Macdonald
University of Nottingham, UK

Dr Helen Roche
Trinity College, Dublin, Ireland

Public Health Nutrition
Editor-in-Chief
Professor Michael J Gibney
Trinity College, Dublin, Ireland

Professor Barrie Margetts
University of Southampton, UK

Professor Lenore Arab
University of North Carolina, USA

Dr John Kearney
Dublin Institute of Technology, Ireland

Clinical Nutrition
Editor-in-Chief
Professor Michael J Gibney
Trinity College, Dublin, Ireland

Professor Marinos Elia
University of Southampton, UK

Professor Olle Ljungqvist
Ersta Hospital, Karolinska Institute, Sweden

Julie Dowsett
Trinity College, Dublin, Ireland

www.nutritiontexts.com

A unique feature of the Nutrition Society Textbook Series is that each chapter will have its own web pages, accessible at www.nutritiontexts.com. In the course of time, each will have downloadable teaching aids, suggestions for projects, updates on the content of each chapter and sample multiple choice questions. With input from teachers and students we will have a vibrant, informative and social website.

The Human Nutrition Textbook Series comprises:

Introduction to Human Nutrition

Introduction to Human Nutrition: a global perspective on food and nutrition
Body composition
Energy metabolism
Nutrition and metabolism of proteins and amino acids
Digestion and metabolism of carbohydrates
Nutrition and metabolism of lipids
Dietary reference standards
The vitamins
Minerals and trace elements
Measuring food intake
Food composition
Food policy and regulatory issues
Nutrition research methodology
Food safety: a public health issue of growing importance
Food and nutrition: the global challenge

Nutrition and Metabolism

Core concepts of nutrition
Molecular nutrition
Integration of metabolism 1: Energy
Integration of metabolism 2: Protein and amino acids
Integration of metabolism 3: Macronutrients
Pregnancy and lactation
Growth and ageing
Nutrition and the brain
The sensory systems: taste, smell, chemesthesis and vision
The gastrointestinal tract
The cardiovascular system
The skeletal system
The immune and inflammatory systems
Phytochemicals
The control of food intake
Overnutrition
Undernutrition
Exercise performance

Public Health Nutrition

An overview of public health nutrition
Nutrition epidemiology
Food choice
Assessment of nutritional status at individual and population level
Assessment of physical activity
Overnutrition
Undernutrition
Eating disorders, dieting and food fads
PHN strategies for nutrition: intervention at the ecological level
Food and nutrition guidelines
Fetal programming
Cardiovascular disease
Cancer
Osteoporosis
Diabetes
Vitamin A deficiency
Iodine deficiency
Iron deficiency
Maternal and child health
Breast feeding
Adverse outcomes in pregnancy

Clinical Nutrition

Principles of clinical nutrition
Nutritional assessment
Overnutrition
Undernutrition
Metabolic disorders
Eating disorders
Adverse reactions to foods
Nutritional support
Ethics and nutrition
The gastrointestinal tract
Nutrition in liver disease
Nutrition and the pancreas
The kidney
Blood and bone marrow
The lung
Nutrition and immune and inflammatory systems
The heart and blood vessels
The skeleton
Nutrition in surgery and trauma
Infectious diseases
Malignant diseases
Pediatric nutrition
Cystic fibrosis
Water and electrolytes
Illustrative cases

Contents

The colour plate section falls after page 240.

Series Foreword

The early decades of the twentieth century was a period of intense research on constituents of food essential for normal growth and development and saw the discovery of most of the vitamins, minerals, amino acids, and essential fatty acids. In 1941, a group of leading physiologists, biochemists, and medical scientists recognized that the emerging discipline of nutrition needed its own learned society and The Nutrition Society was established. Our mission was, and remains, 'to advance the scientific study of nutrition and its application to the maintenance of human and animal health'. The Nutrition Society is the largest learned society for nutrition in Europe and we have over 2000 members worldwide. You can find out more about the Society and how to become a member by visiting our website at www.nutsoc.org.uk.

The ongoing revolution in biology initiated by large-scale genome mapping and facilitated by the development of reliable, simple-to-use molecular biological tools makes this a very exciting time to be working in nutrition. We now have the opportunity to get a much better understanding of how specific genes interact with nutritional intake and other lifestyle factors to influence gene expression in individual cells and tissues and, ultimately, effects on health. Knowledge of the polymorphisms in key genes carried by a patient will allow the prescription of more effective, and safe, dietary treatments. At the population level, molecular epidemiology is opening up much more incisive approaches to understanding the role of particular dietary patterns in disease causation. This excitement is reflected in the several scientific meetings which The Nutrition Society, often in collaboration with sister learned societies in Europe, organizes each year. We provide travel grants and other assistance to encourage students and young researchers to attend and to participate in these meetings.

Throughout its history a primary objective of the Society has been to encourage nutrition research and to disseminate the results of such research. Our first journal *The Proceedings of The Nutrition Society* recorded, as it still does, the scientific presentations made to the Society. Shortly afterwards, *The British Journal of Nutrition* was established to provide a medium for the publication of primary research on all aspects of human and animal nutrition by scientists from around the world. Recognizing the needs of students and their teachers for authoritative reviews on topical issues in nutrition, the Society began publishing *Nutrition Research Reviews* in 1988. More recently we launched *Public Health Nutrition,* the first international journal dedicated to this important and growing area. All of these journals are available in electronic, as well as in the conventional paper, form and we are exploring new opportunities to exploit the web to make the outcomes of nutritional research more quickly and more readily accessible.

To protect the public and to enhance the career prospects of nutritionists, The Nutrition Society is committed to ensuring that those who practice as nutritionists are properly trained and qualified. This is recognized by placing the names of suitably qualified individuals on our professional registers and by the award of the qualification Registered Public Health Nutritionist (RPHNutr) and Registered Nutritionist (RNutr). Graduates with appropriate degrees but who do not yet have sufficient postgraduate experience can join our Associate Nutritionist registers. We undertake accreditation of university degree programs in public health nutrition and are developing accreditation processes for other nutrition degree programs.

Just as in research, having the best possible tools is an enormous advantage in teaching and learning. This is the reasoning behind the initiative to launch this series of human nutrition textbooks designed for use worldwide. The Society is deeply indebted to our former President, Professor Mike Gibney, for his foresight, and to him and his team of editors for their innovative approaches and hard work, in bringing this major publishing exercise to successful fruition. Read, learn and enjoy.

John Mathers
President of the Nutrition Society 2001–2004
Newcastle upon Tyne

Preface

This volume completes the suite of four textbooks in nutrition organized by The Nutrition Society and it is worthwhile revisiting the origins of these publications. Human nutrition has grown dramatically in the last few decades and many new graduate and undergraduate courses have been established. The days when one textbook could adequately cover all the needs of such students is long gone and specialist textbooks are needed at all levels.

The present suite can be considered as individual textbooks but their main objective is to function together as a complete series for students of nutrition. The introductory book, *Introduction to Human Nutrition*, can be used by various groups of students, some of whom will have nutrition as a minor subject. The second, *Nutrition and Metabolism*, provides the bedrock of physiology and biochemistry on which the science of nutrition is built, while the third, *Public Health Nutrition*, discusses the broad spectrum of issues related to nutrition in the public health field. This current textbook is intended for those with an interest in nutrition in the clinical setting, whether they are dietitians or medics, nursing staff or other allied health professionals. Although overlap across the four textbooks is inevitable, the editors have worked hard to minimize and rationalize these overlaps.

Clinical Nutrition starts by setting the scene in assessing nutritional status and discusses the clinical consequences and current management options with under- and overnutrition and eating disorders and metabolic disease. Most of the later chapters then deal with the different organ systems of the body, setting out the most up-to-date thinking on the role of nutrition, whether it involves nutritional support, nutritional education, or a combination of the two.

At this point I would like to thank most sincerely not only the editors and authors of this volume, but also the entire team involved in this very ambitious project: all of the authors, all of the editors, The Nutrition Society, and the team at Blackwell Scientific. Start thinking of the second editions now!

Sadly, we must again record the death of two authors: Professor Vernon Young of MIT, author of two chapters; and Professor Clive West of Nageningen University, who also contributed two chapters to this series of books.

Michael J Gibney
Editor in Chief

Contributors

Simon Allison
Dept Clinical Nutrition
University Hospital
Queen's Medical Centre
Nottingham, UK

Zaira Aversa
Department of Clinical Medicine
University 'La Sapienza'
Rome, Italy

Karin Barndregt
University Hospital Maastricht
Dietetics Dept
Maastricht, The Netherlands

Bruce Bistrian
Beth Israel Deaconess Medical Centre
Boston, USA

Federico Bozzetti
Instituto Nazionale per lo Studio e la
    Cura dei Tumori
Milan, Italy

Eduard Cabré
Dept of Gastroenterology
Hosp. Universitari Germans Trias I
    Pujol
Barcelona, Spain

Julie Dowsett
Department of Nutrition and Dietics
St Vincent's University Hospital
Dublin, Ireland

Marinos Elia
Faculty of Medicine, Health and
    Biological Sciences
Institute of Human Nutrition
Southampton General Hospital
Southampton, UK

Filippo Rossi Fanelli
Department of Clinical Medicine
University 'La Sapienza'
Rome, Italy

Kenneth Fearon
Department of Clinical and Surgical
    Sciences (Surgery)
The Royal Infirmary of Edinburgh
Edinburgh, UK

Guzman Franch
Dept of Surgery
Hospital de Figueres
Universitat Pompeu Fabra
Barcelona, Spain

Gema Frühbeck
Dept of Endocrinology
Clínica Universitaria de Navarra
School of Medicine, University of
    Navarra
Pamplona, Spain

Miguel A Gassull
Dept of Gastroenterology
Hospital Universitari Germans Trias
    I Pujol
Barcelona, Spain

Meritxell Girvent
Facultat de Ciencies Experimental I
    de la Salut
Universitat Pompeu Fabra
Barcelona, Spain

Gabriella Grieco
Department of Clinical Medicine
University 'La Sapienza'
Rome, Italy

Bob Grimble
Institute of Human Nutrition
School of Medicine
University of Southampton
Southampton, UK

Gianfranco Guarnieri
Professor of Internal Medicine
Director, Division of Internal Medicine
University of Trieste
Cattinara Hospital
Trieste, Italy

Aref Haffejee
Department of Surgery
Faculty of Health Sciences
Nelson R. Mandela School of Medicine
University of Natal
Congella, South Africa

Marietjie Herselman
Department of Human Nutrition
Faculty of Health Sciences
University of Stellenbosch
Tygerberg, South Africa

Khursheed Jeejeebhoy
St Michael's Hospital
Toronto, Canada

Mark Kearney
Dept of Cardiology
Guy's, King's & St Thomas' School of
    Medicine
King's College
London, UK

Mary Keith
Research Associate
Division of Cardiovascular and
    Thoracic Surgery
St. Michael's Hospital
Toronto, Canada

Anura Kurpad
Dean, Institute of Population Health
    & Clinical Research
St. John's National Academy of Health
    Sciences
Bangalore
Karnataka, India

Demetre Labadarios
Department of Human Nutrition
Faculty of Health Sciences
University of Stellenbosch
Tygerberg, South Africa

Roderick Little
MRC Trauma Group
University of Manchester
Manchester, UK

Olle Ljungqvist
Professor of Surgery
Karolinska Institute
Centre for Surgical Sciences, and
Head of Centre for Gastrointestinal
    Disease
Ersta Hospital
Stockholm, Sweden

John Macfie
Consultant Surgeon
Dept of Surgery
Scarborough Hospital
Scarborough, UK

Simon Murch
Professor of Paediatrics and Child
    Health
Warwick Medical School
Clinical Sciences Research Institute
Coventry, UK

Tara Murphy
Dept Psychological Medicine
Great Ormond Street Hospital for
    Children
London, UK

Maurizio Muscaritoli
Department of Clinical Medicine
University 'La Sapienza'
Rome, Italy

Brian Noronha
Dept of Cardiology
Guy's, King's & St Thomas' School of
    Medicine
King's College
London, UK

Nicholas Paton
MRC Clinical Trials Unit
London, UK
and
Department of Infectious Diseaes
Tan Tock Seng Hospital
Singapore

Christine Rodda
Paediatric Endocrinology and
    Diabetes Unit
Honorary Senior Lecturer
Dept Biochemistry and Molecular
    Biology
Monash University
Clayton, Australia

Jean-Marc Schwartz
Dept of Nutritional Sciences and
    Toxicology
University of California, Berkeley
Berkeley, USA

Annemie Schols
University Maastricht
Dept of Pulmonology
Maastricht, The Netherlands

Roberta Situlin
Assistant Professor of Nutrition
University of Trieste
Cattinara Hospital
Trieste, Italy

Peter Soeters
Professor of Surgery
Academic Hospital Maastricht
Maastricht, The Netherlands

Antonio Stiges-Serra
Dept of Surgery
Hospital Universitari del Mar
Barcelona, Spain

Luc Tappy
Department of Physiology
Faculty of Biology and Medicine
Lausanne University
Lausanne, Switzerland

Gabriele Toigo
Associate Professor of Clinical
    Nutrition
Director, Division of Geriatrics
University of Trieste
Ospedale Maggiore
Trieste, Italy

Janet Treasure
Department Academic Psychiatry
Guys Campus
London, UK

Olive Tully
Dept Nutrition & Dietetics/National
    Referral Centre for Adult CF
St Vincent's University Hospital
Dublin, Ireland

Christo Van Rensburg
Department of Internal Medicine
Gastroenterology Unit
Faculty of Health Sciences
University of Stellenbosch and
    Tygerberg Academic Hospital
Tygerberg, South Africa

Stephen Wheatcroft
Dept of Cardiology
Guy's, King's & St Thomas' School of
    Medicine
King's College
London, UK

Anthony F Williams
Division of Child Health
Department of Clinical
    Developmental Sciences
St Georges Hospital Medical School
London, UK

EFM Wouters
Professor and Chairman
Department of Pulmonology
University Hospital Maastricht
The Netherlands

Jean Fabien Zazzo
Surgical Intensive Care Unit
Hopital Antoine Beclere
Clamart, France

1
Principles of Clinical Nutrition: Contrasting the practice of nutrition in health and disease

Marinos Elia

Key messages

- To understand how to best meet the nutritional needs of an individual, the distinction between physiology in health and pathophysiology in disease needs to be carefully considered.
- For some groups of patients the requirements are higher than those in health, while for other groups of patients they are lower. If recommendations for healthy individuals are applied to patients with certain types of diseases, they may produce harm.
- In health, only the oral route is used to provide nutrients to the body. In clinical practice other routes can be used. The use of the intravenous route for feeding raises a number of new issues.
- Alterations in nutritional therapy during the course of an acute disease may occur because the underlying disease has produced new complications or because it has resolved. Similarly, in more chronic conditions there is a need to review the diet at regular intervals.

1.1 Introduction

Clinical nutrition focuses on the nutritional management of individual patients or groups of patients with established disease, in contrast to public health nutrition, which focuses on health promotion and disease prevention in the general population. The two disciplines overlap, however, especially in older people, who are often affected by a range of disabilities or diseases. Working together, instead of independently, the two disciplines are more likely to facilitate successful implementation of local, national, and international policies on nutrition. To understand the overlap between them, it is not only necessary to consider some of the principles of nutrition that apply to health, but also special issues that apply to the field of clinical nutrition. These include altered nutritional requirements associated with disease, disease severity and malnutrition, and non-physiological routes of feeding using unusual feeds and feeding schedules. This introductory chapter provides a short overview of these issues partly because they delineate qualitative or quantitative differences between health and disease, and partly because they form a thread that links subsequent sections of this book, which is divided into discrete chapters that deal with specific conditions.

It is now possible to feed all types of patients over extended periods of time, including those who are unconscious, unable to eat or swallow, or have little or no functional gastrointestinal tract. It is possible to target specific patient groups with special formulations, and to even change the formulation in the same patient as nutritional demands alter during the course of an illness. Since some of these formulations may be beneficial to some patient groups and detrimental to other groups or to healthy subjects, the distinction between physiology in health and pathophysiology in disease needs to be considered carefully. It is hoped that some of the principles outlined here will help to establish a conceptual framework for considering some of the apparently diverse conditions discussed in this textbook.

1.2 The spectrum of nutritional problems

Clinical nutrition aims to treat (and prevent) suffering from malnutrition. However, there is no universally accepted definition for 'malnutrition' (literally 'bad nutrition'). The following definition, which encompasses both under- and overnutrition, is offered for the purposes of this chapter.

> Malnutrition is a state of nutrition in which a deficiency or excess (or imbalance) of energy, protein, and other nutrients causes measurable adverse effects on tissue/body function (shape, size, and composition) and function, and clinical outcome.

In this chapter and elsewhere, however, the term malnutrition is mainly used to refer to under- rather than overnutrition.

Both under- and overnutrition have adverse physiological and clinical effects. Those relating to undernutrition (Table 1.1) are diverse, which explains why malnourished patients may present to a wide range of medical disciplines. Several manifestations may occur simultaneously in the same individual, although some predominate, such as those that have a contribution from independent causes. Specific nutrient deficiencies may also have diverse effects, affecting multiple systems, but it is not entirely clear why the same deficiency can present in a certain way in one subject and a different way in another. For example, it is not entirely clear why some patients with deficiency of vitamin B_{12} present to the hematologist with megaloblastic anemia, others to the neurologist with neuropathy and other neurological manifestations (e.g. subacute combined degeneration of the cord), and yet others to the geriatrician with cognitive impairment or dementia.

The spectrum of presentations is more diverse than the above would indicate because protein–energy malnutrition frequently coexists with various nutrient deficiencies. For example, patients with gastrointestinal problems are frequently underweight and at the same time exhibit magnesium, sodium, potassium, and zinc deficiencies, due to excessive losses of these nutrients in diarrhea or other gastrointestinal effluents. There may also be problems with absorption. For example patients with Crohn's disease affecting the terminal ileum, where vitamin B_{12} is absorbed, are at increased risk of developing B_{12} deficiency. Patients who have had surgical removal of their terminal ileum or stomach, which produces the intrinsic factor necessary for B_{12} absorption, also fail to absorb vitamin B_{12}. Isolated nutrient deficiencies may also occur, for example iron deficiency due to heavy periods in otherwise healthy women.

Another complexity is the interaction between nutrients, which may occur at the level of absorption, metabolism within the body, or excretion. One nutrient may facilitate the absorption of another, for example glucose enhances the absorption of sodium (on the glucose–sodium cotransporter). This is the main reason why oral rehydration solutions to correct salt deficiency due to diarrhea (or fluid losses due to other gastrointestinal diseases) contain both salt and glucose. In contrast, other nutrients compete with each other for absorption. For example, because of competition between zinc and copper for intestinal absorption, administration of copper may precipitate zinc defi-

Table 1.1 Physical and psychosocial effects of undernutrition

Adverse effect	Consequence
Physical	
Impaired immune responses	Predisposes to infection
Reduced muscle strength and fatigue	Inactivity, inability to work effectively, and poor self-care. Abnormal muscle (or neuromuscular) function may also predispose to falls or other accidents
Reduced respiratory muscle strength	Poor cough pressure, predisposing to and delaying recovery from chest infection
Inactivity, especially in bed-bound patient	Predisposes to pressure sores and thromboembolism
Impaired thermoregulation	Hypothermia, especially in the elderly
Impaired wound healing	Failure of fistulae to close, un-united fractures, increased risk of wound infection resulting in prolonged recovery from illness, increased length of hospital stay, and delayed return to work (Haydock and Hill, 1987)
Fetal and infant programming	Predisposes to common chronic diseases, such as cardiovascular disease, stroke, and diabetes in adult life
Growth failure	Stunting, delayed sexual development, reduced muscle mass, and strength
Psychosocial	
Impaired psychosocial function	Even when uncomplicated by disease, undernutrition causes apathy, depression, self-neglect, hypochondriasis, loss of libido, and deterioration in social interactions (Keys *et al.*, 1950). It also affects personality and impairs mother-to-child bonding (Brozek, 1990)

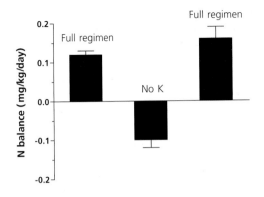

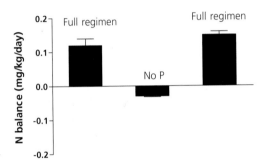

Figure 1.1 Effect of omitting potassium (K) and phosphate (P) from a parenteral nutrition regimen on the nitrogen (N) balance of depleted patients receiving hypercaloric feeding. Adapted from Rudman *et al.* (1975) with permission.

ciency, especially in those with borderline zinc status. Other nutrients interact with each other during tissue deposition. Accretion of lean tissue requires multiple nutrients, and lack of one of them, such as potassium, phosphate, and possibly other nutrients contained within lean tissue, can limit its deposition, even when adequate amounts of protein and energy are available (Figure 1.1). This emphasizes the need to provide all necessary nutrients in appropriate amounts.

1.3 Nutrient requirements

Effect of disease and nutritional status

Fluid and electrolytes

The principles of nutrient requirements in healthy individuals are described in *Introduction to Human Nutrition*, an earlier volume in this textbook series. The average nutrient intake refers to the average intake necessary to maintain nutrient balance. The reference nutrient intake (RNI) refers to the intake necessary to satisfy the requirements of 97.5% of the population (+ 2 standard deviations from the average nutrient intake). In patients with a variety of diseases the requirements are more variable (Figure 1.2). For some groups of patients the requirements are higher than those in health, while for other groups of patients they are lower. For example, in patients with gastrointestinal fluid losses, the requirement for sodium may be double the reference nutrient intake, while in patients with severe renal or liver disease who retain salt and water, the requirements may be well below the average nutrient requirement for healthy subjects ingesting an oral diet. Therefore, if recommendations for healthy individuals are applied to patients with certain types of diseases, they may produce harm. A general guide to the requirements of sodium and potassium in patients with gastrointestinal fluid loss (above those for maintenance) is provided in Table 1.2, which shows the electrolyte content of various fluids. A person with a loss of 1.5 liters of small intestinal fluid may require

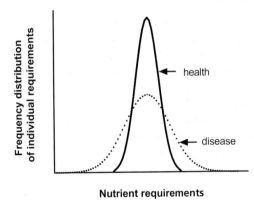

Figure 1.2 Frequency distribution of nutrient requirements in health and disease.

Table 1.2 Electrolyte contents of some body secretions (mmol/l)

Secretion/excretion	Na	K
Gastric	60	10
Pancreatic	140	5
Biliary	140	5
Small intestinal	100	10
Diarrhea	60[a]	20
Feces	25	55
Sweat: insensible	10	10
visible	60	10

[a] Variable (30–140 mmol/l)

~150 mmol of sodium above maintenance (the RNI for sodium is 70 mmol/day according to UK reference standards), whereas loss of the same volume of nasogastrically aspirated fluid requires only ~90 mmol extra sodium. Note that the requirements for potassium in patients losing gastrointestinal fluid are generally much lower than for sodium (Table 1.2).

Excessive salt and fluid administration can be just as detrimental as inadequate intake, causing fluid retention and heart failure in some individuals. Fluid retention is often detected clinically by noting pitting edema at the ankles or over the sacrum, but edema can also affect internal tissues and organs, causing a variety of problems. Some of these problems are shown in Table 1.3. A recent study has questioned the routine clinical practice of administering large amounts of fluid in the early postoperative period in an attempt to reduce the risk of hypotension. In a randomized controlled trial carried out in Denmark, routine fluid administration was compared with a fluid-restricted regimen that aimed to approximately maintain body weight. In those receiving routine fluid therapy, not only did body weight increase significantly more than in the fluid-restricted group, but it significantly increased a variety of complications, including tissue-healing and cardiopulmonary complications. It also increased mortality, but this did not reach statistical significance, possibly because only a small number of subjects died during the course of the study. Acute accidental and elective surgical trauma is associated with a tendency to retain salt and water, at least partly because of increased secretion of mineralocorticoids and antidiuretic hormone. Therefore, administration of excess salt and water as in protein-energy malnutrition may lead to fluid retention that would not occur in normal subjects.

Table 1.3 Problems caused by edema

Site of edema	Consequence
Liver	Abnormal liver function tests
Gastrointestinal tract	Impaired gastric motility with subsequent delay in the time taken to tolerate oral food and recover from abdominal surgery
Brain	Impaired consciousness in those with a head injury, which is associated with some pre-existing cerebral edema
Wounds	Delayed healing

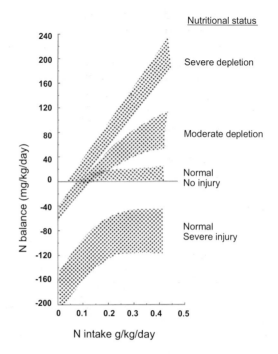

Figure 1.3 Effect of increasing protein (N) intake on N balance in depleted, healthy, and catabolic patients close to energy balance.

Protein

Another difference between nutritional requirements in health and disease concerns body composition and nutrient balance. In healthy adults, nutritional intake aims to maintain body composition (lean body mass and fat mass) within a desirable range, but this may not be the case in disease and malnutrition. Consider the effect of increasing protein intake in normal, depleted, and catabolic subjects (severe acute disease), all of whom are close to energy balance (Figure 1.3). In healthy subjects nitrogen (N) (1 g N = 6.25 g protein) balance is achieved with an intake close to 0.1 g N/kg/day (the RNI is ~0.12 g N/kg/day according to UK reference data, although other more recent data suggest the need for a small revision upwards). Increasing the N intake above this amount leads to little or no further net protein deposition. Depleted subjects continue to deposit protein (positive N balance) when intake is increased above 0.1 g N/kg/day, while catabolic patients show a negative N balance, which shows little improvement above an intake of ~0.25 g N/kg/day. With this in mind, protein requirements take into account the need to limit, but not necessarily abolish, N losses in catabolic patients, and the need to replete tissues in malnourished patients so that their function improves. These criteria differ from those in healthy well-functioning adults, who have no need to change their body composition. In contrast, in healthy children it is necessary to cater for growth and development, which is associated with deposition of tissue and a positive N balance. Similar considerations apply to calculating the requirements of other nutrients and of energy, but metabolism in health and disease differs in a number of ways which affects concepts about requirements.

Energy

In healthy subjects the energy requirements necessary to maintain energy stores are often calculated as multiples of basal metabolic rate (BMR). However, in many acute diseases (Figure 1.4) and a number of chronic diseases, BMR was found to be increased, which led to the view that the energy requirements in such states were also usually increased. This conclusion failed to take into account the decrease in physical activity that occurs as a result of many diseases and disabilities. This decrease counteracts or more than counteracts the increase in BMR, so that total energy expenditure in most disease states (and hence the energy intake necessary to maintain balance) is actually close to normal or even decreased. As indicated above, there is also the need to consider changes in energy stores. In obese individuals it is desirable to reduce the energy stores by providing hypocaloric feeding, and in depleted patients to increase energy stores by providing hypercaloric feeding. In both cases it is usually better to do this during the recovery phase of illness rather than the acute and more unstable phase of illness (see below).

In estimating energy requirements of the hospitalized patient it is worth considering the energy contribution from non-dietary sources, such as intravenous dextrose 5% (~200 kcal/l), dialysate, and fat-based drugs such as propofol (~1.1 kcal/ml).

Metabolic blocks and nutritional requirements

Inborn errors of metabolism

When there is a block in a metabolic pathway that involves conversion of substance A to B, there is accumulation of substance A, which may be toxic (either directly or via its products), and a depletion in substance B, which needs to be either formed within the

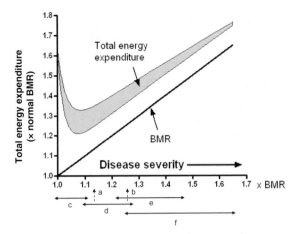

Figure 1.4 Effect of acute disease severity (expressed as multiples of normal basal metabolic rate (BMR)) on total energy expenditure (shaded area). The difference between total energy expenditure and BMR is due to physical activity (and some thermogenesis, which typically accounts for ~10% of energy intake). The increase in BMR is counteracted by a decrease in physical activity. (a) Infection, persistent fever (1°C); (b) infection, persistent fever (2°C); (c) burns 10% (1st month), single fracture (1st week), postoperative (1st 4 days); (d) burns 10–25% (1st month), multiple long bone fractures (1st week); (e) severe sepsis/multiple trauma (patient on respirator); (f) burns 25–95% (1st month).

body by alternative pathways or provided by the diet. An alternative strategy is to replace the enzyme responsible for the block, for example by organ transplantation, although this has only used for a few metabolic disorders. One of the best known examples of a metabolic block occurs in phenylketonurea (PKU), due to deficiency of the enzyme phenylalanine hydroxylase, which is located on chromosome 12 (12q). In the absence of phenylalanine hydroxylase, which normally converts the amino acid phenylalanine to tyrosine in the liver, there is accumulation of phenylalanine and its metabolites, which causes brain damage, mental retardation, and epilepsy. Tyrosine, which is distal to the block, is provided by the diet. The treatment for PKU is to ingest a low-phenylalanine diet (some phenylalanine is required for protein synthesis) (see later section for duration of treatment). The diet, which is not found in nature, is specifically manufactured to restrict the intake of phenylalanine. Other metabolic blocks may require exclusion of other individual nutrients, for example restriction of galactose and lactose in children with galactosemia. Some diets may exclude whole proteins, which may cause food allergy or sensitivity. In the case of celiac disease, which is responsible for a small bowel enteropathy with malabsorption, this means avoiding gluten, which is found in wheat and wheat products (see Chapter 7). However, the problem here is not due to a block in a metabolic pathway, but to an abnormal reaction to food, which appears to be acquired.

Acquired metabolic blocks

Not all metabolic blocks are inherited as inborn errors of metabolism. For example, deficiency of phenyl-alanine hydroxylase can occur as a result of cirrhosis. Since in healthy subjects tyrosine can be formed from phenylalanine, some feed manufacturers felt that they could add little or no tyrosine to parenteral nutrition regimens, especially since tyrosine has a low solubility. However, a few patients with severe liver disease lose their ability to synthesize tyrosine, with the result that it becomes rate limiting to protein synthesis, even in the presence of all other necessary amino acids (i.e. the enzymatic deficiency is ultimately responsible for the metabolic block in protein synthesis, which can be reversed by administering tyrosine). Other examples of acquired metabolic blocks due to amino acids involve histidine in some patients with renal disease, and cystine in liver disease. It is therefore essential that these amino acids (described as conditionally essential) are provided in the diet (oral or intravenous) of such patients even though they are not essential for healthy subjects.

Acquired metabolic blocks may involve pathways other than those of amino acids. An interesting example concerns vitamin D, which is hydroxylated in the liver to produce 25-hydroxy vitamin D and further hydroxylated in the kidney to produce the active metabolite 1,25-dihydroxy vitamin D (Figure 1.5). Some patients with chronic renal failure are unable to produce sufficient amounts of 1,25-dihydroxy vitamin D, due to loss of activity of the enzyme 1 alpha hydroxylase in the kidney. Such patients may suffer from metabolic bone disease, which is at least partly due to deficiency of 1,25-dihydroxy vitamin D. This metabolic block can be bypassed by providing either synthetic 1,25-dihydroxy vitamin D or synthetic 1-hydroxy vitamin D, which is converted to 1,25-dihydroxy vitamin D in the liver (Figure 1.5). Such therapy differs from that used in treatment of PKU in at least two ways: it involves administration of substance distal to the block (cf. restriction of phenylalanine, which is proximal to the block) and it is not found in the normal diet in any significant amounts. It is an example of nutritional pharmacology involving administration of a bioactive substance.

A variety of other bioactive substances have been used in clinical nutrition with the aim of improving outcome. Some products of metabolism require more than one class of substrates for their synthesis. For example hemoglobin (Hb) comprises a variety of amino acids and iron, which forms part of the heme component. All the substrates may be available in adequate quantities, but a block in Hb synthesis may still occur as a result of a deficiency of erythropoietin. This is a bioactive substance produced by the kidney that stimulates Hb synthesis. Erythropoietin synthesis is upregulated during hypoxia, which explains the high Hb concentrations in people living in high altitudes. In contrast, lack of erythropoietin leads to anemia. One of the features of end stage renal failure is severe anemia, which is at least partly due to the inability of the damaged kidney to produce enough erythropoietin. Traditionally, this anemia was treated by repeated blood

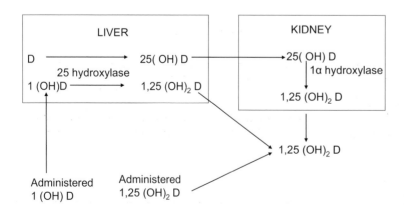

Figure 1.5 Metabolism of vitamin D in the liver and kidney. In renal failure the formation of 1,25-dihydroxy vitamin D (1,25 (OH)$_2$ D) in the kidney may be inadequate and therefore 1,25-dihydroxy vitamin D or 1-hydroxy vitamin D (25 (OH) D) can be prescribed.

transfusions. Now that recombinant erythropoietin is available it can be used to treat this anemia and to eliminate or dramatically reduce the need for repeated blood transfusions, which carry risk of transmitting infections, such as HIV and hepatitis, and which requires admission of patients to special health care facilities to provide the transfusions. Importantly, injections of recombinant erythropoietin have also been shown to improve quality of life. Other examples of nutritional pharmacology, shown in Table 1.4, are divided into those involving administration of prenutrients, pharmacological doses of normal nutrients, and bioactive substances (see table for the rationale for specific types of nutritional pharmacology).

The uncritical use of bioactive substances can produce unpredictable serious side effects, including death. An example involves injections of pharmacological doses of growth hormone (GH) in critically ill patients. It was thought that GH might be beneficial by limiting the marked N loss that frequently occurs in such patients (equivalent to overcoming a metabolic block in net protein synthesis). GH is known to stimulate protein synthesis, and had previously been shown to improve N balance in a wide range of clinical conditions. However, in a large multicenter trial involving patients admitted to intensive care units, pharmacological doses of GH doubled mortality compared with the placebo group (from about 20% to 40%), sending signals to the scientific and clinical community about the dangers of such interventions, especially when the mechanisms of action had not been previously evaluated.

The mechanism(s) responsible for the increased mortality with GH is still uncertain, but several suggestions have been made. One is that large doses of GH have detrimental effects on immune cells, which play a key role in host defense in critical illness. Another concerns the fluid-retaining properties of GH (see above for detrimental effects of fluid overload). Yet another concerns the protein-stimulating properties of GH, which was, paradoxically, the main reason for using GH in the first place. Since muscle is thought to be a major site of action of GH it is possible that stimulation of protein synthesis here may limit the availability of amino acids, including glutamine, to other tissues. These amino acids would normally be used for synthesis of proteins, for example the acute phase proteins in the liver, which participate in the response to infection and inflammation. They are also normally used as fuels for a variety of cells including immune cells (some

Table 1.4 Some examples of nutritional pharmacology

Type I (prenutrients)	
Organic phosphates	The amount of calcium and phosphate that can be added to parenteral nutrition solutions is limited by the solubility of calcium phosphate, which can precipitate. Organic phosphates, such glycerol-phosphate or glucose-phosphate, are soluble and do not precipitate in the presence of calcium. The organic phosphate is hydrolysed within the body to yield free phosphate
Dipeptides	Glutamine degrades during heat sterilization and storage of parenteral amino acid solutions. It can be provided as a dipeptide (e.g. alanylglutamine), which is stable and can be stored for extended periods of time. Poorly soluble amino acids can be provided as soluble dipetides, such as glycyltyrosine or alanylcystine. The dipeptides are hydrolysed within the body to yield free amino acids
Type II (pharmacological doses)	
Glycerol	Free glycerol is used as an emulsifying agent in intravenous fat solutions
Medium-chain triglycerides	Medium-chain triglycerides (up to 50% of total lipid) may be better absorbed and tolerated than long-chain triglyceride. In intravenous use may avoid infusional hyperlipidemia
Glutamine	Glutamine may be given in large amounts (12–30 g) with the aim of improving clinical outcome (e.g. in intensive care units)
Oligofructose	Bifidobacteria or oligofructose, which is a fermentable bifidogenic substrate, can be given orally with the aim of changing intestinal microflora and reducing the growth of potentially pathogenic organisms
Type III (bioactive substances)	
Erythropoietin	See text
1,25-dihydroxy and 1-hydroxy vitamin D	See text
Growth hormone	see text

preferentially utilizing glutamine as a fuel), which play an important role in combating infection.

It has also been suggested that some of the detrimental effects of GH are due to cardiac arrhythmias from high concentrations of non-esterified fatty acids produced by the lipolytic effect of GH. Another suggestion is that the mortality is partly due to disturbances in glucose homeostasis, since GH produced significantly higher circulating glucose concentrations than the placebo.

The importance of strict glucose homeostasis in critically ill patients is demonstrated by another large study involving about 1500 patients, who were randomized to receive insulin to control their plasma glucose concentrations strictly between 4.4 and 6.1 mmol/l, or to receive standard therapy, in which a circulating concentration of 10.0–11.1 mmol was considered acceptable. In the strictly controlled group there was a two-fold reduction in mortality and a two-fold reduction in the number of transfusions and critical care polyneuropathy.

Effect of route of feeding on nutrient requirements

In health, only the oral route is used to provide nutrients to the body; in clinical practice other routes can be used. Before discussing their effect on nutrient requirements it is necessary to briefly consider the type of nutritional support and feeding route. In general, food is the first line of treatment, but if this is inadequate to meets the needs of patients, supplements may be used, followed by enteral tube feeding and then intravenous (parenteral nutrition). However, this linear sequence to the decision-making process is inadequate in a number of situations. The first-line treatment for someone who has acutely developed the short bowel syndrome is parenteral nutrition, not oral nutrition, oral supplements, or even enteral tube feeding. Similarly, tube feeding may be the first-line treatment for a patient with a swallowing problem – not oral food or supplements, which can cause detrimental effects. In some situations (e.g. cerebral palsy) oral feeding is possible but this can take several hours per day and so it may be more practical to tube feed. In essence, the simplest, most physiological, and safest route to provide a patient's nutritional requirements should be sought, while taking into account the practicalities of feeding. Occasional unusual and unsuspected routes

deliver nutrients into the body (see below). The route of feeding can have major effects on nutrient requirements, particularly parenteral nutrition.

Parenteral nutrition

The use of the intravenous route for feeding raises a number of new issues, especially in relation to nutrients that are poorly absorbed by the gut. For some nutrients, such as sodium, potassium iodide, fluoride, and selenium, which are well absorbed, the intravenous requirements are similar to the oral requirements. For nutrients that are poorly absorbed, such as iron, calcium, and especially chromium and manganese, the intravenous requirements are considerably lower than the oral requirements, sometimes up to 10-fold lower (Figure 1.6). If the doses of some of these trace elements or minerals recommended for oral nutrition were used intravenously over prolonged periods of time, they would probably produce toxic effects.

This consideration highlights the key role of the gut in regulating the amount of micronutrients absorbed in health. Sometimes the gut plays the only important role in controlling the status of nutrients within the body. For example, there is no effective physiological

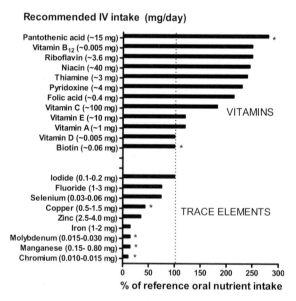

Figure 1.6 Recommended doses of vitamins and trace elements for intravenous (IV) nutrition expressed as a percentage of the recommended nutrient intake (UK values). Those marked with an asterisk indicate nutrients for which there was inadequate information to establish a reference nutrient intake (RNI). For these nutrients the midpoint of the estimated average oral intake is used for comparative purposes.

way of eliminating excess iron once it is within the body. In contrast to the recommended intakes of intravenous trace elements, those for intravenous vitamins are usually higher than the RNI for oral nutrition (Figure 1.6). There are several reasons why this is so. First, patients receiving parenteral (intravenous) nutrition usually have severe disease, which may increase the requirements for some vitamins. Secondly, patients are often affected by pre-existing malnutrition and are in need of repletion. Thirdly, the prescribed nutrients may not be delivered to the patient because they are lost during preparation or storage (e.g. vitamin C may be oxidized by oxygen present in the bag, a process catalysed by copper; some nutrients may be adsorbed on to the plastic bag containing the parenteral nutrition solution).

Gastric and jejunal feeding
Feed may be delivered directly into the stomach using a nasogastric tube, or a gastrostomy tube for long-term feeding in patients with swallowing difficulties. Jejunal feeding (e.g. jejunostomy or nasojejunal tube feeding) can be used in patients with poor gastric emptying, those at risk of regurgitation and aspiration pneumonia, and those with abnormal gastric anatomy and function. Nutrient requirements associated with these routes of feeding when the bowel is functioning normally, are generally similar to those for oral feeding, although many patients on long-term tube feeding are physically inactive due to the underlying disease, and therefore their energy requirements may be less than in healthy subjects. An unusual complication of enteral tube feeding concerns the neurological control of eating. A few children who start tube feeding when young and continue receiving it for prolonged periods, may 'forget' how to eat. They may have to re-learn how to eat when tube feeding is terminated. In contrast, some patients with dementia appear to forget how to eat, have difficulty in re-learning, and may need to start tube feeding.

Subcutaneous
Subcutaneous infusions of saline/dextrose may be given to maintain comfort and hydration in some terminally ill patients requiring palliative care, who cannot drink or eat and who have poor venous access.

Rectal
One of the physiological functions of the large bowel is to absorb salt and water, a property that can be utilized by a rectal infusion of saline in terminally ill patients who are unable to eat/drink and have poor venous access. In the past, rectal feeding has been used to provide a range of other nutrients, including alcohol, which is relatively well absorbed from the large bowel. In 1881, American President James A. Garfield received rectal feeding, which included alcohol, during his terminal illness following a gunshot wound inflicted by an assassin.

Skin
Essential fatty acid deficiency can be treated or prevented by topical skin application of corn oil or safflower oil, which allows sufficient uptake of essential fatty acids into the body. These observations are of more scientific/historical than practical clinical interest, since essential fatty acids can usually be delivered into the gut or directly into veins. Irradiation of the skin with ultraviolet light can also be used to prevent vitamin D deficiency in housebound patients not exposed to direct sunlight. Alternatively, vitamin D tablets can be prescribed, especially since the amount of vitamin in the normal diet is unlikely to contain sufficient amounts to meet the RNI (10 µg/day for subjects aged over 50 years, according to UK recommendations).

Peritoneal
During peritoneal dialysis with solutions of hypertonic glucose, which can cross the peritoneal membrane, several hundred calories may enter the systemic circulation. This is a side effect of treatment which is often not appreciated.

It is useful to remember that tissues that are used to provide nutritional access to the body can also be sites of abnormal nutrient losses, e.g. loss of protein, trace elements from burned skin, loss of protein from the kidney of patients with nephrotic syndrome, and loss of a variety of nutrients from the gut in patients with inflammatory bowel disease or diarrhea.

Effect of phase of disease on nutritional requirements

One of the first steps in the management of patients with severe acute disease is to resuscitate them to establish adequate oxygenation and acid–base status, as well as cardiovascular and metabolic stability. This may involve correcting dehydration or overhydration, and treating any hypoglycemia or hypothermia. Aggressive nutritional support before this stability is established can precipitate further problems with adverse clinical outcomes. For example, a common consequence of major abdominal surgery or systemic illness is ileus or slow gastric emptying. To facilitate oral feeding after surgery, several actions are useful. These include:

- using appropriate analgesia including local anesthetics given via a continuous epidural catheter during the first few days after surgery (this minimizes the need for opiates that have inhibitory effects on gastrointestinal motility);
- avoiding overhydration, which predisposes to postoperative ileus;
- ensuring that the patient is fully informed that they should eat.

For some patients there are risks with giving normal food or oral nutrition shortly after surgery. Aggressive feeding by mouth or by a nasogastric tube may still lead to gastric pooling, predisposing to nausea, vomiting, regurgitation, or aspiration pneumonia. This is more likely to happen in patients who have swallowing problems, pre-existing reflux problems (e.g. in association with a hiatus hernia), or are nursed in a horizontal position.

Aggressive intravenous nutrition with copious amounts of glucose in the early phase of an acute illness, when there is insulin resistance, can result in hyperglycemia, hyperosmolarity, and exacerbation of existing metabolic instability. During the early phase of a severe acute illness it may therefore sometimes be necessary to start with hypocaloric nutrition and increase it over a period of time. This is to ensure metabolic stability and tolerance to nutrients, while maintaining adequate tissue function and limiting excess N loss.

Tissue repletion is mainly recommended during the recovery phase of an acute illness. Similarly, in obese patients the focus on long-term weight loss usually occurs after the acute phase of illness.

The World Health Organization has provided a ten-step guide to the nutritional management of malnourished children, which re-emphasizes the need to consider nutritional support according to the phase of disease. Again, this begins with the stabilization phase, which is associated with resuscitation, followed by the rehabilitation phase, which can take several weeks, and finally the follow-up phase (Figure 1.7). It is notable that the guidelines suggest withholding iron supplementation during the early phase of illness. This is because of concern about the possible adverse effect of iron, which has pro-oxidant properties that facilitate formation of free radicals, which in turn produce cellular damage. The risk is considered to be greater during the early phase of disease, when oxidant stresses are high and antioxidant defences are frequently low as a result of pre-existing malnutrition.

A particular complication of aggressive refeeding of malnourished individuals is the refeeding syndrome. Rapid refeeding of such individuals can precipitate respiratory, cardiovascular, and metabolic problems

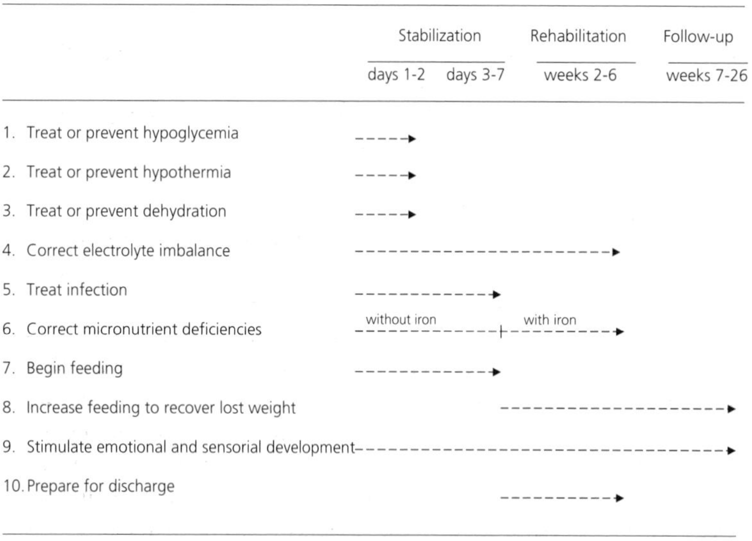

	Stabilization		Rehabilitation	Follow-up
	days 1-2	days 3-7	weeks 2-6	weeks 7-26
1. Treat or prevent hypoglycemia	----▸			
2. Treat or prevent hypothermia	----▸			
3. Treat or prevent dehydration	----▸			
4. Correct electrolyte imbalance	-------------------------▸			
5. Treat infection	--------------▸			
6. Correct micronutrient deficiencies	without iron --------⊢	with iron -------▸		
7. Begin feeding	------------▸			
8. Increase feeding to recover lost weight			-------------------▸	
9. Stimulate emotional and sensorial development	--▸			
10. Prepare for discharge			----------▸	

Figure 1.7 Time frame for the management of the child with severe malnutrition (the 10-step approach recommended by the World Health Organization). Reproduced from WHO (2000) with permission.

that may result in sudden death. For example, sudden death was reported when victims of World War II concentration camps were rapidly re-fed, especially with high carbohydrate diets. The metabolic abnormalities of the refeeding syndrome include low circulating concentrations of potassium, magnesium, and phosphate, which enter lean tissue cells during the process of repletion under the influence of insulin. The low circulating concentrations of these nutrients can precipitate cardiac arrhythmias and sudden death. Slow initial refeeding while monitoring the circulating concentration of these nutrients can reduce the risk of them developing the refeeding syndrome. Precise feeding schedules vary from center to center, although they may begin with half, or less than half of the requirements in severely depleted individuals.

Alterations in nutritional therapy during the course of an acute disease may occur because the underlying disease has produced new complications or because it has resolved. Similarly, in more chronic conditions there is a need to review the diet at regular intervals. A therapeutic diet lacking particular dietary components may no longer be needed if, for example, a specific food allergy or sensitivity has resolved. Another consideration is whether a vulnerable developmental period has passed. It used to be thought that cerebral damage due to phenylketonurea did not occur after the early developmental period so that it would be possible to replace the phenylalanine-poor diet with a more normal diet during later childhood, despite persistence of the underlying metabolic abnormality. Children who reverted to a normal diet, especially during early childhood, however, were found to be particularly vulnerable to regression of the developmental quotient (IQ) and development of other neurological symptoms. Children who stopped the phenylalanine-poor diet at or after the age of 15 have generally not been affected in this way, but few long-term follow-up studies (e.g. 20–30 years) have examined effects on IQ. Many centers therefore recommend some restriction of phenylalanine throughout life.

Feeding schedules

In healthy people, food is normally ingested during a small number of meals, usually 1 to 3 meals per day, although additional snacks may also be taken. Most patients with disease follow similar patterns of eating, but some may require different feeding schedules. For example, children with certain forms of glycogen storage disease need to ingest small, frequent meals rich in carbohydrate to prevent hypoglycemia. In patients receiving artificial nutritional support (enteral tube feeding or parenteral nutrition), less physiological feeding schedules may be employed, either because of necessity or convenience. Continuous feeding over prolonged periods of time, up to 24 hours per day, is simple and convenient to carers managing bed-bound patients, including those who are unconscious. Continuous feeding over prolonged periods may also be necessary when only slow rates of feeding are tolerated. For example, patients with certain intestinal problems, such as the short bowel syndrome, may be able to tolerate and absorb sufficient nutrients to meet their needs only if the gut is infused slowly with nutrients over a prolonged period of time during the day and night. Such an enteral feeding schedule may avoid the need for parenteral nutrition, which is less physiological, more costly, and often associated with a greater number of serious complications.

Many patients on home parenteral nutrition and enteral tube feeding may be able to receive adequate amounts of feed during 12–16 hours per day. This means that they receive continuous pump-assisted infusion during the night (and part of the day), which is again unphysiological. During the day such patients can disconnect themselves from the feeding equipment to undertake activities of normal daily living, including exercise. This practice can have both physical and psychological benefits. It is also associated with some disadvantages, however, including dependency on the feeding equipment and in some cases abnormal appetite sensations. Although lack of appetite is typical during acute illness, some patients with little or no inflammatory disease who are on long-term artificial nutrition may suffer from hunger and desire to eat, even when sufficient nutrients are delivered artificially by tube into the stomach or by catheter into a vein. These abnormal and sometimes distressing and persisting appetite sensations may be due to provision of liquid rather than solid food, to bypassing part of the gut (gastric feeding) or the entire gut (parenteral nutrition), to lack or reduced gastric distension. They may also be the result of psychosocially conditioned responses, such as those stimulated by observing others eating. The physiological responses to normal food intake, which are associated with fluctuating hormonal and substrate responses, are either attenuated or absent when continuous feeding is provided. The clinical significance of these changes is unclear.

Structure and function

Several bodily functions are related to body composition, specifically, the mass of tissue or tissue components. For example, the risk of fracture is greater in individuals with a low bone mineral mass (osteoporosis). Muscle strength is related to muscle mass and body mass index (BMI = (weight in kg)/(height in m)^2) has been found to be a useful marker for a wide range of bodily functions and wellbeing, including quality of life. Repletion of tissues is often associated with improvements in bodily functions, including muscle strength and fatigue, reproductive function, and psychological behavior. However, improvements in physiological function and clinical outcome can also occur in the presence of little or no change in gross body composition, and vice versa. Nutritional intervention during key phases of an illness can have an important effect on outcome. Examples include fluid restriction (compared with high fluid intake in the early postoperative period; see above), glucose administration in the perioperative period, and control of blood glucose concentration with insulin in critically ill patients (see above). The administration of growth hormone to critically ill patients to improve N balance has been associated with detrimental effects, illustrating a dissociation between gross body composition and function.

1.4 Management pathways

Although resources vary in different countries, in different places in the same country, and at different times in the same place in the same country (e.g. during famines), there are common overarching management pathways. These begin with nutritional screening and assessment, which should be linked to care plans (Figure 1.8). The care plans may involve different health care settings (e.g. hospital, community care homes). Since the time spent in hospital may be short (<5% of the duration of an acute illness from onset to complete recovery), treatment initiated here may need to continue and be assessed in the community. It is disturb-

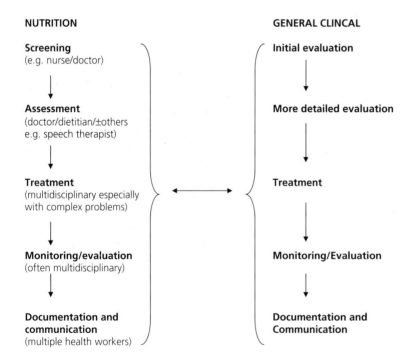

NUTRITION

Screening
(e.g. nurse/doctor)

Assessment
(doctor/dietitian/±others
e.g. speech therapist)

Treatment
(multidisciplinary especially
with complex problems)

Monitoring/evaluation
(often multidisciplinary)

**Documentation and
communication**
(multiple health workers)

GENERAL CLINCAL

Initial evaluation

More detailed evaluation

Treatment

Monitoring/Evaluation

**Documentation and
Communication**

Figure 1.8 Similarity in nutritional and general clinical management pathways and interaction between the two. Adapted from Elia (2003) with permission of BAPEN.

ing that malnutrition is underrecognized and under-treated, and that there is frequent lack of continuity of care. The initial recognition of malnutrition or risk of malnutrition is an essential first step in the management pathway.

For practical reasons, nutritional screening is often distinguished from nutritional assessment.

- *Nutritional screening* is a simple, quick, and general procedure used by nursing medical or other staff, often at first contact with a patient, to detect significant risk of nutritional problems, so that a clear action can be implemented. This may involve referral to a dietitian or another expert.
- *Nutritional assessment* is a more detailed, more specific evaluation of a patient's nutritional status, usually by an individual with some nutritional expertise (e.g. dietitian, clinician with an interest in nutrition, or nutrition nurse specialist). Assessment is usually carried out when serious nutritional problems are identified by the screening process, or when there is uncertainty about the appropriate course of action. It allows specific nutritional care plans to be developed for individual patients. It can also be used to identify micronutrient status, although this frequently requires confirmation by laboratory investigations.

It is also important to distinguish between a nutritional screening test and program:

- A *screening test* refers to the test that is used to identify a disease or a condition (e.g. malnutrition or obesity).
- A *screening programme* refers to the full range of activities from identification of risk using a screening test, to definitive diagnosis and treatment of the disease or condition.

The screening test (or screening tool) should be simple, and quick to perform, valid, reliable and acceptable to both patient and health worker. Since nutritional problems involve different care settings, it is an advantage to be able to use the same tool (or at least the same principles) for all types of patients, even those that cannot be weighed or have their height measured) in all care settings. It is also advantageous if the tool can be used by different health workers (e.g. nurses, doctors, dietitians, health care assistants, social workers, students) to detect both under- and overnutrition for both clinical and public health purposes, and be adapted to care plans according to local policy.

The 'Malnutrition Universal Screening Tool' ('MUST') was developed in the UK with these aims in mind. It is used here to illustrate the principles that have a resonance with general clinical care. They involve a consideration of the past (history of weight loss), current weight status (BMI), and likely future weight change during the course of a disease (Figure 1.9). This process complements the nutritional management structure, which has similarities in clinical care. In order to be rapid and applicable to different care settings, usually no blood tests are used in the initial screening procedure. Chapter 25 illustrates through case studies how the nutritional screening test becomes an integral part of management. The next chapter discusses potential methods for assessing nutritional status in more detail.

1.5 Perspectives on the future

The science of clinical nutrition is rapidly expanding and includes an appreciation of medicine, pharmacology, and nursing disciplines. As you will read, you will appreciate the link between nutritional needs and outcome, including quality of life in a wide range of disease states. It is essential that clinicians provide education and nutrition support to patients centered on the most up-to-date and sound evidence-based practices.

Whether physiological or non-physiological interventions are used, the practice of clinical nutrition is guided by improvements in bodily functions and clinical outcomes, especially if these are also cost-effective.

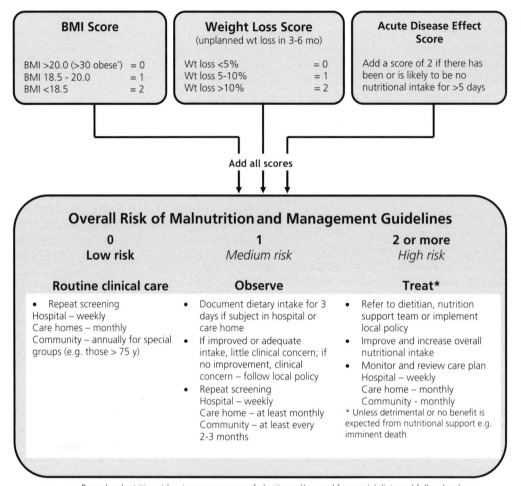

Figure 1.9 Example of a nutrition screening tool, the 'Malnutrition Universal Screening Tool' ('MUST') for adults. Adapted from Elia (2003) with permission of BAPEN.

References and further reading

Brandstrup B, Tennesen H *et al*. Effect of intravenous fluid restriction on post-operative complications: comparison of two perioperative fluid regimens. *Ann Surg* 2003; 238: 641–648.

Brozek J. Effects of generalized malnutrition on personality. *Nutrition* 1990; 6: 389–395.

Elia M (chairman & editor) The 'MUST' report. Nutritional screening for adults: a multidisciplinary responsibility. Development and use of the 'Malnutrition Universal Screening Tool' ('MUST') for adults. A report by the Malnutrition Advisory Group of the British Association for Parenteral and Enteral Nutrition, 2003.

Haydock DA, Hill GL. Improved wound healing response in surgical patients receiving intravenous nutrition. *Br J Surg* 1987; 74: 320–323.

Keys A, Brozek J *et al*. *The Biology of Human Starvation*, Vol. 1, pp. 81–535. Minneapolis, MN: University of Minnesota Press, 1950.

Leyton GB. The effects of slow starvation. *Lancet* 1946; ii: 73–79.

Rudman D, William JM *et al*. Elemental balanced during intravenous hyperalimentation of underweight adult subjects. *J Clin Invest* 1975; 55: 94–104.

Stratton RJ, Green CJ *et al*. *Disease-related Malnutrition. An evidence-based approach to treatment*. Oxford, CABI Publishing, 2003.

van den Berghe G, Wooters P *et al*. Intensive insulin therapy in critically ill patients. *N Engl J Med* 2001; 345: 1359–1367.

WHO (World Health Organization). *Management of Severe Malnutrition: A manual for physicians and other senior health workers*. Geneva: WHO, 1999.

WHO. *Management of the Child with Serious Infection or Severe Malnutrition*. Geneva: WHO, 2000. Available from http://www.who.int/child-adolescent-health/publications/referral_care/homepage.htm

2
Nutritional Assessment

Khursheed N Jeejeebhoy and Mary E Keith

Key messages

- The evaluation of nutritional status in the clinical setting is not an exact science, due to the interactive parameters of disease and nutrition. The clinical methods available to assess nutritional status include clinical and physical examination as well as Subjective Global Assessment (SGA), biochemical, anthropometric, laboratory immunologic, and functional indices of nutritional status.
- The SGA encompasses historical, symptomatic, and physical parameters in order to identify malnourished patients as those who are at increased risk of medical complications and could benefit from nutritional therapy.

- At present, there is no gold standard for evaluating nutritional status. Several of the parameters used in the determination of nutritional status may be influenced by malnutrition but also by the underlying disease or other factors.
- Nutritional assessment should involve a careful clinical evaluation with additional laboratory data to determine specific nutrient deficiencies or severity of illness. This information should be used in a prognostic way to determine which patients may benefit from nutritional therapy.

2.1 Introduction

Nutritional health is maintained by a state of equilibrium in which nutrient intake and requirements balance. Malnutrition occurs when net nutrient intake (nutrient intakes corrected for abnormally large fecal or urinary losses) is less than requirements. Malnutrition leads to a succession of metabolic abnormalities, physiological changes, reduced organ and tissue function, and loss of body mass. Concurrent stress such as trauma, sepsis, inflammation, and burns accelerates loss of tissue mass and function. Ultimately, critical loss of body mass and function occurs, resulting in death (Table 2.1).

The evaluation of nutritional status is a broad topic, and to be of clinical importance the ideal method should be able to predict whether the individual would have increased morbidity and mortality in the absence of nutritional support. In short, can it predict the occurrence of nutrition-associated complications (NACs) and thus predict outcome? Unfortunately, disease and nutrition interact so that disease in turn may cause secondary malnutrition, or malnutrition may adversely influence the underlying disease. Thus,

patient outcomes are multifactorial and any attempt to formulate the influence of malnutrition based on outcomes of single parameters or simple models will fail to consider the many interacting factors. This complexity has been recognized in the recent recommendations of the American Dietetic Association.

In this chapter, we will discuss and evaluate the clinical methods available to assess nutritional status, including clinical and physical examination as well as Subjective Global Assessment (SGA), biochemical, anthropometric, laboratory immunologic, and functional indices of nutritional status. The ability of each of these methods to predict nutritional risk will be discussed, as well as their ability to respond to nutritional therapy.

2.2 Clinical assessment of nutritional status

Clinical and physical assessment

A detailed nutritional history and physical examination provide the first step in the assessment of the indi-

Table 2.1 Clinical assessment of nutritional status

Complete medical history	Weight history
	Recent change in weight
	Nature of weight change
	Presence of food aversions
	Food intake patterns
	Appetite rating
	Nausea and vomiting
	Satiety
	Easily satiated
	Physical limitations
	Dentures
	Poor dentition
	Swallowing difficulties
	Use of alternative medicines
	Herbal remedies
	Vitamin supplements
	Chelation therapy
	Bowel habits
	Previous and concurrent illness
	Family history
	Social support
	Socioeconomic factors
Complete physical examination	
Anthropometric	Weight for height
	Evidence of fat and muscle wasting
	Loose skin folds
	Bony outlines
	Presence of subcutaneous fat
	Hollow cheeks/buttocks
	Temporalis, deltoids, and quadriceps
	wasting
Assessment of muscle function	Hand grip strength
	Walking tests
	Pulmonary function tests
	Cardiac muscle function
Fluid status	Evidence of dehydration
	Hypotension, tachycardia, dry skin
	Evidence of fluid overload
Evaluate specific nutrient deficiencies	Rash
	Stomatitis, glossitis
	Bitot's spots

the moment of measurement but provides a picture of current nutritional status and insight into the patient's future status. The clinical assessment of nutritional status involves a focused history and physical examination in conjunction with selected laboratory tests aimed at detecting specific nutrient deficiencies and patients who are at high risk for future nutritional abnormalities.

A complete medical history should be taken and include information on any changes in weight and if the weight change was voluntary or involuntary. In what direction is the weight loss/gain progressing? In addition to weight loss, specific aversion to specific foods or food groups should be identified as this may suggest specific nutrient deficiencies. Information on the size and number of meals can also indicate whether a diet is balanced or is restrictive. In addition, an assessment of appetite and satiety indices may provide information on an individual's desire to eat. Contributing to this is the ability to chew and swallow a normal diet. This is particularly important in elderly patients who may have difficulty with normal foods due to dental problems. Is there any pain associated with the ingestion of food, which may indicate stricture or obstruction. Nausea and vomiting following the consumption or during the preparation of food should also be investigated. Information regarding the use of any nutritional supplements or herbal preparations should be included in the nutritional history. Changes in bowel habits as well as changes in neuromuscular activity can also provide important information. Finally, a complete medical history with regard to previous or current illness and surgical procedures, family history, medications, and socioeconomic status should be included.

Physical examination

The physical examination corroborates and adds to the findings obtained by history (see Table 2.1).

(1) *Anthropometric assessment.* Current body weight should be compared with previously recorded weights, if available. Weight for height should be compared with standard normal values. A search for evidence demonstrating depletion of body fat and muscle masses should be made. A general loss of adipose tissue can be judged by clearly defined bony, muscular, and venous outlines, and loose skinfolds. Pinching a fold of skin between the

vidual and permit a global assessment of malnutrition as well as identifying any potential nutritional deficiencies (Table 2.1). The clinical assessment of nutritional status attempts to identify the initial nutritional state as well as the interplay of the factors influencing the progression or regression of nutritional abnormalities. Therefore, a clinical nutritional assessment is a dynamic process which is not limited to a single 'snapshot' at forefinger and thumb can detect the adequacy of subcutaneous fat. The presence of hollow cheeks, buttocks and perianal area suggests body fat loss. An examination of the temporalis, deltoids, and quadriceps muscles should be made to search for muscle wasting.

(2) *Assessment of muscle function.* Strength testing of individual muscle groups should be made to evaluate for generalized and localized muscle weakness. In addition, a general evaluation of respiratory and cardiac muscle function should be made.

(3) *Fluid status.* An evaluation for dehydration (hypotension, tachycardia, postural changes, mucosal xerosis, dry skin, and swollen tongue) and excess body fluid (edema, ascites) should be made.

(4) *Evaluation for specific nutrient deficiencies.* Physical examination for the presence of edema and skin lesions can suggest specific nutrition-related syndromes; for example, a scaly red rash around the mouth and nasolabial folds may suggest zinc deficiency. The signs and symptoms of vitamin and trace element deficiency should also be kept in mind during the physical exam; the presence of stomatitis, glossitis, or conjuctivitis may reflect specific nutritional deficiencies. Is there a history of night blindness or the presence of plaques on the conjunctiva (Bitot's spots), suggesting vitamin A deficiency? Signs of bone disease may be assessed by the presence of bone pain or tenderness and kyphosis. Finally, changes in the cardiorespiratory and nervous system should be assessed as thiamin deficiency can present as symptoms similar to congestive heart failure – dyspnea, edema, and tachycardia. Peripheral neuropathy is a symptom of Wernicke–Korsakoff syndrome and again may be related to thiamin deficiency. Vitamin E deficiency, vitamin B_{12} deficiency, hypomagnesemia with hypocalcemia and hypokalemia are also associated with changes in the nervous system.

Subjective Global Assessment

A clinical method for evaluating nutritional status, termed the Subjective Global Assessment (SGA), encompasses historical, symptomatic, and physical parameters. This approach defines malnourished patients as those who are at increased risk for medical complications and who will presumably benefit from nutritional therapy. The basis of this assessment is to determine whether nutrient assimilation has been restricted because of decreased food intake, maldigestion, or malabsorption, whether any effects of malnutrition on organ function and body composition have occurred, and whether the patient's disease process influences nutrient requirements. A form listing the specific features of the history and physical examination used in the SGA is shown in Box 2.1.

Box 2.1 Subjective Global Assessment rating form

A. History
1. Weight change and height :
    Current height _____ cm, Weight _____ kg.
    Overall loss in past 6 months: _____, kg _____ %
    Change in past two weeks (use + or –): _____ kg, _____ %
2. Dietary intake change (relative to usual intake)
    No change
    Change duration = _____ days.
    Type: Suboptimal solid diet
               Hypocaloric liquids
               Starvation
               Supplement: (circle)   nil   vitamin   minerals
3. Gastrointestinal symptoms that persisted for >2 weeks
    None
    Nausea
    Vomiting
    Diarrhea
    Pain   At rest   On eating
4. Functional capacity
    No dysfunction
    Dysfunction: duration _____ days
    Type: Working suboptimally
               Ambulatory but not working
               Bedridden
5. Disease and its relation to nutritional requirements
    Primary diagnosis _____
    Metabolic demand (stress):
        No stress
        Moderate stress
        High stress (burns, sepsis, severe trauma)

B. Physical status
(for each trait specify: 0 = normal, 1= mild deficit, 2 = established deficit)
        Loss of subcutaneous fat
        Muscle wasting
        Edema
        Ascite
        Mucosal lesions
        Cutaneous and hair changes
SGA Grade _____

The history used in the SGA focuses on five areas. The percentage of body weight lost in the previous six months is characterized as mild (<5%), moderate (5–10%), and severe (>10%). The pattern of loss is also important and it is possible for a patient to have significant weight loss but still be considered well-nourished if body weight (without edema or ascites) recently increased. For example, a patient who has had a 10% body weight loss but regained 3% of that weight over the past month would be considered well-nourished. Dietary intake is classified as normal or abnormal as judged by a change in intake and whether the current diet is nutritionally adequate. The presence of persistent gastrointestinal symptoms, such as anorexia, nausea, vomiting, diarrhea, and abdominal pain, which have occurred almost daily for at least two weeks, is recorded. The patient's functional capacity is defined as bedridden, suboptimally active, or full capacity. The last feature of the history concerns the metabolic demands of the patient's underlying disease state. Examples of high-stress illnesses are burns, major trauma, and severe inflammation, such as acute colitis. Moderate-stress diseases might be a mild infection or limited malignant tumor.

The features of the physical examination are noted as normal, mild, moderate, or severe alterations. The loss of subcutaneous fat is measured in the triceps region and the mid-axillary line at the level of the lower ribs. These measurements are not precise, but are merely a subjective impression of the degree of subcutaneous tissue loss. The second feature is muscle wasting in the temporal areas and in the deltoids and quadriceps, as determined by loss of bulk and tone detectable by palpation. A neurologic deficit will interfere with this assessment. The presence of edema in the ankle and sacral regions and the presence of ascites are noted. Coexisting disease such as renal or congestive failure will modify the weight placed on the finding of edema. Mucosal and cutaneous lesions are recorded, as are color and appearance of the patient's hair.

The findings of the history and physical examination are used to categorize patients as being well-nourished (category A), having moderate or suspected malnutrition (category B), or having severe malnutrition (category C). The rank is assigned on the basis of subjective weighting. Equivocal information is given less weight than definitive data. Fluid shifts related to onset or treatment of edema or ascites must be considered when interpreting changes in body weight. In general, a patient who has experienced weight loss and muscle wasting but is currently eating well and is gaining weight is classified as well-nourished. A patient who has experienced moderate weight loss, continued compromised food intake, continued weight loss, progressive functional impairment, and has a 'moderate-stress' illness is classified as moderately malnourished. A patient who has experienced severe weight loss, continues to have poor nutrient intake, progressive functional impairment, and muscle wasting is classified as severely malnourished independent of disease stress. Investigators have reported that the SGA results are reproducible with a greater than an 80% agreement when two blinded observers assessed the same patient.

2.3 Anthropometric assessment of nutritional status

Anthropometric assessment of nutritional status can be divided into two main categories: the assessment of growth and the assessment of body composition. The assessment of growth includes the evaluation of head circumference, weight, and length as well as allowing for the correction of these parameters for age. Assessment of nutritional status based on body composition involves detecting the loss (or gain) of body components relative to previous measurements and relating the values in a given patient to normal standards. The former is affected by the reproducibility and error in the measurements themselves, while the latter is dependent upon the normal range of values. A person who starts off at the upper end of the normal range may be classified as 'normal' despite considerable changes in the measured value. Therefore, it is possible for a person to be in a negative nutritional state for a long time before anthropometric measurements fall below normal.

Anthropometric assessment of growth

Head circumference
Head circumference is important as it is linked with brain size. It can also be used to identify children with conditions associated with a large head (macrocephalic) or small head (microcephalic). Care must be taken in completing this measurement and the results are compared with age-corrected standards. Head circumference for age can be used as an index of malnutrition

during the early years of life; however, since changes in head circumference occur relatively slowly, this technique will generally only identify severe chronic malnutrition.

Length/height

Children under two years of age generally are measured for recumbent length; children over two and adults are measured in the standing position. Weight for height can be used when age is not available and is a sensitive indicator of current nutritional status. Wasting can be identified as a very low weight for a given height. One disadvantage is that poor linear growth can be classified as normal if weight is appropriate for height. Height for age can also be calculated, although this index is more often used as an indicator of the nutritional status of populations rather than individuals. More importantly, it is different for different ethnic groups and a European standard is quite inappropriate for other populations.

Body weight and weight loss

Body weight for age can be used as an index of acute malnutrition, especially when determining length is difficult. However, the results must be interpreted with caution as body weight is a simple measure of total body components and growth, and, therefore, changes in body weight do not provide any insight into the relative changes in each component. Body weight is generally compared to an 'ideal' or desirable weight. This comparison can be made by using formulas such as the Hamwi formula or tables. In addition to the use of tables, several indices have been proposed including the Ponderal Index (height/cubed root of weight) as well as the simple height/weight ratio. However, a simple approach which gives as much information as tables is the calculation of the body mass index (BMI) or Quetelet index. BMI is calculated as weight in kilograms divided by height in meters squared.

The interpretation of different BMIs can be found in Table 2.2. A BMI of 14–15 is associated with significant mortality. However, measurements of body weight in patients in hospital intensive care units or those with liver disease, cancer, or renal failure are confounded by changes in body water due to underhydration, edema, ascites, and dialysate in the abdomen. In addition, the BMI must be interpreted with caution in the young, the elderly, and in athletes. In short, a simple snapshot of BMI cannot be interpreted in terms of the future risks

Table 2.2 Health risk classification according to body mass index (BMI)

Classification	BMI category (kg/m²)	Risk of developing health problems
Underweight	<18.5	Increased
Normal weight	18.5–24.9	Least
Overweight	25.0–29.9	Increased
Obese class I	30.0–34.9	High
Obese class II	35.0–39.9	Very high
Obese class III	≥40.0	Extremely high

The classifications for BMI as reported by Health Canada (2003). Reproduced with the permission of the Minister of Public Works and Government Services Canada 2004. These are applicable to the developed world but may not apply to underdeveloped countries.

of developing NACs unless the direction of loss and the interplay of factors causing the loss are evaluated. Is it simply a lack of food? Is there a problem of intake and/or digestion? Is the BMI low because of previous problems and now these are corrected the individual is gaining weight?

Thus changes in body weight may provide some useful information in the clinical setting. Changes in body weight can be expressed as percentage of usual weight, percentage of weight loss as well as rate of weight loss. Unintentional weight loss of greater than 10% is thought to be a good prognosticator of clinical outcome. However, it may be difficult to determine true weight loss and the accuracy of determining weight loss by history has been found to be only 0.67 and the predictive power 0.75. Hence 33% of patients with weight loss would be missed and 25% of those who have been weight-stable would be diagnosed as having lost weight. Furthermore, the nutritional significance of changes in body weight can again be confounded by changes in hydrational status, presence of ascites, edema, or massive tumor growth. In these circumstances, changes in body water may mask underlying weight loss and additional anthropometric measurements would be required in the assessment of nutritional status.

Anthropometric assessment of body composition

Anthropometric measures can be used to estimate the relative proportions of fat and lean tissue in an individual (see chapter 2 in *Introduction to Human Nutrition* in this series). Measurements of skinfold thickness provide an estimate of the subcutaneous fat deposit and therefore can be used to estimate the amount of total body fat. There are five sites that are routinely used to estimate body fat: triceps, biceps, subscapular, supra-iliac, and mid-axillary. Measurements are best done using precision skinfold calipers. Skinfold measures are subject to both inter and intra-examiner error. Although single measures have been used to estimate body fat, multiple measures are more advisable. Once the fat mass has been estimated the fat-free mass can be estimated by subtraction.

The waist–hip ratio, which is simply the waist circumference divided by the hip circumference, has been used to look at the distribution of body fat. A waist–hip ratio of >1 for men and >0.8 for women is suggestive of increased risk for cardiovascular complications and related death.

The fat-free mass is a combination of lean tissue (protein), water, and minerals. Since muscle is the major protein store it has been used to estimate the protein reserves of the body. Mid-arm muscle circumference and mid-arm muscle area provide a measure of muscle mass which is correlated with measures of total muscle mass and therefore protein status. A decrease in mid-arm muscle circumference may reflect changes in nutritional status, specifically protein reserve, and has been used to monitor the effects of nutrition therapy. Mid-arm muscle circumference is derived from the measurement of the mid-arm circumference and the tricep skinfold thickness and is calculated using the following equation:

Mid-arm muscle circumference =

$$\text{mid-arm circumference} - (\pi \times \text{tricep skinfold thickness})$$

The mid-arm muscle area is thought to be a more accurate index of total body muscle mass as it more accurately reflects changes in muscle tissue. Mid-arm muscle area is estimated using the following equation:

Arm muscle area =

$$\frac{\left[\text{mid-arm circumference} - (\pi \times \text{tricep skinfold thickness}) \right]}{4\pi}$$

The equation is based on numerous assumptions including that the mid-arm cross-section is circular, that the triceps skinfold is twice the average fat rim diameter, that bone atrophies in proportion to muscle wastage during protein energy malnutrition. The estimated coefficient of variation reported for the determination of mid–arm muscle area by trained examiners has been reported to be 7%, therefore small changes in nutritional status will not be detected with this measure.

Anthropometric measures of body composition must be compared with standards in order to evaluate an individual's nutritional status. The most commonly used standards for triceps skinfold thickness and mid-arm muscle circumference are those reported by Jelliffe, which are based on measurements of European male military personnel and low-income American women, and those reported by Frisancho, which are based on measurements of white men and women participating in the 1971–1974 United States Health and Nutrition Survey. The use of these standards to identify malnutrition in many patients is problematic because of the restricted database and the absence of correction factors for age, the effects of hydrational status and physical activity on anthropometric parameters. Several studies have demonstrated that 20–30% of healthy control subjects would be considered malnourished based on these standards and that there is poor correlation between the Jelliffe and Frisancho standards in classifying patients.

Although attempts have been made to create standards for diseases such as dialysis patients, the validity of standards have been questioned and interpretation of the data may be limited by inter-rater variability. In addition, considerable inconsistencies in results have been reported when anthropometric measurements were performed by three different observers. The coefficient of variation was 4.7% for arm circumference and 22.6% for triceps skin fold thickness. Therefore, a change in arm muscle circumference (arm circumference minus triceps skinfold thickness) of at least 2.68 cm was needed to demonstrate a true change in a given patient. These considerations in particular apply to patients in ICUs, and those with liver and renal disease, where edema is a major problem in assessing skinfolds and arm circumference.

Laboratory assessment of body composition

The body consists of compartments or components. There are over 35 well-recognized components and these are organized into five levels of increasing complexity: atomic, molecular, cellular, tissue system, and whole body. In healthy weight-stable subjects there are relatively constant relationships between these components which are correlated with each other. For example, the atomic level component nitrogen is 16% of the molecular level component protein.

Isotope dilution

Total body water, measured by isotope dilution, is usually the largest molecular level component. Water maintains a relatively stable relationship to fat-free body mass and thus measured water isotope dilution volumes allow prediction of fat-free body mass and fat (i.e. body weight minus fat-free body mass). The relationship between total body water and other body composition components may change with disease and this should be considered when interpreting data from hospitalized or chronically ill patients. The usual approach is to measure a dilution volume using one of three isotopes, tritium, deuterium, or ^{18}O-labeled water. This first step allows estimation of a dilution volume of one of the three isotopes. In the second step it is assumed that the proportion of fat-free body mass as water is constant at 0.732. This allows calculation of fat-free body mass and fat. The relationship of this measurement to outcome has not been studied.

Bioimpedance analysis

Bioimpedance analysis (BIA) is a method of estimating body fluid volumes by measuring the resistance to a high-frequency, low-amplitude alternating electric current (50 kHz at 500–800 mA). The amount of resistance measured (R) is inversely proportional to the volume of electrolytic fluid in the body and to a lesser extent on the proportions of this volume. A regression equation is then developed based on a reference measurement of fat-free body mass (i.e. isotope dilution) and the measured R, height, and other variables.

Recently, the difference in the conductive properties of extra- and intracellular fluid has resulted in the development of bioimpedance spectroscopy (BIS). Direct current will pass through extracellular fluid but will not traverse the lipid membrane of cells. As the frequency of the applied current increases the cell membranes act as the dielectric of capacitors and the alternating current will pass partly and easily through the extracellular fluid and with greater resistance through the cells. The total impedance to the current is defined by an equivalent circuit of a resistance and a reactance through a capacitor. As the frequency of the alternating current increases, the reactance at first increases and then decreases until at very high frequencies there is little impedance to the passage of the current through cells. An analysis of the reactance to different frequencies is used to calculate extra- and intracellular water. In healthy adults, it is possible to predict total body water to within 2–3 liters. Much more variable results are observed in diseased patients, owing in part to the population-specific nature of BIA. To date, no relationship between BIA and outcome has been studied in hospitalized patients and the method is not yet fully validated for use in all disease states.

Dual-energy X-ray absorptiometry

Dual-energy X-ray absorptiometry (DXA) is a method developed originally for the measurement of bone density and mass. Systems today also quantify soft tissue composition, and it possible to measure total and regional fat, bone mineral, and bone mineral-free lean components with DXA. The method is based on the attenuation characteristics of tissues exposed to X-rays at two peak energies. Mathematical algorithms allow calculation of the separate components using various physical and biological models. Software can be used to measure regions separately if desired. A typical whole-body scan takes approximately 30 minutes and exposes the subject to ~1 mrem radiation. The method provides the first accurate and practical means of measuring bone mineral mass and offers a new opportunity to study appendicular muscle mass. Again there are no data indicating whether DXA can predict outcome in hospital patients.

Whole-body counting/neutron activation

Potassium, nitrogen, phosphorus, hydrogen, oxygen, carbon, sodium, chloride, and calcium can be measured with a group of techniques referred to as whole-body counting/*in vivo* neutron activation analysis. Shielded whole-body counters can count the gamma-ray decay of naturally occurring ^{40}K. The method is safe and can be used in children and pregnant women. The ^{40}K counts can be used to estimate total body potassium, which in turn can be used to calculate body cell mass and fat-free body mass. Prompt gamma neutron activation analysis can be used to measure total body nitrogen and hydrogen. Nitrogen can be used to calculate total body protein. Delayed gamma neutron activation measures total body calcium, sodium, chloride, and phosphate. These elements can be used to calculate bone mineral mass and extracellular fluid volume. Lastly, inelastic neutron-scattering methods measure total body oxygen and carbon. Carbon is useful in models designed to quantify total body fat.

Whole-body counting/neutron activation methods are important because they provide a means of estimating all major chemical components *in vivo*. These methods are considered the standard for evaluating the body composition components of nutritional interest, including body cell mass, fat, fat-free body mass, skeletal muscle mass, and various fluid volumes. Refeeding the malnourished subject by mouth or by total parenteral nutrition (TPN) results in a rapid increase in total body potassium (TBK) but not total body nitrogen (TBN). In animal studies it has been shown that this increase in TBK is the result of improved membrane voltage and an increase in the intracellular ionic potassium. The findings are consistent with improved cell energetics as demonstrated by nuclear magnetic resonance (NMR) spectroscopy as well as improved muscle function shown concurrently. Loss of TBK is a good predictor of poor outcome in a variety of conditions associated with malnutrition.

Computerized axial tomography and magnetic resonance imaging

These methods measure components at the tissue system level of body composition, including skeletal muscle, adipose tissue, visceral organs, and brain. Computerized axial tomography (CT) systems measure X-ray attenuation as the source and detector rotate in a perpendicular plane around the subject. Magnetic resonance imaging (MRI) systems measure nuclear relaxation times from nuclei of atoms with a magnetic moment that are aligned within a powerful magnetic field. Clinical systems are based on hydrogen, although it is possible to create images and spectrographs from phosphorus, sodium, and carbon. The collected data are transformed into high-resolution images, and this allows the quantification of whole or regional body composition. A large number of studies in phantoms, cadavers, and *in vivo* validate these methods. There are no studies of imaging methods in relation to outcome.

Body composition and outcomes

Although the above methods of body composition measurement can accurately assess different compo-

nents, they are difficult to apply in the clinical setting except in specialized units. The only method which is available for wide clinical application in nutritional assessment is BIA or BIS. Using these methods there have been few data on their ability to predict outcome. In patients on renal dialysis it has been shown that a reduction of the reactance from 70 ohms to 43 ohms increased morbidity by 9% and to 31 ohms by 14%. In cancer patients, a lean body mass by BIA below the normal range was associated with increased morbidity.

2.4   Biochemical indices of nutritional status

Creatinine–height index (CHI)

The excretion of creatinine in the urine is related to muscle mass. Normalized for height the 24-h creatinine excretion is an index of muscle mass. In theory it is a good and simple way of assessing the lean body mass. However, it is dependent upon complete 24-h urine collections and urinary losses or oliguria may result in an inappropriate diagnosis of malnutrition. Patients on diuretics such as those with cardiac and liver failure and those with renal disease are especially likely to have low excretions of creatinine.

Nitrogen balance

Nitrogen balance measures net changes in body protein mass and is based on the assumption that nearly all of the total body nitrogen is incorporated into protein. Since protein contains 16% nitrogen, protein content can be calculated. Nitrogen balance is said to be positive when nitrogen intake is greater than nitrogen losses and negative when nitrogen losses exceed intake. Nitrogen balance can be calculated using the following equation:

$$\text{Nitrogen balance} = I - (U - U_c) + (F - F_c) + S$$

where I is equal to intake of nitrogen (protein (g)/6.25); U is urinary nitrogen, U_c is endogenous urinary nitrogen; F is nitrogen voided in the feces; F_c is endogenous fecal nitrogen losses; and S is dermal nitrogen losses.

The determination of nitrogen balance in the clinical setting is therefore quite complex, limiting its utility, and measures of losses can be difficult.

Urinary excretion of hydroxyproline and 3-methylhistidine

Hydroxyproline is a product of collagen metabolism and is excreted in reduced amounts by malnourished and protein-depleted patients. However, collagen ingestion, sex, age, and the presence of certain diseases can make interpretation of hydroxyproline difficult. Disturbances in collagen metabolism because of diseases such as rheumatoid arthritis also affect circulating levels. In order to try to control for age and sex the hydroxyproline:creatinine ratio has been used as well as a hydroxyproline index which tries to correct for body weight.

3-Methylhistidine is an amino acid found mainly in the actin of muscle fibers. It is released during the breakdown of muscle protein and is excreted in the urine, its excretion thus giving information about muscle mass and breakdown rates. However, in order to interpret this measure accurately, subjects must have been on a meat-free diet for at least three days prior to its measurement. In addition, the effect of sex, age, hormonal status, fitness level, and disease on urinary excretion levels is unclear. Finally, there is little support for the relationship between changes in urinary 3-methylhistidine excretion and morbidity or mortality indices. As a result, the use of 3-methylhistidine as a marker of muscle mass is not recommended.

Serum albumin

Serum albumin is one of the most extensively studied proteins and over the past 30 years there have been about 19 000 citations to it in the Index Medicus! Several studies have demonstrated that a low serum albumin concentration correlates with an increased incidence of medical complications. In addition, low serum albumin is associated with increased mortality in general, especially in elderly nursing home patients and dialysis patients. An understanding of albumin physiology clarifies why serum albumin concentration correlates with disease severity in hospitalized patients but may be inappropriate as a measure of nutritional status *per se*.

The concentration of serum albumin represents the net sum of albumin synthesis, degradation, losses from the body, and exchange between intra- and extravascular albumin compartments, as well as the volume in which albumin is distributed. Albumin is highly water soluble and resides in the extracellular space. The total body pool of albumin in a normal 70-kg man is ~300 g (3.5–5.3 g/kg). Approximately one-third of the total pool constitutes the intravascular compartment and two-thirds the extravascular compartment. The concentration of albumin in blood is greater than that in lymph or other extracellular fluids, and the ratio of intravascular to extravascular albumin concentration varies from tissue to tissue. Within 30 min of initiating albumin synthesis, the hepatocyte secretes albumin into the bloodstream. Once albumin is released into plasma, its half-life is 20 days. During steady-state conditions ~14 g of albumin (200 mg/kg) are produced and degraded daily. Thus, each day ~5% of the total albumin pool is degraded and replaced by newly synthesized albumin.

Equilibration of albumin in the intravascular compartment is rapid and occurs within minutes after albumin enters the bloodstream. Equilibration between intra- and extravascular albumin occurs more slowly. Every hour ~5% of the plasma albumin pool exchanges with extravascular albumin so that the total plasma albumin mass exchanges with extravascular albumin each day. Because the rate of equilibration varies among tissues, complete equilibration may take 7–10 days.

Protein–energy malnutrition causes a decrease in the rate of albumin synthesis because adequate nutrient intake is important for polysomal aggregation and maintenance of cellular RNA levels needed for protein synthesis. Within 24 h of fasting, the rate of albumin synthesis decreases markedly. However, a short-term reduction in albumin synthesis has little impact on albumin levels because of albumin's low turnover rate and large pool size. Indeed, plasma albumin concentration may actually increase during short-term fasting because of contraction of intravascular water. Even during chronic malnutrition, plasma albumin concentration is often maintained because of a compensatory decrease in albumin degradation and a transfer of extravascular albumin to the intravascular compartment. Prolonged protein–calorie restriction induced experimentally in human volunteers or observed clinically in patients with anorexia nervosa, causes marked reductions in body weight but little change in plasma albumin concentration. A protein-deficient diet with adequate calories in elderly people causes a decrease in lean body mass and muscle function without a change in plasma albumin concentration.

Hospitalized patients may have low levels of plasma albumin for several reasons. Inflammatory disorders cause a decrease in albumin synthesis, an increase in albumin degradation, and an increase in albumin transcapillary losses. Gastrointestinal and some cardiac diseases increase albumin losses through the gut, while renal diseases may cause considerable albuminuria. Wounds, burns, and peritonitis cause major losses from the injured surface and in certain circumstances an increase in albumin losses through the gut, kidneys, or damaged tissues. Because the exchange between intra- and extravascular albumin is so large, even small changes in the percentage of exchange can cause significant changes in plasma albumin levels. The normal rate of albumin exchange between intra- and extravascular compartments is more than 10 times the rate of albumin synthesis or degradation.

During serious illness vascular permeability increases dramatically. Albumin losses from plasma to the extravascular space were increased two-fold in patients with cancer cachexia and three-fold in patients with septic shock. Plasma albumin levels will not increase in stressed patients until the inflammatory stress remits and they are not affected by nutritional intake. For example, albumin levels fail to increase in patients with cancer after 21 days of intensive nutritional therapy and in nursing home patients after enteral feeding through a gastrostomy.

Prealbumin

Prealbumin is a transport protein for thyroid hormones and exists in the circulation as a retinol-binding protein (RBP)–prealbumin complex. The turnover rate of this protein is rapid with a half-life of 2–3 days. It is synthesized by the liver and is catabolized partly in the kidneys. Protein–energy malnutrition reduces the levels of prealbumin and refeeding restores levels. However, prealbumin levels fall without malnutrition in infections and in response to cytokine and hormone infusion. Renal failure increases while liver failure may cause decreased levels. Although prealbumin is responsive to nutritional changes, it is influenced by several disease-related factors, making it unreliable as an index of nutritional status in patients.

Serum transferrin

Transferrin is a protein synthesized by the liver and used to carry iron. Transferrin has a much shorter half-life than albumin at 8–10 days and a much smaller body pool and therefore may respond more rapidly to changes in protein status. Unfortunately there is a wide range of transferrin levels associated with malnutrition and, like albumin, serum concentrations are affected by a variety of diseases including hepatic failure, congestive heart failure, and inflammation. In addition, since transferrin is linked with iron metabolism, changes in iron status can affect transferrin levels. For example iron deficiency observed often in pregnancy results in an increased level of transferrin in response to increased iron absorption.

Transferrin has been correlated with poor outcomes in children with kwashiokor but there is no widespread agreement on its relationship with morbidity or mortality.

Serum retinol-binding protein and thyroxine-binding prealbumin

Retinol is carried in the body by retinol-binding protein (RBP). This complex travels with one molecule of thyroxine-binding prealbumin (TBPA) and therefore both of these molecules may be measured as an indicator of nutritional status. The half-life of RBP is short at about 12 h, thereby making it more responsive to protein and energy deprivation as well as to dietary intervention. Unfortunately, as we will see with most serum markers of nutritional status, RBP lacks specificity and is reduced in acute catabolic states, liver disease, and during hyperthyroidism. In addition, it is linked with vitamin A status and is reduced in vitamin A deficiency due to a lack of need for the transport protein.

TBPA is required for the transport of thyroxine. Its half-life is approximately two days, making it a more sensitive index than albumin or transferrin. However, like RBP TBPA is affected by other diseases and even minor stress or inflammation can markedly affect circulating levels.

Serum cholesterol

Low levels of cholesterol are seen in malnourished patients. However, very low levels are seen in patients with liver disease, renal disease, and malabsorption. In addition, low levels of serum cholesterol have been correlated with mortality.

2.5 Immunologic assessment of nutritional status

Malnutrition and its associated nutrient deficiencies is associated with impaired immunological responses which have been reversed with nutritional repletion. Therefore, immunocompetence has been used as a functional index of nutritional status. The limitation of this method lies in its inability to detect individual nutrient deficiencies and therefore must be used as part of a multi-assessment plan in order to assess malnutrition. Nearly all aspects of the immune system have been shown to be affected by malnutrition, but just two tests are most commonly used to determine the adequacy of the immune response.

Lymphocyte count

The measurement of white blood cells is routinely done in hospitalized patients and since lymphocytes generally comprise 20–40% of the total leukocytes their measurement can be used as an index of malnutrition. The total lymphocyte count is determined by dividing the percentage of lymphocytes multiplied by the white blood cell count by 100. A percentage change can be used to identify marginal, moderate, or severe malnutrition. The use of the total lymphocyte count is limited as stress, neoplasia, infection, and sepsis can affect it independent of the nutritional status. In addition, the relationship of the total lymphocyte count to patient prognosis is unclear.

Delayed cutaneous hypersensitivity

Immune competence, as measured by delayed cutaneous hypersensitivity (DCH), is affected by severe malnutrition. While it is true that immune competence as measured by DCH is reduced in malnutrition, several diseases and drugs influence this measurement, making it a poor predictor of malnutrition in sick patients.

The following factors non-specifically alter DCH in the absence of malnutrition:

- Infections (viral, bacterial, and granulomatous)
- Uremia, cirrhosis, hepatitis, trauma, burns, and hemorrhage
- Steroids, immunosuppressants, cimetidine, warfarin, and perhaps aspirin
- General anesthesia and surgery.

Hence, in the critically sick patient many factors can alter DCH, making its use of questionable value in assessing the state of nutrition. Meakins *et al.* (1979) have shown that simply draining an abscess can reverse anergy. Immunity is therefore neither a specific indicator of malnutrition nor is it easily studied.

2.6 Functional tests of malnutrition

SGA identifies patients at risk of complications by clinically assessing changes in intake of food, in body composition, and in function. Functional impairment in malnutrition has been previously studied by examining changes in immune function, ability to perform work in an ergometer and in changes of heart rate during maximal exercise. With the exception of extreme wasting, there are no data showing a relationship between anthropometric features and the development of NACs. In contrast several studies have shown that altered function is associated with poor outcome. For example:

- There is evidence that the strength of the hand grip is predictive of the development of postoperative complications.
- Nutritional manipulation has been shown to rapidly change function before restoration of body composition.
- In elderly subjects a maximum grip strength of greater than or equal to 5 kg was the most sensitive and specific cut-off point to separate survival from death, with a sensitivity of 0.81, specificity of 0.92.
- In a randomized controlled trial, supplementary nutrition had a dramatic effect on the ability to walk in patients with lung disease.
- Muscle function, including hand grip, respiratory muscle strength, and relaxation rate of the adductor pollicis, have been shown to be the main indicators of surgical complications rather than weight loss.
- In patients with inflammatory bowel disease it has been demonstrated that muscle function is restored before body composition.

Effect of malnutrition on body composition and muscle function

A lack of nutrient intake results in a loss of body fat and lean tissue. Therefore, the effects of nutritional depletion and repletion with refeeding have been judged by changes in body composition, especially of lean tissue. One of the elements responding to nutrient intake is body potassium, which has been used as an index of body cell mass, the metabolically active component of the lean tissue. In contrast to body nitrogen, body potassium responds rapidly to feeding by both oral and intravenous routes. These changes have been interpreted as being due to changes in lean body mass. However, the early restitution of body potassium without a rise in body nitrogen indicates that cell ion uptake occurs earlier than protein synthesis with nutritional support. In support of this conclusion, it has been shown, using ion-selective electrodes, that hypocaloric feeding results in a fall in muscle membrane potential and in the concentration of intracellular ionic K^+. The changes were specifically related to nutrient deprivation as they could not be reversed by potassium supplementation *per se*.

Since five molecules of adenosine triphosphate (ATP) are required for the incorporation of one molecule of amino acid into protein, and 77% of the free-energy change of ATP hydrolysis is used to maintain the Na–K gradient across the cell membrane, and energy intake limits nitrogen retention, these find-ings suggest that nutritional support initially alters cell energetics rather than mass. In addition, Z band degeneration and calcium accumulation occur with hypocaloric feeding in humans at a time when body weight and total body nitrogen are within the normal range. These myofibrillar effects are related to changes in cell energetics. Therefore the critical cellular changes with nutritional manipulations are, in effect, related to cell function.

Assessment of muscle function

Traditionally, muscle performance is assessed by tests that involve voluntary movement such as fatigue during endurance exercise, rapidity and force of isometric contraction as well as grip strength. In addition involuntary function measurements can be done using muscle stimulation. Two key elements of the muscle response to involuntary nerve stimulation are a change in the force frequency response of muscle (Figure 2.1a) and the relaxation rate of muscle (Figure 2.1b). These two variables have been shown to be related to metabolic and nutritional changes.

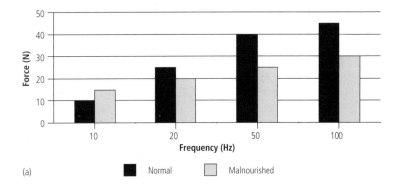

(a)

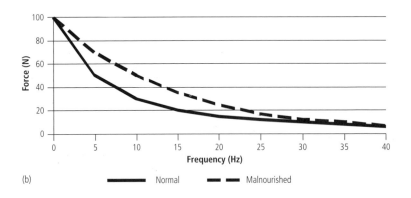

(b)

Figure 2.1 Change in the (a) force frequency response of muscle and (b) the relaxation rate of muscle seen in malnutrition.

Mechanism of changes in muscle function and ways to assess the effect of refeeding on mitochondrial energetics

Studies using ^{31}P-NMR (nuclear magnetic resonance spectroscopy) have given insight into the effect of protein–energy malnutrition on skeletal muscle function. The essential abnormality was related to deficient oxidative phosphorylation in the mitochondria.

Since ^{31}P-NMR studies showed that muscle function abnormalities in malnutrition are likely to be the result of mitochondrial dysfunction resulting in reduced oxidative phosphorylation, studies were performed to measure the effect of malnutrition on enzyme complexes controlling oxidative phosphorylation. In hypocalorically fed rats there was a significant fall in complex I, II, and III but not in complex IV. These changes were specifically reversed by feeding protein. Of greater interest was the finding that the changes in muscle were mirrored in blood mononuclear cells. In humans with malnutrition, mitochondrial complex abnormalities were demonstrated and were corrected by refeeding (Table 2.3). From this it is clear that complex I activity is reduced in malnourished patients, and is restored before other parameters.

2.7   Nutritional assessment tools in clinical decision making

The goals of nutritional assessment are to define accurately the nutritional status of an individual patient, to identify clinically relevant malnutrition, and to use assessment tools to monitor changes in nutritional status during nutritional support. As stated in the introduction, this is the state in which the nutritional status is associated with increased NACs. Nutritional assessment can be determined based on single anthropometric, biochemical, or immunological measures. However, the ideal test of nutritional status must be sensitive and specific enough to be unaffected by factors that are not related to nutrition and must respond to nutritional repletion. Given the dynamic nature of disease, finding one test that meets this criteria is unlikely.

In view of this limitation, a nutritional index that is an aggregate of several individual nutritional indices needs to be devised in order to provide an overall picture of a patients' nutritional status. The following three assessment indices are examples of this approach of using multiple parameters:

- Prognostic Nutritional Index (PNI)
- The Hospital Prognostic Indicator (HPI)
- Subjective Global Assessment (SGA)

Finally, health care professionals can rely exclusively on clinical assessment to judge the presence or absence of malnutrition.

Prognostic Nutritional Index (PNI)

Buzby *et al.* developed the PNI, calculated retrospectively from multiple parameters, to predict the occurrence of complications. The PNI depends on four indices: serum albumin, serum transferrin, triceps skinfold, and DCH and is largely used to predict risk.

$$PNI\,(\%) = 158 - (16.6 \times albumin) - (0.78 \times TSF) - (0.2 \times TFN) - (5.8 \times DCH)$$

where albumin is serum albumin concentration (g/dl); TSF is triceps skinfold (mm); TFN is transferrin concentration (g/dl), and DCH is delayed cutaneous hypersensitivity (grade of reactivity to any of three anti-

Table 2.3 Effect of feeding on mononuclear cell mitochondrial complex

	Weight	BMI	LBM	kcal/kg	Albumin	Complex I	Citrate S
D0	47.2 (10.5)	17.3 (3.6)	34.4 (8.1)	14.6 (12.3)	26 (7)	1.7 (0.9)	19 (11.3)
D7	47.3 (9.8)	17.3 (3.2)	33.7 (6.1)	30.4* (14.7)	26 (4)	2.6** (1.4)	29.2* (13.9)
D14	45.3 (10.6)	16.3 (3.6)	33.6 (6.0)	42.4* (11.6)	25 (2)	2.6** (1.1)	22.9*** (11.6)

*$P < 0.01$, **$P < 0.03$ and ***$P = 0.02$ vs. D0 (Wilcoxon test).
The standard nutritional assessment is compared to changes in mitochondrial complex activity on D0 (prefeeding) and D7 (1 week refed) and D14 (2 weeks refed) in malnourished patients. It is clear that complex I activity is reduced in malnourished patients and is restored before other parameters.
Reproduced from Briet *et al.* (1999) with permission from the American Gastroenterological Association.

gens: 0 non-reactive, 1 <5 mm reactivity, and 2 >5 mm reactivity).

A PNI of <40% is considered low risk, 40–50% is considered high risk, and >50% is very high risk. The PNI has been criticized as the factors are not independent of one another and may be affected by non-nutrition related factors thereby making the separation of the effects of nutritional deficiency from the disease process itself difficult.

The Hospital Prognostic Indicator (HPI)

The Hospital Prognostic Indicator (HPI) has also been proposed to be useful in the clinical setting. This index relies on serum albumin, delayed hypersensitivity responses, clinical status (defined as septic or non-septic), and the presence or absence of cancer. The equation has an overall predictive value for mortality of 71%, a sensitivity of 74%, and a specificity of 66%. However, the HPI has not been widely used in the clinical setting.

Subjective Global Assessment (SGA)

Subjective Global Assessment (SGA) is based on a carefully performed medical history and physical examination and has been proposed as an alternative measurement of nutritional status. The question remains 'how does SGA compare with traditional methods described above?' To make a meaningful comparison, the predictive accuracy of the different techniques done on the same individuals has been compared in a prospective analysis of 59 surgical patients. In this study, preoperative SGA was a better predictor of postoperative infectious complications than serum albumin, serum transferrin, DCH, anthropometry, creatinine–height index, and the PNI. Combining SGA with some of the 'traditional' markers of nutritional status increased the ability to identify patients who developed complications (from 82% to 90%) but also increased the percentage of patients identified as 'malnourished' but who did not develop a postoperative complication (from 25% to 30%). Therefore, increasing assessment sensitivity also increases the number of patients who might receive unnecessary nutrition support.

How does SGA perform in predicting complications in conditions other than preoperative patients? Several studies have reported successful use of the SGA to predict complications in general surgical patients, patients on dialysis, and liver transplant patients.

Currently there is no 'gold standard' for evaluating nutritional status and the reliability of any nutritional assessment technique as a true measure of nutritional status has never been validated. An unresolved problem with all prognostic nutritional indices is that several of the parameters used may be influenced not only by malnutrition, but also by the underlying disease. No prospective controlled clinical trials have demonstrated that providing nutrition support to patients judged to be malnourished influences clinical outcome. However, a retrospective subgroup analysis of a large multicenter trial found that parenteral nutrition given preoperatively to patients diagnosed as severely malnourished by SGA or a nutritional risk index (based on serum albumin and body weight change) decreased postoperative infectious complications We recommend that nutritional assessment should involve a careful clinical evaluation with additional laboratory studies as needed to help determine specific nutrient deficiencies or severity of illness. This information should be used in a prognostic fashion to decide which patients might benefit from nutritional therapy.

2.8   Perspectives on the future

The term malnutrition is a continuum which starts when the patient fails to eat enough to meet their needs and progresses through a series of functional changes that precede any changes in body composition which are related to the duration of reduced intake and its severity. To base the definition of malnutrition on any one of these changes is inappropriate. Only by recognizing the different facets of malnutrition can we define its various manifestations in relation to our clinical objectives. SGA combined with selected objective parameters at this moment provides the best clinical way of meeting these objectives. In the future, muscle function may be useful in determining optimal nutrient intake early in the course of feeding. Techniques such as BIA, DXA, and MRI combined with spectroscopy may provide powerful tools in the future.

References and further reading

American Dietetic Association. ADA's definition for nutrition screening and assessment. *J Am Diet Assoc* 1994; 94: 838–839.

Briet F, Twomey C, Jeejeebhoy KN. Effect of feeding malnourished patients for 1 mo on mitochondrial complex I activity and nutritional assessment measurements. *Am J Clin Nutr* 2004; 79: 787–794.

Briet F, Twomey C, Jeejeebhoy KN. Refeeding increases mitochondrial complex activity in malnourished patients. Evidence for a sensitive nutritional marker. *Gastroenterology* 1999; 116: A541.

Buzby GP, Mullen JL, Matthews DC, Hobbs CL, Rosato EF. Prognostic nutritional index in gastrointestinal surgery. *Am J Surg* 1980;139(1): 160–7.

Edwards RHT. Physiological analysis of skeletal muscle weakness and fatigue. *Clin Sci Mol Med* 1978; 54: 463–470.

Fritz T, Hollwarth I, Romaschow M, Schlag P. The predictive role of bioelectrical impedance analysis (BIA) in postoperative complications of cancer patients. *Eur J Surg Oncol* 1990; 16: 326–331.

Health Canada. *Canadian Guidelines for Body Wright Classification in Adults*, 2003. Available from http://www.hc-sc.gc.ca/hpfb-dgpsa/onpp-bppn/weight_book_e.pdf

Ikizler TA, Wingard RL, Harvell J, Shyr Y, Hakim RM. Association of morbidity with markers of nutrition and inflammation in chronic hemodialysis patients: a prospective study. *Kidney Int* 1999; 55: 1945–1951.

Meakins JL, Christou NV, Shizgal HM, MacLean LD. Therapeutic approaches to anergy in surgical patients. *Ann Surg* 1979; 190: 286–296.

Mijan de la Torre A, Madapallimattam A, Cross A, Armstrong RL, Jeejeebhoy KN. Effect of fasting, hypocaloric feeding, and refeeding on the energetics of stimulated rat muscle as assessed by nuclear magnetic resonance spectroscopy. *J Clin Invest* 1993; 92: 114–121.

Prealbumin in Nutritional Care Consensus Group. Measurement of visceral protein status in assessing protein and energy malnutrition: standard of care. *Nutrition* 1995; 11: 169.

Russell, DMcR, Walker PM, Leiter LA *et al.* Metabolic and structural changes in skeletal muscle during hypocaloric dieting. *Am J Clin Nutr* 1984; 39: 503–513.

Twomey C, Jeejeebhoy KN. Impaired lymphocyte mitochondrial complex activity in malnourished patients with significant weight loss. *Gastroenterology* 1999; 116: A582.

Veterans Affairs Total Parenteral Nutrition Cooperative Study Group. Perioperative total parenteral nutrition in surgical patients. *N Engl J Med* 1991; 325: 525–532.

3
Overnutrition

Gema Frühbeck

Key messages

- The World Health Organization (WHO) has declared obesity as the largest global chronic health problem in adults, which by 2025 will emerge as a more serious world problem than malnutrition.
- Currently, it is estimated that over 300 million people worldwide are obese, while more than one billion suffer from overweight.
- Many factors contribute to the development of overweight and obesity, including energy intake and expenditure, genetic factors, endocrine disorders, environmental factors, psychosocial influences, and other factors to a greater or

lesser extent.
- The hazards of excess body weight have been clearly established by epidemiological and clinical studies, highlighting the need for careful diagnosis and effective treatment programs.
- A multidimensional approach involving politicians, medical and health professionals, as well as industry, communities, and individuals is necessary to successfully tackle the obesity pandemic.
- The most effective treatment in the long term is, and will be, obesity prevention.

3.1 Introduction

It is only half a century since obesity was introduced into the International Classification of Diseases (ICD-9 code 278.0). However, in the twenty-first century it has already reached epidemic proportions and will be the leading cause of death and disability in this century world-wide, thus threatening to reverse many of the health gains achieved in the last decades. Surprisingly, obesity is a chronic disease that is often neglected, being frequently not even thought of as a serious, life-threatening disease.

Definitions and classification

The widely used clinical term 'obesity' derives from the Latin *ob*, standing for 'on account of,' and *esum*, meaning 'having eaten.' Strictly speaking, obesity is not defined as an excess of body weight but of body fat, to the extent that health may be adversely affected. Despite this important difference, medical criteria for the diagnosis of overweight and obesity do not rely on the measurement of adiposity. By convention set out in international guidelines overweight and obes-

ity are arbitrarily defined on the basis of the body mass index (BMI) or Quetelet's index (Table 3.1). The index is calculated by dividing the individual's weight (expressed in kilograms) by the square of his or her height (expressed in meters). A graded classification is valuable to diagnose individuals, to establish meaningful comparisons of weight status within and between populations, to identify intervention priorities as well as to provide a firm basis for evaluating treatments and interventions. Although the BMI is widely used as

Table 3.1 WHO classification of overweight and obesity in adults according to body mass index (BMI)

Classification	BMI (kg/m²)	Risk of comorbidity
Underweight	<18.5	Low[a]
Normal range	18.5–24.9	Average
Overweight	25.0–29.9	Increased
Obesity	≥30.0	
Class I	30.0–34.9	Moderate
Class II	35.0–39.9	Severe
Class III (morbid)	≥40.0	Very severe

[a]Low for the non-communicable diseases associated with obesity, but increased mortality due to cancer and infectious diseases.
Reproduced with permission from World Health Organization (1998).

a simple surrogate measure of body fat and has been shown to correlate closely with adiposity, it does not provide an exact description of body composition. The principal limitation of the BMI as a measure of body fat is that it does not distinguish fat mass from fat-free mass.

The classification of overweight and obesity in children and adolescents is especially complicated by the continually changing height and body composition. During these developmental periods the changes often take place at different rates and times in diverse populations, making the agreement over the diagnosis of overweight and obese children and adolescents difficult to establish. Pediatricians in the US have classically used the 85th and 95th centiles of BMI for age and sex based on US nationally representative survey data as cut-off points to identify overweight and obesity. However, by choosing percentile values, any public health analyses and comparison purposes are minimized due to the fact that cut-off points vary between populations and over time. Recently a standard definition for child overweight and obesity cut-off points for BMI based on international data and linked to the widely accepted adult cut-off points of 25 and 30 kg/m² has been established.

The scale of the problem

The obesity epidemic rolls on without signs of abatement (see *Public Health Nutrition*, chapter 9). The World Health Organization (WHO) has declared obesity as the largest global chronic health problem in adults, which by 2025 will emerge as a more serious world problem than malnutrition. Currently, it is estimated that over 300 million people worldwide are obese, while more than one billion suffer from overweight. While in 1980, 6% of men and 8% of women in Britain were clinically obese, by 1998, those figures had ballooned to 17% of men and 21% of women, and by now, the numbers have continued to increase to 22% of men and 24% of women (Figure 3.1). About a fifth of the population is obese and nearly two-thirds of men and over a half of women in England are either overweight or obese. If this progression continues, more than a quarter of adults will be obese by 2010. The growth of obesity in England reflects a worldwide trend. In 1991, 12.0% of US adults were clinically obese (defined as a BMI ≥30.0 kg/m²). By 2000, those figures had grown to 19.8%, representing a 65% increase in a

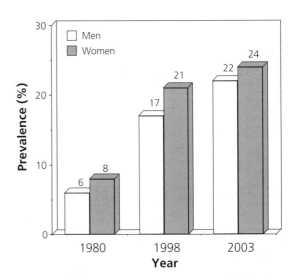

Figure 3.1 Increase in the prevalence of obesity in the UK in the last two decades.

decade. In 1999, an estimated 61% of US adults were overweight or obese, along with 13% of children and 14% of adolescents. During the past two decades, the percentage of children and adolescents who are overweight has nearly doubled and almost trebled, respectively. Disparities in overweight and obesity prevalence exist in many segments of the population based on race and ethnicity, gender, age, and socioeconomic status. In general, the prevalence is higher in women who are members of racial and ethnic minority populations and those with a lower family income.

Economic impact and global burden

Economic evaluation of health care is the generic term referring to the various methods used to make the costs and benefits associated with any change in health service delivery explicit, while burden and cost of illness studies estimate the absolute amount of resources used in treating a disease over a given period. Unfortunately, the consequences of overweight and obesity are more far-reaching than mere esthetic problems (Tables 3.2 and 3.3). Excess body weight puts patients at a higher risk of heart disease, hypertension, diabetes mellitus, dyslipidemia, stroke, osteoarthritis, sleep apnea, certain cancers, and other serious associated diseases. The problems linked to obesity cause in the UK an estimated human cost of 18 million sick days a year and 30 000 deaths a year, with an estimated direct cost of US$0.91

Table 3.2 Reported economic costs of obesity

| Country | Year | Cost | | Health care expenditure (%) |
		Direct	Indirect	
Netherlands	1989	$0.5 billion		2.4
New Zealand	1991	$208 million		>2
France	1992	$69.7 million	$ 0.69 million	4
Australia	1996	$1.13–1.89 billion		
Canada	1997	$1.11–4.56 billion		
Spain	1999	$1.68 million		
USA	2000	Included in indirect	$117 billion	6–7
UK	2003	$0.91 billion	$3.63 billion	>1.5

Adapted from Caterson *et al.* (2004).

billion a year in treatment costs to the NHS, accounting for an indirect cost of US$3.63 billion a year to the UK economy. In 2000 the total direct and indirect costs attributed to overweight and obesity amounted to US$117 billion in the US.

In addition to the serious life-threatening diseases associated with obesity, a range of debilitating conditions such as osteoarthritis, respiratory difficulties, gallbladder disease, infertility, psychosocial problems, etc., which lead to reduced quality of life and disability, are extremely costly in terms of both absence from work and use of health resources, accounting for approximately 9.4% of US health care expenditures. Each year, an estimated 300 000 US adults die from illnesses caused or worsened by obesity, a death toll that may soon overtake tobacco as the chief cause of preventable deaths. Importantly, the risk increases throughout the range of moderate and severe overweight for both men and women in all age groups.

3.2 Etiology

Remarkable new insights into the mechanisms controlling body weight are providing an increasingly detailed framework for a better understanding of the pathogenesis underlying weight gain. Key peripheral signals have been linked to hypothalamic neuropeptide release, and the anatomic and functional networks that integrate these systems have begun to be elucidated. Obesity is a multifactorial disease influenced by both genetic and environmental factors (Figure 3.2). Since obesity has reached epidemic proportions the epidemiologic triad of host, agent, and environment can be used to consider causal factors.

The agent, by definition, is energy imbalance, where energy intake exceeds energy expenditure. This thermodynamic mismatch is determined by both genetic and environmental components. In the epidemiologic triad, features of the host affect obesity in ways that are

Table 3.3 Diseases used in studies of costs of obesity and the relative risks (RR) utilized.

Frequency of use	Disease	RR range
Invariably	Type 2 diabetes mellitus	2.9–27.6
Frequently	Hypertension	2.5–4.3
	Coronary heart disease	1.7–3.5
	Gallbladder disease	1.9–10
	Cancer	1.2–1.5
Often	Dyslipidemia	1.4–1.5
	Stroke	1.1–3.1
	Osteoarthritis	1.8
Occasionally	Gout	2.5
	Venous thrombosis	2.4

From Caterson *et al.* (2004).

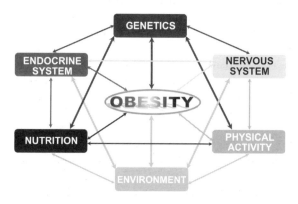

Figure 3.2 Schematic representation of the multifactorial factors influencing the development of obesity.

not well understood. Some individuals appear to be more susceptible than others to weight gain. Genetic factors impinge on appetite, food choices, endocrinology, metabolism, activity, and how the body fine-tunes the balance between energy intake and expenditure. In the last years an alphabet soup of genes has been found to influence everything from food intake to how fat is stored in the body. The third entity that facilitates an epidemic is the environment, by bringing the susceptible host and the agent together.

Environmental factors include our increasingly sedentary lifestyles as well as social and cultural values. Evidence for a genetic component to obesity is multiple and includes twin studies, adoption studies, familial aggregation, complex segregation analysis, monogenic syndromes, and gene variants that affect the obese phenotypes. Quantitating the exact genetic contribution to a predisposition to obesity has proved difficult. Great progress has been made in understanding the molecular mechanisms underlying phenotypes of altered body weight, adiposity, and fat distribution.

The energy balance equation

Energy balance regulation is an extremely complex process composed of multiple interacting homeostatic and behavioral pathways aimed at maintaining constant energy stores. It is now evident that body weight control is achieved through highly integrated interactions between nutrient selection, organoleptic influences, and endocrine responses to diet, as well as being influenced by genetic and environmental factors. The brain is known to play a critical role in maintaining whole-body energy balance by regulating energy intake and expenditure in accordance with afferent and efferent signals. Regulation of body weight was once considered a simple feedback control system, in which the hypothalamus modulated food intake to compensate for fluctuations in body weight. The existing body of evidence has fostered the transition from the classic 'lipostat' to a multifactorial model, including factors emerging from several different organs.

From an evolutionary point of view, animals feed to satisfy their immediate caloric and nutritional requirements from meal to meal, but also to allow energy and nutrients to be stored in anticipation of high energy demands or seasonal food shortages. Thus, food intake control involves the integration of external environmental cues with multiple internal physiological signals as well as external social elements and hedonic influences. An obese phenotype, which ultimately expresses a heterogeneous group of conditions with multiple causes, can only occur when energy intake exceeds energy expenditure for an extended period of time. The sustained energy balance displacement incontrovertibly leads to changes in body energy stores.

Energy intake

The amount of food consumed represents a major contributor to the control of body weight and consequently to obesity development. The biobehavioral food intake control system includes orosensory, gastrointestinal, circulating, nutritional, metabolic, and central influences, which interact to elicit facilitatory or inhibitory signals. The main food and nutrient influences affecting the human appetite system are summarized in Table 3.4. Multiple systems ranging from elaborated cognitive influences to purely chemical signals work at different levels to maintain a functional cascade of sequential physiological events to regulate hunger and satiety. Feeding patterns including the amount, kind, and composition of food consumed are governed by a pleiad of influences from quite diverse anthropologic spheres.

In the last decade, with the identification of leptin, research into appetite control has progressed at a

Table 3.4 Main influences affecting the human appetite system

Influence	Examples
Cognitive	Restraint, emotions, previous experiences, conditioned associations
Sociocultural	Religious beliefs, education, tradition, learned experiences, economy-acquisition level
Gustatory	Palatability, learned/innate preferences, food-specific satiety, nutrient-associated sensory stimuli, cephalic phase events
Neuroendocrine	Orexigenic and anorexigenic peptides, entero-insular axis, adipostatic signals, sympathetic/parasympathetic balance
Gastrointestinal	Nutrient composition, water content, energy density, digestibility, pH, osmolarity, peptidic/hormonal/neural release, stomach size, mechanical distension, emptying rate, absorption
Metabolic	Nutrient partitioning/flux, nutrient–genotype interactions, hepatic metabolism
Behavioral	Age, sex, socioeconomic status, occupation, meal patterns, physical activity level, pathophysiology/developmental stage

Orexigenic	Anorexigenic
Agouti-related protein (AGRP)	Amylin
Beacon	Alpha-melanocyte-stimulating hormone (α-MSH)
Dynorphin	Bombesin
Endocannabinoids	Brain-derived neurotrophic factor (BDNF)
Gamma-aminobutyric acid (GABA)	Calcitonin-gene related peptide (CGRP)
Galanin	Cholecystokinin
Glucocorticoids	Ciliary neurotrophic factor (CNTF)
Ghrelin	Cocaine- and amphetamine-related transcript (CART)
Growth hormone-releasing hormone (GHRH)	Corticotropin-releasing hormone (CRH)
Interleukin 1 receptor antagonist	Enterostatin
Melanin-concentrating hormone (MCH)	Gastrin-releasing peptide (GRP)
Motilin	Glucagon
Neuropeptide Y (NPY)	Glucagon-like peptide 1 and 2 (GLP-1, GLP-2)
Noradrenaline (α_2 receptor)	Histamine
Opioid peptides (β-endorphin)	Insulin
Orexins/hypocretins	Interleukin 1, interleukin 2
	Leptin
	Neurotensin
	Norepinephrine (β receptor)
	Oxytocin
	Oxyntomodulin
	Peptide YY$_{3-36}$
	Pituitary adenylate cyclase-activated peptide (PACAP)
	Prolactin-releasing peptide
	Serotonin
	Somatostatin
	Thyrotropin-releasing hormone (TRH)
	Tumor necrosis factor alpha (TNFα)
	Urocortin
	Xenin

Table 3.5 Hormones, neurotransmitters, and peptides implicated in food intake control

phenomenal rate (see chapter 3 in *Nutrition and Metabolism*). A complex network of synchronous, redundant, and counterbalancing peptide signals has been identified. These interactions are mainly mediated in the hypothalamus, where orexigenic and anorexigenic signals regulate feeding behavior via effects on hunger and satiety (Table 3.5). The means by which the body strives to defend fat stores in the face of large variations in day-to-day energy intake and expenditure is a topic of paramount biomedical importance. In this sense, it can be stated that not all peptides are 'equal,' which implies that the adaptive responses to weight gain and loss are critical and have evolved differentially over time based on teleological reasons. Thus, the efficiency of the peptides and systems aimed at defending the organism against starvation is more important than the anorexigenic pathways.

Progress in understanding the contribution of energy intake to the etiology of obesity has been seriously confounded by underreporting, averaging about 30%

of energy consumption in obese subjects. Whether this phenomenon takes place consciously or subconsciously has not been established. Several causes may underlie underreporting, ranging from changes in eating habits subsequent to the pressure of recording food intake to underestimation of portion size and inadequate knowledge of food composition as well as forgetfulness. In addition, individual macronutrients are known to exert different effects on eating behavior as a consequence of their diverse satiating ability.

Based on experiments with manipulated foods and retrospective analyses of dietary records, protein has been suggested to be the most satiating macronutrient, while fat appears to have the weakest effect, which provides support for subjects readily overeating in response to high fat foods. However, other factors such as energy density have also to be taken into consideration, since under conditions of isoenergetically dense diets the high fat hyperphagia does not occur. The role played by sensory preferences for particular food groups in association with obesity has also been addressed; however, the high intersubject variability may mask any potential obese–lean differences. Initially, some epidemiological studies suggested that individuals reporting eating a greater number of small meals had a lower relative weight than those eating fewer but large meals. A review of the literature failed to find any significant association between the eating frequency and obesity development.

Energy expenditure

Total energy expenditure (TEE) reflects the sum of three major components, namely basal metabolic rate (BMR), thermogenesis, and physical activity (Figure 3.3). The BMR represents 60–75% of the total energy expenditure in sedentary people. It represents the energy required to maintain the basic physiological functions such as respiration, circulation, cellular homeostasis, and tissue regeneration. The BMR can be measured following highly standardized conditions, including the determination early in the morning, with the subject in a complete rest, in a thermoneutral environment, and after an overnight fast. Approximately 80% of the interindividual variance in BMR can be accounted for by age, fat-free mass, and gender. Potential mechanisms for the remaining variance can be attributed to differences in sympathetic nervous system activity and skeletal muscle metabolism. Although this leaves some scope, which may predispose

subjects with a relatively low BMR to obesity development, BMR studies have conclusively shown that obese individuals have an increased BMR relative to their lean counterparts.

The thermogenesis compartment comprises the heat production specifically generated for body temperature maintenance (thermoregulatory thermogenesis), the obligatory heat loss associated with the absorption, transport, and metabolism of recently ingested food (diet-induced thermogenesis, DIT) as well as the heat production switched on in order to dissipate excess dietary energy as heat (adaptive thermogenesis or luxus consumption). In humans, due to the large body size and subsequent low surface area:volume ratio, thermoregulatory thermogenesis is usually of minor importance. In addition, clothing and heating have minimized the thermogenic challenge of cold stress. The DIT, also termed postprandial thermogenesis, is mostly obligatory but does also contain a so-called 'facultative' fraction, which is non-obligatory and is stimulated by the sympathetic nervous activity.

The capacity for facultative thermogenesis has been suggested to explain the differential propensity to weight gain during periods of overfeeding. Under carefully controlled experimental conditions and with rigorous determination techniques any significant role for this energy compartment in the modulation of energy balance during overfeeding has been discarded. However, in the last years evidence that the best predictor of interindividual differences in fat gain during overeating is the so-called non-exercise activity thermogenesis (NEAT) has been provided. NEAT encompasses, besides the calorie expenditure of activities of daily living, the energy costs of all non-volitional muscle activity such as muscle tone, posture maintenance, and fidgeting. Interestingly, changes in NEAT have been reported to account for differences in fat storage between individuals, suggesting that as humans overeat, activation of NEAT dissipates excess energy to preserve leanness, and that failure to activate NEAT may lead to weight gain. Since thermogenesis accounts only for a fraction of TEE (about 10%) the potential for a significant contribution in humans is relatively small, though not negligible.

The most variable component of energy expenditure is represented by physical activity, which may account for 20–50% of TEE. It consists of the sum of all gross muscular work involved in body displacement, including all minor movements, as well as in performing

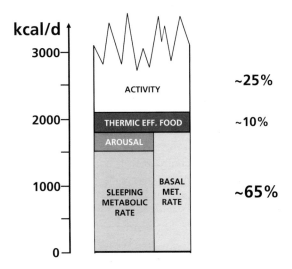

Figure 3.3 Major components of daily energy expenditure in humans (example for a 70-kg man).

physical work. The ratio of TEE/BMR gives an index of the activity of an individual, the physical activity level (PAL). In humans the freedom to undertake exercise and everyday lifestyle physical activities accounts for a further high interindividual variability in this energy fraction. Physical work can be divided into weight-independent and weight-dependent activities. Consequently, the energy cost of weight-bearing exercises is highly correlated with body mass and is, therefore, much higher in obese individuals. Moreover, activity can be further divided according to whether it is essentially obligatory or discretionary. In modern societies mechanization has replaced most manual labor. Therefore, leisure time physical activity is gaining a dominant role in determining energy expenditure. In this respect, the general secular trend towards less active lifestyles in affluent countries appears as the major contributor to the obesity epidemic.

Genetic factors

Although the search for genes responsible for human obesity has experienced outstanding advances, the genetic explanation for, or susceptibility to, obesity in the vast majority of patients has not been identified. In some rare cases of severe childhood-onset obesity, single gene defects have been accounted for. Further evidence for a genetic component to obesity is derived from twin studies, adoption studies, familial aggregation, complex segregation analysis, monogenic syndromes, and gene variants that affect the obese phenotypes. Quantitating the exact genetic contribution to a predisposition to obesity has proved difficult. Great progress has been made in understanding the molecular mechanisms underlying phenotypes of altered body weight, adiposity, and fat distribution by creating transgenic animal models. A role of utmost importance for genetic factors in body weight regulation seems difficult to reconcile with the burgeoning of human obesity in the past decade. Available evidence supports the fact that obesity is an oligenic disease, whose expression can be modulated by numerous polygenic modifier genes interacting with each other and with environmental factors such as food choices, physical activity, and smoking (Figure 3.4).

Genetic epidemiology
Genetic epidemiology studies are useful for addressing specific questions pertaining to the extent of famil-

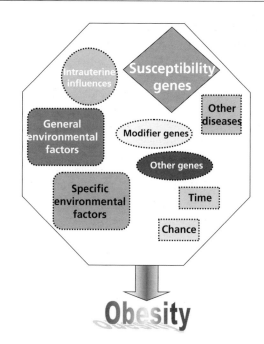

Figure 3.4 Obesity represents a complex oligogenic disease.

ial aggregation in obesity, the relative contribution of non-genetic vs. genetic factors, paternal vs. maternal transmission, contribution of shared genetic and environmental factors to covariation among phenotypes, etc. Monozygotic twins (MZ) share 100% of their genes while dizygotic twins (DZ) twins share on average half of them. Therefore, twin studies allow for separation of the genetic component of variance. Nonetheless, twins may also share common environmental influences thus masking the real genetic component. Heritability estimates for BMI derived from twin studies typically cluster between 50 and 80%. The correlations of MZ twins reared apart provide a direct estimate of the genetic effect, given the fact that members of the same pair were not placed in similar environments, that behavioral characteristics were different, and that intrauterine factors did not affect long-term variation in BMI. The heritability of BMI under these circumstances would be in the range of 40–70%.

Adoption studies represent a useful tool for quantifying the contribution of the common environmental effects by exposing adoptive parents and their offspring (and adopted siblings) to the same environmental sources of variation, while the adoptees and biological parents share only genetic sources of variance. It has to be taken into consideration, however, that selective and late placement in the adoptive home may result in inflated common environmental estimates (translating to reduced heritability estimates) if the placement is based in part on genetic similarity between the biological and adoptive parents. Heritability estimates for the BMI tends to cluster around 30%, with all the remaining variance attributable to non-shared individual environmental factors.

Comparison of resemblance in pairs of spouses, parents, children, brothers, and sisters, including sometime MZ and DZ twins, for body weight, BMI, and selected skinfold thicknesses have been approached in family studies. As would be expected the highest familial correlation appears among MZ twins (0.73), whereas the average correlation is lowest among spouses (0.13). In an intermediate position are the parent–offspring, sibling, and DZ twin correlations, with 0.22, 0.28, and 0.27, respectively. In the Quebec Family Study, based on 1698 members and 409 families and including nine types of relatives by descent or adoption, a total transmissible variance across generations for the BMI of about 35%, but a genetic effect of only 5% was observed. It can be concluded that the heritability of obesity phenotypes is highest with twin studies, intermediate with nuclear family data, and lowest when derived from adoption data. When several different types of relatives are used jointly in the same design, the heritability estimates typically cluster around 25–40% of the age- and gender-adjusted phenotype variance. In addition, they always tend to be slightly higher for fat distribution phenotypes than for overall body fat, reaching a value of about 50% for abdominal visceral fat.

In segregation analysis, the phenotype is assumed to be influenced by the independent and additive contributions from the major gene effect, a multifactorial background due to polygenes, and a unique environmental component (residual). An overview of the segregation analysis studies for obesity phenotypes provided evidence for the segregation of a recessive locus with a frequency of about 0.2 and accounting for 35–45% of the variance, with a multifactorial component accounting for 40–45% of the variance. Taken together, the several different existing segregation studies quite consistently indicate that body fat and adbominal visceral fat are influenced by the segregation of a recessive locus explaining up to about 65% of the variance in addition to a multifactorial component accounting for 20–40% of the residual variance. These observations

provide evidence for the existence of a subset of obese families in which some genes appear to be more important than others in the genetic etiology of obesity.

Another interesting topic is the genetic covariation between obesity and comorbidities. Multivariate genetic studies try to address whether or not, and to what extent, the associations between overweight and its associated comorbidities share common genetic and/or environmental etiologies. In this regard, the Quebec Family Study examined the hypothesis of a shared genetic basis between measures of body fat and other traits of the metabolic syndrome, showing that adiposity and glucose and insulin concentrations are influenced by specific genetic and environmental factors. Furthermore, shared genetic and environmental factors were shown to contribute to explain the common variance ranging from 5 to 25% between indicators of body fat and insulin within individuals. The obtained results illustrated that there is a shared genetic basis between the two traits with a bivariate heritability estimate of about 10%. Other studies have investigated the cross-trait familial resemblance between measures of body fat and cardiovascular elements (blood pressure, cholesterol, triglycerides, waist-to-hip ratio, etc.).

In summary, the multivariate genetic studies strongly support the presence of familial aggregation in the clustering of obesity and most of its comorbidities, with family studies showing a common familial basis for the covariation between insulin and body fat, adiposity distribution, blood pressure, lipidemia, and high-density lipoprotein (HDL) fractions as well as of HDL particle size. Nevertheless, the shared genetic variance between body fat phenotypes and circulating concentrations of cholesterol and lipoproteins may be lower than for other manifestations of the metabolic syndrome.

Molecular epidemiology

The identification of genes and mutations predisposing to obesity has been principally based on linkage and association studies with candidate genes. Both strategies rely on the principle of co-inheritance of adjacent DNA markers. Linkage studies analyze the cosegregation between a marker locus and a trait within families, whereas association studies test in the population for the co-occurrence of an allele at a marker locus and a trait in unrelated individuals. Candidate genes can be selected on the basis of several approaches:

- observed influence of the trait in animal models – candidate genes by mutation;
- known chromosomal locations physiologically or metabolically relevant for the obesity phenotype – functional candidate genes;
- position in a region of the genome – positional candidate genes, near a Mendelian obesity syndrome, within a quantitative trait locus (QTL) homologous to a locus linked to obesity in animal models or identified through human genome-wide scans.

Single gene mutation mouse models
So far, a small number of single genes with spontaneous mutations have been observed to be responsible for mouse models of obesity. These mutations are listed in Table 3.6. Most human linkage and association studies of the cloned genes from obesity mouse models have yielded negative results with only a small number of cases of human obesity related to the specific mutations mentioned. Nevertheless, these candidate genes have been extremely useful to gain more insight into the understanding of the molecular basis of human body weight control. This is extraordinarily evident in the case of leptin and how it has contributed to the unravelling of new pathways in the regulation of food intake and energy balance.

Functional candidate genes
The last update of the human obesity gene map, incorporating published results through October 2002 as well as related websites (http://obesitygene.pbrc.edu; http://www.obesity.chair.ulaval.ca/genemap.html) show the number of genes and DNA sequence variations known to be associated and/or linked with obesity-related phenotypes together with the exact chromosomal location of the gene. As of October 2002, 222 studies have reported positive associations with 71 candidate genes. Putative loci have been found on all

chromosomes except Y. More than 300 genes, markers, and chromosomal regions have been associated and/or linked with human obesity phenotypes such as increased BMI or adiposity. Interestingly, the positive findings of the large number of genes identified has not always been replicated in independent populations. Potentially, candidate genes can be defined on the basis of an impact on body mass, adiposity, fat distribution, food intake, satiety signals, energy expenditure, diet-induced thermogenesis, physical activity, nutrient partitioning, and comorbidities, among others.

A recent review of the evidence for the presence of an association between markers of candidate genes with BMI, body fat, and other obesity-related phenotypes has identified 51 genes. From all those genes only the ADRB2, GNB3, LDLR, LEP, LEPR, PPARG, TNFA, UCP2, and UCP3 genes have been shown to be associated with obesity-related phenotypes in at least five different studies.

Positional candidate genes
Positional candidate genes of obesity are considered those for which their position in the human genome maps to a chromosomal region containing genes or loci that could influence obesity. Undoubtedly, Mendelian syndromes of obesity represent a good example of positional candidate genes. Although it has been observed that overweight and obesity runs in families, most cases do not segregate in families according to a clear pattern of Mendelian inheritance. Nonetheless, some rare Mendelian disorders with obesity as a clinical feature have been described and are summarized in Table 3.7. The Prader–Willi syndrome is the most common of the listed disorders, with an estimated prevalence of 1:25 000.

Most of the disorders listed share some other clinical features, in addition to obesity, such as mental retardation, delayed growth and maturation, hypogonad-

Table 3.6 Single-gene mutations of mouse models of obesity and their corresponding chromosomal regions in the human genome

Mutation	Gene product	Genetic effect	Chromosome Mouse	Human
Obese (ob)	Leptin	Recessive	6 (10.5)	7q31.1
Diabetes (db)	Leptin receptor	Recessive	4 (46.7)	1p31
Agouti yellow (A^y)	Agouti signaling peptide	Dominant	2 (89.0)	20q11.2
Fat (fat)	Carboxypeptidase E	Recessive	8 (32.6)	4q32
Tubby (tub)	Insulin signaling protein	Recessive	7 (51.5)	11p15.5
Mahogany (mg)	Attractin	Recessive	2 (73.9)	20p13

Table 3.7 Disorders with Mendelian inheritance in humans with obesity as clinical feature

Inheritance	Disorder	Mapping
Autosomal dominant	Achondroplasia	4p16.3
	Adiposis dolorosa (Dercum disease)	NA
	Albright hereditary osteodystrophy	
	AHO	20q13.2
	AHO2	15q
	Posterior polymorphous corneal dystrophy	20q11
	Morgani–Stewart–Morel syndrome	NA
	Momo syndrome	NA
	Prader–Willi syndrome	15q11.2–12
	Angelman syndrome	15q11-q13
	Ulnar-mammary Schnizel syndrome	12q23–24.1
	Familial partial lipodystrophy	1q21-q22
	Insulin resistance syndromes	19p13.3
	Thyroid hormone resistance syndrome	3p24.3
	Polycystic ovarian syndrome	NA
Autosomal recessive	Alström syndrome	2p13-p12
	Bardet–Biedl syndrome	
	BBS1	11q13
	BBS2	16q21
	BBS3	3p13-p12
	BBS4	15q22.3–23
	BBS5	2q31
	BBS6	20p12
	Berardinelli–Seip congenital lipodystrophy	9q34
	Biemond syndrome	NA
	Cohen syndrome	8q22–23
	Carbohydrate-deficient glycoprotein syndr. t IA	16p13
	Fanconi–Bickel syndrome	3q26.1–26.3
	Cushing disease	NA
	Macrosomia adiposa congenita	NA
	Pickwickian syndrome	NA
	Urban–Rogers–Meyer syndrome	NA
	Short stature–obesity syndrome	NA
	Summit syndrome	NA
X-linked	Börjeson–Forssman–Lehman syndrome	Xq26.3
	Choroideremia with deafness and obesity	Xq21.1-q21
	Mehmo syndrome	Xp22.13-p21
	Chudley mental retardation syndrome	NA
	Wilson–Turner syndrome	Xq21.1–22
	Simpson–Golabi–Behmel syndrome	
	SGBS1	Xq26
	SGBS2	Xp22

NA, not available.

ism, as well as dysmorphic characteristics affecting the facies and limbs, making them difficult to distinguish and sometimes leading to missclassifications. In this sense, the Laurence–Moon and the Bardet–Biedl syndromes have long been considered a single entity (Laurence–Moon–Bardet–Biedl syndrome) because of the presence of mental retardation, hypogenitalism, and pigmentary retinopathy in both syndromes. However, the Laurence–Moon syndrome can not be considered as an obesity syndrome, since obesity is not present in all cases, while it is a characteristic feature of the Bardet–Biedl syndrome. Similarly, the Carpenter syndrome resembles the Summit syndrome, but obesity is only developed in older patients.

For most of the listed syndromes the specific genetic or molecular defect is unknown. Only about a third, mainly belonging to the autosomal dominant and X-linked syndromes, have been mapped.

Furthermore, positional candidate genes of obesity can be identified from genomic scans with a set of evenly spaced genetic markers covering the entire genome. Box 3.1 lists the nine relevant genome-wide scans of obesity carried out and reported to date, while Table 3.8 shows the genomic regions with obesity quantitative trait loci (QTLs) identified at least in two studies. QTLs represent regions of the genome containing markers that have shown significant evidence of linkage with obesity phenotypes. Although the ethnic groups, sampling strategies, density of the markers, phenotypes selected as well as the analytical strategies vary across the different studies the information obtained suggests that there are most probably some common genes and sequence variants involved in the genetic predisposition to obesity among a whole variety of populations or ethnic groups. Moreover, it appears that the predisposition to obesity might be also influenced by other genes and alleles whose prevalences and effect sizes vary from population to population.

Table 3.8 Genomic regions with obesity quantitative trait loci (QTLs) found in at least two of the studies

Gene	Evidence in
1p11–31	PFS, QFS
2p21	PLFS, SAFHS
7q31	OOAP, QFS
8q11–23	HERITAGE, SAFHS
9q22–34	HERITAGE, QFS
10p12–15	HERITAGE, OOAP, PLFS
14q11–31	HERITAGE, OOAP
17q11–21	QFS, SAFHS
18q12–21	PFS, FFS, QFS
20q11–13	PFS, UPFS

The genetic and molecular epidemiology studies carried out over the last decade have considerably enhanced our understanding of the genetic factors contributing to the development of obesity and involved in shaping interindividual differences not only in body weight or adiposity, but also in the susceptibility to response to energy balance challenges as well as the development of several obesity-associated comorbidities. Under way are linkage and association studies in various populations to identify these genes together with the analysis of a variety of obesity subphenotypes, the exploration of the interactions between gene–gene/gene–nutrient/gene–environment. In addition, new technological aids as embodied by the application of microarrays will further contribute to broaden our knowledge in this complex field.

Endocrine disorders

While genetic factors cause obesity mainly through endocrine mechanisms, most endocrinologic changes taking place in obese patients are due to obesity itself. Primary endocrine causes of obesity encompass hypothalamic structural lesions due to tumors (craniopharyngioma, pituitary macroadenoma with suprasellar extension) as well as other space-occupying lesions produced by trauma, infiltration, inflammation, or iatrogenic damage through surgery or radiotherapy. Panhypopituitarism, growth hormone (GH) deficiency, and hypogonadism represent further contributing factors of primary endocrine obesity. Among the recently described monogenetic syndromes of obesity with hypothalamic dysfunction the mutations in leptin, leptin receptor, pro-opiomelanocortin, prohormone convertase 1, and melanocortin-4 receptor (MC4R) need to be mentioned. These are extremely rare syndromes in everyday clinical practice, except for the MC4R mutation, which has been reported to appear in approximately 4% of morbidly obese patients.

Endocrinopathies

Contrary to common belief, primary endocrine disorders are not the underlying cause in most cases of human obesity. However, a number of known endocrinopathies causally associated with obesity in their clinical presentation should be taken into consideration. The diagnostic process should explore the potential presence of adrenocortical, thyroid, ovarian, and pancreatic diseases. The hypercortisolemia characteristic of Cushing's syndrome (due to primary adrenal disease, increased pituitary stimulation or from ectopically secreted adrenocorticotropic hormone (ACTH)) is accompanied by an enlarged visceral adipose tissue depot as well as all the features of the metabolic syndrome. Hypothyroidism may lead in about 60% of patients to weight gain. Since the prevalences of hypothyroidism and obesity are about 4% and 15%, respectively, it is feasible that both conditions will coexist in some patients.

The exact mechanisms linking the polycystic ovary syndrome (PCOS) with obesity have not been completely established. The hyperandrogenism with chronic anovulation is not always accompanied by increased body weight, while the insulin resistance is universal and independent of the effect of obesity. Pancreatic insulin-secreting tumors are extremely rare (with an approximate incidence of 1:1 000 000) with the spontaneous hyperinsulinism producing recurrent hypoglycemia leading to hyperphagia and subsequent weight gain.

Endocrine changes as a consequence of obesity

Adipose tissue has been shown to release a number of hormones, cytokines and factors collectively termed as adipokines, such as tumor necrosis factor alpha (TNFα), interleukin 6 (IL-6), leptin, resistin, adiponectin, etc., with known effects on insulin secretion and/or action. Overweight and obesity are characterized by hyperinsulinemia and increased insulin response to an oral glucose load. Hepatic insulin extraction is decreased, particularly in central obesity, contributing further to insulin resistance and finally leading to type 2 diabetes mellitus. Obese individuals display elevated plasma fatty acid concentrations, which impair insulin-stimulated skeletal muscle glucose uptake and oxidation as well as insulin-mediated hepatic glucose output suppression. The main disturbances of the principal endocrinological axes associated with obesity are summarized in Table 3.9, while Figure 3.5 illustrates the endocrine consequences of increased adiposity.

The dysregulation of the hypothalamic–pituitary axis (HPA) in obesity is characterized by a centrally driven altered ACTH secretory dynamics and hyperresponsiveness together with a peripheral elevation of cortisol production and local response at the adipocyte level. The association of increased activity of the HPA with central obesity is based on the effect of elevated cortisolemia on visceral adipose tissue, which

Table 3.9 Disturbances in the main hormonal axes in obesity

Axis/circumstance	Finding
Hypothalamic–pituitary–adrenal	Normal plasma and urinary cortisol concentrations
	Normal 24 h ACTH/cortisol levels
	Increased cortisol production and breakdown
	Decreased daytime cortisol changes and reduced morning peaks
	Increased ACTH pulse frequency + decreased pulse amplitude
	Impaired cortisol suppression after dexamethasone challenge
	Increased stress-induced ACTH secretion
	Elevated adrenal androgen production
Growth hormone–insulin-like growth factor 1	Decreased GH concentrations, reduced pituitary secretion
	Elevated GHBP release
	Decreased IGFBP-1 and IGFBP-3
	Blunted response to stimuli
Hypothalamic–pituitary–gonadal	
In men	Decreased total and free testosterone
	Reduced C19 steroids
	Elevated estrogen production
	Potential aromatase activity alteration
	Decreased LH secretion
	Reduced SHBG levels
In women	Increased free testosterone fraction
	Elevated estrogen production
	Normal gonadotropin secretion
	Reduced SHBG synthesis and levels
	Elevated SHBG-bound and non-bound androgen production
With PCOS	Elevated adrenal androgen secretion
	Increased ovarian testosterone release
	Elevated estrone/estradiol ratio
	Increased androstendione aromatization
	Elevated free steroid levels
	Reduced SHBG
	Decreased IGFBP-1
	Insulin resistance, metabolic syndrome

ACTH, adrenocorticotropic hormone; GH, growth hormone; GHBP, growth hormone-binding protein; IGFBP, insulin-like growth factor-binding protein; LH, luteinizing hormone; SHBG, sex hormone-binding globulin; PCOS, polycystic ovary syndrome.

exhibits a high density of glucocorticoid receptors. Elevated receptor binding together with low circulating binding globulins may lead to an accelerated clearance

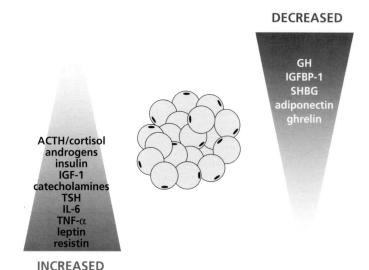

DECREASED

GH
IGFBP-1
SHBG
adiponectin
ghrelin

ACTH/cortisol
androgens
insulin
IGF-1
catecholamines
TSH
IL-6
TNF-α
leptin
resistin

INCREASED

Figure 3.5 Main endocrine changes associated with increased adiposity.

of cortisol. Increased expression of 11-β-hydroxysteroid dehydrogenase in visceral adipocytes may further contribute to exaggerated local cortisol production, thereby leading to central obesity.

In women, increased body fat is associated with hyperandrogenism and ovulatory dysfunction, often leading to infertility. Circulating testosterone and androstenedione levels are usually increased in obese women, whereas sex hormone-binding globulin (SHBG) concentrations are decreased, with an elevated estrone/estradiol plasmatic ratio. The low SHBG activity facilitates accelerated testosterone clearance rates, resulting in an elevated proportion of unbound testosterone available for hepatic extraction and clearance. In obese men, a decrease in circulating levels of total and free testosterone as well as SHBG are observed.

The hypothalamic–pituitary–thyroid axis (HPT) exerts a relevant role on energy homeostasis, as evidenced by adaptive changes taking place during the course of overfeeding and fasting periods. Despite the observation of normal free thyroid hormone concentrations in obese adults, other studies have suggested a central upregulation based on increased TSH and decreased prolactin responses to TRH. While overfeeding increases total thyroid hormone concentrations and decreases reverse T3 levels, fasting has been shown to be accompanied by low free T3 and T4 concentrations in obese individuals. The changes in the pituitary–thyroid axis involve the action of leptin in the arcuate nucleus on neuropeptide Y (NPY) and pro-opiomelanocortin (POMC)-expressing neurons.

The alterations present in the growth hormone/insulin-like growth factor (GH/IGF) axis of obese subjects include a nutrient and neuroendocrine-induced inhibition of secretion as well as increased binding and clearance, which lead to decreased GH concentrations. Hyposecretion of GH depends more on pulse amplitude decrease than on reduced pulse frequency. Elevated concentrations of GH-binding protein further contribute to the low GH levels observed in obesity. The increased circulating free fatty acids present in obese individuals downregulate pituitary GH secretion, while a dysregulated hypothalamic glucose sensing with a blunted inhibitory effect of glucose on GH secretion takes place in obesity.

Given the suppressing effect of insulin on GH secretion, the hyperinsulinemia characteristic of obesity further contributes to decreases in its secretion. Elevated IGF-1 resulting from adipose mass enlargement contributes to GH hyposecretion via a negative feedback on pituitary cells. Recently, the decreased ghrelin concentrations observed in obesity have been also suggested as a potential mechanism of reduced GH secretion.

Environmental factors

Recent trends indicate that the primary causes of obesity lie in environmental or behavioral changes, since the escalating rates of obesity are ocurring in a relatively constant gene pool and, hence, against a constant metabolic background. In their elegant study, Prentice and Jebb (1995) clearly showed that in the past 20 years average recorded energy and fat intake in Britain had declined substantially, so that at the population level energy intakes had fallen, while obesity rates experimented a continous escalation.

The paradox of increasing obesity in the face of decreasing food intake can only be explained if levels of energy expenditure have declined faster than energy intake, thus leading to an overconsumption of energy relative to a greatly reduced requirement. The implication is that levels of physical activity, and hence energy needs, have declined even faster than intake. Furthermore, the development and use of new forms of technology that affect everything from housing to transport as well as clothing, communications, and an increasingly larger scope of factors has led to a postindustrial society in which lower energy expenditure by humans through improved insulation and automatization cause less energy to be spent in human activities.

Over the last decades for many people leisure time pursuits are dominated by TV viewing and other inactive pastimes. Proxy measures of physical inactivity such as car ownership and TV viewing have rocketed. The rapid rise in childhood obesity has been mirrored by an explosion of non-active leisure pursuits for children such as computers and video games. Currently, evidence suggests that modern inactive lifestyles are important determinants in the etiology of obesity, possibly representing the dominant factor.

Due to the fact that obesity is intricately bound up with the individual's lifestyle, a number of public sector agencies play a potentially significant role in reshaping what can be called as an 'obesogenic' environment (Figure 3.6), in which sedentarism and cheap, high-fat foods dominate over active leisure-time occupations and healthy food choices. However, successful efforts must focus not only on individuals, but also on group, institutional, and community influences, as well as public policy. A multidimensional approach understands that individual changes can only occur in a supportive environment with accessible and healthy food choices, opportunities for engaging in regular physical activity and access to adequate medical treatment. The environment has to be considered to encompass not just the physical environment, such as the layout of the cities, but the environment of economic and social organization and cultural values. In this sense, the public health would benefit from going beyond a narrowly mechanistic focus on energy intake and physical activity and examine the economic, social, and cultural context more broadly.

Clinical medicine and public health agencies have to face preventing obesity with new partners, including food marketers and manufacturers, public and private health care purchasers, large employers, transportation agencies, urban planners, and real-estate developers. All of them will play a key role in shaping and supporting social and environmental policies that can help the population, in general, and children, in particular, improve their diet and become more physically active.

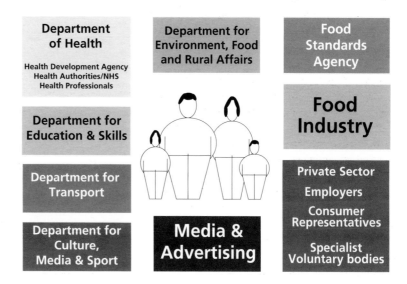

Figure 3.6 Multifaceted influences and institutions in the UK impinging on the family and the individual with a potential impact on reversing the current obesogenic environment.

Psychosocial influences

Obesity is a dynamic, multidimensional biosocial phenomenon exerting a complex synergistic interaction between pathophysiology and the social world. For this reason, excess body weight has to be studied within its particular cultural and historical circumstances. The main social characteristics of individuals known to be associated with body weight regulation include sex, age, race, education level, type of occupation, employment, income, marital status, household size, parenthood, residential density, and geographical region. In addition, psychological factors focusing on the association between overnutrition and behavioral, cognitive as well as emotional processes, which may be under genetic or environmental influence, have to be taken into consideration. Large-scale comparative studies using objective measures of personality or psychiatric disorder are necessary to provide a scientific basis for the relation between emotional disorders and obesity. In general, community studies fail to find a higher prevalence of psychiatric disorders among obese patients compared with normal weight individuals. However, some disorders – in particular depression and anxiety – do appear to be overrepresented among a subset of obese adults who also report binge eating.

The psychosomatic model of obesity proposes that certain personality characteristics or types accompanied by higher than normal levels of emotional distress and lower self-esteem are linked to the development of obesity. Although this may be the case among specific subgroups, such as severely obese patients and obese binge eaters, no clear-cut evidence of the association of any particular personality type with a higher risk of obesity has been established. Nevertheless, personality and emotional distress may play an important role in the response to treatment, especially in failure to comply to dietary indications. The role of dietary restraint in the understanding of obesity suggests that in susceptible subjects it may precipitate eating disorders, while in other individuals it may represent an effective strategy for body weight regulation. The psychobiological model suggests that obese individuals are particularly responsive to external food cues or have a diminished responsiveness to internally generated satiety cues.

Community studies have identified a prevalence of binge eating disorder as high as 2.5% in the general population, reaching about 20–30% rates among obese patients. Emotional eating resulting from arousal is caused by disinhibition of restraint and represents a less severe form of binge eating. Food addictions, especially craving for specific items or macronutrients such as chocolate or carbohydrates, suggest that self-control might be impaired because of biologically based drives for intake. Volitional control of food intake may be difficult for some individuals since hunger is a powerful drive leading to food seeking and consumption. However, specific experimental evidence to support the addiction theory is required to exclude conditioned effects. In addition, food consumption implies a reward experience, which has also to be taken into account. Cognitive behavior specialists have recognized the beneficial effect of decreasing body image dissatisfaction among obese individuals to reduce distress and improve treatment.

Miscellaneous causes

Several different causes of either physiological, sociological, behavioral, pharmacological, or pathological nature covering a broad spectrum of human conditions are able to impact on the complex mechanisms implicated in energy homeostasis. Viruses have been suspected of being involved in obesity in humans. Whether this represents an important mechanism for the induction of obesity, remains, as yet, unclear.

Under normal circumstances in developed countries mean gestational weight gain in normal-weight, healthy, well-nourished women with uncomplicated pregnancies ranges from 11 to 16 kg with approximately 25% of the increase being attributable to fat deposition in maternal adipose tissue. Reports showing a net increase in BMI with sucessive pregnancies provide evidence for a positive correlation between raising body weight and parity. Changes derived from lactation, dietary habits, and physical activity levels related to child-rearing rather than to child-bearing may underlie the excess weight gain associated with parity. Confounding variables that need to be taken into consideration when studying the relation between parity and weight gain include age, education, initial body weight, marital status, health status, smoking, drinking habits, and dieting.

Pregnancy does not lead to obesity in the majority of women; most regain their pre-pregnant weight within around 12 months after delivery. Nevertheless, about 10–15% of women weigh at least 5 kg more after pregnancy compared with their preconception body weight. Risk factors for maternal obesity development include those associated with the period of pregnancy itself (weight gain and smoking cessation during pregnancy), factors common to both the pregnancy and postpartum periods (changes in body image, energy intake and eating patterns, dieting or attitudes towards weight gain), as well as elements specific to the postpartum period (breastfeeding and psychosocial factors, such as stress, self-esteem, and social support).

Middle-aged and older smokers have been shown to weigh on average around 3–4 kg less than non-smokers of a similar age. In contrast, among adolescents and young adults weight differences are small or non-existent, with smoking initiation not evidencing an association with weight loss. However, a number of large prospective studies have observed that smoking cessation is accompanied by a weight gain of about 2–4 kg that is more evident in women, younger people, black people, people of lower prior weight, and heavy smokers. In general approximately 20% of quitters experience a postcessation weight gain of about 10 kg. An increase in energy intake together with the loss of the potentially acute metabolic-enhancing actions attributed to nicotine may contribute to a shift in the balance equation towards weight gain. Undoubtedly, the benefits of quitting smoking outweigh the detrimental effects associated with weight gain and, therefore, should not discourage smoking cessation attempts.

The incidence of weight gain during treatment with several different frequently prescribed drug groups (Table 3.10) has been clearly established. Among the antidepressant medication, the tricyclic drugs are effective for normal mood restoration, but their use is accompanied by a noticeable weight gain, which may sometimes affect medication compliance. The mechanisms of action by which tricyclics promote weight gain have not been completely disentangled but certainly reflect changes in energy balance due to a decrease in energy expenditure related to a reduced sympathetic nervous activity and, to a smaller extent, an increase in caloric intake.

The serotonin-specific reuptake inhibitors represent an alternative antidepressant treatment option usually without the side effect of excessive weight gain due to the lack of influence in increasing appetite and at the same time exerting a potential enhancement of resting energy expenditure. Weight gain has been reported in relation to the use of older monoamine oxidase inhibi-

Table 3.10 Drugs commonly associated with weight gain

Pharmacological group	Drugs
Adrenergic antagonists	Alpha and beta blockers
Anticonvulsants	Valproate, carbamazepine, vigabatrin
Antidepressants	Amitriptilin, imipramine, doxepine, fenelzine, amoxapine, desipramine, trazodone, tranilcipromine, lithium
Antidiabetics	Insulin preparations, sulfonylurea agents, glitazones, tiazolidinediones
Antimigraine drugs	Flunarizine, pizotifen
Antipsychotics	Chlorpromazine, chlordiazepoxide, thioridazine, trifluoperazine, mesoridazine, promazine, mepazine, perphenazine, prochlorperazine, loxapine, haloperidol, thiothixene, fluphenazine, clozapine, olanzapine, risperidone, quetiapine, sertindole
Antiserotoninergics	Cyproheptadine, sanomigran, loratadine, astemizole
Steroids	Glucocorticoids, estrogens (at pharmacological doses), megestrol acetate, tamoxifen
Others	Some antineoplastic agents and immunosuppressants

tors; however, with the newer generation of drugs this side effect appears to be less important. Lithium treatment is commonly followed by weight gain, especially in already overweight patients, in relation to increased food and fluid intake, as well as a hypothyroidism-related decreased energy expenditure.

Antipsychotics are known to promote weight gain during prolonged treatment. The effect is more evident among the conventional drugs than among the novel antipsychotics. An increased energy intake together with reduced physical activity have been proposed to be the apparent mechanisms of this medication-induced weight increase. A commonly described side effect of epilepsy and mania treatment includes weight gain. This effect can be especially pronounced in susceptible subjects with an increase of up to 15 kg over a few months due to a marked influence on food intake.

Anxiolytics, such as benzodiazepine and its derivatives, are not likely to produce a significant weight change in clinical practice, although an increase in body weight has been observed in short-term administration in rodents due to an effect on dopamine D2 receptors or gamma-aminobutyric acid neurons, whereas no influence in long-term experiments was shown.

The combined antihistaminergic and serotoninergic effect of cyproheptadine and pizotifen probably lead to early but rather modest weight gain attributable to an increase in appetite. The non-sedating antihistaminergic compounds loratadine and astemizole induce weight gain too, but to a smaller degree than the older drugs. The appetite-inducing effect of these compounds has been tried in patients with anorexia nervosa and cancer cachexia, but without successful results. Flunarizine, a calcium antagonist applied in migraine prophylaxis, promotes a dose-dependent increase in body weight of up to 4 kg during the first months of treatment by stimulating food intake. The use of non-specific beta-blockers has been associated with a modest but sustained weight gain due to a decrease in energy expenditure, including facultative thermogenesis.

Intensive insulin therapy for the treatment of either type 1 or type 2 diabetes mellitus has been shown to promote weight gain attributable to reduced glucosuria and decreased energy expenditure by the reversal of the catabolic metabolism. Metformin treatment for obese type 2 patients was not accompanied by significant changes in body weight compared with the conventional control group, while a more favorable outcome as regards diabetes complications and mortality were evident. However, the newer glitazones have been reported to be associated with a modest though significant weight gain, which needs to be verified in long-term studies.

A common adverse effect of long-term glucocorticoid therapy is weight gain, which clearly has an impact on body fat distribution by predominantly increasing the abdominal fat depot as well as inducing insulin resistance. The underlying mechanisms of action seems to be related to centrally mediated effects increasing NPY activity and a pronounced decrease in uncoupling proteins expression. Women using oral contraceptives often find that they gain weight, while postmenopausal women following hormone replacement therapy also report an impact on body weight control. High to moderate doses of megestrol acetate produce an increase in appetite and, consequently, in body weight, while tamoxifen, a partial estrogen receptor antagonist, also induces weight gain. Some other non-hormonal antineoplastic drugs, such as cyclophosphamide and fluorouracil, have been associated with weight increase through an unknown mechanism.

3.3 Clinical presentation

The hazards of excess body weight have been clearly established by epidemiological and clinical studies. Although obesity can be easily identified and several different assessment methods are available (Table 3.11), patients who are mildly or moderately overweight may be overlooked. Recent studies have shown that about 25% of overweight patients were thought to be of normal weight by their primary care physicians. It is, however, worrisome that obesity itself is being underestimated by health care professionals. In spite of the high prevalence of this chronic disease it is documented by physicians only in a small proportion of patients, indicating that this life-threatening condition is considerably underreported in medical records.

Similarly, a retrospective analysis has observed an apparently low rate of obesity in hospital outpatient departments treating obesity-related conditions (4% cardiology, 5% rheumatology, and 3% orthopedics), when compared to the true prevalence (30% cardiology, 20% rheumatology, and 25% orthopedics). The large disparity between apparent and true prevalence clearly shows that opportunities for obesity diagnosis and treatment are being missed.

Table 3.11 Methods for the assessment of overweight and obesity

Measurement	Methods
Energy intake	24 h dietary recall
	72 h diet recall
	Food frequency questionnaire
	Macronutrient composition record
Energy expenditure	Indirect calorimetry
	Physical activity level questionnaire
	Movement detector
	Heart rate monitoring
	Doubly labeled water
Body composition	Body mass index
	Skinfold thickness
	Bioelectrical impedance
	Near infrared interactance
	Dual-energy X-ray absorptiometry (DXA)
	Air-displacement plethysmography (BOD-POD)
	Underwater weighing
	Isotope dilution
Regional fat distribution	Waist circumference, waist-to-hip ratio
	Computerized axial tomography
	Ultrasound
	Magnetic resonance imaging

Body composition

The BMI is an accepted index to define differing levels of overweight and obesity, and clinical protocols can be easily adapted to record weight, height, and the resulting BMI calculation. However, obesity is defined by an excess body fat not simply by an increased body weight relative to height. It is well known that neither body weight nor BMI provide an exact description of body composition. Therefore, a further step needs to be taken by drawing attention not only to weight but to body composition itself (see chapter 3 in *Introduction to Human Nutrition*). The principal limitation of the BMI as a measure of body fat is that it does not distinguish fat mass from fat-free mass. Even more, when lifestyle interventions are introduced, measured body fat and BMI can travel in opposite directions. When patients follow a calorie-restricted diet only, body fat may increase despite the weight lost if the majority of the decrease is at the expense of lean body mass. In contrast, an increase in physical activity accompanied by a decrease in energy intake may lead to an increase in total body weight due to the fact that the reduced total fat may be masked by the incremented lean body mass, resulting in a satisfactory and clinically relevant change in percentage fat and hence obesity-associated risk factors. It is therefore important to measure the body compartment that actually creates the health risks, namely body fat. This challenge, together with the effect of therapeutical interventions to alter adiposity distribution, has relevant implications for clinical practice and research.

In the context of tissue, total body weight can be divided into adipose tissue, skeletal muscle, skeleton, and the remaining organs and viscera. The classical methods of body composition estimation are based on a two-compartment model, in which the body is divided into fat and fat-free mass (FFM), the latter including water, protein, glycogen, and mineral. This model assumes that the densities of adipose and lean tissue are constant, namely 0.9 and 1.1 kg/liter, respectively. Table 3.12 summarizes the characteristics of the currently available methods for the estimation of body fat. The selection of the most appropriate method varies according to the specific circumstances and aims (cross-sectional vs. longitudinal assessment; clinical vs. laboratory studies; special subpopulations, etc.). Simple and cheap anthropometric methods are useful for epidemiological surveys of large populations, while more sophisticated and expensive techniques are reserved for research studies aimed at gaining insight into the pathophysiological basis underlying body weight homeostasis.

Further relevant issues to take into consideration are the cost, facilities, and time associated to the use of each of the methods as well as the need for cooperation of the subjects and expertise of the staff. One of the difficulties in evaluating *in vivo* body composition methods is the lack of a true optimal technique. Body composition techniques are frequently compared using correlation analysis. This provides only partial information since methods may show a good relationship with each other, but may not always agree or be equally inaccurate. Therefore, it is of utmost importance to

Table 3.12 Characteristics of body fat estimation methods applied to obesity

Method	Practicality	Accuracy	Sensitivity to change	Cost
Skinfold thickness	++++	++	+	$
Circumference	++++	++	+	$
Body mass index	+++++	+	++	−
Bioelectrical impedance	+++	+	++	$
Near infrared interactance	+++	+	+	$
Total body electrical conductivity	+++	+	+	$
Underwater weighing	+	+++++	++++	$$$$$
DXA	++	+++	++	$$$$
Potassium-40 counting	+	+++	+	$$$$$
Computerised tomography	++	+++++	++++	$$$$$
Magnetic resonance imaging	++	+++++	++++	$$$$$
BOD-POD	+++	+++++	++++	$$$
Multicompartment models	+	++++	++	$$$

DXA, dual-energy X-ray absorptiometry; BOD-POD, air-displacement plethysmography.

validate the data obtained against a reference method and also in a similar population. This is especially true in overweight and obese individuals in whom body fat lost is being monitored.

Up-to-date underwater weighing is considered the traditional 'gold standard' but is impractical for its widespread application at the clinical level. In the last years air-displacement plethysmography (BOD-POD) has been reported to agree closely with the reference hydrodensitometry underwater weighing method, showing that the plethysmographic technique predicts fat mass and FFM more accurately than dual-energy X-ray absorptiometry (DXA) and bioelectrical impedance.

Fat distribution

Regional distribution of body fat is known to be an important indicator for metabolic and cardiovascular alterations, providing an explanation for an inconstant correlation between BMI and these disturbances in some individuals. The observation that the topographic distribution of adipose tissue is relevant to understanding the relation of obesity to disturbances in glucose and lipid metabolism was formulated before the 1950s. Since then, numerous prospective studies have revealed that compared with the 'gynoid or female-type obesity' fat distribution with a predominantly lower body, gluteofemoral, or peripheral fat deposition, 'android or male-type obesity' (also termed central or abdominal obesity), characterized by an increased fat in the upper body, correlates more

often with an elevated mortality and risk for the development of diabetes mellitus type 2, dyslipidemia, hypertension, and atherosclerosis.

The waist-to-hip circumference ratio (WHR) represents a simple, convenient, and useful anthropometric measurement for the estimation of the proportion of abdominal or upper-body fat. However, the WHR does not distinguish between accumulations of deep (i.e. visceral) and subcutaneous abdominal fat. In this sense, imaging techniques, especially computed tomography and magnetic resonance, allow the topographical differentiation of the fat depots showing that the detrimental metabolic and cardiovascular influences of abdominal obesity are mediated by the intra-abdominal fat accumulation.

Comorbidities

Obesity has been reported to cause or exacerbate a large number of health problems (Figure 3.7), which are known to impact on both life expectancy and quality of life. The association between increased body weight and the main systemic comorbidities extending across most major medical specialities are summarized in Table 3.13. Obesity is accompanied by important pathophysiological alterations as a consequence of metabolic and/or mechanical effects associated with excess body weight such as type 2 diabetes mellitus, dyslipidemia, cardiovascular disease, hypertension, stroke, gallbladder disease, infertility, respiratory difficulties, sleep apnea, certain forms of cancer, osteoarthritis, psychosocial problems, etc., which lead to reduced quality of

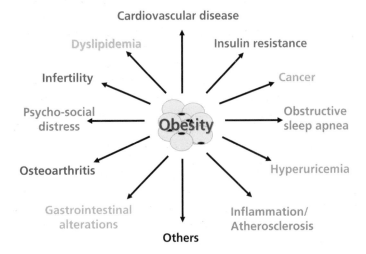

Figure 3.7 Main comorbidities associated with obesity.

Table 3.13 Association of systemic comorbidities with overweight and obesity

System	Pathology/effect
Metabolic	Hyperinsulinism, hyperglycemia
	Insulin resistance, type 2 diabetes mellitus
	Dyslipidemia
	Hyperuricemia, gout
	Syndrome X
Cardiovascular	Hypertension
	Left ventricular hypertrophy, congestive heart failure
	Arrhythmias, sudden death
	Cerebrovascular disease, stroke
	Endothelial dysfunction
	Low-grade chronic inflammation
	Increased sympathetic activity
Hematologic	Impaired fibrinolysis
	Procoagulant state
	Hyperviscosity
	Atherothrombosis, thrombophlebitis
Endocrine	Hirsutism
	Elevated adrenocortical activity
	Disturbances in circulating sex steroids and binding globulins
	Infertility
	Polycystic ovary syndrome
	Breast cancer
Gastrointestinal	Hiatus hernia
	Gastroesophagic reflux
	Gallstone formation, gallbladder hypomotility and stasis
	Gallbladder carcinoma
	Steatosis, cirrhosis
	Colorectal cancer
Respiratory	Restrictive ventilatory pattern, decreased FRC, FVC, and TLC
	Dyspnea/shortness of breath in exercise and/or at rest
	Obesity hypoventilation syndrome
	Obstructive sleep apnea
Renal	Proteinuria, albuminuria
	Enhanced sodium retention
	Renin–angiotensin–aldosterone system stimulation
	Disturbed Na/K ATPase activity, Na/K cotransport
Genitourinary	Incontinence
	Prostate/endometrial/ovarian cancer
Locomotor	Nerve entrapment
	Low back pain, joint damage
	Osteoarthritis
Dermatologic	Increased sweating
	Oppositional intertrigo
	Wound dehiscence
	Lymphoedema
	Acanthosis nigricans

FRC, functional residual capacity; FVC, forced vital capacity; TLC, total lung capacity.

life, decreased life expectancy, and increased mortality. The comorbidities directly causing mortality encompass cancer and cardiovascular disease (see chapters 13 and 14 in *Public Health Nutrition*).

In a recent large prospective cohort study, high BMI values were shown to be associated with increased mortality from cancer for overweight individuals. The underlying biologic mechanisms that have been regularly invoked to explain the association between adiposity and cancer involved mainly steroid hormones and the insulin-like growth factor system. However, recent evidence provided by an extensive study reported an increase in all cancer mortality, suggesting the contribution of further adipocyte-related factors to mutagenesis.

In response to the emerging body of scientific medical data linking excess adiposity to coronary heart disease (CHD), the American Heart Association reclassified obesity as a major, modifiable risk factor for CHD in 1998. The pathophysiological relevance of adipocyte-derived molecules resides in the participation of some of these factors beyond body weight control in vascular homeostasis through effects on blood pressure, fibrinolysis, coagulation, angiogenesis, insulin sensitivity, proliferation, apoptosis, and immunity, among others. In this respect, adipokines have been shown to be implicated either directly or indirectly in the regulation of several processes that regulate the development of inflammation, atherogenesis, hypertension, insulin resistance, and vascular remodeling. Cardiovascular disorders weaken the heart and tire the patient, thus leading to inactivity and weight gain. Similarly, cardiovascular-related target-organ damage alters endothelial, vascular, and renal functions, thereby worsening hypertension. In addition, obesity *per se* can lead to hypertension, thus completing a 'vicious triangle,' which perpetuates the phenomenon.

Cardiac alterations in obese patients reflect an integrated response to multiple hemodynamic, structural, functional, biochemical, metabolic, and endocrine derangements. An elevated BMI results in an increase in blood volume, as well as in sympathetic activity. In addition to increased blood pressure, obese individuals show elevated viscosity and risk factors, such as fibrinogen, plasminogen activator inhibitor type 1 (PAI-1), C-reactive protein, etc., which alter the rheological properties, adding further to the pressure load of the heart. Thus, pressure and volumen load take place simultaneously. Consequently, structural changes to the heart take place. Cardiac mass and geometry alterations lead to left ventricular (LV) hypertrophy. LV wall thickness and myocardial remodeling result in a progressive impairment in LV filling, conducing to a high risk of diastolic dysfunction. Alterations in systolic function may also become evident. In particular, long-standing obesity may result in a decrease in mid-wall fiber shortening and ejection fraction.

In addition to heart failure, arrhythmias take place. Particularly, ventricular ectopic beats in relation to a concentric pattern of LVH, and atrial fibrillation due to atrial enlargement. In synergy, these maladaptive changes increase the risk of cardiovascular death.

Other conditions such as type 2 diabetes, syndrome X, dyslipidemia, atherothrombosis, hypertension, and pulmonary alterations are responsible for the direct morbidity related to obesity, at the same time as contributing indirectly to mortality. While osteoarthritis, gallstone formation, gastrointestinal alterations, and psychosocial problems represent disturbances more likely to cause morbidity rather than mortality. Since these topics are extensively reviewed in chapter 16 of *Public Health Nutrition* as well as in Chapter 5 of this volume, the reader is referred to these specific chapters for a more detailed information.

3.4   Clinical assessment

Given the escalating prevalence rates, obesity will be the leading cause of death and disability in this century word-wide. The rapid increase of obesity to epidemic proportions collides with a scenario where, paradoxically, preoccupation with body weight, fitness, and diet pervades today's society in the developed world. The hazards of excess body weight have been clearly established by epidemiological and clinical studies, highlighting the need for programs for early competent diagnosis, treatment, and prevention. Interestingly, obesity has not until recently featured strongly in medical training, with medical school curricula not even addressing obesity as a disease. Moreover, it has been reported that health professionals hold negative views of overweight and obese patients. Negative attitudes have been observed in medical students, qualified practitioners, nurses as well as dietitians, and may lead to beliefs about the usefulness of intervention, thus representing a barrier to good practice.

A thorough clinical evaluation of the overweight or obese patient includes a medical history and physical examination, with the review-of-systems section specifically addressing the identification of the etiological factors mentioned above as well as providing particular emphasis to the assessment of risk factors and the presence of comorbidities. The history should focus on age of onset of obesity, minimum body weight in adulthood, special events related to weight gain and loss (in women: menstrual history, pregnancies, age at menopause), previous weight loss attempts, treatment modalities, outcomes, and complications. A dietetic history including usual eating pattern, current physical activity level (type and regularity), habitual lifestyle as well as family and social constellation of the patient should be obtained. Smoking history as well as alcohol and substance abuse need also to be asked about.

It is also important to get a clear picture about the nutritional knowledge of the patient since it will determine whether a basic or more sophisticated level of nutrition education will be applied in the sessions. As described earlier, several different medications are known to promote weight gain and should be recorded and, if possible, changed to plausible alternatives with a lower impact on body weight. With the current high prevalence rates of obesity, easily obtained non-prescription weight loss products are an appealing alternative on the increase. Because over-the-counter weight control products, cold remedies, and dietary supplements are generally regarded as safe by the general population, many patients do not inform their physicians about the use of these products. However, due to the possibility of herb–drug and drug–drug interactions physician's should ask their patients about the use of non-prescription weight loss products as well as other supplements.

It is noteworthy that in the group of people using non-prescription weight loss products individuals with uncontrolled or undiagnosed diabetes, hypertension, heart disease, and other weight-related health conditions may be frequent. In this group of patients the use of the mentioned non-prescription products, in general, and of ephedra and ephedrine, in particular, may result in especially adverse effects.

Height and weight should be determined and the resulting BMI calculated. Waist circumference, WHR, and neck circumference should be measured with a tape. Depending upon availability of resources, the physician should try to get information on body composition and fat distribution. Blood pressure should be checked with an appropriately sized cuff. Any evidence of cardiac and pulmonary alterations as well as signs of hyperlipidemia, thyroid disease, and other endocrinopathies should be investigated. The clinician should search for all of the aforementioned obesity-associated complications. Signs and symptoms of these conditions may have been overlooked by the patient and not related to obesity itself and, therefore, should be carefully screened by the physician.

The third part of the clinical evaluation encompasses the laboratory tests, which are relevant for risk assessment and decision making. These include fasting plasma glucose (if needed, confirmation of impaired glucose tolerance or type 2 diabetes by a 2-hour value after an oral glucose tolerance test; in already diagnosed diabetic patients a glycated hemoglobin HbA1c determination), lipid profile (cholesterol-total, LDL, HDL, and triglycerides), basal insulin (may allow to apply several insulin sensitivity/insulin resistance indices), liver function tests for steatohepatitis, thyroid-simulating hormone (TSH) to discount a potential hypothyroidism, and prostate-specific antigen (PSA)

in men as a screening test for prostate cancer. In some specialized centres analysis of known cardiovascular risk factors such as fibrinogen, homocysteine, C-reactive protein, PAI-1, etc. are also carried out.

According to the outcome of the medical history and physical examination a number of complementary explorations may be indicated such as an ophthalmic evaluation in diabetes or sustained hypertension, referral to the cardiologist for a potential echocardiogram, a polysomnographic study in heavy snorers, sleep apnea, nighttime awakening, daytime fatigue with episodes of sleepiness and/or morning headaches, mammography and gynecological screening tests, evaluation of gastroesophageal reflux/hiatus hernia in patients complaining about indigestion, or an ultrasound of the gallbladder in case of abdominal pain.

Several different algorithms have been outlined to help in identifying and managing these complicated patients (Figure 3.8a–d). Most of them are based on BMI assessment and quantification of additional comorbidities in order to apply the most appropriate treatment options for both weight and risk factor man-

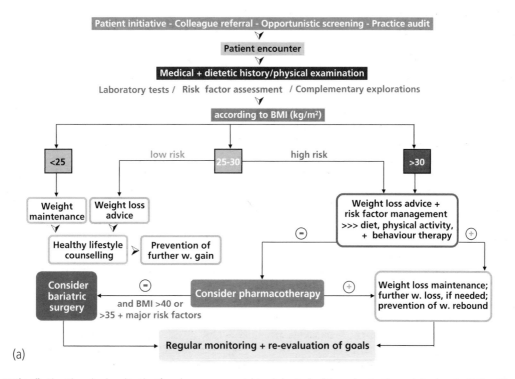

(a)

Figure 3.8(a–d) Algorithms developed to identify and manage overweight and obesity. (b–d) Reproduced with permission from the National Heart, Lung, and Blood Institute (NHLBI) of the National Institutes of Health Obesity Education Initiative (OEI). (*Continued.*)

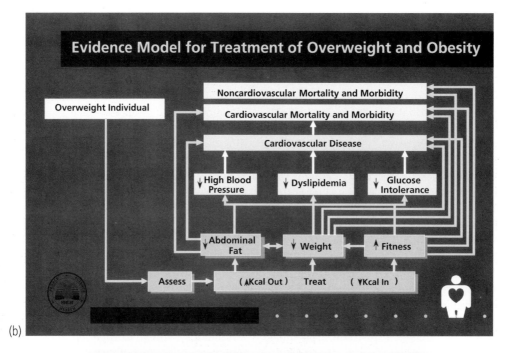

(b)

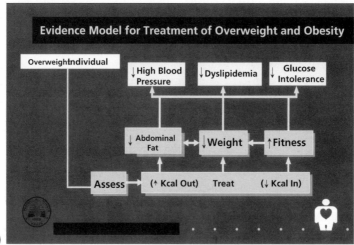

(c)

Figure 3.8(a–d) (Continued.)

agement. Before starting any treatment both patient and physician should have realistic expectations. It may be useful to instruct patients about what can be considered a successful outcome and the time-scale needed to reach it. Once the original therapeutic goal has been achieved, it is also important to provide weight maintenance programs and continuous follow-up since obesity has to be considered a chronic disease.

3.5 Treatment approaches

Obesity is a particularly challenging medical condition to treat that goes beyond the mere cosmetic problem. From all the above, it becomes evident that obesity requires a coordination of care from multiple health care providers with a multidisciplinary group with varied expertise working together as a team to assist

Treatment Algorithm *

Each step (designated by a box) in this process is reviewed in this section and expanded upon in subsequent sections.

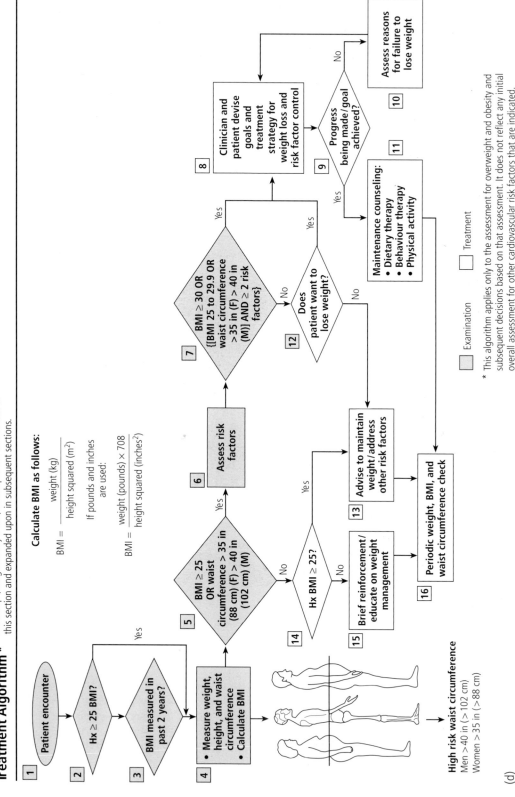

Calculate BMI as follows:

$$BMI = \frac{weight\ (kg)}{height\ squared\ (m^2)}$$

If pounds and inches are used:

$$BMI = \frac{weight\ (pounds) \times 708}{height\ squared\ (inches^2)}$$

High risk waist circumference

Men >40 in (>102 cm)
Women >35 in (>88 cm)

* This algorithm applies only to the assessment for overweight and obesity and subsequent decisions based on that assessment. It does not reflect any initial overall assessment for other cardiovascular risk factors that are indicated.

(d)

Figure 3.8(a–d) (Continued.)

patient care. There are three recognized approaches to the treatment of the complex etiology and multifactorial nature of obesity: lifestyle changes, pharmacotherapy, and bariatric surgery, which should be applied either alone or in combination according to the characteristics of the patients.

General principles

Information lies at the foundation of developing effective strategies to successfully tackle excess body weight. As described above, weight gain represents the consequence of many interacting processes, and, as such for a disease with a multifactorial etiology there will be different approaches to its management that will be more or less effective to different individiuals. Undoubtedly, any intervention achieving a negative energy balance over an extended time period will result in weight loss. In this sense, it is important to inform patients about the rationale and beneficial effects of the different recommendations and treatment strategies.

Lifestyle changes

The most successful weight-reduction programs are those that combine diet with exercise within a matrix of behavior modification. The main modifiable factors affecting energy balance are dietary energy intake and energy expended through physical activity. Treatment of obesity is most successful if realistic goals are set, a balanced diet is stressed, and a safe rate of weight loss per week is achieved through a combination of moderate caloric intake reduction (diet) and increased energy expenditure (physical activity).

Dietary management

It is worth remembering the word 'diet' originally comes from the Greek *diaita*, meaning 'manner of living,' and it is truly this that the obese patient must change. Fad diets promising a quick fix should be avoided. Unlike drugs, which must go through stringent clinical testing before they are licensed, fad diets can be promoted without being put on a trial. Diets with altered levels of protein, carbohydrate, or fat are very popular with the dieting public, which is desperate to find 'new' strategies for successful weight loss and maintenance.

The Nutrition Committee from the American Heart Association has published a statement for health care professionals analyzing the frequently followed high-protein diets. The Science Advisory concludes that high-protein diets are low-calorie diets, even though none is advertised as such. In obese individuals macronutrient composition of the diet has little effect on the rate or magnitude of weight loss unless nutrient composition influences caloric intake. The amount of protein recommended in high-protein diet regimens exceeds established requirements and may impose significant health risks. Animal proteins, rather than plant-based ones, are generally advocated leading to increased intake of purines and saturated fat, ultimately resulting in raised uric acid and LDL cholesterol concentrations, elevating the risk of gout and cardiovascular disease in susceptible individuals. By omitting certain foods, and sometimes entire food groups, the diets are deficient in fiber and carbohydrates, as well as some vitamins, minerals, and protective phytochemicals, with detrimental effects on cancer development and osteoporosis.

High-protein, high-fat diets induce ketosis and are initially attractive because they promote a quick weight loss attributable to water loss and glycogen depletion, which engenders a false sense of accomplishment. If the imbalance is maintained, loss of appetite associated with ketosis results in lower total caloric intake potentially leading to muscle breakdown and, consequently to increased per cent body fat. It is concluded that high-protein diets are not recommended because they restrict healthful foods that provide essential nutrients with potential cardiac, renal, skeletal muscle, bone, and liver abnormalities. Similarly, the promotion of eating certain foods in a specific order, at concrete times, or in purposeful combinations has no nutritional–medical basis.

Physical activity

Together with energy intake, the other main modifiable factor affecting the energy balance equation is energy expended through physical activity. The addition of exercise to a diet program is important because it determines the composition of weight loss. Two meta-analyses pooling data from 74 published trials have found that exercise is able to attenuate fat-free mass loss. Interestingly, it has been shown that in previously sedentary people, a lifestyle physical activity intervention is as effective as and has similar effects to a structured exercise program in improving physical activity itself, cardiorespiratory fitness, systolic and diastolic blood pressure as well as insulin sensitivity, serum triglycerides, and total cholesterol concentrations. Moreover, physical activity has been shown to be of utmost importance for long-term weight management. Therefore, patients should be urged to cut down on sedentary activities while increasing everyday lifestyle activities. In fact, less than one-third of the general population meets the recommendations to engage in at least 30 min of moderate physical activity five days per week, while 40% of adults engage in no leisure-time physical activity at all.

Pharmacotherapy

In comparison with other diseases, at present there is a paucity of drug therapy options for obesity influenced by a history of past failures in trying to overcome the regulatory requisites of safety and efficacy that are defined for an acceptable weight loss product. Since effective pharmacotherapy for obesity is likely to require long-term application; it is essential to outweigh potential risks, side effects, and costs against benefits. No prospective randomized controlled trials have evaluated the efficacy of currently approved antiobesity drugs for longer than two years. Treatment discontinuation should be considered in non-responders after an unsuccessful one-month period.

Two products are currently available in the market: orlistat and sibutramine. Orlistat is a lipase inhibitor working peripherally in the digestive tract to prevent breakdown, and hence absorption, of approximately 30% of dietary fat. The standard dose of 120 mg three times daily taken with the main meals has been evaluated in seven prospective randomized controlled trials, showing that at one year about twice as many patients treated with orlistat lost 10% or more of their initial body weight as those in the placebo group while one-third more patients taking orlistat lost 5% or more of their initial body weight compared with placebo-treated individuals. Successful weight loss was more difficult to achieve in patients with associated risk factors like coronary heart disease and type 2 diabetes mellitus.

Volunteers enrolled in a trial conducted within a primary care setting with no dietitian or behavior modification counseling were less successful in achieving weight loss. Four trials included a second-year extension of the one-year studies with the aim of preventing weight regain, rather than inducing further weight loss.

Due to its mechanism of action, orlistat may be associated with unpleasant side effects, including the production of oily stools, abdominal pain, flatulence, fecal urgency, and incontinence when ingested with high-fat diets. In one- and two-year trials about 70–80% of volunteers treated with orlistat experienced one or more gastrointestinal events compared with approximately 50–60% of subjects treated with placebo. Gastrointestinal side effects usually occurred within the first month and were of mild to moderate intensity. About 4% of orlistat-treated subjects vs. 1% of placebo-treated volunteers withdrew from the study because of gastrointestinal complaints.

Many of the gastrointestinal side effects of orlistat can be prevented by concomitant therapy with a gel-forming fiber (psyllium mucilloid). Inhibition of fat digestion prevents fatty acid release into the lumen, which is needed to stimulate cholecystokinin secretion and gallbladder contraction, thus laying the base for an increased risk of gallstone formation by orlistat. However, orlistat administered with meals of varying fat content reportedly did not reduce gallbladder motility and no evidence of increased gallstone formation in all trials has been observed. In addition, the increased delivery of fat to the colon has raised a concern of a potential increased risk of colon cancer. However, orlistat administration in volunteers has been shown not to increase colonocyte proliferation, and no increased incidence of colon cancer in the different clinical trials has been noticed.

Long-term orlistat treatment can affect the homeostasis of fat-soluble vitamin. It has been observed that concentrations of vitamins D, E, and beta-carotene decreased below normal limits in around 5% more orlistat- than placebo-treated volunteers, which normalized rapidly with vitamin supplementation. Therefore, it is recommended that all patients treated with orlistat should be given a daily multivitamin supplement that is taken at a time when orlistat is not being ingested.

It is important to bear in mind that orlistat may interfere with the absorption of lipophilic drugs when taken simultaneously. A few cases of subtherapeutic circulating concentrations of cyclosporine in organ transplant recipients starting orlistat treatment for obesity have been reported. Orlistat should not be taken for at least 2 h before or after ingestion of lipophilic drugs and circulating drug concentrations should be followed to ensure appropriate dosing if needed. Pharmacokinetic studies suggest that orlistat does not interfere with absorption of selected drugs with a narrow therapeutic index like warfarin, digoxin, and phenytoin, and other products that are likely to be taken simultaneously with the lipase inhibitor like glyburide, oral contraceptives, furosemide, captopril, nifedipine, atenolol, and alcohol.

Sibutramine is a mixed serotonin–noradrenaline reuptake blocker leading to increased levels of neurotransmitters, which cause a decrease in food intake. In addition, the inhibition of the reuptake of noradrenaline has, on the one hand, the added effect of increasing resting energy expenditure, and on the other hand, side effects related to increased heart rate and blood pressure. Sibutramine treatment at doses between 1 and 30 mg per day for six months have shown a dose-dependent weight loss effect, amounting for 0.9% and 7.7% of initial body weight for placebo and 30 mg/day, respectively. The current recommended starting dose is 10 mg/day, which can be increased by 5 mg if needed.

The efficacy of sibutramine therapy in producing and maintaining weight loss has been evaluated in two prospective one-year randomized controlled trials. Interestingly, it has been shown that weight loss was equivalent in intermittent (15 mg/day given during weeks 1–12, 19–30, and 37–48) or continuous sibutramine treatment. The evaluation of sibutramine therapy in long-term weight management after an already achieved weight loss shows that approximately 43% of sibutramine-treated and 16% of placebo-treated volunteers maintained 80% or more of their original weight loss.

Mild and usually transient side effects associated with sibutramine are dry mouth, headache, constipation, and insomnia. More importantly, sibutramine has been reported to cause a dose-related increase in heart rate and blood pressure. On average, an increase of 2–4 mmHg in systolic and diastolic blood pressure accompanied by an elevation of 4–6 beats/min have been observed at a dose of 10–15 mg/day. However, some patients have suffered much larger increases in both heart rate and blood pressure, requiring dose reduction or treatment discontinuation. Sibutramine therapy is contraindicated in patients with poorly controlled hypertension. The risk of adverse effects was not increased in patients with controlled hypertension compared with normotensive volunteers.

Recently, the Italian regulatory authorities have suspended the sales of sibutramine after reports of serious cardiac alterations, including two deaths, in patients taking the product. Authorities in England, Germany and France have not suspended sales of sibutramine but are reviewing the evidence.

Pharmacological treatment of obesity is currently approved for use in adults with a BMI above 30 or over 27 kg/m^2 with comorbidities. Surprisingly, in the time period between 1996 and 1998 only about 10% of women and 3% of men with a BMI 30 kg/m^2 reported to have used prescription weight loss medication. With the actual high prevalence rates of obesity, non-prescription product use is on the increase. Easily obtained non-prescription weight loss products are an appealing alternative. From 1996 to 1998 in a multistate survey with a population-based sample of 14 679 adults, 7% reported overall non-prescription weight loss product use, 2% declared phenylpropanolamine (PPA) use, and 1% reported ephedra consumption. In addition, among prescription weight loss product users, 33.8% also took non-prescription agents.

PPA, the main ingredient in the over-the-counter (OTC) weight loss aids reported in the mentioned study, is a synthetic ephedrine alkaloid with stimulant properties reducing appetite. Case reports of adverse cerebrovascular and cardiac events and a study showing an increased risk of stroke resulted in the voluntary withdrawal of all OTC PPA products from the market in November 2000. Dietary supplements are generally regarded as safe and are regulated as foods rather than drugs. In addition, there can be a discrepancy between the actual composition or potency of a product and the specifications on the label. In this sense, 55% of ephedra supplements tested failed to list the ephedrine alkaloid content on the label or had more than a 20% difference between the actual amount and the amount listed on the label.

Unfortunately, 'non-traditional' or 'alternative' treatments are extremely popular and widely used. However, there is no clear support by existing data in the peer-reviewed literature concerning their efficacy and safety. Of 18 methods/products advocated as potential anti-obesity/fat-reducing agents none was convincingly demonstrated to be safe and effective in two or more peer-reviewed publications of randomized double-blind placebo-controlled trials conducted by at least two independent laboratories.

Bariatric surgery

Bariatric surgery is a term derived from the Greek words for 'weight' and 'treatment.' Bariatric surgical procedures are major gastrointestinal operations that (a) seal off most of the stomach to reduce the amount of food one can eat, and (b) rearrange the small intestine to reduce the calories the bodies can absorb. There are several different types of bariatric weight loss surgical procedures, but they are known collectively as 'bariatric surgery.'

Bariatric surgery should be considered for morbidly obese (BMI above 40 or over 35 kg/m^2 with comorbidities), well-informed, and motivated patients, with previous failure to conventional treatment, fulfilling the established selection criteria in whom the operative risks are acceptable. Candidates for surgical procedures should be selected carefully after evaluation by a comprehensive, multidisciplinary team with medical, surgical, nutritional, and psychiatric expertise working in a clinical setting with adequate support for all aspects of management and assessment providing both preoperative and postoperative counseling and support. In this context, it is important to bear in mind that effectiveness of surgery does not necessarily need to be circumscribed to body weight alone but may focus on beneficial effects on obesity-associated diseases.

The aim of surgery is to produce a dramatic decrease in energy intake, which can be achieved by triggering an early and enhanced satiety sensation, reducing hunger signals as well as through bypassing relevant parts of the gastrointestinal system, thereby allowing rapid transit via the digestive tract, and partly a subsequent malabsorption resulting from undigested food quickly shunted into the large intestine.

According to the underlying mechanism of action bariatric procedures can be classified into restrictive, malabsorptive, and mixed techniques. Restrictive procedures increase esophageal and gastric distension, producing an early satiety sensation. The placement of an adjustable gastric band represents a purely restrictive procedure, producing a small gastric pouch and a narrow passage into the remainder of the stomach. The partitioning of the stomach into two parts (either vertically or horizontally) producing a slow emptying into the digestive tract is known as gastroplasty. Malabsorptive techniques involve bypassing large parts of the absorptive gastrointestinal tract. Exclusively malabsorptive procedures like the jejuno-ileal bypass are

no longer performed and have been replaced by mixed techniques combining restriction and malabsorption.

The proximal Roux-en-Y gastric bypass leaves a small stomach pouch near the oesophagogastric junction excluding the major curvature, thus bypassing most of the stomach and duodenum. Like the gastric bypass the biliopancreatic diversion is also a mixed intervention. However, the latter technique consists in a subtotal horizontal gastrectomy leaving on average a 200-ml upper gastric remnant and involves a more extensive malabsorptive element as the gastric pouch is connected to the final segment of the intestine, completely bypassing the duodenum and jejunum.

Traditionally, gastric surgery was carried out as an open procedure, but today all techniques can be performed via laparoscopy. The results from initial large series and a randomized controlled trial show that weight loss is the same using the open or laparoscopic approach. However, the laparoscopic access for bariatric surgery has proved to reduce postoperative pain, recovery time, and perioperative complications.

Complications related to bariatric surgery include early hemorrhage problems, gastrointestinal leakage leading to peritonitis, splenic laceration with potential need of splenectomy, subphrenic abscesses, wound infection, wound seromas, pulmonary embolism, and late complications derived from stomal stenosis, marginal ulcers, staple line disruption, dilation of the bypassed stomach, internal hernias, torsion of the intestinal limb, closed loop obstruction, cholelithiasis, vomiting, dumping syndrome, and specific nutrient deficiencies.

The impaired absorption and decreased intake are responsible for the appearance of certain nutrient deficiencies, especially of iron, calcium, folic acid, and vitamin B_{12}. Nonetheless, these deficiences can be easily prevented by starting prophylactic vitamin and mineral supplementation after surgery. The perioperative mortality rate after open obesity surgery taking into account studies including large numbers of patients is usually less than 1.5%. Approximately 75% of the deaths are caused by anastomotic leaks and peritonitis while 25% are due to pulmonary embolism. Recent series evaluating the laparoscopic gastric bypass alone establish the perioperative mortality around 1%, and the risk of early postoperative complications about 10%.

The clinical effectiveness of bariatric surgery has been compared with conventional therapy as well as by assessing the outcomes of different types of surgery in 17 randomized clinical trials and one non-randomized clinical trial. Comparing horizontal gastroplasty with a very low-calorie diet, no significant difference in weight loss at 12 months was observed (23 vs. 18 kg), although at 24 months patients undergoing gastroplasty had lost significantly more weight (32 vs. 9 kg) with about 58% of gastroplasty patients exhibiting less than 40% overweight compared with only 7% of non-surgical patients. In the Danish Obesity Project trial comparing jejunoileostomy with medical management, surgically treated patients had also lost significantly more weight at two years (42.9 vs. 5.9 kg). In the Swedish Obese Subjects (SOS) cohort study (the most extensive study in terms of sample size and years of follow-up performed so far) comparing bariatric surgery (vertical banded gastroplasty, gastric banding and gastric bypass, $n = 1210$) with conventional treatment ($n = 1099$), patients treated surgically had lost significantly more weight after two years than conventionally managed obese subjects (−23 vs. 0% weight loss). All patients treated surgically exhibited significant improvements in all health-related quality-of-life measures at two years compared with patients on conventional treatment. At eight years patients in the surgical group had a 16.3% weight loss compared with a 0.9% weight gain in the conventional treatment group.

Among the three different bariatric surgery procedures the gastric bypass group patients had a lower weight at eight years than gastroplasty and gastric banding patients. Moreover, in the SOS beneficial effects of surgical treatment over 10 years have been observed with respect to body weight, diabetes, triglycerides, HDL-cholesterol, uric acid, and quality of life but not necessarily as regards total cholesterol or blood pressure.

Four prospective, randomized trials comparing vertical-banded gastroplasty with gastric bypass have further shown that weight loss was greater with the latter, with an average loss of excess weight of 42 vs. 68% at one year, and about 35 vs. 62% after a three-year follow-up period. Moreover, average weight loss after gastric bypass has been reportedly maintained up to 14 years after surgery.

The majority of surgeons contend that gastric bypass is the bariatric procedure of choice for most patients with severe obesity. Although it is a technically complex operation, needing experienced professionals, the physical, psychological, and social benefits outweigh the low perioperative risk. High-risk morbidly obese patients with multiple comorbidities may in particular benefit from a less invasive approach because they are more vulnerable to cardiopulmonary and wound-related complications.

Recently, a bariatric surgery algorithm taking into consideration variables of BMI, age, gender, race, body habitus, comorbidities, and outcomes provided a logical framework for selection of the appropriate bariatric operation for each patient. It has to be stressed that gastrointestinal surgery is an effective last resort remedy in morbidly obese patients with previous failure to conventional treatment. A weight loss of 50–70% of excess body weight has been reported with surgical treatment. More importantly, long-term weight loss has been shown to extend to ten years and longer. The importance of carefully reviewing patients' treatment expectations and setting realistic goals should not be underscored since many patients who seek bariatric surgery often have unrealistically high weight loss expectations. The assessment of the efficacy of gastric surgery requires evaluation beyond weight loss variables alone.

The long-term benefits of bariatric surgery are more fully characterized by its ability to reduce or eliminate comorbid diseases and their associated morbidity and mortality. Significant improvements in diabetes and hypertension as well as in pulmonary function, cardiovascular risk factors, osteoarthritis, reproductive performance, self-esteem, sick leave, and quality of life among others have been extensively reported. In any case, after gastrointestinal surgery patients have to undergo lifelong medical follow-up and surveillance.

Gradually more insurers are beginning to cover bariatric operations, recognizing that this kind of surgery can have powerful medical benefits saving money in the long run. Surgical therapy in patients with morbid obesity is significantly more effective at producing and maintaining weight loss than medical and psychosocial approaches and, hence, more convenient from a cost-effectiveness, cost-utility, and cost-benefit analysis perspective. Contrary to what would be expected according to the existing evidence in terms of weight loss and impact on obesity-related comorbidities, bariatric surgery is underutilized, with only a small fraction of eligible patients being referred to the specialist. Given the favorable long-term outcomes of surgery for the treatment of morbid obesity and the current underprovision of services and skills to support bariatric surgery via laparoscopy, detailed implementation strategies to mainstream this surgical approach in carefully selected patients should be considered by health systems.

Other options

Since morbid obesity is not showing signs of abatement and gastroplasty and gastric bypasses represent ablative, irreversible surgical procedures, new, minimally invasive, and reversible approaches are constantly being sought.

Intragastric balloon

Intragastric balloon (IGB) therapy is a non-surgical attempt to induce early satiety by placing a silicone elastic balloon with a self-sealing radio-opaque valve into the body of the stomach endoscopically, under sedation. After placement the device is inflated under direct vision. The IGB should be viewed as a temporary treatment option that achieves moderate weight loss (around 15 kg). It is rarely successful if not associated with dieting and behavior modification. Peptic ulceration or a large hiatus hernia preclude insertion of the balloon. Major complications of this procedure include balloon displacement resulting in intestinal obstruction and balloon deflation at around 3–4 months. A 5% risk of laparotomy for major complications associated with the balloon and a 1.4% conversion rate for gastric banding have been observed.

In the early days, commercial suppliers recommended a three-month limit for balloon placement. At the end of 1999 new designs prompted the recommendation by the manufacturers of balloon placements for up to six months. Ulcer prophylaxis with a proton pump inhibitor for the duration of IGB therapy has proved useful in avoiding peptidic ulceration or gastrointestinal bleeding. Strict and regular follow-up together with removal of the device between three and six months is essential to avoid potentially serious complications. The utility of the IGB has been advocated in relation to desirable BMI reduction and, hence, operative risk reduction before embarking on definitive bariatric surgery. However, to date no evidence for this application has been provided by studies especially designed for this purpose.

Gastric pacing

Gastric pacing represents a novel, potential therapy for the treatment of obesity that showed promising results in experimental animal models. Preliminary effects of the application of an implantable gastric stimulator in 24 morbidly obese patients included a significant weight loss of an average 4.7 BMI units reduction over nine months, due to an increased satiety conducive to a reduced food intake. The electrical stimulator system is composed of a bipolar electrocatheter (the gastric lead), which is tunneled intramuscularly at the lesser curve of the anterior gastric wall (upper third of the antrum), and a gastric pacemaker (a microcircuit with a battery), connected to the lead and located outside the abdomen. The electrical stimulator system can be implanted either laparoscopically or using open surgery under general anesthesia. Intraoperative fiber optic flexible endogastroscopy is usually performed to ensure that the mucosa has not been damaged during electrode implantation as well as to warrant that no intracavity penetration has taken place. After placement of the lead, the gastric pacer is located in a subcutaneous pocket created in the anterior abdominal wall.

In a recent study gastric pacing has been reported to elicit a 20% excess weight loss after six months, accompanied by a decrease in plasma concentrations of cholecystokinin (CCK), somatostatin, glucagon-like peptide 1 (GLP-1), and leptin. The safety and efficacy of gastric pacing is being evaluated in clinical trials in many countries and still requires the analysis of long-term effects.

3.6 Prevention

The relevance of obesity prevention becomes evident not only for health professionals, but also to politicians given the far-reaching medical, social, and economic consequences of having to deal with the ill consequences and difficulties associated to its management. To some extent past and recent prevention efforts may have been inhibited by a number of external factors, ranging from the lack of acceptance of obesity as a serious health problem to the commercial interests of the food industry in continuing with a blossoming market.

Childhood obesity

Obesity prevention in children is a key factor in urging a strong response to the current epidemic. General practitioners and pediatricians, therefore, need to provide a much more prevention-oriented, systematic, and vigorous weight loss approach. Health professionals should be especially alert in early identification of overweight and obese children at the same time as being less complacent and more active in starting their treatment. Not surprisingly, obesity in childhood is associated with many of the same diseases observed in adults such as hypertension, sleep-disordered breathing, dyslipidemia, and insulin resistance, accompanied also by social stigmatization.

The rapid rise in childhood obesity has been mirrored by an explosion of non-active leisure pursuits for children such as computers and video games. Television watching represents the principal source of inactivity for most children in developed countries and has been linked to the prevalence of obesity. Substantial declines in physical activity have been reported to occur during adolescence in girls and have been shown to be associated with higher BMI. Public health approaches in schools should extend beyond education to include the physical and social environment together with school policy and links to family and community. Age-appropriate and culturally sensitive instruction develops the knowledge, attitudes, and behaviors needed to adopt healthy lifestyle changes. Increased general activity and play rather than competitive sport and structured exercise appear to be more effective. Adherence may be improved by making the activity enjoyable, increasing the choice over type and level of activities as well as by providing positive reinforcement of even small achievements.

Initiatives in key settings

To halt the drift from healthy weight into overweight and obesity diverse initiatives have identified activities and interventions in five key settings (families and communities, schools, health care, media and communications, and worksites). Individual behavioral change obviously lies at the core of all strategies to reduce excess body weight. Clinical medicine and public health agencies have to face preventing obesity at multiple levels with new partners, including food marketers and manufacturers, agricultural, nutritional

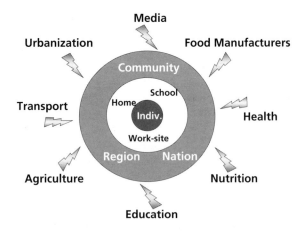

Figure 3.9 Multidimensional approach to target the obesity epidemic.

and educational authorities, public and private health care purchasers, mass media and opinion leaders, large employers, transportation agencies, urban planners, and real-estate developers (Figure 3.9). All public and private sector stakeholders with the potential to influence lifestyle and body weight will play a key role in shaping and supporting social and environmental policies that can help citizens improve their diet and become physically active.

Additionally, physicians play a key role in the correct diagnosis and management of overweight and obesity with a particular need to focus on children and adolescents whose excess weight and sedentary lifestyle will form the basis for a lifetime of preventable morbidity and increased premature mortality.

3.7 Perspectives on the future

We are currently facing a paradoxical situation in which high prevalence rates of obesity and overweight collide with a scenario where clear opportunities for diagnosis and effective treatment are being missed. Information lies at the foundation of developing evidence-based strategies to successfully tackle the obesity epidemic. Physiological and genetic studies are improving our understanding of the complex mechanisms controlling appetite and energy expenditure. Overweight and obesity can no longer be viewed as strictly a personal matter; it is everybody's responsibility since health problems resulting from this disease are threatening the health gains achieved in the last decades world-wide.

The hazards of excess body weight have been clearly established by epidemiological and clinical studies, highlighting the need for careful diagnosis and effective treatment programs. Overweight and obesity are serious health issues that will only worsen without thoughtful and evidence-based interventions. Numerous weight loss strategies have been proposed over the past decades, making the task of obesity management evaluation daunting.

Undoubtedly, to persuade politicians, medical and health professionals, as well as industry, communities, and individuals, it is necessary to successfully tackle the obesity pandemic. It is important to bear in mind that actions to reduce overweight and obesity will fail without a multidimensional approach. Moreover, special attention should be paid to the role played by physicians since lack of motivation to work with overweight and obese patients owing to negative peceptions of the efficacy of treatments or adherence to treatment may be an important barrier to successfully implement interventions in the health care setting. According to the particular characteristics of the patient either lifestyle changes, pharmacotherapy, surgery, or a combination should be applied. In morbidly obese patients refractory to diet and drug therapy, a substantial and sustained weight loss after bariatric surgery is obtained. However, the most effective treatment in the long term is, and will be, obesity prevention.

References and further reading

The information has been obtained from the existing textbooks and PubMed searches of obesity-related topics as well as from the websites of the most relevant international health institutions such as the World Health Organization (WHO), the National Audit Office (NAO), and the National Institute of Clinical Excellence (NICE), the National Institutes of Health (NIH), which have convened expert panels to carry out comprehensive and critical evaluations of multiple clinical trials in an effort to establish evidence-based guidelines.

Björntorp P (ed) *International Textbook of Obesity*. Chichester: John Wiley & Sons, 2001.

Blackburn GL, Kanders BS (eds) *Obesity: Pathophysiology, Psychology, and Treatment*. Chapman & Hall Series in Clinical Nutrition. New York: Chapman and Hall, 1994.

Bray GA, Bouchard C (eds) *Handbook of Obesity. Clinical Applications*, 2nd edn. New York: Marcel Dekker, 2004.

Bray GA, Bouchard C (eds) *Handbook of Obesity. Etiology and Pathophysiology*, 2nd edn. New York: Marcel Dekker, 2004.

British Nutrition Foundation Task Force. *The Report of the British Nutrition Foundation Task Force. Obesity*. Oxford: Blackwell Science, 1999.

Caterson ID, Franklin J, Colditz GA. Economic costs of obesity. In: *Handbook of Obesity. Etiology and Pathophysiology*, 2nd edn (GA Bray, C Bouchard, eds), pp. 149–156. New York: Marcel Dekker, 2004.

Kopelman PG (ed) *Management of Obesity and Related Disorders*. London: Martin Dunitz, 2001.

Kopelman PG, Stock MJ (eds) *Clinical Obesity*. Oxford: Blackwell Science, 1998.

Lean M (ed.) *Clinical Handbook of Weight Management*. London: Martin Dunitz, 1998.

Medeiros-Neto G, Halpern A, Bouchard C (eds) *Progress in Obesity Research*, Vol 9: *Proceedings of the 9th International Congress on Obesity, Sao Paulo, 2002*. Surrey: John Libbey Eurotext, 2003.

Prentice AM, Jebb SA. Obesity in Britain: gluttony or sloth? *BMJ* 1995; 311: 437–439.

World Health Organization (WHO). *Obesity. Preventing and Managing the Global Epidemic. Report of a WHO consultation on obesity*. WHO/NUT/NCD/981. Geneva: WHO, 1998. Available from www.who.int/nut/obs.htm.

Websites of interest

Agency for Healthcare Research and Quality. U.S. Preventive Services Task Force recommendations on screening adults for obesity. http://www.ahrq.gov/research/dec03/1203ra34.htm

International Association for the Study of Obesity. www.iaso.org

International Obesity Task Force. www.iotf.org

Medical Research Council, Human Nutrition Research. http://www.mrc-hnr.cam.ac.uk/downloads/ALeanerFitterFuture.pdf

National Audit Office. Tackling Obesity in England. Report by the Comptroller and Auditor General HC 220 Session 2000–2001: 15 February 2001. www.nao.gov.uk/publications/nao_reports/00-01/0001220.pdf

National Center for Chronic Disease Prevention and Health Promotion. http://www.cdc.gov/nccdphp/dnpa/obesity/trend/prev_reg.htm

National Heart, Lung, and Blood Institute (NHLBI) of the National Institutes of Health (NIH) Obesity Education Initiative (OEI). http://www.nhlbi.nih.gov/about/oei/oei_pd.htm

National Institute for Clinical Excellence (NICE). Clinical and cost effectiveness of surgery for people with morbid obesity. www.nice.org.uk/Docref.asp?d=28703

NICE. Surgery to aid weight reduction for people with morbid obesity: final appraisal determination. www.nice.org.uk/article.asp?a=32081

Office of Disease Prevention and Health Promotion, Centers for Disease Control and Prevention, National Institutes of Health. The Surgeon General's call to action to prevent and decrease overweight and obesity, 2001. www.surgeongeneral.gov/library

WHO Global Strategy on Diet, Physical Activity and Health. http://www.who.int/dietphysicalactivity/en/

4
Undernutrition

Anura V Kurpad

Key messages

- Acute undernutrition is suspected when an involuntary weight loss of greater than 10% of the body weight occurs over the preceding 3–6 months.
- Chronic undernutrition is similar to chronic energy deficiency; this is characterized by a low body mass index in weight-stable individuals.
- Undernutrition that is uncomplicated by disease is associated with several nutrient-saving and homeostatic responses.
- When disease and undernutrition coexist, the adaptive nutrient-saving responses are generally reversed, such that the depletion of body nutrient stores and tissue is accelerated.
- Nutritional screening is a rapid generic procedure, often undertaken by non-specialist health professionals to identify individuals at risk of undernutrition. Assessment is a more in-depth evaluation of nutritional status, which is normally undertaken by a specialist in nutrition such as a dietitian, and is specific to the disease and the patient.
- The assessment of undernutrition can be made clinically using simple clinical techniques. More complex techniques for measuring depletion and body composition or function are also available.
- Nutritional support in undernutrition should be tailored to the clinical situation; in any case, a modest and balanced diet should be instituted as soon as possible. Monitoring the nutritional support given is essential for a successful outcome.
- There are dangers associated with aggressive and unbalanced diet administration.

4.1 Introduction

Undernutrition is a term that is often used generically to describe a variety of nutrient deficiencies. The common way to think of undernutrition is in terms of body weight; this has often led to the terms underweight and undernourished being used interchangeably. Undernutrition is caused by a less than adequate intake of nutrients, most of which are related to the energy intake. In adults, this has led to the term 'energy deficiency,' with a further subclassification into acute, which is sudden, and associated with a declining body weight, and chronic, which occurs over a long period of time, such that the body weight over the preceding few months may be low, but stable.

The consequences of undernutrition can be physical, psychological, and behavioral. Examples of these are shown in Table 4.1.

4.2 Pathophysiology of undernutrition

Body composition

Body weight loss on starvation is initially rapid (up to 5 kg over a few days), due to the emptying of glycogen reserves, the utilization of body protein and the accompanying water loss. The later loss of body tissue that accompanies negative energy balance is primarily fat, although varying amounts of lean tissue are lost as well. This is demonstrated in a classic study on the effect of long-term semi-starvation on healthy men done by Keys and co-workers about 50 years ago. During their six-month semi-starvation study, the lean tissue loss observed in the subjects represented about half of the total weight loss. Although physical activity would be expected to maintain muscle mass in such a situation, it is clear that lean tissue is also catabolized to provide energy in the face of large energy deficits. The

Table 4.1 Some of the functional consequences of undernutrition

Physical	Muscle strength and fatigue
	Hypothermia
	Reduced respiratory muscle function and reduced cough pressure, predisposing to chest infections
	Immobility predisposing to venous thrombosis and embolism
	Impaired immune function
	Reduced wound healing
	Reduced final height in women leading to small pelvic size and small birth weight infants
Psychological and behavioral	Depression
	Anxiety
	Reduced will to recover
	Self-neglect
	Poor bonding with mother and child
	Loss of libido

composition of weight loss is dependent on different conditions under which the negative energy balance is imposed: in healthy, normal young men, the weight loss is composed of fat and fat-free mass, while in obese individuals it may be primarily fat mass.

Energy metabolism

Accompanying the changes in body composition during acute negative energy balance, are adaptive changes in energy expenditure. These changes in energy expenditure could occur in one or more of the components of energy expenditure. These components are the basal metabolic rate (BMR), thermogenesis, or the production of heat by the body in response to various stimuli, and the physical activity of the individual (Figure 4.1).

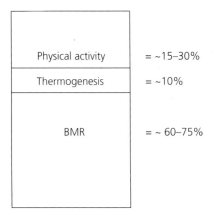

Figure 4.1 Components of total 24-h energy expenditure.

Reductions in the BMR are partly mediated through weight loss itself, in which metabolically demanding tissues of the body are reduced in size, and partly through reductions in the metabolic activity of these tissues. In the semi-starvation study referred to before (Keys *et al.*, 1950), the subjects' BMRs decreased by about 25% when expressed per kilogram of their fat-free mass (or metabolically active tissue). This decline was most rapid in the first two weeks, indicating that the reduced metabolic activity of the fat-free tissue occurred quickly in response to energy deficiency.

The factors underlying the decrease in the activity of the fat-free mass include reduced activity of the sympathetic nervous system, which is a part of the autonomic nervous system and which partly drives the heat-producing activity of the fat-free mass. Other factors include altered peripheral thyroid metabolism and lowered insulin secretion, along with substrate utilization designed to maintain glucose production and maximize fat usage. Leptin (the *ob* gene product), which is expressed in adipose tissue and secreted into the circulation, acts at the hypothalamic level as a lipostatic mechanism through modulation of satiety and the activity of the sympathetic nervous system. Leptin levels are low in anorexia nervosa, suggesting that leptin may be important in undernourished, low fat mass states as a potential modulator of the energy-sparing response to energy deficiency.

An additional modulator of the response to underfeeding is the genetic makeup of the individual. In an interesting study on monozygotic twin pairs (Bouchard and Tremblay, 1997), the body weight and compositional change was studied after 93 days of negative energy balance induced by increased exercise with constant dietary intake. The within-pair variation was much less than the between-pair variation for loss of weight, body fat, visceral fat, and respiratory exchange ratio during exercise (see Figure 4.2 for weight change), showing that subjects with the same genotype were more alike in responses than subjects with different genotypes.

On the other hand, there are also findings of an increased BMR per kg body weight in a number of clinical studies arising from energy deficiency, and it is possible that these conflicting findings are due to several factors, such as whether the patient was in a state of recovery or not, or due to methodological errors during the conduct of BMR measurement. The increased

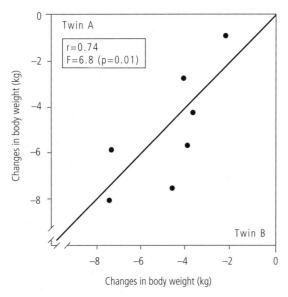

Figure 4.2 Changes in body weight with negative energy balance in seven pairs of twins. Twin A on the ordinate, and twin B on the abscissa. Reproduced from Bouchard and Tremblay (1997) with permission.

BMR could also be due to the stress imposed by illness in clinical situations (see below).

Changes in thermogenesis could also account, in part, for decreased total energy expenditure in response to total or semi-starvation, although these are not as consistent or dramatic as the fall in BMR in acute negative energy deficiency. The thermogenic response to a cold stimulus has been demonstrated to be lower in elderly undernourished women who were admitted into hospital with fractured femurs.

Even with otherwise healthy individuals, semi-starvation or starvation leads to a reduction in physical activity. From the behavioral viewpoint, the imposition of an acute energy deficiency also causes apathy, with a marked reduction in spontaneous activity. A decrease in food intake results in a change in selection of discretionary activity patterns, such that lower activity discretionary patterns are selected. These behavioral changes are obviously designed to maximize the chances of survival under conditions of acute energy deficiency.

Overall therefore, it appears that energy deficiency is associated with body weight loss, along with changes in body composition, as well as a reduced BMR and physical activity. Figure 4.3 shows how these factors interact with each other to attain lower energy expenditure when an acute negative energy balance exists.

If the lowered energy expenditure is adequate to compensate for the decreased energy intake that caused the negative energy balance, and allows for a new neutral energy balance to be achieved, the person can survive, albeit at a lower plane of nutrition. This leads to a chronic energy deficiency (CED), which is discussed below. If a homeostatic response is not possible due to a severe energy deficit, body energy and muscle stores continue to be lost until a lethal weight loss occurs, usually when body weight or fat free mass has fallen to about half its original value.

Protein metabolism

When nitrogen (protein) intake is reduced, the nitrogen output also decreases, although this could take

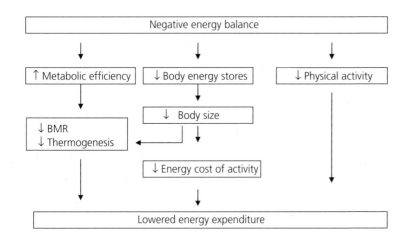

Figure 4.3 Interaction between factors leading to lowered energy expenditure as a result of negative energy balance. BMR, basal metabolic rate.

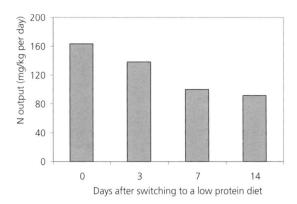

Figure 4.4 Rate of change in N excretion after changing from a high to a low protein intake. Redrawn from Quevedo *et al.* (1994).

some days to occur. In subjects who are put on low protein diets, some 7–14 days may be required for the nitrogen (N) output to stabilize at a new lower level (Figure 4.4). This is important when assessing N balance particularly over a short time period since the previous N intake influences the amount of N output.

This adaptation spares body protein and preserves essential functions in the body, since the protein loss never reaches zero, there will be losses of protein from the body, primarily from the skeletal muscle mass. In more chronic undernutrition (but not starvation), the relatively greater loss of muscle mass leads to an increase in the viscera to skeletal muscle mass ratio of the fat-free mass. An important point is that when the protein intake is acutely reduced, there is a transient loss of N over a period of days. This has been attributed to a 'labile' pool of body protein, which contracts when protein intake is reduced (and conversely, expands when protein intake is increased), but the identity of this pool of body protein has not been established in humans.

The adaptive reduction in N output during protein deprivation can be mediated though a decrease in amino acid oxidation, or due to reduced formation of ammonia in the kidney, or due to a reduced formation of glucose (gluconeogenesis) in the liver. The need for glucose, which in conditions of starvation is met by proteolysis, is primarily to provide glucose to tissues that need it, particularly the brain. Although ketoacids, which derive from fat, become important fuels for the brain as starvation progresses, they do not eliminate brain glucose requirements. Increasing the energy intake will improve N balance, just as increasing the N

intake would, and when both N and energy are provided at their minimum requirement level, the N balance would be expected to be zero. Thus, energy can be said to have a protein-sparing effect in the submaintenance range of protein intakes. The effect of N and energy intake on N balance is interdependent and complex. The level of N intake determines the change in N balance that can be achieved with an increase in energy intake. On the other hand, the effect of energy intake on N balance depends on the intake range within which alterations in energy intake occur, and a value of 7.5 mg N/kcal energy has been reported for submaintenance energy intakes of up to about 15 kcal/kg (Figure 4.5).

About one-third of the variation in N balance can be attributed to variations in energy intake relative to the requirement, and 1–1.5 mg N/kg body weight would be gained (or spared) per extra 1 kcal/kg body weight of energy intake at maintenance levels of intake. This has led to the suggestion that in undernutrition the high slope of the N balance to energy intake relationship is due to replenishment or maintenance of the body cell mass, while at high energy intakes the N retained may be needed to support the extra energy retained as fat.

The type of energy source (carbohydrate or fat) is also important in determining the influence of energy on N balance. In the submaintenance range of protein intakes, it has been shown that carbohydrate is more effective than fat, possibly because of the greater insulinogenic influence of carbohydrate. At maintenance intakes, as well as in the clinical setting, both carbohy-

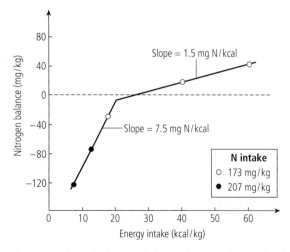

Figure 4.5 Relationship between N balance and energy intake. Reproduced from Elwyn *et al.* (1980) with permission.

drate and fat have been found to be equally effective, although some studies suggest that a high-fat/glucose regimen is better than a low-fat/glucose regimen (Mc-Cargar *et al.*, 1989). The message from these observations is that energy spares protein, and 100–150 g of glucose per day has been described to be effective in reducing urea N excretion by about half.

Measurements of the rate of protein turnover show that this changes little if at all with moderate reductions in protein intake, although with severe protein deficiency there is a reduction in whole body protein turnover. Whole body protein synthesis does not appear to change with feeding, and changes in proteolysis appear to mediate most of the acute regulatory changes associated with feeding and fasting. While whole body protein synthesis rates are relatively unchanged, there may be differences in tissue-specific protein synthesis rates. In rats given a low protein intake, rates of protein synthesis are reduced in the muscle, but increased in the liver. The rate of synthesis of albumin is also decreased with a low protein intake; however, this is followed by a decrease in the rate of catabolism as well after a few days. In addition, there is also a transfer of albumin from the extravascular to the intravascular pool, thus preserving serum albumin concentrations. Similarly, a relatively low protein intake does not change the concentrations of other liver secretory proteins, such as retinol-binding protein and transferrin.

There are other nutrients that are important in the maintenance of the fat-free mass. Intracellular constituents such as potassium or phosphorus are also important in maintaining a positive N balance when a diet adequate in protein and energy is given to malnourished patients. Diets lacking in potassium or phosphorus lead to negative N balances even when all other nutrients are adequate, while a diet lacking in sodium reduces the extent of the observed positive N balance in malnourished patients receiving an otherwise adequate diet.

Hormonal mediators

During starvation, the maintenance of blood glucose levels is paramount for the organism. Thus starvation is associated with a decrease in the hypoglycemic hormone insulin, and an increase in counter-regulatory hormones that aim to increase glucose, including glucagon, which promotes hepatic glucose production. The lowered insulin concentrations also allow for a reduced peripheral utilization of glucose, and an in-

creased mobilization of fat. Thus, fatty acids become an important oxidative fuel for peripheral tissues during starvation. Thyroid hormone levels also show changes in that the active form of the hormone (T_3) is reduced while the inactive form (reverse T_3) is increased in the serum. The activity of the sympathetic nervous system is also reduced, as are serum concentrations of catecholamines. The implication of a decrease in these hormones in nutritional terms is that energy expenditure decreases, thus reducing the magnitude of the negative energy balance.

Immune function in undernutrition

The immune system depends on cellular and secretory activities that require nutrients in much the same way as other processes in the body. Severe protein–calorie malnutrition causes a decline in immune function, in terms of lymphocyte number, cell-mediated immunity, antibodies, and phagocytosis, and therefore an increase in infective morbidity. The levels of other immune mediators, including most complement factors (complement is an important mediator of inflammation that is activated by antibodies) are also decreased in protein–energy malnutrition. The decreased immunocompetence seen with undernutrition is a type of acquired immunodeficiency, and several adverse clinical effects such as opportunistic infections, marked depression of the delayed cutaneous hypersensitivity response, and an increased frequency of septicemia occur. A low protein intake also results in a decline in both cell-mediated and antibody-based immunity.

Although single nutrient deficiencies are rare in humans, experimental evidence is available for the importance of several nutrients such as vitamins (vitamins A, C, E, pyridoxine, and folate), and minerals such as zinc, iron, copper, and selenium. Some amino acids such as arginine and glutamine, and other nutrients such as *n*-3 polyunsaturated fatty acids, are important for specific immune functions such as T cell immunity, and may be beneficial in wound healing and resistance to infections and tumorigenesis as well.

4.3 Pathophysiology of undernutrition complicated by stress

The coexistence of undernutrition and the stress of an injury or infection will lead to a potentiation of the

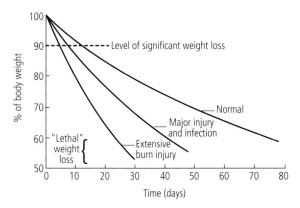

Figure 4.6 Effect of infection and injury on weight loss. Reproduced from Souba and Wilmore (1998).

rate at which nutritional depletion occurs. This is illustrated in Figure 4.6, which shows that a reduction in body weight occurs much faster if starvation is associated with injury or infection.

Energy metabolism

During injury or infection there is an increased BMR, and this increase is dependent on the severity of the injury. Thus the BMR may even double with burns of more than 40% of the body surface, whereas it may only increase by about 25% in patients with long bone

fractures, and even less after surgery (Figure 4.7). If there is fever associated with the injury, the metabolic rate will increase concomitantly. However, this does not necessarily mean that the energy requirements of a patient are raised dramatically. In sick patients who are likely to be in bed, the increase in the BMR due to the stress imposed by the disease may be offset by the decrease in physical activity, such that the total daily energy expenditure may not change drastically.

Protein metabolism

With injury, nitrogen loss also occurs and this may be extensive enough to lead to muscle wasting and muscle weakness. The amount of N lost varies depending on the severity of injury, but in general, there is always an increased N loss. This contrasts with the picture of reduced N losses due to adaptation to low protein intake as shown in Figure 4.4. There is an increase in protein synthesis rates associated with an even greater increase in protein breakdown rates leading to net N loss. The prior nutritional status of the patient is important in determining their muscle mass, and possibly the amount of N that is lost from muscle after injury. The amino acids that are released from the muscle in response to injury do not match the composition of the muscle that is broken down, and alanine and glutamine represent about 60% of the amino acids released from muscle

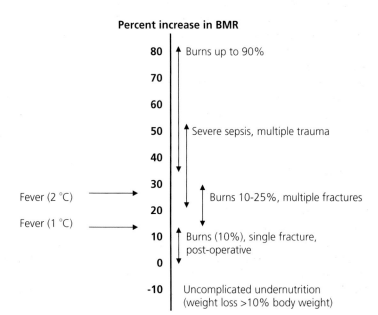

Figure 4.7 The effect of disease and malnutrition on the basal metabolic rate (BMR). Modified from Elia (1991).

after injury. While glutamine is taken up by the kidney for ammonia generation and by the gut as an oxidative fuel, alanine is taken up by the liver for glucose synthesis. In addition, the outflow of amino acids from muscle also serves to fuel the acute phase protein synthesis in the liver. In an undernourished or starved patient, this loss will be magnified because of an inability to replenish the protein breakdown which is required to fuel these processes. A depleted muscle can then no longer provide enough substrates for the splanchnic organs to maintain intestinal integrity and to maintain a high immunocompetence, thereby creating a vicious cycle. It is not known how fast depleted muscle can be restored in undernourished patients, and it is likely that depleted muscle will be restored back to normal only very slowly depending on activity and exercise during rehabilitation.

Hormonal mediators

There are several hormonal and cytokine mediators of the catabolic response to injury. Elevated levels of catecholamines and cortisol are characteristic, in contrast to what is seen in uncomplicated starvation, and promote an increased energy expenditure, nitrogen loss, and glucose production along with the mobilization of free fatty acids. Insulin levels are reduced in the early response to injury, but are raised later in the course of the injury response as insulin resistance appears, probably mediated by cortisol and catecholamines. Glucagon levels are also increased to facilitate glucose production. Proinflammatory cytokines such as tumor necrosis factor-alpha (TNFα), interleukin 1 (IL-1), and interleukin 6 (IL-6) are also important in stimulating acute phase protein synthesis (which is in turn fueled by amino acids from muscle), increased loss of muscle protein, increased lipolysis, and fever, leading to an increased energy expenditure.

If the increased metabolic response continues along with undernutrition, it results in cachexia, which is characterized by extreme weight loss, tissue wasting, and anorexia. The latter contributes in turn to the wasting by a vicious cycle. Cachexia can occur in chronic illnesses as well as cancers and AIDS.

4.4 Chronic undernutrition

Chronic undernutrition or chronic energy deficiency (CED) is a weight-stable condition, in the presence of lower than normal energy intakes. This state is achieved by the presence of low body weight and fat stores, but the individual's health is normal and body physiological function is not compromised to the extent that the individual is unable to lead an economically productive life. While this condition exists to a very small extent in developed countries, between 25% and 50% of adults from developing countries can be described as having CED.

The consequence of an inadequate energy intake during the childhood and adolescence of an individual is a reduced body size and a low BMI. In individuals with CED, there is also stunting due to the presence of low energy intakes and concomitant repeated infections in childhood and adolescence. Both the body fat and the fat-free mass are decreased when compared with normally nourished individuals. Within the fat-free mass, relatively more muscle is lost, which means that the viscera to muscle ratio is increased. It is important to note that in individuals with chronic undernutrition, the BMR expressed per kg body weight or fat-free mass, may not be decreased as it is in individuals with acute undernutrition. When the relationship between BMR and body weight is examined, it shows a line with a positive slope. When this line is extended back to a zero body weight, the BMR does not drop to zero as one would expect with a simple ratio relationship, but has a positive intercept on the y-axis. Therefore, a simple expression of the BMR per kg body weight may not be the best way to look for differences in BMR between normal and undernourished individuals.

However, there may also be a physiological explanation for the conflicting findings of an increase in the BMR per kg body weight or fat-free mass, which can partly be explained by the relatively higher contribution of the viscera to the metabolic rate. Similarly in terms of their protein turnover, these individuals have an increase in the rate of protein turnover expressed per kg body weight, and although the relation between protein turnover and body weight will also have a positive y-intercept, a physiological explanation for the higher protein turnover is the relative loss of slowly turning over tissues such as muscle, compared with the preservation of the more rapidly turning over proteins of the viscera.

Chronic marginal malnutrition is also associated with reduced grip strength and studies have shown that adults with CED have lower handgrip strengths, in absolute terms, as well as when corrected for forearm muscle area in comparison with well-nourished subjects. In addition, it has been found that CED subjects also fatigue faster when subjected to standard laboratory isotonic and isometric exercise protocols than their well-nourished counterparts, although some studies could not find any differences in endurance between undernourished and normal individuals. Taken together, individuals with CED have reduced skeletal muscle performance that is largely explained by the reduction in muscle mass, but may also be partly due to functional changes in skeletal muscle.

4.5 Undernutrition in elderly individuals

There is an increase in the number of elderly people in most populations due to a longer life expectancy, but little data on the effects of undernutrition on such individuals in the long term, or in chronically energy-deficient elderly subjects. The total daily energy expenditure of elderly individuals reduces with progressive age, by about 0.4 MJ/day/decade. A reduction in BMR and physical activity largely accounts for this change, with smaller changes in thermogenesis. The elderly individual also loses muscle mass, a process called sarcopenia, which is also associated with a reduction in skeletal muscle strength. The reduction in skeletal muscle mass has been linked at least in part to suboptimal intakes of protein and the availability of amino acids. In elderly women, consumption of energy-adequate but protein-deficient diets resulted in significant decreases in adductor pollicis function, while in supplemented elderly people on a resistance exercise schedule, muscle mass increased. Aging is also associated with a decline in immune function, which compounds the problem in a clinical situation, and an adequate nutritional intake can modify this decline in immunity.

A three-week underfeeding trial of elderly subjects by about 3.4 MJ/day showed that they reduced their resting and total energy expenditure to the same degree as normal young subjects subjected to an energy restriction of similar magnitude. The decline in resting energy expenditure was greater than what would have been expected from the weight loss alone, as is expected in acute undernutrition, but this decline was smaller than what was observed in the younger adults. A longer term study of underfeeding by about 3.7 MJ/day for six weeks showed that the older individuals lost greater amounts of weight than their younger counterparts and reported a significantly lower frequency of hunger during underfeeding. When they were followed up over a period of six months of normal unrestricted feeding, they did not regain their lost weight. It is thought that aging is associated with a significant impairment in the control of food intake in response to prior changes in energy intake.

Hospitalized elderly patients have a high prevalence of malnutrition, with adverse outcomes related to complications, mortality, and length of stay in hospital. These patients need to be identified, and nutritional support can improve the clinical outcome in them. There are also beneficial effects of nutritional support on the readmission rate in to hospital and the ability of the elderly patient to be maintained at home, although the regaining of depleted muscle mass seems unlikely. There is a case for adequate nutrition to be given to elderly patients; a study on malnourished elderly patients with hip fractures showed that their ability to walk after surgery was improved after nutritional support; however, strong evidence is still unavailable for many other outcomes in these patients, particularly on morbidity and mortality.

4.6 Assessment of undernutrition

A distinction should be made between nutritional screening and nutritional assessment. The first is a rapid generic procedure, often undertaken by non-specialist health professionals, to identify individuals at risk of undernutrition. Nutritional assessment is an in-depth evaluation of nutritional status, which is normally undertaken by a specialist in nutrition, such as a dietitian, and is specific to the disease and patient.

The assessment of undernutrition has to be viewed from two perspectives. From a nutritional and physiological viewpoint, one would like to know the consequences of undernutrition on body composition and function. From the clinical perspective, one would like to know the predictive value of the assessment, particularly in judging what the clinical outcome would be. In addition, the clinical perspective would also place a value on those assessments that provide an early diagnosis of undernutrition, so that nutritional support can be started promptly. It would seem ideal to have a single test or index that would provide a specific and sensitive nutritional assessment, as well as predictive information on the clinical outcome. In practice this is not so, and simple clinical assessments of the nutritional state have proved as useful as complex sophisticated tests in defining the nutritional status for clinically useful purposes. A good nutritional assessment is also important in deciding the nutrient requirements of the individual (see Chapter 2).

4.7 Treatment

The aim of treatment of undernutrition in the clinical setting is two-fold; there is a need to prevent undernutrition from progressing (to prevent weight loss and maintain body weight) and to provide nutrients for nutritional repletion (weight gain) to occur. Equally, the provision of nutrients to sick undernourished patients is unlikely to be effective in terms of clinical outcome in the presence of sepsis and altered metabolism such as insulin resistance and cytokine-mediated events, unless the underlying pathology is addressed. The first step is to assess the nutritional requirements of the patient, followed by decisions on how to deliver these nutrients to the patient.

Assessment of energy and protein requirements

The assessment of the energy requirement in an undernourished patient is based on the energy expenditure. As Figure 4.1 shows, the major component of the energy expenditure is the BMR, which can either be measured by indirect calorimetry or can be predicted by equations that use easily measurable parameters such as the body weight, height, and age of the patient. The actual measurement of the BMR requires several conditions to be met in healthy individuals, including a state of fast, complete rest when awake, and thermoneutrality of the environment. These conditions are unlikely to be met in the clinical state, and a measurement of the metabolic rate under these conditions can at most be called a resting metabolic rate (RMR). The prediction of BMR can be made through the use of age- and gender-based predictive equations, which were recommended by the FAO/WHO/UNU (1985).

A single equation that incorporates weight, height, and age for each gender is the Harris–Benedict equation. This states that the energy requirement (kcal/day) can be calculated by:

For men: Energy requirement =
$(13.7 \times W) + (5.0 \times H) - (6.8 \times A) + 66$

For women: Energy requirement =
$(9.6 \times W) + (1.9 \times H) - (4.7 \times A) + 65.5$

where W is weight in kg, H is height in cm, and A is age in years.

Some error would be expected with the use of these equations, and these are of the order of 10–20%. If there is a coexisting illness, this will cause the BMR to be increased and an appropriate stress factor for the illness will have to be multiplied into the BMR. For instance, if the measured BMR is 1200 kcal/day, and the stress factor related to illness is 1.3; the BMR becomes $1400 \times 1.3 = 1560$ kcal/day.

Once the BMR is known, the total energy expenditure can be obtained by the use of factors representing the other components that are multiples of the BMR. In general, since the other major component of energy expenditure is the physical activity, only this needs to be taken into consideration for practical purposes. The physical activity factor depends on whether the patient is confined to bed, or moving around. The total energy expenditure based on the activity ranges from about 1.3 to 1.5 times the BMR (Figure 4.8).

The decrease in physical activity during illness usually offsets any increase in the BMR due to stress, and overall, it is usually never necessary to provide any more than a modest energy intake. The use of hyperalimentation or the feeding of large amounts of energy to sick patients has no evidence to support its use.

The requirement of protein is to some extent dependent on the energy provided; however, the actual

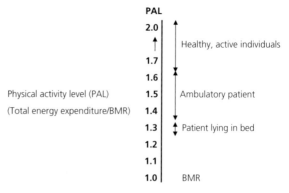

Figure 4.8 Physical activity levels (PAL). This factor is multiplied into the basal metabolic rate (BMR) to obtain total energy expenditure.

protein requirement must be met in undernourished patients. As stated above, the energy requirement is usually not increased, and simply providing an excess of energy will not promote a positive N balance if the protein intake is less than adequate. The normal protein intake that is considered safe, in the sense that it meets the requirements of 95% of the population, is 1 g/kg per day. This protein also needs to deliver essential amino acids in amounts that are adequate. Recent data (which are still the matter of debate) on essential amino acid requirements indicate that this is higher than what was earlier thought, and would need the inclusion of good-quality protein in the diet. Thus, proteins from cereals given alone are likely to be limiting in lysine, and appropriate complementary foods to cereals, such as legumes or animal protein sources, should also be provided in the diet. When protein accretion is the goal of nutritional therapy, the protein intake will have to be raised to about 1.5 g/kg per day, but should ideally not exceed 2 g/kg per day, since there may be a diminished ability of the kidney and liver to tolerate a high amino acid load. Expressed as a percentage of the energy given, the protein intake should be about 15%.

This does not mean that the non-essential amino acids are not important. These amino acids are now recognized to have important roles in the maintenance functions of the body, such as those involved in defense of the body as well as movement and absorption of nutrients. These include skeletal muscle, immune, and intestinal function, which are particularly important during stress (Table 4.2). At a requirement level of intake, given the recent data on essential amino acid requirements, the non-essential amino acids would constitute about 70% of the total amino acid intake.

In disease states, certain amino acids may become essential, and this is called conditional essentiality. Glutamine is an example of a conditionally essential amino acid; it acts as the preferred respiratory fuel for lymphocytes, hepatocytes, and intestinal mucosal cells. Low concentrations of glutamine in plasma reflect reduced stores in muscle and this reduced availability of glutamine in the catabolic state seems to correlate with increased morbidity and mortality. Adding glutamine to the nutrition of clinical patients, either in enteral or parenteral feeds, may reduce morbidity, and several clinical trials have evaluated the efficacy and feasibility of the use of glutamine supplementation. Similarly, arginine may limit immune function and thus be conditionally essential; nutrition that is enhanced in specific nutrients designed to boost immunity is called immunonutrition. Critically ill patients fed a high-protein diet enriched with arginine, fiber, and antioxidants were found to have a significantly lower catheter-related sepsis rate, although there were no differences in mortality or hospital length of stay. The response of undernourished patients to such immunonutrition is dependent on their prior level of antioxidants and perhaps their genotype as well.

Requirements for other nutrients

The provision of adequate energy and protein to the patient must be accompanied by other nutrients such as micronutrients and electrolytes. When tissue depletion occurs in undernutrition, fluid and electrolyte shifts occur that can cause problems on feeding the patient (discussed under refeeding syndrome). As stated earlier, diets that are lacking in potassium or

Table 4.2 Non-essential amino acids in maintenance functions of the body

System	Function	Product	Precursor
Intestine	Energy	ATP	Glu/Asp/Gln
	Growth	Nucleic acids	Gln/Asp/Gly
	Protection	Glutathione	Cys/Glu/Gly
		Nitric oxide	Arg
Muscle	Energy	Creatine	Gly/Arg
Nervous	Transmitters	Glutaminergic	Glu
		Glycinergic	Gly
		Nitric oxide	Arg
Immune	Peroxidative	Glutathione	Cys/Glu/Gly
	Lymphocytes		Glu/Arg/Asp
Cardiovascular	Blood pressure regulation	Nitric oxide	Arg

Modified from Reeds (2000).
Glu, glutamate, Asp, asparate, Gly, glycine, Cys, cysteine, Arg, arginine, Gln, glutamine

Table 4.3 Clinical manifestations of micronutrient deficiencies

Micronutrient	Symptom/sign
Thiamine (B_1)	Beriberi, Wernicke's encephalopathy
Riboflavin (B_2)	Glossitis, cheilosis
Pyridoxine (B_6)	Dermatitis, neuropathy
Niacin[a]	Pellagra
Folic acid	Megaloblastic anemia,
Cobalamine	Megaloblastic anemia, glossitis, diarrhea, neuromyopathy
Ascorbic acid	Scurvy
Vitamin A	Xerophthalmia, night blindness, infections
Vitamin D	Osteomalacia
Vitamin K	Clotting abnormalities
Iron	Anemia
Zinc	Rashes, anorexia, growth retardation, alopecia
Iodine	Hypothyroidism
Selenium	Cardiomyopathy, myositis
Copper	Anemia, neutropenia, infections

[a]Niacin equivalents

phosphorus lead to negative nitrogen balances even when all other nutrients like energy and protein are adequate, while a diet lacking in sodium can reduce the extent of a positive nitrogen balance in malnourished patients receiving an otherwise adequate diet. Zinc levels also fall when malnourished patients are fed, and energy supplements to children with protein–energy malnutrition are not effective in the absence of zinc. Zinc is also an important micronutrient in diarrhea and surgical stress. Iron is an important micronutrient in anemic patients. Table 4.3 shows the symptoms and signs caused by the deficiency of vitamins and minerals in the body. In disease, requirements of vitamins and minerals are likely to increase. Overall, it is very important to provide a diet that is balanced in all nutrients, and unbalanced nutrient intakes can often happen in situations where artificial feeding is instituted by the use of elemental mixtures or in situations where energy supplements are given without attention to protein and micronutrients.

4.8   Potential problems with nutritional supplementation in undernutrition

Several complications are possible when delivering nutrients to patients. These range from problems related to aggressive feeding and overfeeding (see below), to those associated specifically with enteral and parenter-

al nutrition. Gastric retention and the hazard of aspiration of the gastric contents is a complication of enteral feeding. A slow rate of administration of calories is important, as is the evaluation of the food residue in the stomach, particularly in the early stage of feeding. In order to avoid this problem, nasoenteral tubes are used. Another problem linked to enteral feeds is diarrhea, with associated cramps and nausea. Important reasons for this may be bacterial contamination of feeds or a rapid rate of infusion of the feed. Electrolyte disturbances arising secondary to the diarrhea should also be investigated.

When total parenteral nutrition (TPN) is given, it is through a central vein, and there are several technical problems that arise with insertion of the catheter. Catheter insertion is best done by someone who is experienced in this procedure, and it is also important to ensure that the catheter is used only for delivering nutrition, and not for withdrawing blood. Catheter sepsis is a serious complication of TPN, and can negate all the benefits derived from the nutrition, as well as adding significantly to the costs of care, thus, no effort should be spared in adhering to the correct guidelines for catheter care. A low-grade fever or a fever spike is an indication that catheter sepsis may have occurred. Metabolic complications like hyperglycemia can occur due to the administration of glucose at a faster rate than can be cleared by the body. In addition, illness by itself can also decrease the body's ability to utilize glucose. Other metabolic complications related to electrolyte disturbances can also occur, and these are discussed below.

The metabolic complications of overfeeding can be curtailed by identifying patients at risk, providing adequate assessment, coordinating interdisciplinary care plans, and delivering timely and appropriate monitoring and intervention.

Monitoring the nutritional support given is essential to maintain metabolic stability and promote recovery. Complications should be documented, and interventions and the outcomes of clinical care evaluated on a regular basis to assess the appropriateness of the nutritional support that is given.

Refeeding syndrome

When severely undernourished patients are given nutritional repletion, an expansion of the extracellular volume occurs, due to a positive sodium and water balance, which can create dependent edema. When depleted patients are given energy and protein supplements, there is a stimulation of glycogen storage and N retention with cellular protein synthesis and the movement of water into cells. When carbohydrates are administered as the main source of energy, insulin secretion is stimulated, leading to an enhanced cellular uptake of glucose, phosphorus, water, and other minerals such as potassium and magnesium. An expanded extracellular and circulatory volume with refeeding also can result in stress of the still depleted cardiac muscle in such patients.

It is important to be aware of the refeeding syndrome when starting nutritional therapy for the undernourished patient. Energy and protein feeding, and the restoration of circulatory volume should be instituted slowly, and electrolytes, particularly phosphorus, potassium, and magnesium, should be monitored for abnormalities, especially in the first week. It is also worth administering vitamins routinely and restricting sodium intake. The axiom 'A little nutrition support is good, too much is lethal' is apt in this situation, and the goals for nutrition support should be instituted accordingly. In the short term, it is unlikely that protein accretion will take place to a clinically observable extent; what is more important is that previously lost function, such as muscle strength, will return, and this is what is required immediately. Overfeeding with energy in an attempt to make the patient gain weight will result only in fat deposition (see below) and clinical complications.

Nutritional supplementation in chronic undernutrition

It is well known that the refeeding of semi-starved individuals leads to an increase in body weight, particularly fat, as was described in the semi-starvation study of Keys *et al.* (1950). Studies on energy repletion (with low protein supplements) of individuals with a low BMI for about six weeks showed that the body weight increased, but also that a large part of the weight gain was fat. This pattern of weight gain is altered when these individuals are given additional protein repletion in addition to their energy replete diets, where an increase in protein intake to about 2 g/kg per day (compared with about 0.6 g/kg per day in their habitual diets) in addition to the increased energy intake led to an increase in the fat-free mass, in terms of both

muscle and visceral mass. While body fat continued to increase, its rate of increase relative to the body weight change was slower. This suggests that a healthier pattern of weight gain can be achieved by attention to protein intake. Significant improvements in $Vo_{2\,max}$ after protein and energy feeding has also been observed, due to an improvement in muscle mass, however this is not observed with energy supplementation alone. It is also important that an appropriate level of physical activity is followed for regaining muscle mass.

The potential for the increase in fat stores on refeeding raises important public health issues related to the epidemic of type 2 diabetes and coronary heart disease (CHD) in transitioning populations in developing countries. Asians and Mexican Americans seem to have a higher amount of body fat at a given BMI, and it is thought that insulin resistance is related to circulating concentrations of the proinflammatory cytokines secreted by adipose tissue such as TNF , and, in conditions where there is a higher possibility of subclinical infections, this may be a significant factor in the development of insulin resistance. There is also preliminary evidence that adipose tissue, in addition to secreting cytokines and leptin, also elaborates a protein named resistin, which may have a role in increased insulin resistance.

A common thread that runs through these observations is the role of accumulated body fat in general, which points to a dual problem particularly in developing countries: while CED will remain a major public health problem, economic growth and development may lead to an equally large burden of chronic disease. Appropriate preventive measures that avoid excessive nutrient intake as well as the aggressive promotion of healthier lifestyles will be needed.

4.9 Prevention

It is relatively common for patients who are admitted into hospital to become undernourished. There are several reasons why undernutrition can occur: this could be due to a reduced food intake or due to increased requirements for nutrients. The questions that need to be asked are whether undernutrition affects the patients' clinical outcome, and therefore, should it be treated? Further, does treating malnutrition have a beneficial effect on the clinical outcome? There is little doubt that undernutrition affects the clinical outcome in terms of recovery, lower morbidity, hospital stay, and even quality of life in undernourished patients, and therefore, little doubt that this should be treated. A further question is how much a lack of feeding can be tolerated without ill-effect, in both normally nourished and undernourished patients. For the latter group, it seems clear that feeding should be instituted as quickly as possible, building up rapidly to full-strength feeding. In normally nourished patients, it appears that a week of a low nutrient intake can be tolerated without ill-effect, and this could happen, for instance, during the course of elective surgery. However, it should be reiterated that it is best to feed patients as soon as it is possible to do so.

The beneficial effect of nutritional support in patients is more difficult to establish, given that studies are done over short periods of time in heterogeneous patient populations with different treatment regimens. For many diseases complicated by malnutrition, strong data are still lacking in terms of the beneficial effect of nutritional support on disease outcome, and this is due to the many confounders that exist when such clinical trials are done. This task becomes even more difficult with seriously ill patients. However, there is evidence available to suggest that nutritional intervention in undernourished patients is beneficial in changing their clinical outcome. Studies on perioperative nutritional support have shown benefits in terms of postoperative outcomes, and malnourished patients with fractured hips have also been demonstrated to recover their postoperative ability to walk sooner when they were given nutritional support. The clear course to follow clinically is to institute nutritional support promptly, in a moderate and balanced manner, after an assessment to define what the goals of nutrition are, and to follow this up with careful monitoring of the patient to prevent complications.

4.10 Future perspectives

What is the future for the problem of undernutrition? A challenge that still exists is to be able to diagnose the functional consequences of undernutrition at an early stage. For example, while tests for muscle functions exist, there is a need to assess if cognitive functions are impaired and a need to validate these tests as specific for undernutrition.

There are several functional nutritional supplements becoming available based on physiological evidence for the requirement of specific nutrients in specific situations. Novel methods for the delivery of nutrients such as glutamine, through the use of dipeptides is another area of development. However, the administration of individual specific nutrient substrates (arginine, glutamine, different types of triglycerides and short-chain fatty acids) has the potential to produce a variety of metabolic responses that could be both beneficial and harmful. These effects depend on the type and quantity of substance infused, the quality of methodology in the study, as well as the disease and clinical condition of the patient. For example, immunonutrition with arginine, glutamine, nucleotides or ω-3 fatty acids either alone or in combination is said to decrease infectious complication rates. However, it has also been suggested that severe systemic inflammation might even be intensified by arginine and unsaturated fatty acids, by their direct effect on cellular defense and the inflammatory response; therefore caution should be exercised when using immune-enhancing substrates that may actually aggravate systemic inflammation. The same reasoning is true for those substances such as growth hormone and insulin-like growth factor type 1 (IGF-1) that are being evaluated for their effects in improving protein accretion and the immune response of the body.

While the development of new substrates, modulators, and pharmaconutrition is likely to improve the outcome for many patients, overall, for a clinical benefit, one must differentiate between information about the effects of individual substrates on the metabolic response to illness and information on clinical outcomes, particularly in the long term. Another issue of importance is the need for information that will define the cost efficacy of artificial nutrition across a broad spectrum of clinical practice.

More studies are required to evaluate the interaction between an individual's genotype of relevance to the response to injury and infection, nutrients, and prior nutritional status. It can be anticipated that an optimal mixture of glucose, fat, and protein, along with specific nutrients and modulators (to create something like a dream diet) will prove beneficial for specific conditions, but it is prudent to evaluate these in terms of specific beneficial and adverse clinical outcomes since, with many novel nutrients, there is perhaps the danger of creating specialized fads in the place of specialized foods.

Nutritional support to the undernourished has the possibility of adverse effects. This is well documented clinically and in acute undernutrition. The effect of nutritional supplementation particularly in adult chronic undernutrition needs to be evaluated for its potential long-term adverse effects, since it seems likely that a large part of the weight gain is fat.

References and further reading

Akner G, Cederholm T. Treatment of protein–energy malnutrition in chronic nonmalignant disorders. *Am J Clin Nutr* 2001; 74: 6–24.

Bouchard C, Tremblay A. Genetic influences on the response of body fat and fat distribution to positive and negative energy balances in human identical twins. *J Nutr* 1997; 127: 943S–947S.

Chandra RK, Kumari S. Effect of nutrition on the immune system. *Nutrition* 1994; 10: 207–210.

Detsky AA, McLaughlin JR, Baker JP *et al.* What is subjective global assessment of nutritional status? *JPEN J Parenter Enteral Nutr* 1987, 11: 8–13.

Elia M. Organ and tissue contribution to metabolic rate. In: *Energy Metabolism. Tissue determinants and cellular corollaries* (JH Kinney, H Tucker, eds), pp. 61–80. New York: Raven Press, 1991.

Elwyn DH. Nutritional requirements of adult surgical patients. *Crit Care Med* 1980; 8: 9–20

FAO/WHO/UNU. Energy and protein requirements. Report of a Joint FAO/WHO/UNU Expert Consultation. *World Health Organ Tech Rep Ser* 1985; 724: 1–206.

Gonzalez-Gross M, Marcos A, Pietrzik K. Nutrition and cognitive impairment in the elderly. *Br J Nutr* 2001; 86: 313–321.

Grimble RF. Nutritional modulation of immune function. *Proc Nutr Soc* 2001; 60: 389–397.

Heymsfield SB, Wang Z, Baumgartner RN *et al.* Human body composition: advances in models and methods. *Annu Rev Nutr* 1997; 17: 527–558.

Jeejeebhoy KN. Nutritional assessment. *Gastroenterol Clin North Am* 1998; 27: 347–369.

Jensen GL, McGee M, Binkley J. Nutrition in the elderly. *Gastroenterol Clin North Am* 2001; 30: 313–334.

Keys A, Brozek J, Henschel A, Mickelson O, Taylor HL. *The Biology of Human Starvation*. St Paul, MN: University of Minnesota Press, 1950.

McCargar LJ, Clandinin MT, Belcastro AN, Walker K. Dietary carbohydrate-to-fat ratio: influence on whole-body nitrogen retention, substrate utilization, and hormone response in healthy male subjects. *Am J Clin Nutr.* 1989; 49: 1169-78.

National Advisory Group on Standards and Practice Guidelines for Parenteral Nutrition. Safe practices for parenteral nutrition formulations. *JPEN J Parenter Enteral Nutr* 1998; 22: 49–66.

NIH Technology Assessment Conference Statement. Bioelectrical impedance analysis in body composition measurement, 1994.

Reeds PJ. Dispensable and indispensable amino acids for humans. *J Nutr* 2000; 130: 1835S–1840S.

Quevedo MR, Price GM, Halliday D, Pacy PJ, Millward DJ. Nitrogen homoeostasis in man: diurnal changes in nitrogen excretion, leucine oxidation and whole body leucine kinetics during a reduction from a high to a moderate protein intake. *Clin Sci* 1994; 86: 185–93.

Souba WW, Wilmore DW. *Modern Nutrition in Health and Disease*. Philadelphia: Lippincott, Williams and Wilkins, 1998.

Waterlow JC. Metabolic adaptation to low intakes of energy and protein. *Annu Rev Nutr* 1986; 6: 495–526.

Young VR, Borgonha S. Adult human amino acid requirements. *Curr Opin Clin Nutr Metab Care* 1999; 2: 39–45.

5
Metabolic Disorders

Luc Tappy and Jean-Marc Schwarz

Key messages

- The prevalence of non-transmissible diseases such as cardiovascular diseases, cancer, diabetes, and obesity has increased substantially in European and North American populations.
- A similar trend is now being observed in many countries of Africa and South-East Asia and appears to be related to improvements in average income and industrialization/urbanization.
- Morbidity is positively correlated with body mass index, even within the normal range of 20–25 kg/m². The hypothesis that a low energy intake is associated with an increased lifespan is corroborated by animal studies.
- The concomitant occurrence of obesity, impaired glucose tolerance or type 2 diabetes, hypertension, and dyslipidemia has been named the 'metabolic syndrome', or syndrome X. Insulin resistance is a common observation with each of these clinical conditions.
- These metabolic disorders, or diseases of affluence, can be attributed not only to dietary factors, but also to decreased physical activity and other environmental factors. It is also likely that the genetic background of individuals plays an important role.

5.1 Introduction

The average life expectancy of European and North American populations has increased drastically during the second half of the twentieth century. This is essentially attributable to a marked reduction of the mortality associated with infectious diseases. In contrast, the prevalence of and mortality associated with non-transmissible diseases, such as cardiovascular diseases, cancer, diabetes, and obesity has increased substantially. A similar trend is presently observed in many countries of Africa and South-East Asia and appears to be related to improvements in average income and industrialization/urbanization. This epidemiologic evolution suggests that the development of these diseases is strongly dependent on the way of life of affluent societies.

The wealth of a nation impacts indisputably on the way of life of its population. As a result of industrialization, individuals switch from physically active rural occupations to more sedentary factory and office jobs. The higher income associated with these jobs also promotes the use of automated housework devices, cars, etc. This leads to a substantial reduction of physical activity. Simultaneously, the mode of feeding and the type of macronutrients consumed are altered as a consequence of urban living, changes in market food availability, and the more frequent consumption of meals in restaurants and fast foods. The urban feeding pattern is associated with a decrease in the consumption of high-fiber/high-carbohydrate foods and an increase in the proportion of fat consumed when compared with traditional, rural diets.

These changes in the way of life are thought to be involved in the pathogenesis of non-transmissible diseases. As an example, obesity has dramatically increased over the past century. While rare at the beginning of the twentieth century, it now affects 20–50% of European and North American populations. The development of obesity has been shown to be generally associated with ingestion of a high-fat diet. There is evidence, however, that the amount of food calories consumed per capita has decreased from the 1950s until now at the same time as the prevalence of obesity increased. This clearly indicates that the amount of energy expended in physical activity dropped during this period, but was not compensated by a proportional reduction of food intake.

In addition to nutritional changes and alterations of physical activity, other factors also intervene in affluent societies to change the pattern of diseases. Traffic casualties are clearly the consequence of our way of life. There is also an important increase in the consumption of alcohol and other addictive substances, which can be viewed as a consequence of affluence. Chapter 4 deals with overnutrition; this chapter will essentially focus on the effects of caloric intake on health and its role in the pathogenesis of metabolic disorders (obesity-related metabolic alterations, type 2 diabetes, and hypertension). In addition, the effects of alcohol as a source of calories will be considered.

5.2   Energy intake, health, and longevity

In individuals who maintain a constant body composition, energy intake has to be in balance with energy expenditure. The latter is proportional to body mass (or more specifically to lean body mass) and hence is increased in obese patients. This simply means that obese patients have high energy intakes and lean patients low energy intakes. Obviously, ad libitum energy intake is frequently excessive, both in humans and in animals when food is available in profusion. Excessive intake has clearly deleterious effects on health which may be direct and/or indirect. This is illustrated by the very significant association between body mass index (BMI), an index of adiposity, and morbidity for various diseases. At the other end of the spectrum, a very low energy intake, as observed in people unable to feed themselves because of disease or physical incapacities, is associated with muscle and organ wasting, and immune dysfunction and hence with adverse health outcomes. Between these two extremes of obesity and cachexia, there is however a full range of energy intakes which allow the maintenance of an individual BMI between 19 and 25 kg/m^2. This wide variation illustrates that a normal body weight and food intake is not easily defined. It appears, however, that morbidity is positively correlated with BMI even within the normal range of 20–25 kg/m^2.

The hypothesis that a low energy intake (but above the starvation threshold) is associated with an increased

lifespan is corroborated by animal studies. In protozoans, insects, rodents, and non-human primates, energy restriction reduces the incidence of diseases and extends lifespan. This strongly suggests that the level of energy intake and/or metabolic factors modulates the aging process. Several hypotheses can be proposed to explain these effects of caloric restriction. A low energy intake reduces body weight and the weight of most individual organs (with the exception of the brain). In some studies, energy restriction lowers the rate of oxygen consumption per kilogram of lean body weight, indicating that tissue metabolism is reduced. In relation with this lowering of tissue metabolic rate, energy restriction decreases the synthesis of reactive oxygen species, and hence the oxidative stress imposed on the organism. The reactive oxygen species generated during oxidative stress cause enzyme deactivations, induce DNA mutations, or alter cell membranes (Figure 5.1).

Energy restriction may also act through a reduction in plasma glucose and insulin concentrations, and an improved insulin sensitivity. In this context, it is of interest that a gene associated with longevity in *Caenorhabditis elegans* belongs to the family of the insulin receptor gene. Energy restriction has also been shown to be associated with induction of DNA repair systems. Aging and energy restriction have opposite effects on tissue gene expression: aging is associated with an increased expression of genes involved in the stress response in the skeletal muscle of mice. These include acute phase proteins, inflammatory mediators, and

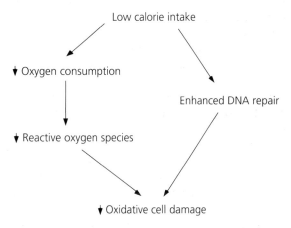

Figure 5.1 Putative mechanisms linking caloric intake with longevity.

inducible DNA repair systems. Energy restriction has the opposite effects. This suggests that there is induction of a stress response as a result of damaged proteins during aging. This response may be secondary to a decrease in cellular systems involved in turnover of cellular constituents. Energy restriction, by increasing the expression of genes coding for biosynthetic processes, may attenuate the effects of aging.

5.3 The metabolic syndrome

Obesity, impaired glucose tolerance or type 2 diabetes, hypertension, and dyslipidemia are diseases of major importance in western societies (Box 5.1). Nutritional imbalances and, more specifically, excess calorie intake are recognized as playing a role in the pathogenesis of each of these conditions taken separately. Furthermore, these metabolic diseases often appear in cluster, with two or more of them being present in the same individual. The concomitant occurrence of these alterations therefore has been renamed the metabolic syndrome, or syndrome X. Additional features of the syndrome are hyperuricemia and impaired fibrinolysis secondary to high plasminogen activator inhibitor concentrations in blood.

The habitually concomitant occurrence of obesity, hypertension, dyslipidemia, and impaired glucose tolerance/diabetes has led to the search for a common factor at the origin of each of them. This led to the recognition that hyperinsulinemia was usually present in each of these clinical conditions. The hypothesis of a role of hyperinsulinemia in the syndrome was further strengthened by the recognition that fasting plasma insulin concentrations represent an independent risk

factor for the development of cardiovascular diseases in cohort studies.

In all these conditions, hyperinsulinemia is the consequence of insulin resistance. Furthermore, insulin resistance *per se* has also been identified as an independent risk factor for the development of cardiovascular diseases in large cohort studies. This suggests that insulin resistance may be the common link between obesity, dyslipidemia, hypertension, impaired glucose tolerance/type 2 diabetes, and impaired fibrinolysis.

5.4 Pathophysiology of insulin resistance

Insulin exerts several different actions at the level of various tissues. Regulation of glucose metabolism is a major action of insulin. In skeletal muscle, adipose tissue, fibroblasts, and several other tissues, insulin increases glucose uptake, oxidation, and storage. These effects are largely secondary to the effect of insulin on specific proteins involved in the facilitated diffusion of glucose from the interstitial space into the cells. In tissues whose glucose metabolism is not dependent on insulin concentrations, cells constitutively express on their cell surface glucose transporter proteins isoforms (e.g. GLUT1, GLUT3). The permanent presence of these proteins on the cell membrane ensures a continuous entry of glucose into the cells. Insulin-sensitive tissues (skeletal muscle, adipose tissue, etc.) express a specific isoform of glucose transporter GLUT4. GLUT4 has the special feature that it can be essentially sequestered into the cells when insulin receptors are not occupied by insulin. When insulin concentrations increase, as after a carbohydrate meal, stimulation of insulin receptors on the surface of the cells triggers the rapid translocation of GLUT4 to the plasma membrane. This allows a rapid, several-fold increase in the number of glucose transporters present at the cell surface, and hence the entry of glucose into the cell.

In addition, insulin activates or inhibits several key intracellular enzymes involved in glucose, fat, or amino acid metabolism. At the level of liver cells, it inhibits glucose production. Some of these effects are due to the interaction of insulin with insulin receptors at the target cell surface and activation of complex intracellular transduction mechanisms. A substantial number of these actions on glucose metabolism can be attributed, however, to indirect effects of insulin (i.e. actions exerted on other cell types, which in turn regulate glucose

---

Box 5.1 The metabolic syndrome

Main features:

- Obesity
- Dyslipidemia (high LDL cholesterol, low HDL cholesterol, high triglycerides)
- Type 2 diabetes/insulin resistance
- Hypertension
- Hyperuricemia
- High fibrinogen

Associated with hyperinsulinemia/insulin resistance

metabolism in distinct cells). Thus, the decrease in free fatty acids produced by insulin contributes substantially to increase glucose oxidation in skeletal muscle and to inhibit glucose production in the liver.

Insulin also regulates lipid metabolism. In adipose tissue, it inhibits lipolysis and free fatty acid release. In skeletal muscle, it decreases lipid oxidation by inhibiting the transport of acyl CoA into the mitochondria. In hepatocytes, it suppresses ketogenesis. Insulin also exerts regulatory effects on protein metabolism by stimulating whole body protein synthesis and inhibiting protein breakdown. In addition to its metabolic actions, insulin also affects a number of other processes: it stimulates Na reabsorption by the kidney, decreases K⁺ concentrations through an activation of Na/K AT-Pase, produces vasodilation in skeletal muscle, increases the sympathetic nervous system activity, and exerts growth-promoting effects.

Insulin affects these different processes with various levels of effectiveness (Figure 5.2). Inhibition of lipolysis and ketone bodies production is already half-maximal at insulin concentrations about twice basal values. Stimulations of vasodilation and sympathetic nerve activity are also attained at low insulin concentrations. In contrast, half-maximal stimulation of glucose transport and oxidation requires higher insulin concentrations (about 10–20 times basal concentrations).

Sensitivity to insulin of various processes

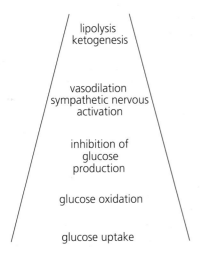

Figure 5.2 Insulin concentrations required to half-maximally effect various metabolic steps. This illustrates differential insulin sensitivity of various tissues.

5.5 Insulin resistance

Insulin resistance corresponds to blunted insulin actions in the presence of normal or increased insulin concentrations. When insulin resistance is mentioned, it usually means a decreased stimulation of glucose metabolism in response to a given concentration of insulin. It can be documented *in vitro* (decreased insulin-induced glucose transport on isolated cell preparation) or *in vivo* (decreased whole body glucose utilization in response to insulin infusion). Insulin resistance has been reported in various clinical conditions: obesity and type 2 diabetes mellitus, dyslipidemia, essential hypertension, and many others. Even in healthy individuals, a wide range of insulin sensitivity is observed, and a substantial portion of the normal population can be considered as 'insulin resistant.' Several factors may be involved in insulin resistance (Box 5.2). Body fat mass is a strong determinant of insulin sensitivity, and obese patients generally have a substantial decrease in insulin responsiveness.

In healthy individuals, insulin sensitivity is a familial trait, which suggests that genetic (as yet unidentified) factors are involved. Ethnic factors (possibly in part on a genetic basis) are also involved: obese Black Africans, Asian, and Hispanic Americans tend to have a more severe insulin resistance than Caucasians of comparable BMI. Dietary factors are also involved. Excess energy intake leads to obesity and insulin resistance. In addition, high-fat diets or high-fructose diets can lead to the development of insulin resistance in rodents and/or humans. Finally, physical fitness and habitual physical activity are important factors which modulate insulin sensitivity. Physical training clearly improves insulin actions through uncompletely understood and probably multiple mechanisms. A lower body fat mass, an increased skeletal muscle mass, and alterations of muscle oxidative enzymes induced by training may all be involved.

Insulin resistance appears to affect specific insulin-sensitive pathways, but to leave other pathways unaf-

Box 5.2 Factors involved in insulin resistance

- Familial/genetic factors
- Obesity
- High (saturated) fat diet
- Low physical activity

fected. Thus, it has been shown that insulin-mediated glucose utilization is impaired in obese patients, while the antilipolytic effects of insulin (decreased lipolysis per unit fat mass) remain little affected. Similarly, stimulation of kidney Na reabsorption and possibly of sympathetic nervous system activity may not be impaired. Since feedback regulatory mechanisms lead to an increased insulin secretion and the development of hyperinsulinemia in insulin-resistant individuals, this differential tissue insulin resistance may lead to overstimulation of some insulin-sensitive processes by hyperinsulinemia. This may account for the increased muscle sympathetic nerve activity and kidney Na reabsorption in obese hyperinsulinemic individuals, for instance.

The molecular mechanisms responsible for a decreased insulin effectiveness remain unknown. A decreased translocation of GLUT4 in response to insulin may be involved and may be the consequence of alterations in the insulin receptor signaling cascade. In addition, there is evidence that insulin resistance in skeletal muscle, which accounts for the major portion of the decreased insulin-mediated glucose disposal in obese diabetic patients, may be secondary to alterations of adipose tissue metabolism. This concept is supported by the observation that elevated free fatty acid concentrations acutely decrease insulin sensitivity in humans by decreasing muscle glucose transport and oxidation. In addition, activation of peroxidase proliferator-activated receptor gamma (PPARγ), which is essentially expressed in adipose cell, increases insulin sensitivity *in vivo*.

5.6   Role of affluence in diabetes, dyslipidemia, and essential hypertension

These disorders are treated in detail in specific chapters of this textbook. We will therefore only review briefly the role of nutritional changes associated with affluence and insulin resistance in their pathogenesis.

Type 2 diabetes mellitus

Until now this disorder has been highly prevalent in Europe and North America, but uncommon in emergent countries. Recent evolution, however, indicates a sharp increase of this disorder in Africa and South-East Asia. Type 2 diabetes is a complex disease, in which ge-

netic factors, nutritional factors, and environment are involved. It is frequently, but not invariably, associated with overweight or obesity. The development of hyperglycemia in type 2 diabetes results in an increase in fasting glucose production and a decreased postprandial glucose utilization. The latter is the consequence of impaired glucose-induced insulin secretion and of insulin resistance (Box 5.3). Nutritional factors may impact on both processes.

Insulin secretion is not abolished in type 2 diabetes, and plasma insulin and C peptide concentrations may be found decreased, normal, or even increased. The first phase of insulin secretion in response to intravenous glucose, however, is abolished while insulin secretion after oral glucose is delayed. When insulin secretion is related to plasma glucose concentration, a decreased glucose-induced insulin secretion is observed. The mechanism at the origin of a decreased insulin secretion in type 2 diabetes remains unknown. Based on the observation that a low glucose-induced insulin secretion is a familial trait, genetic factors can be suspected. Several monogenic forms of diabetes are due to a reduced insulin secretion secondary to mutations of beta cell transcriptional factors (HNF1α, HNF4α, HNF4β, PDX-1). It is therefore possible that alterations of other transcription factors are involved in type 2 diabetes as well, but have not yet been identified.

Nutritional factors may also be involved. There is considerable evidence that fatty acids are involved in the control of insulin secretion. Long-chain fatty acids increase insulin secretion of islet cells *in vivo* and *in vitro* in the short term. This effect is due to a stimulation of insulin release by long-chain fatty acid CoA. In contrast, incubation of islet cells in the presence of elevated levels of fatty acid over several days impairs insulin release. This effect is concomitant with accumulation of triglyceride in the islet cells. It is therefore possible that energy and fat overfeeding decrease insulin secretion through a lipotoxicity on islet beta cells.

Insulin resistance is observed at various degrees in type 2 diabetes. It is severe in obese patients, and moderate to low in lean patients. The inhibition of insulin

---

Box 5.3 Pathogenesis of hyperglycemia in type 2 diabetes

- Impaired glucose-induced insulin secretion
- Insulin resistance (skeletal muscle, adipose tissue)
- Increased endogenous (hepatic) glucose production

actions may in part be genetically determined. There is evidence, however, that a large portion of it is acquired. Weight loss significantly improves insulin resistance in obese type 2 diabetic patients. Energy restriction rapidly enhances insulin sensitivity, before any significant changes in body composition take place. This indicates that energy intake may be as important or more important than body fat in determining insulin actions.

Part of the insulin resistance observed in obese type 2 diabetes may be related to their increased free fatty acid concentrations. As a consequence of increased body fat mass, the rate of whole body lipolysis is increased in obese patients, resulting in elevated free fatty acid concentrations. Elevated free fatty acid concentrations in turn inhibit insulin-mediated glucose disposal by decreasing insulin-mediated glucose transport and oxidation. The exact mechanisms by which fatty acid exerts these effects is not known. Nonetheless, a role of fatty acid in the insulin resistance of obese type 2 diabetic patients is substantiated by the observation that antilipolytic agents improve their insulin sensitivity.

Infusion of lipid emulsion, which increases free fatty acid concentrations, acutely inhibits insulin-mediated glucose disposal, and hence produces insulin resistance in humans. No such effect is observed after addition of fat to a carbohydrate meal. This can be explained by the fact that dietary lipids reach the circulation as chylomicrons which are hydrolyzed locally in adipose tissue capillaries. The free fatty acids liberated are essentially used for triglyceride resynthesis in the adipocyte, and the plasma free fatty acid concentrations do not increase. High fat feeding is nonetheless associated with the development of insulin resistance in animal models and in humans. The mechanisms remain unclear. A high intake in saturated fat may increase intracellular lipid stores, particularly in skeletal muscle. Alternatively, it has been proposed that changes in plasma membrane lipid composition may be involved.

Apart from its actions on intracellular metabolism, insulin also produces vasodilation in skeletal muscle and adipose tissue. This effect is mediated by an endothelial release of nitric oxide (NO). NO is produced by endothelial cells from arginine through the action of endothelial nitric oxide synthase in response to various local stimuli, including shear stress. The released NO diffuses within the vascular wall and is a major factor relaxing vascular smooth muscle cells. It may participate in the stimulation by insulin of glucose metabolism by increasing the delivery of glucose and insulin itself to insulin-sensitive tissues. The vasodilatory effects of insulin are decreased in obese and type 2 diabetic patients, which may contribute to their insulin resistance. Here again, a role of free fatty acids has been postulated in this impairment of NO synthesis by endothelial cells of obese patients.

Insulin resistance and dyslipidemia

Overweight and obesity are frequently associated with elevated plasma triglyceride concentrations and decreased HDL concentrations. Similar changes in plasma lipid profile can be induced by high carbohydrate feeding. It appears that insulin resistance may play a role in the pathogenesis of these alterations. In insulin-resistant obese subjects, free fatty acids are released from the adipose tissue as a result of both insulin resistance in adipose tissue and enhanced body fat mass. Activation by insulin of lipoprotein lipase is reduced, resulting in decreased clearance of triglyceride-rich lipoprotein particles. Insulin resistance also results in increased insulin secretion and hyperinsulinemia. At the level of liver cells, high insulin concentrations in the presence of increased free fatty acid supply leads to increased triglyceride synthesis and secretion of very low density lipoproteins (VLDLs). In addition, insulin may stimulate hepatic *de novo* lipogenesis from carbohydrate.

Dietary management of the metabolic syndrome

Given the key role played by insulin resistance in the pathogenesis of this syndrome, its dietary management and that of directly related metabolic disorders are essentially aimed at improving insulin sensitivity (Box 5.4).

The keystone of this dietary management is to avoid overweight and hence to provide a daily amount of energy corresponding to the energy need of the individual at his/her 'ideal body weight,' i.e. the weight for which the epidemiological studies have shown the lower mortality and morbidity. Tables such as those established by the Metropolitan Life Insurance Company list ideal body weights according to the sex and height of the individual. It is important to note that an obese individual expends substantially more energy than an individual of similar height and sex at his/her ideal body weight, and hence will progressively lose weight if fed the corresponding amount of energy.

Box 5.4 Dietary management of the metabolic syndrome

- Prevent overweight/reduce excess body weight
- Provide energy intake required to maintain an 'ideal body weight'
  - Male: Resting metabolic rate (kcal) = 879 + 10.2 kg body weight
  - Female: Resting metabolic rate (kcal) = 795 + 7.2 kg body weight (Owen, 1988)
  - Total energy intake = resting metabolic rate × 1.4–1.7 according to the level of habitual physical activity
- Avoid diets associated with low insulin sensitivity
  - favor complex carbohydrate and dietary fibers
  - favor monounsaturated fats
  - limit saturated fat intake
- Encourage regular physical activity.

Diet composition also affects insulin sensitivity. A diet high in simple carbohydrates is associated with high postprandial plasma glucose and insulin concentrations and with a low insulin sensitivity. Excessive amounts of simple sugars such as sucrose and fructose are associated with the development of insulin resistance, dyslipidemia, and hypertension. On the other hand, diets high in saturated fat also induce the development of insulin resistance and dyslipidemia. The current concepts favor two alternative approaches, i.e. high-carbohydrate, fiber-rich diets, or high-monounsaturated fat diets, the relative benefits of which remain debated. A low-saturated fat intake is the common denominator of these two diets and appears of importance to prevent insulin resistance.

Encouragement of regular physical activity should be an integral part of the dietary management of the metabolic syndrome. The improved physical fitness associated with physical activity leads to enhanced insulin sensitivity, increased levels of protective HDL cholesterol, and assist in preventing overweight.

Insulin resistance and hypertension

Hypertension is frequently encountered in insulin-resistant patients. Moreover, essential hypertension (but not secondary hypertension) is associated with decreased insulin sensitivity even in lean individuals. Several mechanisms may possibly be involved to increase blood pressure in insulin-resistant patients. Hyperinsulinemia stimulates muscle sympathetic nerve activity, and this may increase arterial vasoconstrictive tone. Hyperinsulinemia also stimulates Na$^+$ reabsorption in the kidney, which may contribute to the pathogenesis of hypertension. Finally, as mentioned in the previous section, insulin resistance is often associated with increased plasma fatty acid concentrations. Such increased fatty acid concentrations have been observed to produce endothelial dysfunction, and may be responsible for the absence of insulin-induced vasodilation. This mechanism may contribute to insulin resistance. In addition, endothelial dysfunction may be responsible for enhanced pressor responses to sympathetic stimulations, such as mental stress, and hence participate in the pathogenesis of hypertension (Figure 5.3).

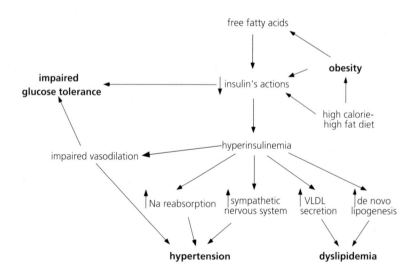

Figure 5.3 Possible mechanisms linking insulin resistance with the metabolic syndrome.

5.7 Alcohol

As a consequence of affluence the consumption of drugs, tobacco, and alcohol increases. This is likely to have a deep impact on public health. Alcohol consumption shows large interindividual variability, ranging from zero to more than 100 g/day. On average, however, it represents up to 10% of total calorie intake in many European countries. Alcohol is essentially metabolized in the liver, where it can be converted into acetaldehyde through the actions of three distinct enzymatic systems: alcohol dehydrogenase, the microsomial ethanol oxidizing system, and catalase. In most non-habitual drinkers, alcohol dehydrogenase represents the major pathway for alcohol metabolism. In usual drinkers the contribution of the microsomial ethanol oxidation system increases, however, due to its induction by ethanol itself. Metabolism of ethanol by catalase remains quantitatively minor.

After ethanol administration, plasma ethanol concentration increases rapidly, then decreases more or less linearly, indicating a constant rate of conversion into acetaldehyde and acetate. The average rate of alcohol metabolism is about 100 mg/kg per hour, but shows considerable interindividual variability.

Excess ethanol intake has well-known deleterious effects on the liver, resulting in hepatic steatosis, steatohepatitis, and alcoholic liver cirrhosis. Alcohol consumption is also associated with gastritis and peptic ulcer disease, and can lead to acquired cardiomyopathy, myopathy, and neuropsychiatric disorders. The reader is directed to specialized chapters about clinical medicine for these specific, alcohol-related diseases. We will deal here briefly with the effect of alcoholic calories consumption on body weight control and cardiovascular risk factors.

Alcohol and body weight

The net effect of alcohol consumption on body weight remains poorly understood. Both restrospective dietary survey and experimental prospective studies indicate that addition of alcoholic calories to the diet does not inhibit consumption of non-alcoholic calories. As a consequence, alcohol consumption is estimated to increase total calorie intake. On the other hand, epidemiological studies show no clear association between alcohol intake and excess body weight. Some studies show even a negative correlation between alcohol intake and body weight in women. This discrepancy may suggest that alcohol calories are not efficiently utilized and may be wasted as heat losses. If this were the case, one would expect that energy expenditure would increase unduly after alcohol consumption. Experimental studies, however, do not support this concept. The increase in energy expenditure observed after ingestion of alcohol corresponds to about 20% of its energy content. This can largely be attributed to the expected energy cost of alcohol metabolism. There is indeed an obligatory consumption of ATP for conversion of alcohol into acetaldehyde. Based on this ATP consumption, it can be calculated that the thermic effect of alcohol metabolism through the alcohol dehydrogenase pathway is about 15% and through the microsomial ethanol oxidizing system about 30%. The measured thermic effect of alcohol falls between these two values, suggesting that there are no significant additional heat losses. This indicates that alcoholic calories are used efficiently to provide energy to the organism.

Further studies indicate that alcoholic calories essentially replace fat as a fuel source when available. The absence of relationship between alcohol intake and body weight therefore remains a mystery. It is possible that alcohol consumption stimulates the energy expended in physical activity, or exerts other, unrecognized, effects on energy intake or expenditure.

Alcohol and blood lipids

Moderate alcohol consumption increases plasma HDL cholesterol concentrations through unknown mechanisms. This effect improves the atherogenic risk profile, and may be involved in the reduction of cardiovascular and overall mortality observed in moderate drinkers.

Alcohol consumption has also been associated with increased plasma triglyceride levels. This effect is particularly observed in overweight individuals. The rise in triglycerides is mainly associated with the VLDL fraction. The exact mechanism remains unknown, but is thought to involve increased free fatty acid re-esterification and VLDL secretion in hepatocytes. Decreased VLDL clearance may also be involved. Alcohol consumption also stimulates *de novo* fatty acid synthesis in the liver, but this pathway represents only a minor portion of alcohol metabolism.

Alcohol and glucose metabolism

Acute alcohol administration has been shown to impair glucose tolerance in healthy individuals. Acute ethanol intoxication has even been associated with overt diabetic decompensation in predisposed individuals (presumably with latent diabetes or low insulin secretory response). This appears to be due to an alcohol-induced inhibition of insulin sensitivity, the mechanism of which remains unknown. Alcohol has also been associated with hypoglycemia. This may be due to potentiation by alcohol of the hypoglycemic effect of drugs (insulin or sulfonylureas), or may occur in fasting individuals, particularly after carbohydrate deprivation. Acute inhibition of hepatic gluconeogenesis is the main mechanism responsible for this effect.

Alcohol and blood pressure

Administration of a single dose of ethanol produces vasorelaxation, and induces a modest drop in blood pressure. In contrast, heavy habitual alcohol consumption produces a dose-dependent increase in blood pressure. The mechanisms remain disputed but may involve a stimulation of the sympathetic nervous system.

5.8 Perspectives on the future

This is ample evidence that the western mode of life is associated with an increased risk for major non-communicable diseases. This can be attributed not only to dietary factors, but also to decreased physical activity and other environmental factors. It is also likely that the genetic background of individuals plays an important role. Genetic factors may possibly explain why some individuals increase their cardiovascular risk factors or develop diseases as a consequence of their mode of life while other individuals do not. In the future, it is very likely that identification of the genes involved will lead to novel, possibly individualized, therapeutic and preventive strategies. Meanwhile, it appears reasonable to provide guidelines aimed at increasing physical activitiy and preventing excess calories and saturated fat intake.

References and further reading

Blundell JE, Lawton CL, Cotton JR, Macdiarmid JI. Control of human appetite: implications for the intake of dietary fat. *Annu Rev Nutr* 1996; 16: 285–319.

Felber JP, Acheson KJ, Tappy L. *From Obesity to Diabetes.* Chichester: John Wiley & Sons, 1992.

Flegal KM. Trends in body weight and overweight in the U.S. population. *Nutr Rev* 1996; 54: S97–S100.

Hellerstein M, Schwarz J, Neese R. Regulation of hepatic de novo lipogenesis in humans. *Annu Rev Nutr* 1996; 16: 523–557.

Jéquier E, Tappy L. Regulation of body weight in humans. *Physiol Rev* 1999; 79: 451–480.

Manson JE, Willett WC, Stampfer MJ *et al.* Body weight and mortality among women. *N Engl J Med* 1995; 333: 677–685.

McGarry JD, Dobbins RL. Fatty acids, lipotoxicity and insulin secretion. *Diabetologia* 1999; 42: 128–138.

Moore H, Summerbell C, Hooper L *et al.* Dietary advice for treatment of type 2 diabetes mellitus in adults. *Cochrane Database Syst Rev* 2004; CD004097.

Owen OE. Resting metabolic requirements in men and women. *Mayo Clin Proc* 1988; 65: 503–510.

Pi-Sunyer FX. Short-term medical benefits and adverse effects of weight loss. *Ann Intern Med* 1993; 119: 722–726.

Reaven GM, Lithell H, Landsberg L. Hypertension and associated metabolic abnormalities – the role of insulin resistance and the sympathoadrenal system. *N Engl J Med* 1996; 334: 374–381.

Spiegelman BM. PPAR-gamma: adipogenic regulator and thiazolidinedione receptor. *Diabetes* 1998; 47: 507–514.

Storlien LH, Pan DA, Kriketos AD, Baur LA. High fat diet-induced insulin resistance. Lessons and implications from animal studies. *Ann NY Acad Sci* 1993; 683: 82–90.

Suter PM, Schutz Y, Jéquier E. The effect of ethanol on fat storage in healthy subjects. *N Engl J Med* 1992; 326: 983–987.

Weindruch R, Sohal RS. Caloric intake and aging. *N Engl J Med* 1997; 337: 986–994.

Westerterp KR, Prentice AM, Jéquier E. Alcohol and body weight. In: *Health Issues Related to Alcohol Consumption* (Macdonald I, ed.), pp. 104–123. Brussels: ILSI Europe, 1999.

Wright J, Marks V. Alcohol. In: *The Metabolic and Molecular Basis of Acquired Disease* (Cohen RD, Lewis B, Alberti KGMM, Denman AM, eds), pp. 602–633. London: Baillière Tindall, 1990.

6
Eating Disorders

Janet Treasure and Tara Murphy

Key messages

Anorexia nervosa

- The *Diagnostic and Statistical Manual of Mental Disorders* (DSM-IV) distinguishes between restricting and binge–purge anorexia nervosa. Restricting anorexia nervosa is characterized by low weight and a severe restriction of food, whereas the binge–purge subtype is noted for purging behaviors such as vomiting and laxative use in addition to low weight.
- Anorexia nervosa is one of the most common chronic disorders in adolescence, prevalence is between 0.1% and 1% in young females in western countries.
- Research into the etiology of anorexia nervosa has included genetic, biological, and psychosocial factors.
- Treatments found to have the best outcome include cognitive behavioral therapy, cognitive analytical therapy, motivational enhancement therapy, and family therapy.
- The prognosis for people with anorexia nervosa is varied: one-third of patients make a full recovery, one-third continue with maintenance of the illness, and one-third remain very ill or die.

Bulimia nervosa

- The diagnosis of bulimia nervosa was introduced in 1979. The main features of the condition are recurrent episodes of binge eating followed by purging behaviors.
- The prevalence of bulimia nervosa is 1–3% in young females. The annual incidence is 12/100 000 amongst the general UK population and a similar figure was found in Holland. There were large increases in the condition in the late 1980s and early 1990s. This may have been due to increased

recognition by the population and health professionals.
- The causes of bulimia nervosa are unknown. Negative self-evaluation, dieting, childhood victimization, and predisposition to a robust appetite and obesity are risk factors.
- Randomized controlled trials have shown that specific treatments such as cognitive behavioral therapy are useful in managing bulimia nervosa but they have their shortcomings. Antidepressant medication has also found to be useful in rehabilitation of bulimia nervosa.
- About a third of people recover from bulimia nervosa, though residual problems with attitudes to food and weight can remain a year after treatment, and approximately 10% have problems at 10 years.

Binge eating disorder

- Binge eating disorder (BED) is the most recently recognized eating disorder to be classified by a psychiatric diagnostic manual (though only as an appendix).
- The causes of BED are similar to those of bulimia nervosa but there may be a greater predisposition to obesity.
- The prevalence of BED is about 2% in the general population. Research suggests that it has a broader demographic distribution than anorexia nervosa or bulimia nervosa.
- Cognitive behavioral therapy is presently the most commonly used treatment for BED; in addition to this, interpersonal psychotherapy and selective serotonin reuptake inhibitors show positive effects in treatment.
- The long-term prognosis for BED has not been established but there is a marked improvement in binging in the short term.

6.1 Introduction

Eating disorders are classified into three variants: anorexia nervosa, bulimia nervosa, and binge eating disorders (BED). These classifications are in turn frequently divided into subtypes. In addition there are are less well researched and less easily defined conditions such as night eating disorder and eating disorder not

otherwise specified (EDNOS). EDNOS is the category used for cases that do not strictly fit strictly into the classification criteria.

Rather than a multiplicity of subcategories it may be more helpful to conceptualize the eating disorders as falling on a spectrum. The spectrum model (Figure 6.1) denotes the continuum on which the eating disorders which we describe in this chapter are seen to

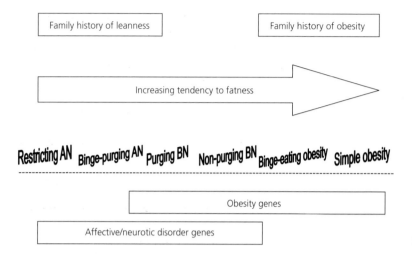

Figure 6.1 The spectrum model.

lie. This model shows the genetic and phenotypic variation between restricting anorexia nervosa, bulimia nervosa, and BED.

Our understanding of etiology, treatment, and outcome in all three conditions is still in the learning stages. The conceptualization of these disorders is that mental health rather than nutritional health is the key element. In this chapter the 'history' of eating disorders is explored, along with the epidemiology of these conditions, the techniques used in management, and their outcome. Present and future research lies in genetic and biological areas as well as focusing on cognitive, emotional, and perceptual understandings. Research into the carers of people with eating disorders and their needs have added to improvements in outcome and coping after inpatient treatment.

Section I: Anorexia nervosa

6.2 History

The cultural framing of anorexia nervosa has led to wide differences in the way that the condition has been managed. Anorexia nervosa was construed as spiritual asceticism in medieval Europe. Later, people with anorexia nervosa were regarded as freaks who defied the laws of science. This culminated in an unfortunate incident in the nineteenth century when Sarah Jacob, the 'Welsh fasting girl', was subjected to the scrutiny of scientific skeptics. The claim that she did not need to eat was put to the test and led to her rapid death.

In Britain, following the medical categorization of the disorder in the late nineteenth century, cases of anorexia nervosa were predominately managed by physicians. Gradually over the last half of the twentieth century, especially after the emergence of bulimia nervosa, psychiatrists started to take over the care. In contrast, in France, psychiatrists have been involved in the management of these cases since the middle of the nineteenth century. This wide cultural variation in the conceptualization and management remains today. For example, in China most cases are still referred to physicians. Most western countries now find it most effective to use a mixture of medical, psychological, and social expertise in the management of anorexia nervosa.

6.3 Etiology

Most explanations of causation are multidimensional, including genetic factors, biological factors, psychological vulnerability, family, and sociocultural setting conditions. However, one of the problems with such an all-encompassing model is that it is very difficult to prove or disprove and it makes any attempts at prevention very difficult, as vulnerabilities have to be remedied on so many fronts. One major flaw in a large proportion of the work on etiology is that there has been a tendency to group anorexia and bulimia nervosa together or to use poorly defined subgroups such as college girls with abnormal eating attitudes as the basis of modeling risk factors. Given the wide difference in the history of the two conditions it would seem wise to regard them as separate entities until proved otherwise.

There are numerous biological models of anorexia nervosa.

Biological factors

There are two domains of interest that may underpin the biological vulnerability. One hypothesis is that there is an abnormal regulation of body composition and appetite. Evidence to support this is the tendency for leanness to run in families of people with anorexia nervosa and the fact that some strains of lean animal are prone to stress-related wasting. A variant of this model is that stress triggers the spiral of weight loss in those with a specific biological vulnerability. An alternative model is that biologically determined temperamental traits such as harm avoidance and persistence (or other components of the obsessive personality) may act as either a risk factor or in a moderating or mediating fashion. None of the models below is mutually exclusive.

Model 1: Genes as a risk factor for eating disorders

Evidence for a genetic component in the etiology of anorexia nervosa has gradually unfolded. Family studies have found that the risk of eating disorders in the female relatives of people with both anorexia nervosa and bulimia nervosa is increased 5- to 7-fold. Twenty per cent of the female relatives of people with anorexia nervosa had some form of eating disorders, compared with 4% of the comparison group with no eating disorder. In twins the concordance rates for anorexia nervosa is high, ranging from 50% to 70% depending on the phenotype. The impact of heritability is estimated to be over 50%. In this area there is the problem of not being able to control for a common emotional environment.

One of the candidate genes for anorexia nervosa is the *5HT52A* promoter region. Several groups have found that the risk of developing anorexia nervosa is twice as likely in people with this gene promoter as in people without it, but there is also evidence in the literature which challenges this. The research in this area is still developing.

Model 2: Leptin: a possible abnormality in the control of body composition

One of the key components in the control of body composition is leptin, a hormone secreted by fat cells. One hypothesis is that abnormal control of leptin regulation underlies the weight loss in anorexia nervosa. When fat cells decrease in size the output of leptin decreases. Less leptin is transported into the brain. Low levels of leptin interfere with reproductive function and should allow the appetite system to be disinhibited, increasing food intake, with an associated decrease in metabolism and activity. The fact that reproductive function is suppressed in anorexia nervosa suggests that the abnormality of appetite and activity is downstream of leptin. Indeed preliminary research does not suggest that there is any abnormality in leptin function in anorexia nervosa. The levels are low when patients are underweight and are increased with weight gain and in the normal range on recovery. However, it is possible that there may be subtle abnormalities in this system

Model 3: An interaction between chronic stress and weight

This theory links the psychosocial aspects of anorexia nervosa with the biology of appetite. Chronic stress may lead to an abnormal form of activation of the hypothalamic–pituitary–adrenal system, which might interfere with the normal homeostatic control of appetite.

Model 4: Serotonin, an abnormality in neurotransmitters

Serotonin is of interest as a potential candidate gene in eating disorders because of its roles in both the physiological and the psychological domains. Serotonin is involved in: eating behavior, animal models of anorexia nervosa, and temperamental traits such as impulsivity compulsivity and emotional reactivity.

There is some evidence of abnormal serotonin function persisting after recovery from anorexia nervosa. It is possible that abnormalities in serotonin regulation predispose people to develop the disorder.

Environmental factors

Various environmental factors may have an influential role in the etiology of anorexia nervosa.

Cultural factors

It is possible that a cultural focus on dieting serves to maintain the illness and may cause the course of the disease to be more severe, accounting for the trend for a higher mortality and increased readmission rates. There is little evidence to suggest that dieting is a risk factor in anorexia nervosa, in contrast to the research on bulimia nervosa. Many feminist writers have suggested that the changing roles of women and the shift in the assumptions of power and control may have led to the emergence of eating disorders. Such arguments are made about eating disorders in general but are probably more relevant to bulimia. Arguments from a feminist/transcultural perspective suggest that a phobia of control may be an appropriate definition of the psychopathology of both anorexia and bulimia nervosa.

The British Medical Association's Report (May, 2000) stated that 'this meeting fears that some forms of advertising may be contributing to an increase in the incidence and prevalence of Anorexia Nervosa [eating disorders in general]. It calls for greater responsibility in the use of such images in the media.' This was followed by a review which described the possible negative influence that the media can have on young people in the development of their self-esteem, eating patterns, and body image.

Although there is evidence that anorexia nervosa develops in all social classes and in people with average intelligence, there is a tendency for women with anorexia nervosa and their families to be engaged in a struggle to attain higher ranking. The conclusion from a recent systematic review about epidemiology in different cultures (time and place) suggest that bulimia nervosa varies in incidence across cultures and is most common in western societies. This variation is less marked for anorexia nervosa, which suggests that bulimia nervosa is more responsive to environmental changes and in particular those related to shape and weight and food availability.

Personal vulnerability factors

The onset of anorexia nervosa and bulimia nervosa usually (in 70% of cases) follows a severe life event or difficulty. There is a tendency for these patients to have a maladaptive coping response to the triggering event, exemplified by avoidance and helplessness. This cognitive and emotional set is present from childhood. Obsessional personality traits associated with self-disgust and sensitivity to criticism may lead to compensatory strategies such as perfectionism and a tendency to please others and submit to their wishes.

6.4 Clinical features

Anorexia nervosa most usually has its onset in the mid-teenage years but it can start as early as age eight. Between 90% and 96% of those affected are young women. Anorexia nervosa is amongst the three commonest chronic disorders in adolescence alongside asthma and obesity. The proportion of males detected in primary care is ten-fold lower than females. The incidence rate falls off rapidly by a factor of 10 in women over the age of 25. It has a large impact in terms of physical (resulting from nutritional deprivation) morbidity and psychosocial impairment. Psychiatric illness is categorized by the use of the *Diagnostic and Statistical Manual of Mental Disorders*, currently in its fourth edition, which is a recorded collection of symptoms of mental illness. The DSM-IV (as it is known) allows health professionals to categorize symptoms of pathology into classified disorders.

There have been recent changes in the DSM-IV criteria for anorexia nervosa, which have divided it into two subtypes (American Psychiatric Association, 1994). The classical form is now termed anorexia nervosa restricting subtype. This is distinguished from the binge–purge subtype, in which there is regular binge eating or purging behavior (i.e. self-induced vomiting or the misuse of laxatives, diuretics or enemas). The diagnostic criteria for anorexia nervosa are listed in Table 6.1. However although these behaviors appear to be reasonable proxy measures of different subsyndromes there are no clear-cut divisions between them. This may have an impact on research and lead to unclearly defined groups of patients in studies. Over time, the diagnostic criteria have also broadened. In DSM-III there had to be a 25% weight loss. This has now decreased to a weight loss below 15% of the matched population, which roughly corresponds to the *International Statistical Classification of Diseases and Related Health Problems*, tenth revision (ICD-10) criterion of a body mass index of less than 17.5 kg/m^2. This minor

Table 6.1 Diagnostic criteria for anorexia nervosa

DSM-IV	ICD-10 (F50)
Refusal to maintain body weight over a minimal norm/leading to body weight 15% below expected	Significant weight loss (BMI <17.5 kg/m^2) or failure of weight gain or growth Weight loss self-induced by avoiding fattening foods and one or more of the following (a) vomiting (b) purging (c) excessive exercise (d) appetite suppressants (e) diuretics
Intense fear of gaining weight or becoming fat	A dread of fatness as an intrusive overvalued idea and the patient imposes a low weight threshold on him- or herself
Disturbance in the way in which one's body weight, size, or shape is experienced, e.g. 'feeling fat' (denial of seriousness of underweight or undue influence of body weight and shape on self-evaluation)	
Absence of three consecutive menstrual cycles	Widespread endocrine disorder (a) amenorrhea (b) raised growth hormone (c) raised cortisol (d) reduced T3

1. Restricting type
2. Binge–purging type: binge eating or vomiting/misuse of laxatives or diuretics

Reproduced with permission from American Psychiatric Association (1994) and World Health Organization (1992).

change in classification illustrates the changing viewpoints of the illness that can challenge consistency in research.

The DSM-IV originates in the United States and the ICD-10 is based in Europe. The criteria are similar in both systems. An approach that views the symptoms on a continuum (Figure 6.1) may be more appropriate, as patients frequently move between diagnostic categories.

The criteria of a disturbed body image was included in the systems of classification used in the 1980s but this was later dropped as it was not always present and was difficult to define. Again, this illustrates the difficulties that have been found in standardizing diagnosis of anorexia nervosa. This feature is probably a metaphor for more abstract discontent and is largely dependent on gender and cultural factors.

6.5 Epidemiology

The incidence of anorexia nervosa is seven new cases presenting for treatment per 100 000 population in western countries. Approximately 4000 new cases arise in the UK every year. The average duration of the disorder is six years. The prevalence in young women ranges from 0.1% to 1%. Although earlier research suggested that the incidence of anorexia nervosa might have increased over the twentieth century, the balance of evidence suggests otherwise. It is possible that the binge–purge subtype of anorexia nervosa, in which there is less severe weight loss, has increased. The number of cases in the community is probably higher than reported or treated as one of the critical clinical criteria is the reluctance to seek help.

6.6 Management of anorexia nervosa

There have been few randomized controlled trials, that is, research which directly compares the benefits of two or more forms of treatment. Those that have been accomplished have had very low power and have included a selected sample. This would suggest that not enough people were included in the studies to assess a realistic view of the outcomes. Also, when the sample is somewhat self-selected it makes it difficult to generalize the results to a larger population.

Nutritional rehabilitation is a part of any good care plan which can help lower the risks of long-term complications, even death. This rehabilitation also provides patients with time to consider more clearly their behavior, gain insights into their condition, and re-establish control over their eating.

The management of anorexia nervosa is based upon clinical pragmatism. The choice of treatment depends upon (1) the patient's age, (2) medical severity, and (3) duration of the disorder. For patients under the age of 17, it is helpful to have their family involved in treatment. Also, if the onset of the illness was in early adolescence – no matter what the patient's chronological age is – it is usually helpful to involve the family in some capacity. Parental counseling, using cognitive behavioral therapy, is useful in helping the family to understand the illness and to deal with the problems it causes.

The efficacy of family work may be enhanced if it is tailored to the developmental stage of the person with a eating disorder. A study involving adolescents with eating disorders and their families found that the level of critical comments about the person with anorexia nervosa had an impact on the chance of recovering from the illness.

Early and mild cases of anorexia nervosa can be treated in the community. General practitioners, community psychiatric nurses, or school counselors trained in the management of eating disorders can provide effective care, offering a collaborative therapeutic relationship, education about the consequences of the disorder and nutrition, and regular weight monitoring. The health professional should also try to engage the family or other carers in the treatment. Families often need support if they are to care effectively for a younger member of the family with anorexia nervosa.

The standard method of treatment endorsed by the American Psychiatric Association Guidelines (2000) and standard psychiatric texts is inpatient treatment. However under the National Institute for Clinical Excellence (NICE) guidelines recently published (www. nice.org) the first choice of treatment is outpatient therapy. Unlike most other psychiatric conditions, in which the use of inpatient beds is rapidly decreasing, admission rates for anorexia nervosa in many countries are increasing. Relapse and readmission is common. However, newer models of treatment are being developed which include alternative forms of management such as day patient and outpatient treatment and stepped care services.

Outpatient psychotherapy or counseling for older patients can be effective if there has not been excessive weight loss (i.e. less than 25%). Self-help books on anorexia nervosa may prove to be of benefit as adjuncts to therapy. In comparison with standard nutritional management, psychotherapy has been found to be more acceptable and efficacious. New models of cognitive behavioral therapy (employing thoughts and feelings) have been developed and are being tested as techniques to prevent relapse. Cognitive analytical therapy and short dynamic therapy (exploring relationships with other people and past experience) have also been found to be useful. Therapy for anorexia often needs to be continued long term. It is important that psychological treatment is supplemented by regular medical monitoring.

People who are admitted for inpatient treatment generally have a poor prognosis. This is because the factors which lead to inpatient care, i.e. clinical severity and poor motivation, are adverse prognostic features. Inpatient treatment combines nutritional management with psychological approaches.

Pharmacotherapies

In the last 40 years a wide variety of pharmacological agents have been tried in the treatment of anorexia nervosa with limited success. Medications have been used to promote weight gain, to treat associated psychiatric comorbidity (such as depression and obsessive–compulsive behavior), medical complications, and in preventing relapse.

Antidepressant medications have been used in a number of treatment trials for anorexia nervosa, based in part on the observed increased prevalence of depression in patients with anorexia nervosa and in their first-degree relatives. Some of the new antipsychotic drugs have been tried, but the results of drug treatment have been disappointing compared with psychotherapy and they are poorly accepted by patients.

Weight-related complications

The complications can be broadly divided into those that relate to starvation and those that are associated with weight control measures.

Skin and hair changes

The skin is dry and fine, downy, lanugo hair develops. There is often loss of head hair and what is left appears thin and lifeless.

Musculoskeletal problems

Individuals with severe anorexia nervosa have poor muscle strength and a decrease in stamina. Proximal myopathy is a useful marker of severe physiological compromise. It can be elicited by asking the patient to stand from a crouched position. This symptom indicates the need for urgent nutritional rehabilitation and inpatient treatment.

Osteoporosis and pathological fractures are the commonest causes of pain and disability in anorexia nervosa. The annual incidence of non-spine fractures of 0.05 per person per year in anorexia nervosa is seven-fold higher than the rate reported from a community sample of women aged 15–34. Risk factors for this complication are a long duration and increased severity of illness.

Effects on the CNS

Brain substance decreases in anorexia nervosa and the ventricular spaces and the sulci increase in size. To a degree these structural abnormalities, such as loss of gray matter, persist despite weight recovery for over a year, which suggests that there may be a degree of irreversible damage even in adolescents with a short history. The cause of the cerebral atrophy is uncertain. It may be a general effect of starvation or may result from the high level of cortisol, which is present in anorexia nervosa and which is known to be toxic to dendrites.

Functional cognitive impairment is seen with deficits in memory tasks, flexibility, and inhibitory tasks persisting despite weight recovery. Women who have recovered from anorexia nervosa have average IQ scores.

Cardiovascular problems

The heart becomes smaller and less powerful because muscle is lost. Blood pressure and heart rate is lowered. This can lead to faints. There is poor circulation in the periphery and this leads to cold blue hands, feet, and nose. At its extreme, this results in chilblains and even gangrene, particularly in children.

Sudden death has been known to occur in anorexia nervosa and may result from arrhythmias. QT prolongation is common in anorexia nervosa and low potassium, which results from many of the methods of weight loss, can exacerbate this problem.

Fertility and reproductive function

Fertility is reduced in women with anorexia nervosa. In part this is due to suboptimal physical recovery. In a follow up of 12.5 years in Denmark the fertility rate was a third of that expected and the perinatal mortality rate was six-fold higher. Women with anorexia nervosa may also have difficulties in feeding their children, who may become malnourished and stunted in growth. It has been found that women with anorexia nervosa have significantly more miscarriages and cesarian deliveries. The offspring of women with anorexia nervosa are significantly more likely to be born prematurely and are of lower birth weight than the offspring of controls.

Endocrine system

The hypothalamic–pituitary–gonadal axis regresses to that of a prepubertal child. The pituitary does not secrete follicle-stimulating hormone (FSH) and lueteinizing hormone (LH) and the ovaries decrease in size. The ovarian follicles remain small and do not produce estrogens or progesterone. By contrast, the hypothalamic–pituitary–adrenal axis is overactive, probably driven by excess corticotropin-releasing factor (CRF), with high levels of cortisol which are not constrained by any feedback.

Gastrointestinal tract

Residual gastrointestinal problems such as irritable bowel syndrome are common after recovery from anorexia nervosa. Functional abnormalities such as delayed gastric emptying and generalized poor motility are related to the degree of undernutrition. Anatomical abnormalities as a result of the trauma of vomiting and overeating or loss of mesenteric fat occur. Structural abnormalities such as ulcers are common. It is important not to overlook the effects of sorbitol present in sugar-free gums and sweets, which can cause abdominal distension, cramps, and diarrhea.

Haematology

All components of the bone marrow are diminished but the order in which this is discernible in the peripheral blood is white cells, red cells, and finally platelets. The level of marrow dysfunction relates to the total body fat mass. The immune system is compromised, with a decrease in CD8 T cells.

Table 6.2 Mineral deficiencies associated with anorexia nervosa

Mineral	Factors associated with the development of the deficiency	Effects of deficiency on the body
Calcium	Excessive exercise at a low weight and absence of dairy products in the diet	Osteoporosis
Iron	Avoidance of red meat in the diet	Iron deficiency anemia
Zinc	Avoidance of red meat	Loss of appetite
		Loss of taste sensation
Potassium and phosphate	Vomiting, laxative and diuretic abuse	Cardiac abnormalities
	Rapid refeeding	Cardiac failure

Nutrients of importance in anorexia nervosa

Table 6.2 shows some of the most common mineral deficiencies seen in anorexia nervosa.

Calcium

Osteoporosis is a severe complication of anorexia nervosa and treatment is uncertain. A diet with adequate amounts of calcium and vitamin D is recommended. The majority of people with anorexia nervosa consume low-fat diets and are likely to be deficient in both.

Potassium and phosphate

Starvation may lead to the depletion of potassium and phosphate, which are imperative in cardiac muscle functioning. The requirements for potassium and phosphate will increase through refeeding and the demands placed on the heart are also increased. Care must be taken when nutritional therapy is instituted to avoid refeeding syndrome (see Chapter 8).

Vitamins

Vitamin deficiency is unusual in eating disorders. Protection from this deficiency usually comes as a result of low-fat diets usually including a large amount of water-soluble vitamins in the form of fruit and vegetables. In anorexia nervosa, metabolic activity is at a minimal level; an example is that the thiamin required for carbohydrate metabolism is required at much lower levels than people on a balanced diet. A general vitamin and mineral supplement is recommended to supplement nutritional rehabilitation.

Section II: Bulimia nervosa

6.7 History

Bulimia nervosa has been described since ancient times. In Ancient Egypt the practice of emesis was described in detail in *Ebers' Papyrus*, the oldest surviving medical document. The papyrus lists several means of emptying the stomach, using anything from cow's milk to concoctions of fennel and honey. From Herodutus we know that the Egyptians used to purge themselves for up to three days every month. They believed that this would help them to preserve health as it was thought that 'all diseases to which men were subject proceed from food itself'.

The word bulimia is derived from the Greek *bous*, meaning ox, and *limos*, meaning hunger, it suggests hunger of such severity that a person had the ability to consume a whole ox, indicating a pathological state of appetite. Throughout the eighteenth and nineteenth centuries self-induced vomiting has been described as being a medical curiosity or symptom of other diseases.

The diagnosis of bulimia nervosa was introduced by Professor Gerald Russell in 1979. He associated the term with a subgroup of patients with anorexia nervosa who displayed a chaotic pattern of eating, with episodes of fasting or extreme weight control, in contrast to patients who restricted their food.

6.8 Etiology

People with bulimia nervosa have an older age of onset, a more chronic outcome, and a higher incidence of premorbid and family obesity. The etiology of bulimia tends to fall into three domains: personal vulnerability, environmental adversity, and dieting risk factors.

Psychological factors

Core beliefs (absolute beliefs about the self, others, and the world) and underlying assumptions (the rules that each individual follows throughout their lives) were compared between a group of people suffering from bulimia nervosa and a group diagnosed with depression. The results showed that although levels of negative self-evaluation were significantly similar, when assumptions based around weight, shape, and eating were investigated, they proved to be very different. The authors suggest that depression in young women is associated with the function that weight and shape play in self-acceptance.

Environmental risk factors

Research reveals a strong link with abusive family experiences. Research has found that women with bulimia nervosa tend to report more troubled childhoods than women from non-morbid control groups. Results suggest that they resemble the results gained from women suffering from depression. Childhood sexual abuse has been identified as a predictor for bulimia, specifically when psychiatric comorbidity exists, though it has not been found to be related to the severity of the condition.

Dieting risk factors

Dietary restraint theory developed during the 1970s suggests that restrained eaters (people who chronically attempt to maintain strict control over their eating) are at high risk for becoming temporarily disinhibited (leading to a binge). A number of studies have detailed the circumstances that can lead to a binge, including negative mood, substance abuse, and cognitive load. Binge eating may be employed as a coping strategy by people with bulimia nervosa when triggers in their lives are activated, though the research suggests that eating does little to combat the feelings of anxiety and is likely to increase it. People with bulimia nervosa have a predisposition to a robust appetite and a tendency to overweight; these are traits that run in their families.

6.9 Clinical features

Bulimia nervosa is defined by binge eating or the excessive intake of food in a brief period of time with a sense that the eating is out of control, counterbalanced by inappropriate compensatory behavior. This may include purging, vomiting, the use of laxatives and diuretics. Alternatively, it may be accompanied by non-purging, fasting, excessive exercise, and with a preoccupation with body shape and weight. It is associated with a fear of becoming fat. The diagnostic criteria included in DSM-IV and ICD-10 are listed in Table 6.3.

In bulimia the criteria relating to the frequency of symptoms and the definition of a binge have become tighter and the forms of weight control behavior have become more explicit.

What is a binge?

Binge eating is used to describe the consumption of an amount of food that is definitely larger than most people would eat during a similar period of time and

Table 6.3 Diagnostic criteria for bulimia nervosa

DSM-IV	ICD-10 (F50.2)
Recurrent episodes of binge eating (rapid consumption of a large amount of food in a discrete period of time)	A preoccupation with food, and an irresistible craving for food; the person succumbs to episodes of overeating in which large amounts of food are consumed in a short period of time.
A feeling of lack of control over eating behavior during the eating binges	The person attempts to 'counterbalance' the 'fattening' effects of food by one or more of the following: self-induced vomiting; purgative abuse; alternating periods of starvation; use of drugs such as appetite suppressants, thyroid preparations, or diuretics
The person regularly engages in either self-induced vomiting, use of laxatives or diuretics, strict dieting or fasting, or vigorous exercise in order to prevent weight gain	
A minimum average of two binge-eating episodes a week for at least three months	The psychopathology consists of a morbid dread of fatness and the person holds him- or herself at a sharply defined weight threshold, well below the premorbid weight that constitutes the optimum or healthy weight in the opinion of the physician
Persistent overconcern with body shape and weight	

Reproduced with permission from American Psychiatric Association (1994) and World Health Organization (1992).

in similar circumstances. The term was recently investigated and it was found in a sample of 60 women diagnosed with BED that 'loss of control' was the sole criterion used to define binge eating by a majority of the sample (82%). In addition to this, the criteria 'large amount of food' and 'eating to relieve negative affect' were reported less frequently as descriptors, though they appear to be important criteria.

6.10 Epidemiology

The short history of bulimia nervosa means that there is much less epidemiological data available than for anorexia nervosa. The incidence of cases presenting to primary care in the UK is 12/100 000 in the population. The incidence of bulimia presenting for medical care increased during the 1980s, and a three-fold increase in detection was reported between 1988 and 1993. In part this may be due to a combination of increased recognition by both patient and doctor. The data from a study examining the lifetime psychiatric history of a cohort of twins suggests that there is an age cohort effect, with a marked increase in the risk in those women born after the 1950s.

The prevalence of bulimia is 1–3% in adolescence and families. Onset occurs typically during the late teens and early adult years. Children under the age of 14, however, have been identified and it has been suggested that the occurrence of bulimia in these young people is increasing.

6.11 Management

A large number of randomized controlled trials have been carried out to evaluate treatment for bulimia. There is confidence that cognitive behavioral treatment is effective for approximately half of the patients treated. Self-help books and CD-ROM treatments have also been employed to deliver cognitive behavioral treatment.

A sequential model of care for bulimia using low intensity models such as psycho-educational or bibliotherapy was recommended in the Royal College of Psychiatrists Report (2001) and several alternative models have been described using the cognitive behavioral treatment model. The advantages of such an approach are that it does not waste resources because those who respond to a minimal intervention are 'filtered out.' One possible adverse effect of sequential treatment is that it can lead to the experience of failure, which may lower the person's already fragile self-esteem and damage the therapeutic alliance.

Antidepressant medication has been found to be somewhat effective for people with bulimia nervosa. Patients with eating disorders are particularly wary of any side effects relating to appetite and weight control. These patients commonly go to the library and read the small print. Many are thus reluctant to take tricyclic antidepressants which have weight gain in their list of possible side effects. Thus the weight loss listed as an effect of selective serotonin reuptake inhibitors may lead to better compliance with this drug.

Complications of weight control strategies

Fluid balance

Low potassium levels can result from vomiting or laxative and diuretic abuse. Usually, this is associated with raised levels of bicarbonate but some laxatives can produce a metabolic acidosis. Many other salts and metabolites are reduced, for example magnesium, phosphate, calcium, sodium, and glucose. Dehydration can also be a problem.

Dental changes

The commonest stigma of persistent vomiting is erosion of dental enamel, in particular from the inner surfaces of the front teeth. Eventually dentine is exposed and the teeth become oversensitive to temperature and caries develops. Complications such as abnormal tooth wear are not limited to the group that vomit, however. Other causes of poor dental health are overconsumption of acidic foods such as fruit and carbonated drinks, or grinding and loosening of the teeth due to osteoporosis of the jaw.

Salivary glands

A non-inflammatory swelling of the salivary glands is frequently found in the parotids of people with bulimia nervosa. In a sample of patients with bulimia it was shown that the parotid gland was 36% larger than that in a sample of matched controls. In the group with bulimia the salivary gland size was significantly correlated with frequency of bulimic symptoms and with serum amylase concentrate. The exact factors underlying salivary gland enlargement in bulimia remains unknown, but it is thought that the increased level of amylase is probably produced by the salivary gland.

Kidneys

The misuse of laxatives and vomiting may affect renal function through hypokalemia and volume depletion. The breakdown of renal function may arise from a reduced glomerular filtration rate (GFR) or renal (kidney) tubular damage (RTD). The term 'renal insufficiency' is used to refer to the mild effect of this condition, while severe dysfunction is termed 'renal failure.'

Gut trauma

Gastric dilatation, if found to be chronic, may cause the stomach to lose contractibility, resulting in venous occlusion and possible gastric perforation. In the initial stages of treatment for this condition reversible changes may be possible, but as the disorder progresses irreversible damage to the gastric wall may occur. This is particularly so if large amounts are consumed after a long period of famine.

6.12 Comorbidity with physical problems

A major management difficulty occurs when eating disorders develop in the context of somatic illness. This is a particular problem with diabetes mellitus. Approximately a third of adolescent girls with diabetes have some form of eating disorder; mainly bulimia nervosa or binge eating disorder. It is common for these patients to omit their insulin as a means of losing weight. The combination of diabetes and an eating disorder may lead to the development of early and severe neurovascular complications, retinopathy (three times as prevalent in patients with highly disordered eating), osteoporosis, and a higher mortality (five times that of anorexia alone and 15 times that of diabetes). Eating disorders also lead to difficulties in the management of Crohn's disease and thyroid disease.

Section III: Binge eating disorder

6.13 History

In 1959 Albert J. Stunkard identified binge eating disorder (BED) as a distinct eating pattern in some people suffering from obesity. This phenomenon received little systematic attention until syndromes around bulimia nervosa were more clearly delineated. Binge eating disorder was added in the appendix in DSM-IV (American Psychiatric Association, 1994). Despite the fact that BED was more common than binge–purge bulimia it was still considered to be a category 'deserving further study' rather than a full syndrome.

The validity of BED as a diagnostic entity has been supported by its strong association with overconcern with weight and shape, impairment in work and social situations, and general psychological comorbidity.

6.14 Etiology

The restraint model of BED has less face validity than it does for bulimia as these people are usually above their set point for weight and are obese. In addition to this it is found that 50% of them begin to binge eat before there is any dieting behavior.

A number of risk factors may contribute to the development of BED. These included specific adverse childhood experiences, parental depression, vulnerability to obesity, and also repeated exposure to negative comments about weight and shape.

A person with BED is more likely than an obese person without BED to start dieting at a younger age, to become overweight at a younger age, and to invest more time in unproductive attempts at weight loss.

6.15 Clinical features of BED

BED is differentiated from non-purging bulimia nervosa through the absence of fasting, intense physical exercise or other purging, compensatory behaviors. Table 6.4 lists the diagnostic criteria for BED.

Epidemiology

Preliminary research suggests that BED has a broader demographic distribution than anorexia or bulimia. During the 1980s, several reports were published detailing moderate or severe binge eating in 20–50% of the British population, which was noted to be similar to that found in the United States.

Table 6.4 Diagnostic criteria for binge eating disorder

DSM-IV
Recurrent binge eating. A feeling of lack of control during binges. Binges associated with at least three of the following features
    Eating very fast
    Eating until feeling uncomfortably full
    Eating large amounts when not feeling physically hungry
    Eating alone because of embarrassment about overeating
    Feeling disgusted, depressed, or guilty about the binges
    Feeling very distressed about the binge eating

Reproduced with permission from American Psychiatric Association (1994).

The prevalence of binge eating behavior in a general female Austrian population was also studied and it was found that 12.2% of the sample ($N = 1000$) fulfilled the diagnostic criteria for binge eating, 8.4% for binge eating syndrome, and 3.3% for BED.

Clinical features

Usually the onset of BED occurs in the mid-twenties or earlier in the teenage years. In community samples the sex ratio appears to be similar. In people attending weight loss classes the female-to-male ratio is 3:2. Research shows that between 2% and 5% have had anorexia, whereas between 5% and 10% have suffered from bulimia. A lifetime history of comorbidity is common, and 50–70% of patients report having suffered from major depression, between 25% and 30% personality disorders, and 70% anxiety disorders.

Complications of BED

Obesity may involve a number of serious medical complications, including high blood pressure, cardiovascular disease, high cholesterol, type 2 diabetes, lower back pain, and arthritis.

For a more comprehensive listing of the medical complications of overnutrition, see Chapter 3.

High blood pressure

High blood pressure is the most common of all cardiovascular diseases in the industrialized world. Consistent high blood pressure forces the heart to work beyond its capacity. If untreated, it can lead to swelling of the optic nerve or hemorrhaging of the retina, heart attack, stroke, and negative effects on the kidneys. If identified, hypertension can be treated effectively and easily.

Cholesterol problems

High levels of low-density lipoprotein (LDL) in the body can cause numerous health problems. LDL cholesterol infiltrates arterial walls, initiating the inflammatory disease known as arteriosclerosis, and possibly in turn heart disease or a stroke. High levels of cholesterol may not have any obvious symptoms but may be risk factors for other conditions such as angina, arteriosclerosis, and other circulatory ailments.

Diabetes mellitus

Diabetes results from the body's inability to process the hormone insulin effectively. Approximately 90% of people with diabetes have the type 2 subtype and a substantial proportion of these people will have BED. Long-term complications of diabetes can damage the eyes, nervous system, kidneys, the cardiovascular and circulatory systems, in addition to hindering the body's overall resistance to infections.

Heart disease

BED increases the risk of coronary heart disease, characterized by blockages in the coronary arteries that lead to a lower level of oxygen-rich blood flow to the heart. This is frequently a result of arteriosclerosis. Diabetes, high blood pressure, being overweight, abnormal fat metabolism, and high levels of cholesterol may all contribute to the development of heart disease.

Treatment of BED

Most treatment for BED has been adapted from therapy for bulimia; it is usually presented in the form of cognitive behavioral therapy or interpersonal psychotherapy (a treatment that focuses largely on the client–therapist relationship). As yet there are no evidence-based guidelines for selecting between them. In reality, choice of treatment is often dictated by local resources and available expertise. The treatment is principally concerned with eliminating binge eating and the associated eating disorder pathology. Self-help forms of cognitive behavioral therapy have proved to be effective in reducing binge eating. One of the greatest difficulties with the treatment of BED is that nothing appears to produce significant weight loss in BED patients.

Antidepressant medication (including selective serotonin reuptake inhibitors) have shown mixed results at best. Results show a rapid relapse in responders following the discontinuation of the drug.

In the short term, traditional behavioral weight loss treatments aimed primarily at weight loss via dietary restraint have also proved effective in reducing binge eating as well as producing weight loss.

6.16 Night eating syndrome

Night eating syndrome was first recorded more than four decades ago. It has never been established whether it is a diagnosed expression of eating disorder or if it is a dimension of behavior. There is much overlap between BED and night eating syndrome. Interestingly, the main difference between the two is that people with night eating syndrome tend to be free of preoccupation with food and dieting.

6.17 Prognosis of eating disorders

A third of patients have a poor prognosis even after 20 years. Treatment in specialized centers probably improves the outcome, as the mortality rate in areas without a specialized service is higher. Even patients with a good outcome often have residual problems such as abnormal attitudes to food and eating. Abnormally low serum albumin levels and a low weight (≤60% average body weight) predict a lethal course. Although depression and other abnormal cognitions exist alongside eating disorders, their presence has not been found to adversely affect prognosis.

Prevention

Various efforts have been made to develop prevention programs for eating disturbances and eating disorders. Usually they have been designed for children at secondary school and college. Although prevention programs are able to increase knowledge about healthy eating, nutrition, body composition, and dieting, changes in eating disorder attitudes and behavior are less marked.

Education has been given in the form of a seminar or a self-help manual. Encouraging self-help is helpful, in particular in the early stages of the illness. Autobiographical books of young people who have recovered and videotapes about the illness and its consequences and treatment modalities can aid this approach.

Future programs may need to be more developmentally appropriate and focused on more general risk factors. They may need to include components to help young people cope with physical, social, and emotional changes during puberty; being teased by peers about shape and appearance; dating, sexuality, and the sudden changes in mood characteristic of this stage of development.

6.18 Perspectives on the future

Eating disorders are psychological illnesses in which distress is manifested in the form of disordered eating patterns. This has damaging effects on nutrition, physical health, mood, and cognition, which serve to reinforce the destructive spiral. A number of epidemiological studies report that mild eating disturbances at a subclinical level exist widely in adolescents in the age range of 11–18 years. Eating disorders rank high amongst the common chronic conditions of childhood.

Much more research is required to develop a better understanding of eating disorders in general. A better knowledge of the biological–environmental interaction is likely to be central to an improved understanding of the etiology and treatment of eating disorders. One of the keys to future research is thought to lie in the collaboration of interdisciplinary teams that bring together specialists with different but effective approaches to the management of these disorders. Research is needed to investigate the biological, psychological, and environmental factors involved in eating disorders in general and work towards evaluating treatments and their outcomes.

References and further reading

Anorexia nervosa

American Psychiatric Association. *Diagnostic and Statistical Manual of Mental Disorders*, 4th edn (DSM-IV). Washington, DC: American Psychiatric Association, 1994.

American Psychiatric Association. Practice guideline for the treatment of patients with eating disorders (revision). American Psychiatric Association Work Group on Eating Disorders. *Am J Psychiatry* 2000; 157: 1–39.

British Medical Association. *Eating Disorders, Body Image and the Media*. London, BMA, 2000.

Bulik CM, Sullivan PF, Wade TD *et al.* (2000) Twin studies of eating disorders: a review. *Int J Eating Disord* 2000; 27: 1–20.

Connan F, Campbell IC, Katzman M, Lightman SL, Treasure J. A neurodevelopmental model for anorexia nervosa. *Physiol Behav* 2003; 79: 13–24.

Fairburn CG, Shafran R, Cooper Z. A cognitive behavioural theory of anorexia nervosa. *Behav Res Ther* 1999; 37: 1–13.

Hebebrand J, Remschidt H. Anorexia nervosa viewed as an extreme weight condition: genetic implications. *Hum Genet* 1995; 95: 1–11.

Jarman M, Walsh S. Evaluating recovery from anorexia nervosa and BN: integrating lessons learned from research and clinical practice. *Clin Psychol Rev* 1999; 19: 773–788.

Treasure J. *Anorexia Nervosa: A survival guide for families, friends and sufferers.* Hove, Sussex: Psychology Press, 1997.

World Health Organization. *International Statistical Classification of Diseases and Related Health Problems* (ICD-10). Geneva: World Health Organization, 1992.

Bulimia nervosa

Cooper M, Hunt J. Core beliefs and underlying assumptions in bulimia nervosa and depression. *Behav Res Ther* 1998; 36: 895–898.

Fairburn CG, Welch SL, Doll HA *et al.* Risk factors for bulimia nervosa: a community based, case-control study. *Arch Gen Psychiatry* 1997; 54: 509–517.

Royal College of Psychiatrists, Council Report, and CR87. *Eating Disorders in the UK: Policies for service devlopment and training.* London: Royal College of Psychiatrists, 2001.

Schmidt U, Treasure J. *Getting better Bit(e) by Bit(e).* Hove, Sussex: Psychology Press, 1993.

Steiner H, Lock J. Anorexia nervosa and bulimia nervosa in children and adolescents: a review of the past 10 years. *J Am Acad Adolescent Psychiatry* 1998; 37: 352–359.

Binge eating disorder

Abbott DW, DeZwann M, Mussell MP *et al.* Onset of binge eating and dieting in overweight women: implications for etiology, associated features and treatment. *J Psychosom Res* 1998; 44: 367–374.

Adami GF, Meneghelli A, Scopinaro N. Night eating and binge eating disorder in obese patients. *Int J Eat Disord* 1999; 25: 335–338.

Fairburn FG, Doll HA, Welch SL, Hay PJ, Davies BA, O'Connor ME. Risk factors for binge eating disorder. A community based, case-controlled study. *Arch Gen Psychiatry* 1998; 55: 425–432.

General reading

Palmer RL. *Management of Eating Disorders.* Chichester: Wiley, 2000.

Trotter K. Nutrition and eating disorders. *Nurs Times* 1997; 7(1): 1–6.

7
Adverse Reactions to Foods

Simon H Murch

Key messages

- An increase in dietary allergies has occurred within the childhood population in recent decades, with an estimated frequency of up to 5% of children demonstrating allergy to cow's milk protein.
- As dietary exposures in early life have broadened for the children of the developed world, previously rare adverse reactions have become increasingly common.
- It is important to differentiate between the different forms of adverse reactions to foods, in particular the difference

between food intolerance and food allergy.
- There are two major classes of food allergic reactions, immunoglobulin E (IgE)-mediated and non-IgE-mediated, and within these classes reactions may be divided clinically into those of quick onset, and those of slow onset.
- Within the last few years, light has been shed onto the role of enterocytes within the mucosal immune system.
- Infant handling at the time of initial colonization may have impact on allergic sensitization.

7.1 Introduction

In recent decades it has become clear that dietary allergies have become increasingly common in the more privileged countries of the world. This increase has been most apparent within the childhood population, with an estimated frequency of up to 5% of children demonstrating allergy to cow's milk protein. In addition to this remarkable increase in frequency, there has been a change in patterns of presentation. As dietary exposures in early life have broadened for the children of the developed world, previously rare adverse reactions to antigens such as peanut and sesame seeds have become increasingly common. There are intriguing geographical differences, such as recent reports of anaphylaxis to birds' nest soup in Singaporean infants. Early life exposures, possibly extending even to prenatal life, have changed substantially for the children of the developed world in the last two generations. It is clear that children born in disadvantaged conditions within the developing world have a much lower incidence of dietary allergies: early life exposures are thus probably the major determinant of allergic sensitiza-

tion worldwide, with genetic predisposition only really coming into the equation once a certain threshold of improved material conditions is passed.

Later in this chapter the evidence for recent demographic shifts in food allergic sensitization will be discussed in the context of advances in understanding of the basic mechanisms of oral tolerance – the phenomenon of specific unresponsiveness to dietary antigens. Because such tolerance is mediated by immunological mechanisms, there will be some overlap with concepts discussed in Chapter 16 on 'Nutrition and Immune and Inflammatory Systems' and elsewhere in this book.

First, it is important to differentiate between the different forms of adverse reactions to foods, in particular the difference between food intolerance and food allergy. Only the latter is mediated by an immune response to dietary antigens, whereas the former may be a consequence of a variety of non-immune mechanisms. There may, however, be an overlap in the symptoms displayed, and an accurate history is thus a vital component of the assessment of a patient suspected of adverse food reactions.

7.2 Food intolerance

This is, by definition, a reproducible adverse reaction to ingested food that is not mediated by immune hypersensitivity. Food intolerance may be in response to the whole food, for example an aversion to its appearance, taste, or smell. It may be a consequence of inability to handle normally specific components of individual foods: the most common worldwide is lactose intolerance due to decreased expression of the enzyme lactase within the intestinal brush border, as lactase expression is genetically programmed to reduce substantially in adulthood in many population groups, particularly those with ancestral origin in southern Europe and Africa. If lactose-containing dairy products are taken above a threshold amount by someone with low lactase levels, the excess lactose cannot be broken down in the small intestine, and is then fermented by the bacteria within the colon to produce gas, water, and acid breakdown products. This usually causes uncomfortable abdominal distension and diarrhea.

Potentially more serious, and thankfully much rarer examples, occur in infants with inborn errors of metabolism, where lack of individual metabolic enzymes leads to damaging build-up of toxic metabolites of initially dietary origin. A good example of this is phenylketonuria, in which brain damage occurs if dietary phenylalanine is not excluded.

A third mechanism of food intolerance may occur when foodstuffs contain components with definite pharmacological effects, such as tyramine in cheeses and red wines: while most people are able to tolerate these, use of certain medications such as monoamine oxidase inhibitors may interfere with innate detoxication mechanisms and lead to potentially dangerous toxicity if these foods are consumed. Some people are sensitive to the histamines naturally occurring in strawberries, and rapidly develop rash or wheezing after eating them – although the symptoms appear similar to immediate allergic reaction, they are mediated by non-immunological mechanisms and are thus due to food intolerance and not allergy.

Direct effects of foods are common, particularly those due to bacterial contamination. In most cases this is sporadic, and clustering only occurs if large numbers of people eat the same contaminated food (e.g. wedding guests, airline passengers). However, the advent of modern food-handling practices increases the potential for very widespread transmission of such infections. This has occurred with recent outbreaks of life-threatening *Escherichia coli* 0157:H7 infections in Europe and North America. While considerable epidemiological detective work is necessary to trace the source of such epidemic food poisoning, there is usually little doubt of the involvement of food ingestion. This may not be so obvious if the foodstuff is contaminated by non-bacterial toxins or chemicals. In recent decades there have been epidemics of irreversible neural damage due to contamination of cooking oils in Spain and mercury poisoning in Japanese fishermen, and in neither case was it initially obvious that food contamination was to blame.

Detection of inborn errors of metabolism in early life is particularly important, as appropriate removal of dietary components in infancy can completely prevent serious brain damage. Recognition of the importance of early diagnosis led to the introduction of routine heel prick testing of all newborn infants for phenylketonuria. Other rare disorders are not routinely tested for, and it is important to consider these diagnoses in any infants with early abnormal symptoms, including vomiting, poor feeding, hepatosplenomegaly, prolonged jaundice, failure to thrive, hypoglycemia, floppiness, or impaired consciousness. The onset of such symptoms after weaning of a breastfed infant to sucrose-containing foods may occur in hereditary fructose intolerance. Rapid diagnosis is the key, and delays usually occur because a metabolic cause is not included in the differential diagnosis of an unwell infant.

7.3 Food allergy

Allergies occur as a consequence of a breakdown in immunological tolerance. The immune system has continually to differentiate between myriad foreign molecules, recognizing and responding to those which pose a threat to the organism – such as pathogens or their toxins – and remaining largely unresponsive (tolerant) to those necessary for survival and health – such as foods and the commensal bacterial flora in the intestine. There is recent evidence to suggest that the role of the bacterial flora in establishing immune tolerance is considerable: this will be discussed in more detail later in the chapter.

Allergies are a varied group of conditions induced by inappropriate immune reactivity to foreign antigens: these are called allergens if they reproducibly cause symptoms on exposure. Food allergic responses by definition require an abnormal immunologically mediated reaction to ingested dietary antigens. However, there may well be overlap in the clinical manifestations of allergies and non-allergic food intolerance, and there is much potential for confusion if true allergy is mistaken for intolerance or vice versa. The nature of an allergic response is that initial sensitization is required, and that the first exposure will not lead to obvious response, but hypersensitivity reactions occur on later challenge. Recent changes in the presentation of infant allergies suggest that such initial sensitization may occur without such an obvious history, and many exclusively breastfed infants have sensitized to minute amounts of dietary antigen passing into their mother's breastmilk.

7.4 Types of food allergy

There are two major classes of food allergic reactions, immunoglobulin E (IgE)-mediated and non IgE-mediated: the former are generally obvious, present soon after ingestion, and are thus relatively easy to investigate and diagnose (Box 7.1). They can be more violent than non-IgE-mediated reactions, and can even cause death through anaphylaxis in severe cases. The latter tend to present rather later and can be more subtle, but may be an important (and often unrecognised) cause of ill-health (Box 7.2). The immunological basis of such reactions is discussed in more depth later in this chapter.

Food allergic reactions may be divided clinically into those of quick onset (within minutes to an hour of food ingestion), and those of slow onset (taking hours or days). In general, quick-onset symptoms tend to be IgE-mediated and slow-onset symptoms non-IgE-mediated. However, this is by no means invariable, and many children with clear quick-onset responses to foods have a low or even undetectable serum total IgE and absent food-specific IgE. It is also notable that genetically engineered 'knockout' mice, totally deficient in IgE, may still suffer anaphylaxis. In such cases it is now thought likely that IgG1 bound to IgG receptors on mast cells may substitute for IgE to induce antigen-specific mast cell degranulation. This may explain discordance between negative radioallergosorbent testing (RAST) and positive skin-prick testing, as the latter is induced by degranulation of cutaneous mast cells and may thus potentially proceed independently of IgE.

Box 7.1 The classical forms of hypersensitivity – after Gell and Coombs (1968)

Type I: Anaphylactic or immediate hypersensitivity
This occurs within minutes of exposure, and is characteristic of quick-onset food allergy. The reaction occurs when an allergen reacts with IgE (or in certain circumstances IgG1) on the surface of activated mast cells. This leads to mast cell degranulation and release of vasoactive agents such as histamine, proteases, and cytokines such as TNFα. Peanut hypersensitivity is a classic type I response.

Type II: Cytotoxic hypersensitivity
This reaction occurs when antibody binds to a cell or tissue component and fixes complement, which leads to complement-mediated cell death. It is thus not usually thought to play a role in food allergic responses, although complement activation itself is seen in some forms of food-induced enteropathy such as celiac disease.

Type III: Immune complex hypersensitivity
In this type of reaction, also known as the Arthus reaction, antigen and antibody (IgG or IgM) form complexes in the presence of antigen excess to induce complement fixation and consequent local inflammatory response, several hours after exposure to antigen. Recent evidence suggests that the Fc receptors for immunoglobulin, rather than complement itself, are important for such tissue damage.

Type IV: Delayed hypersensitivity or cell-mediated immunity
This reaction is mediated by T lymphocytes and macrophages. Much evidence has accrued since the publication by Gell and Coombs to suggest that T cell responses (e.g. T_H1 or T_H2 secretion patterns) may determine overall immunopathology. The classic type IV reaction is a T_H1 response, as in celiac disease, and less is known about T_H2 immunopathology in food allergy.

In a study of 120 London children with multiple food allergies (Latcham *et al.*, 2003), we found overall a significant increase of serum IgE in those children with early-onset symptoms over those with late-onset, but about 30% of the early-onset group showed no elevation of IgE and >10% of the late onset group did have elevated IgE. What we found notable in this study was that the great majority (>90%) of those with early-onset symptoms additionally demonstrated late-onset symptoms and shared with the late-onset group a pattern of immune deviation (elevated IgG1 and B cells, reduced IgG2, IgG4, CD8 and natural killer cells, with low or low-to-normal IgA). This concords with data from an Iceland population survey, in which lower quartile IgA was more predictive of allergy than was IgE, from a Finnish study, where increased B cell and decreased CD8 cell numbers were found in infants with food allergy, and from a study in the UK, where low IgA, IgG2, and IgG4 were frequent findings in infants with

Box 7.2 Forms of food intolerance (non-allergic)

- *Direct toxic effects* – contamination with bacteria, presence of heavy metals or toxins, such as contaminated water, cooking oil, mercury poisoning, or fish neurotoxins, or direct effects of food additives. This may include bacteriological or toxopharmacological responses.
- *Intolerance as a consequence of enzyme deficiency* – may be *inborn*, as in a variety of metabolic enzyme deficiencies (e.g. phenylketonuria, tyrosinemia, galactosemia, urea cycle defects, primary lactase deficiency, glucose–galactose malabsorption, or sucrase–isomaltase deficiency), *developmentally regulated* (adult-type lactase deficiency), or *acquired* as a consequence of small intestinal enteropathy (e.g. downregulated expression of lactase and other hydrolases, the sodium–glucose cotransporter, or fatty acid binding protein). In this last case, the initiating lesion is likely to be immunologically mediated – enteropathy is usually a consequence of activation of T cells within the mucosa – sometimes as a consequence of an adverse response to dietary antigen (e.g. celiac disease, CMSE), sometimes unrelated to foods (e.g. Crohn's disease, giardiasis, tropical enteropathy). Note that the clinical expression may be identical – the presence of lactose intolerance may be as a result of any of these three processes.
- *Symptoms due to pharmacological properties of foods* – tyramine contained in cheese or red wine, histamine in strawberries.

food-sensitive colitis. These data suggest that there may be a consistent pattern of minor immunodeficiency associated with the process of sensitization in early life, and that the manifestation of that sensitization (quick or slow-onset) may depend on whether the child has inherited a tendency to high IgE production. In other words, high IgE does not cause food allergy *per se*, but may determine how that allergy is expressed.

Most of the early literature on food allergy focuses on IgE and quick-onset responses, which is understandable as it is so much more obvious to detect.

7.5 Patterns of food allergic responses

Quick-onset symptoms

These often follow the ingestion of a single food, such as egg, peanut, or sesame. Within minutes the sufferer may notice tingling of the tongue, and there may be the rapid development of skin rash, urticaria, or wheezing. Angioneurotic edema, with swelling of the mucous membranes, can develop extremely fast, and the airway may become compromised. In cases where appropriate therapy is not available, life-saving tracheostomy has even been performed in cases of gross laryngeal

edema. Anaphylactic shock may also occur, with dramatic systemic hypotension accompanying the airway obstruction.

Specific therapy for mild cases of immediate hypersensitivity would include antihistamines such as chlorpheniramine, together with inhaled bronchodilators as appropriate. It is notable that some patients can make a biphasic response, with a relatively modest initial reaction followed several hours later by a more profound and potentially life-threatening response, and thus care should be taken in the assessment to ensure that adequate instructions and therapy are administered before allowing the patient home. The presence of wheezing on examination should suggest caution, and a bronchodilator should certainly be prescribed, and in many cases a few days' course of oral prednisolone.

More severe reactions should be assessed very rapidly, and any evidence of airway obstruction or systemic hypotension warrants the immediate use of intramuscular adrenaline. Use of a preloaded syringe pen, such as a pediatric or adult EpiPen, is generally acceptable and avoids potential dosage errors at such a time of extreme stress. Clearly this necessitates urgent transfer to an appropriate medical setting such as an Accident and Emergency department. There, it is likely that other measures, including oxygen, intravenous hydrocortisone, and intravenous or intramuscular chlorpheniramine should be administered, and the requirement for inhaled beta-adrenergic bronchodilator therapy assessed. Supportive treatment for hypotension or cardiac dysrhythmia may be required, and in the most severe cases the patient may need to be transferred to an intensive therapy unit.

In the follow-up of a patient who has had an immediate hypersensitive response to food antigens, a decision needs to be taken about the level of prophylaxis required, and whether or not to prescribe an adrenaline pen. Clearly the severity of the first response will inform this decision, and it is probably better to err on the side of caution if foods such as peanuts are implicated, because of their propensity for triggering particularly severe episodes. If there is doubt about the food involved, both skin-prick tests and specific IgE tests (RAST tests) may be very helpful: these should be postponed for several weeks after an episode of anaphylaxis as they may be artefactually negative in the immediate aftermath of a severe reaction.

Late-onset symptoms

Symptoms may appear slowly and insidiously and their true allergic nature may not be recognized (Table 7.1). These may include failure to thrive or chronic diarrhea due to enteropathy or colitis, eczema, rhinitis, or rectal bleeding. As these are likely to be mediated by T cells in a delayed hypersensitive reaction, they may not be so clearly linked to food ingestion. More recently the concept of food allergic intestinal dysmotility has been suggested in pediatric patients, with dietary antigen (most commonly cow's milk, soya, or wheat) inducing gastroesophageal reflux (Plate 1 and Figure 7.1) or constipation (Figure 7.2).

On gastrointestinal investigation of children with delayed responses, antigen-induced dysmotility or mucosal pathology such as small intestinal enteropathy or colitis may often be found. However, both skin-prick tests and RASTs may be negative, but it can be shown that food elimination relieves all the symptoms and that challenge with the food causes return of symptoms – if a child with severe eczema, failure to thrive, or intractible reflux has been transformed by an exclusion diet, it may only be the therapeutic pedant who will undertake an early challenge. Much more common is the problem of a patient with a genuine food-induced reaction who is refused appropriate treatment because the 'investigations are negative' (i.e. RASTs or skin-prick tests), and thus it 'can't be allergy.'

Both types of reaction may occur individually or together: as mentioned above, a careful history will usually uncover delayed responses in even the most apparently monosensitized immediate responder. The slow response is likely to be T cell-mediated, and the frequency of patients with low circulating immunoglobulins in the food allergic population means that patients may have clinically important dietary responses without detectable antibodies. *Failure to detect specific antibodies does not rule out food allergy.*

7.6 Diagnostic criteria for food allergy

Whatever the results of tests, an essential criterion for secure diagnosis of food allergy is a response to an elimination diet. Ideally there should be relief of all symptoms, gain in weight, and normal growth. A positive response to challenge is strongly supportive but not always essential in routine practice, particularly when other diagnostic tests were positive at diagnosis.

In childhood allergy there is often reacquisition of tolerance with age, and a challenge may then reasonably be performed when the child is older (usually greater than two years, but often rather later, especially in multiply allergic children). ESPGHAN (the European Society for Paediatric Gastroenterology, Hepatology and Nutrition) has made recommendations for diagnostic criteria (ESPGHAN, 1992).

In children with multiple food allergies the response to elimination of a single antigen may be incomplete, and lengthy inpatient assessment with a very restricted diet is often required. Such situations may become very enmeshed, and it may be difficult to persuade some parents to broaden their child's diet. Particularly if the child is manifesting non-IgE-mediated allergy it may be extraordinarily difficult for anyone concerned (including the allergist) to avoid wood–trees agnosia.

Table 7.1 Clinical manifestations in food allergic responses

1. Quick onset	Wheezing
	Urticaria
	Angioedema
	Rashes
	Vomiting
	Gastroesophageal reflux
	Anaphylaxis
2. Late onset	Diarrhea
	Abdominal pain
	Allergic rhinitis
	Atopic eczema
	Food-sensitive enteropathy or colitis
	Rectal bleeding
	Constipation
	Protein-losing enteropathy
3. Arguable responses	Irritable bowel syndrome
	Chronic fatigue
	Attention deficit with hyperactivity (ADHD)
	Autistic symptoms
4. Secondary general effects	Eosinophilia
	Iron-deficiency anemia

Notes:
A. Those who make a clear quick-onset response may go on to show secondary worsening after a period of some hours, and it is important to institute appropriate medical therapy and/or supervision.
B. The conditions in group 3 are ones in which there are a number of reports of favorable clinical responses to exclusion of dietary antigens, sometimes impressive. However these have yet to be established in the lists of true food allergies, and probably only a proportion of such patients will benefit. An open-minded approach, and joint management with a skilled dietitian, would nevertheless appear reasonable at present. As with every dietary exclusion, the clinical response should be sufficiently good to make it worthwhile continuing with the exclusion, and food challenges performed to confirm a genuine effect.

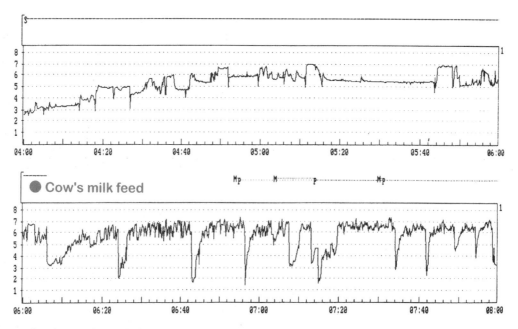

Figure 7.1 Evidence from a 24-h pH study of the triggering of gastroesophageal reflux by cow's milk, in a three-year-old child. Episodes of reflux are seen when the pH dips below 4. During the course of 24 h, the reflux episodes only occurred after milk, and not after taking equal volumes of an amino acid formula.

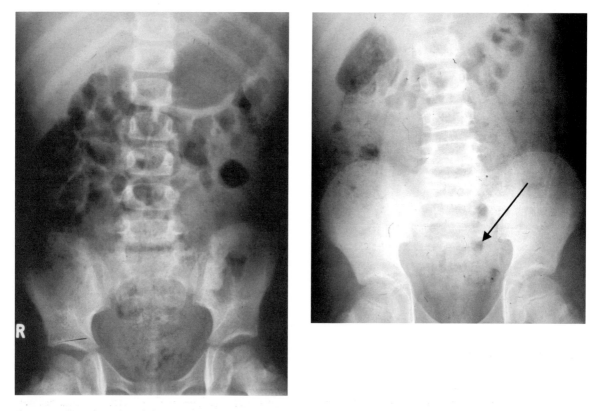

Figure 7.2 Allergic dysmotility with chronic constipation. Abdominal X-ray is often helpful, as the constipation may not be clinically obvious if the characteristic impaction within the rectum (acquired megarectum – arrowed) is the only feature. These cases were chronically unresponsive to conventional therapy, but remitted after cow's milk and wheat were excluded from the diet for a period of several months.

As these children typically worsen in all regards when suffering intercurrent viral infections, and have a propensity for prolonged viral infections related to minor immunodeficiency, it is imprudent to make any definitive statements about the extent of allergies, or even perform food challenges, while the child is unwell.

In cases where there is looming conflict between parent and pediatrician about the current state of allergies, multiple blinded food challenges may be needed. Once again, close teamwork with an experienced dietitian is absolutely required. The 'gold-standard' double-blind placebo-controlled food challenge (DB-PCFC) is a cumbersome and time-consuming intervention that nevertheless may have a very useful and important role in sorting out such cases. If there is real uncertainty about a single food, and the child makes immediate responses, it may be possible to repeat the challenge and withdrawal and truly establish tolerance or persistent reactivity in a way that no other test can. Its value decreases markedly when there are large numbers of foods to be tested, and the child makes delayed responses only. Normal day-to-day variation may then be overinterpreted, the family often become distressed by prolonged incarceration in hospital or the child catches a viral infection from another admitted during a general take, with predictable return of ill-health that is then taken by the zealot (parent or pediatrician) as evidence of allergy, and sometimes very little true advance may be made despite a prolonged admission.

In adult practice, similar principles may apply and indeed similar problems may occur. Food allergy may be invoked as a cause of an almost unlimited spectrum of symptoms, and such beliefs will be given apparent credence by any number of internet websites. Conversely, there are many people with genuine delayed hypersensitive reactions – food allergic dysmotility is a good example – in whom the opportunity for clinical improvement is missed because of a lack of immediate hypersensitive responses and negative skin-prick tests and specific IgE on RAST testing. The time-consuming nature of extensive DBPCFC testing is difficult to reconcile with most full-time occupations.

7.7 Food-sensitive enteropathy

In food-sensitive enteropathy, there is an immunologically mediated abnormality of the small intestinal mucosa, which may include excess lymphocyte infiltration,

epithelial abnormality, or architectural disturbance with crypt lengthening or villous shortening. This may often impair absorption and less commonly causes a frank malabsorption syndrome. This continues while the food remains in the diet and remits on an exclusion diet. In cases of diagnostic uncertainty, it may be necessary to confirm the return of mucosal abnormality by food challenge. This was more common practise in the days (not too many years ago) when the very existence of food-sensitive enteropathies other than celiac disease was questioned by many practitioners.

The most common cause of such enteropathy in childhood is cow's milk, and the evidence of cow's milk sensitive enteropathy (CMSE) was obtained by such serial biopsies. However, improvements in infant formulas have led to a change in the mucosal appearances of CMSE, so that celiac-like villous atrophy is now very rare in the developed world. This places histopathologists in some diagnostic difficulty, and there is no international consensus in the reporting of subtle lesions such as villous blunting or mild increase in mucosal eosinophils (Plate 2).

7.8 Specific food allergies

Allergic responses to many food proteins have been described. The most common in childhood are cow's milk, soya, eggs, and fish, with peanut allergy rapidly becoming more frequent. However, intolerance to fruits, vegetable, meats, chocolate, nuts, shellfish, and cereals have been described. In adult life there is a different spectrum, with allergy to nuts, fruits, and fish relatively more common than in childhood. However, as the dietary exposures of children broaden in the developed world, the range of reported allergens also increases: thus sesame, kiwi fruit, mango, avocado, and other allergies have increased in frequency in the UK. As mentioned in the introduction, such sensitization appears to depend more on genetics, infectious challenges, and patterns of exposure than innate antigenicity of individual foodstuffs, with the possible exception of some highly allergenic foods such as peanuts.

There is no consistent association between any particular food and specific syndromes, although some foods are more likely to induce enteropathy, particularly cow's milk and soya. This may simply be a reflection of the dose ingested. The incidence of gastrointestinal food allergy is greatest in early life and appears to decrease with age. However, analogy with celiac disease, in which late-onset enteropathy is more likely to be clinically subtle, suggests that the increase in colonic salvage that occurs with age may mask true food-sensitive enteropathy. In early life the enteropathy associated with dietary allergy may sometimes be relatively subtle (Plate 3), but may cause profound failure to thrive (Plate 4). However, complex dietary allergy may occur with quite normal growth (Figure 7.3). There are some recent reports suggesting that CMSE may indeed occur in adult life, but the whole area remains understudied.

Cow's milk

Cow's milk hypersensitivity may manifest as described above, either as an immediate response, sometimes even causing anaphylaxis, or with delayed responses within the gut or skin. These sensitizations classically follow an episode of gastroenteritis, so-called post-enteritis syndrome, and are often manifested as 'lactose intolerance.' The point that lactose intolerance in infants and young children is most commonly a secondary consequence of a food-sensitive enteropathy can-

not be emphasized too strongly, and use of a reduced-lactose milk or exogenous lactase simply masks this problem without addressing the basic lesion. Modern adapted feeding formulas are much less sensitizing than the older infant feeding formula (unfortunately still routinely used in much of the developing world), and the severity of CMSE lessened in recent years when such milks were introduced.

Positive cow's milk RASTs are seen in some children with enteropathy but are more typical of quick reactors. Similarly, positive skin-prick tests may be found in CMSE but correlate best with quick-onset syndromes. Elevated titers of IgG and IgM milk antibodies have been described in cow's milk protein intolerance but with a poor clinical correlation. Unlike celiac disease, CMSE is often of variable severity and shows patchy distribution on small bowel biopsy (Plate 3).

CMSE may also induce protein losing enteropathy or iron deficiency anemia. Cow's milk colitis may also occur and induce occult or overt gastrointestinal bleeding. Usually CMSE and cow's milk-induced colitis do not coexist in the same patient. Cow's milk allergy is now recognized to induce esophageal reflux in many

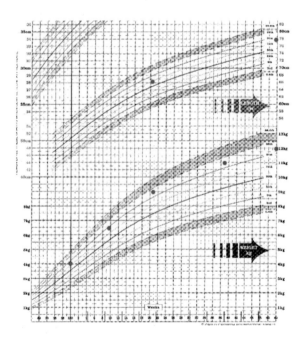
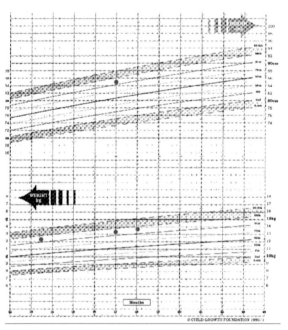

Figure 7.3 Dietary allergy does not always cause failure to thrive. This child, who had both IgE-mediated and non-IgE-mediated allergies to multiple dietary antigens, nevertheless showed good growth despite chronic eczema, colic, gastroesophageal reflux, and constipation. In well-grown children without an IgE-mediated component, who have negative skin-prick tests and RASTs, the diagnosis of allergy is often missed and the mothers labeled 'neurotic' or 'demanding.'

infants, which in severe cases can also induce hematemesis or anemia.

Soya allergy

Soy-based formulas have for some years been used in infants with cow's milk allergy, although not usually by pediatric gastroenterologists or allergists. They appear to be at least as antigenic as cow's milk-based formulas, and there are numerous reports of intolerance to soy protein. Such reactions have varied from anaphylaxis to chronic enteropathy, as well as eczema, asthma, and colitis. Thus the spectrum of abnormalities is largely similar to cow's milk allergy. The high incidence of soy intolerance in infants treated for CMSE makes soya formulas an unsatisfactory first-line treatment for cow's milk allergy, and most specialist units now use hydrolysate formulas.

Egg

In contrast to cow's milk, egg allergy usually presents as an acute response, and there is no real evidence of egg enteropathy. Vomiting within a few minutes to an hour after ingestion is characteristic, but diarrhea, abdominal pain, and nausea may also occur. Delayed responses are most likely to occur in the lungs (asthma) and skin (eczema). RAST and skin-prick responses to egg are more likely to be positive than for many other allergens.

Wheat

While acute allergic reactions to wheat are much more rare, acute wheat anaphylaxis has been described. Delayed hypersensitive reactions are both common and clinically important. Of particular importance is the role of wheat gluten in causing celiac disease (Plate 2), which is not only common (now recognized to occur in >1% of European populations) but very variable in manifestation – from the classic child with profound failure to thrive and malabsorption, to a thriving child with unexplained neurological problems, as described. While in-depth discussion of celiac disease is beyond the scope of this review, it is important to recognize that its incidence is increased in children with other dietary allergies, partly because IgA deficiency is a shared risk factor, and it is advisable that serological testing for celiac disease (currently based on IgG and IgA gliadin

antibodies, and IgA endomyseal and/or ti glutaminase antibodies) should be perfor food allergic patients if blood is being taken tests.

Subtle forms of wheat intolerance

Less well understood is the role of wheat in precipitating intestinal dysmotility, which can manifest as gastroesophageal reflux and particularly constipation. Allergic dysmotility represents part of the spectrum of non-IgE-mediated food allergy, and is receiving increasing recognition. There is now increasing evidence that both gastroesophageal reflux and constipation may be features of the food allergic dysmotility syndrome (Plates 1 and 2; Figures 7.1 and 7.2), which may present as infant colic and then continue well beyond infancy to cause chronic symptoms that may require prolonged dietary exclusions. There are so far few studies of food allergic dysmotility in adults, but this area may become directly relevant to irritable bowel syndrome in atopic patients.

The histological characteristic of food allergic dysmotility is local eosinophilic infiltration (Plate 3). In addition, both wheat and cow's milk may sometimes be implicated in childhood behavioral disturbances, and early reports of improved cognitive responses in children with attention deficit disorder with hyperactivity and autism have been published. The effects of wheat exclusion in such children may sometimes be impressive, but it is mandatory to screen for celiac disease before commencing such a diet. The presence of bioactive morphine analogs in cow's milk and wheat (beta-casomorphine and gliadomorphine) has been suggested as the cause of this striking cognitive effect, and indeed administration of beta-casomorphine to rodents induces marked behavioral change and expression of neural activation genes. Such a response would technically thus be an intolerance rather than true allergy.

Peanuts

Peanut allergy is concerning, because of its rising incidence and its propensity to induce severe anaphylaxis. Even trace amounts of peanut can cause death in those severely sensitized. The reasons for the surge in peanut hypersensitive cases may relate to different patterns of exposure, with sensitization via low-dose exposure in breast-milk or even by the percutaneous route in children with eczema, if skin creams containing peanut-derived oils are used.

In the UK it is now recommended that children, particularly from an atopic background, should not be given peanut products until after the age of six. However, as most children now appear to be sensitized very early in life by non-classical routes, this may not be as effective as hoped. One encouraging point is that around a half of early-sensitized infants may reacquire tolerance to peanuts with age. The skin-prick test is extremely useful in peanut allergy, particularly the size of response: children with a >7 mm wheal have a >95% chance of remaining sensitized, and thus rechallenge is inadvisable. By contrast, those with a <4 mm response have a similar chance of being tolerant. However, peanut challenge should always be undertaken with extreme caution, by experienced personnel with full resuscitation equipment and appropriate drugs to hand.

7.9 Multiple food allergy

Increasing numbers of infants and children develop gastrointestinal and other symptoms related to a wide variety of foods. These may be immediate or delayed, and do not differ significantly from those described above for individual foods. They often have an individual and family history of atopy, and may have increased eosiniphils in peripheral blood with elevated serum IgE and positive RAST and skin-prick tests to specific foods. In this circumstance there is overlap with eosinophilic gastroenteritis, where eosinophils are found within gastric and intestinal biopsies but where a clear history of dietary triggering may not be obtained. Many such cases sensitize by the evolutionarily novel route of maternal breast milk, with the trace amounts of dietary proteins apparently sufficient to sensitize or insufficient to tolerize: a specific defect in oral tolerance for low-dose antigen has been postulated as a cause of this phenomenon, which even now is seen only in privileged children from the developed world.

Diets involving the elimination of single foods are usually ineffective. It was first shown that infants can be sensitized to cow's milk via trace amounts in maternal breast milk when the mother drank cow's milk, and more recently it has become clear that sensitiza-

tion to many other antigens can occur in this way. One important clinical point is that many infants showed continued responses to trace amounts of cow's milk protein in conventional hydrolysate formulas, and may require an amino acid-based formula. Such propensity to sensitize during breastfeeding would clearly have been maladaptive in evolutionary terms, and it is becoming clear that it is the recent change in non-dietary exposures (infective) that may be preventing the normal induction of immune tolerance to low-dose antigens.

Recent evidence of defective production of transforming growth factor beta (TGFβ), the cytokine involved in low-dose oral tolerance, by multiply allergic infants may be relevant in this process. As this appears to represent a fundamental alteration in the pathogenesis and presentation of food allergies, which is presenting increasingly frequently internationally, it is important to explore some recent insights into the nature of dietary tolerance.

7.10 Scientific background: the basic mechanisms of immune response to dietary antigen

Innate immunity and the importance of evolutionary heritage

Much progress has been made in the last three decades in understanding the basic mechanisms of immune responses to dietary components. However, much of the literature is based on phenomenology, and generally biased towards IgE-mediated early responses. This does not provide a secure footing to examine or understand the dramatic recent changes in the incidence and presentation of dietary allergies. Given that early infectious exposures appear to play the most dominant role in determining whether allergic sensitization occurs, it is worthwhile considering the basic mechanisms that are now thought to govern intestinal immune responses.

There is one important difference in the overall setup of the mucosal immune system of the intestine, when compared with the systemic immune system, essentially due to evolutionary longevity. This relates to a relative dominance of primitive or paleoimmune mechanisms. Fossils of early Cambrian hemichordates, from over 600 million years ago, show a recognizable gastrointestinal tract. Thus long before the earliest development of adaptive immune systems, which can recognize antigen in a specific way and respond more vigorously on reacquaintance, the basic mechanisms of host defense through innate immunity were in place within the gut.

The explorations of comparative immunology in primitive organisms by Ilya Metchnikoff in the late nineteenth century established a clear cellular basis for host defense within the gut that has considerably more resonance today than it appeared to have for his peers at the time. Such mechanisms, based on phagocytosis or cytokine secretion by macrophages, which themselves express receptors that recognize cell wall components of potential pathogens, together with production of chemotactic factors and localization of complement, remain central in intestinal homeostasis.

Much current work focuses on the molecules and receptors, such as Toll protein receptors, that integrate initial innate immune responses with a subsequent specific lymphocyte reaction. It was clear from Metchnikoff's studies that the cells lining the gut of some primitive organisms showed functions comparable with both enterocytes and macrophages, and it is now recognized that the enterocytes themselves are very active participants in the immune response to foods.

Primitive lymphocyte populations: the first steps to adaptive immune responses to antigen

The pattern of evolutionary change in the intestine appears to be one of adding-on of new levels of control, rather than abandonment of the older established mechanisms. The intestine contains disproportionately large numbers of primitive lymphocytes, both T cells and B cells, which show some limited antigen-specific adaptive responses, but possess the ability to respond rapidly to infectious threat. The peritoneal B cell population, termed B1 cells, which can usually be recognized because they express a molecule (CD5) normally restricted to T cells, are quite distinct from circulating B cells (B2 cells), in that they produce antibody of broad affinity for bacterial products but generally of low specificity for individual antigens. Little is yet known about the role of this major class of intestinal B cells, although a role in some autoimmune responses appears likely from murine studies. Amongst the T cell population, lymphocytes expressing a T cell receptor

composed of a γ and a δ chain (γδ cells), rather than the α and β chain of circulating and most intestinal T cells, are also highly overrepresented within the intestine. An important role for γδ cells in some food-reactive processes is suggested both by findings of low mucosal IgA in γδ-deficient mice and by increased numbers of intraepithelial γδ cells in celiac disease. However, little is yet known about the role of these numerous cell types in the maintenance of enteric tolerance in humans.

Lymphocytes may differentiate within the intestine

The great majority of circulating T cells mature within the thymus, where cells are selected for death by apoptosis if they either fail to react adequately to self major histocompatibility complex molecules (MHC) or if they overreact to self antigen. In this way, the tendency towards autoimmunity is minimized, although this is clearly unlikely to affect potential reactivity towards dietary antigen. However, it is clear that a very substantial portion of the body's T cells do not undergo this process, but mature instead within the epithelium of the intestine (extrathymic differentiation). Thus T cells may be detected at several stages of immaturity in the epithelium, expressing both CD4 and CD8 molecules (double positive cells), expressing neither CD4 or CD8 (double negative cells) or expressing unusual arrangements of these receptors (CD8 cells containing two α chains – αα homodimers – rather than the α and β chains characteristic of circulating CD8 cells).

It is fair to say that very little indeed is known about the interaction of these cells with dietary antigens – yet given their huge numbers and their situation, right at the very interface with luminal antigens of all types, it is extremely likely that these reactions are very important. It is notable that infants with immunodeficiencies of all kinds have an extraordinarily high incidence of dietary sensitizations, chronic enteropathy, and failure to thrive. This author's prejudice is that future generations of researchers will view the intense focus on IgE in food allergies that has characterized the last decades as quite misguided.

Antigen presentation by the epithelium

In recent years, light has been shed onto the role of enterocytes within the mucosal immune system. Enterocytes line the lumen of the gut and represent the first cellular component of the mucosal barrier to antigens, separating the immune system of the gut from both dietary antigens of all kinds and massive numbers of bacteria. Apart from their function in absorption of nutrients, enterocytes are now recognized for their ability to process and present antigen. They are known to secrete immunoregulatory cytokines, among them TGFβ and the interleukins IL-1, IL-6, IL-8, IL-10, and IL-15, in a pattern distinct from classical antigen-presenting cells. Therefore, a role of intestinal epithelial cells in induction of tolerance has been suggested, and it is suspected that enterocytes are of major importance in downregulating immunologically mediated intestinal inflammation, either by induction of tolerogenic lymphocyte subsets, or through direct effects on lymphocyte activity.

In support of this contention, it is now recognized that disturbed epithelial function leads to immunopathology. Hermiston and Gordon induced focal increase in gut permeability by engineering a dysfunctional cell adhesion molecule, E-cadherin, and were able to demonstrate marked secondary inflammation around leaky epithelium. In the context of allergy, it is notable that sensitization to cow's milk formulas often occurs in the aftermath of gastroenteritis, where epithelial integrity has been damaged by pathogens.

Distribution of T cells within the intestine

It is likely that T cell responses are critical in determining tolerance or sensitization to dietary antigen, and there are intriguing differences in racial susceptibility to sensitization to individual antigens. This is seen particularly well within the Far East and Australasia, although little is still known about these mechanisms in humans.

There are clear differences between the T cells of the lamina propria and the epithelium in the small intestine. CD8 cells may have both suppressor and cytotoxic functions, whereas CD4 cells play a more indirect role in controlling functions of other cell types by secretion of individual cytokines. CD8 cells predominate within the epithelial compartment, where they are known as intraepithelial lymphocytes (IELs), whereas CD4 cells are rarely seen within this compartment. By contrast, CD4 cells predominate within the tissue beneath the epithelium (lamina propria), although CD8 cells are also plentiful. Great advances have been made in dissecting the patterns of secretion of inflammatory messenger molecules (cytokines), and two broad patterns of cytokine production are now recognized. This is of major importance in controlling allergic responses.

The T_H1/T_H2 paradigm of T cell responses and infectious exposures

T helper cells coordinate the immune response by both direct cell–cell contact and secretion of cytokines. Two major groups of T helper cells are now recognized, directing immune reactions towards either a cell-mediated (T_H1) or humorally mediated (T_H2) response. T_H1 cells produce cytokines such as IL-2, interferon-gamma (IFNγ), tumor necrosis factor alpha (TNFα), and TNFβ that induce chronic cell-mediated responses and suppress IgE production. Such reactions occur in Crohn's disease, sarcoidosis, and probably celiac disease. T_H2 cells produce a contrasting combination of cytokines (IL-4, IL-5, IL-6, IL-10, and IL-13) that promote humoral responses, including IgE production, and suppress cell-mediated responses. T_H1 cells differentiate from precursors (T_H0 cells) in the presence of the cytokine IL-12, which enhances IFNγ production and reduces IL-4. IL-12 is itself produced by macrophages in response to bacterial products, which may represent one mechanism by which lack of early infectious challenge may promote allergies (i.e. by skewing responses away from T_H1).

Differentiation towards T_H2 cells occurs in the presence of IL-4, which is produced by a variety of cells, particularly in the presence of helminth infections and almost certainly in response to some viral infections. The increasing use of immunizations, which often induce a T_H2 response rather than the T_H1 response required to clear pathogenic organisms, has been postulated to play a role in the development of allergies. However, the lack of allergies in well-vaccinated developing-world populations and the former Communist countries suggests that other environmental exposures are likely to be dominant in this regard. It is however possible that a lack of appropriate early infectious exposures may increase the chance of aberrant responses to any later immunomodulatory intervention. Recent evidence of significantly reduced allergic responses in Swedish infants brought up in an 'anthroposophic' lifestyle, where all medical interventions were avoided for cultural reasons, or in Italian military recruits with past exposures to a pattern of gut infections suggestive of poor early life hygiene, suggests that the comfortable consensus of the last 20 years may have been inappropriate in the context of allergy. It has been said that the only triumph of Communism was the defeat of allergy, and comparison of the rising incidence of allergies in the Baltic states or former East Germany with unreconstructed Moscow or Bucharest suggests that there is more than a grain of truth in this.

Control of B cell responses, and the importance of mucosal IgA production

Antibodies are produced by plasma cells, terminally differentiated B cells, and this may occur either independently of T cells or following specific interactions between T cells and B cells. Only after such specific interaction can high-affinity antibodies be produced. However, within the intestine there is also large-scale production of T cell-independent antibodies, directed against bacterial components, by the primitive B-1 cell population. It remains unclear whether this response is involved in dietary tolerance.

T cells play an important role in shaping the type of antibody response, and T cell-derived cytokines and surface molecules directly affect the shift in antibody isotype (from the default IgM response) towards either the protective IgA response or the proallergic IgE response. The cytokine TGFβ is highly important in this regard, as a molecule that induces IgA production. As it is also implicated in T cell tolerance mechanisms, it is now thought to be one of the most important molecules in the prevention of allergic responses, and will be discussed in more depth later in this chapter.

The pattern of antibody production within the gut immune system is significantly different from systemic responses, in that IgA predominates, and this is important in protecting the mucosal surface and limiting allergic sensitization. Within the lamina propria, IgA plasma cells dominate, and even in allergic children the number of IgE plasma cells is relatively low. It is secreted actively into the lumen in a dimeric form called secretory IgA, following its complexing with secretory component, a glycoprotein synthesized by the enterocytes. As IgA antibodies complex with luminal antigen, they are important regulators of dietary antigen entry.

Detection of serum IgG antibodies to food antigens implies either that ingested immunogenic molecules have entered the systemic circulation and induced a response there, or that local intestinal skewing towards the IgA isotype has been disrupted. Small amounts of food IgG antibodies, particularly to cow's milk or wheat gliadin, are often found in serum of normal children and may not indicate clinically relevant intolerance, although high titers suggest a problem with mucosal permeability as seen in small intestinal enteropathy.

Skewing of B cells towards IgE

While it is now increasingly accepted that non-IgE-mediated responses to dietary antigen may be an important cause of chronic symptomatology, IgE-mediated mechanisms account for the majority of immediate hypersensitive reactions to foods. Transient IgE responses to foods are seen in normal children, and their clinical relevance is uncertain. By contrast, high level IgE responses are usually pathological and may be important in severe food allergies and anaphylaxis.

Production of IgE is favored by dominance of T_H2 responses, particularly due to IL-4 and IL-13 secretion. The receptors for IL-4 and IL-13 share a common component, the α chain (IL-4Rα), and mutations in IL-4Rα that increase signaling through this receptor have been associated with increased atopy. The response of the cell to IL-4 and IL-13 is dependent on a subsequent signaling pathway in which the molecule STAT-6 (signal transducer and activator of transcription-6) is critical. It is thus notable that mice deficient in either IL-4Rα or STAT-6 cannot mount an IgE response to antigen challenge.

By contrast to T_H2 cytokines, products of T_H1 cells (particularly IFNγ and IL-2) directly inhibit IgE production, as do other T_H1-associated cytokines such as IL-12 and IL-18.

As T_H1 responses are upregulated by infectious exposures, this may partly explain the protection against allergy that childhood within the developing world gives.

Mucosally produced IgE may also be transported into the gut lumen (or airway) as is IgA, but by a mechanism that does not utilize secretory component. Such compartmentalization of response may explain why skin-prick testing or serum-specific IgE (RASTs) may be negative in some cases where there is a clear history of rapid-onset responses to dietary antigens. In addition, there is evidence in rodents of an IgE-independent pathway in which IgG1 may directly induce anaphylaxis.

Mast cells and eosinophils in food allergies

As mentioned above, there is a clear link between food allergic responses within the intestine and the infiltration of eosinophils, white blood cells which produce a number of vasoactive and proinflammatory mediators. Both eosinophils and mast cells, which also produce such mediators, have been particularly implicated in dysmotility responses, and it is likely that these products may directly affect the function of enteric nerves. Elevated levels of eosinophil cationic protein (ECP), along with TNFα, have been detected in the stools of infants with food allergies associated with eczema. However, the time course of fecal ECP production is slow, and it does not appear during immediate hypersensitive responses, although mast cell products such as TNFα and tryptase may be detected.

Thus, although mast cells and eosinophils may produce a similar spectrum of mediators, with similar effects upon gut motility, they may mediate two quite different responses: rapid responses are induced by immediate degranulation of mast cells (which store 'prepacked' mediators in intracellular granules) whereas delayed responses may occur after recruitment of eosinophils from the peripheral circulation.

As eosinophil accumulation within the mucosa is a hallmark of chronic food allergic responses, there has been great interest in their recruitment mechanisms. Two molecules are very clearly implicated, the chemokine (chemotactic cytokine) eotaxin and the cytokine IL-5. The qualifications of eotaxin as a critical mediator of the food allergic response were underlined by an important murine study using 'knockout' technology, where genes of interest are deleted (knocked-out) by genetic manipulation techniques. Ovalbumin-sensitized mice were challenged with oral administration of ovalbumin-coated beads, and mounted an allergen-specific T_H2 response with mucosal eosinophilia and IgE and IgG1 production. Use of eotaxin-deficient mice treated identically gave very different results, with no mucosal eosinophils but increased circulating numbers, whereas IL-5 deficiency led to reduced circulating eosinophils.

In another study, IL-5 mRNA was increased after antigen challenge, leading to mucosal eosinophil recruitment, which could be blocked by anti-IL-5 monoclonal antibody. In humans, there is also evidence of increased IL-5 mRNA in the gut mucosa of food allergic patients, but not in atopic or non-allergic controls.

There is thus increasing evidence for a final common pathway in the mucosal allergic response to dietary antigen, which is dependent on upregulation of IL-5 production and expression of the chemokine eotaxin. These may be amenable to specific therapy in the future.

Oral tolerance to dietary antigens

So this chapter ends on the note where it should logically have started, given that the very nature of food allergy demands that the normal state of immunological tolerance to what we eat has been broken. However, the field of oral tolerance is complex and may not appear immediately relevant to non-immunologists. So what has happened to induce such a dramatic increase in food allergies in the western world, and why do demographics seem to matter so much?

Oral tolerance is an actively maintained phenomenon which extends beyond the confines of the mucosal immune system so that systemic immunological tolerance to an antigen is induced by taking it orally. The molecular mechanisms of oral tolerance to dietary antigens have been the subject of intense study during the last decade. The nature of the antigen is to a certain extent important, and some foods are undeniably more sensitizing than others. However, as in so much of immunology, the most critical components appear to be antigen dosage, timing of first administration, and input from innate immunity.

The dose of ingested antigen appears to be particularly important in determining how tolerance is established. Clearly the bulk of dietary antigen needs to be absorbed by enterocytes for nutritional purposes, and this is presented by the epithelium to the immune system in such a way that lymphocyte reactivity is suppressed, and the lymphocytes are rendered anergic. Potential mechanisms include the known absent expression of costimulatory molecules by enterocytes, or more direct inhibition of the lymphocytes by suppressor cell populations or cytokines. Epithelial barrier function is critical, and this form of tolerance may be abrogated by its breakdown and consequent presentation of dietary antigen by activated antigen presenting cells, in presence of proinflammatory cytokines – hence the post-gastroenteritis sensitization to cow's milk in bottle-fed infants. It has also been demonstrated that feeding extremely high doses of dietary antigen to mice induces cell suicide (apoptosis) of antigen-specific lymphocytes within their Peyer's patches, but this has not yet been demonstrated in humans.

Tolerance to low-dose antigen is thought to be mediated separately, and requires uptake by the antigen-sampling M cells in the epithelium that overlies the organized lymphoid tissue of the Peyer's patches. This process depends on the active generation of suppressor lymphocytes within the Peyer's patches. Two such populations are now recognized, and they appear to be centrally important in maintaining mucosal tolerance. Thus the T_H1/T_H2 paradigm has been extended in a manner that is central to the control of potential food allergic responses. Two cytokines are particularly important, TGFβ and IL-10, produced by T_H3 and T regulator 1 (T_R1) cells respectively. Although probably produced within Peyer's patches, these cells home to the lamina propria and suppress intestinal immune reactivity by a process termed 'bystander tolerance,' in which they release TGFβ or IL-10 upon encountering antigen, thus suppressing potential reactivity of all surrounding lymphocytes. If these cells are not generated, spontaneous gut inflammation may occur in response to the enteric flora, and tolerance cannot be established.

The major clue to the role of infectious challenge in preventing food allergies comes from recognition that both gut colonization and local inflammation appear to be required to establish oral tolerance. Mice maintained germ-free, i.e. without gut colonization, do not establish normal enteric tolerance for antigen, and require about 30% additional calories to gain weight compared with colonized mice. The sheer extent of gene induction within enterocytes by the commensal flora, as demonstrated by multiple array technology, has been an important recent finding that is probably quite central in concepts of mucosal tolerance.

The main question has been whether specific T cell responses to the gut flora are involved in priming of mucosal tolerance, or whether this reflects a necessary input from the ancient innate immune system. The answer was provided by an excellent study using the sophisticated techniques of transgenic technology, where mice were bred that had only one population of T cells which reacted to a specific peptide in hen egg lysozyme. Thus any reaction to the gut flora had to come from innate immune cells such as macrophages. Despite possessing huge numbers of lymphocytes that could react to this egg protein, the animals were entirely tolerant to egg under normal circumstances. However, if the in-flammatory response of macrophages towards the gut flora was blocked – using an inhibitor of prostaglandin E2 (PGE2) production – tolerance was broken and food-sensitive enteropathy followed. This has been an influential study, showing an obligatory input from the gut flora to the innate immune system in the establishment and maintenance of mucosal tolerance, and specifically the unexpected role of PGE2 as a pivotal molecule in oral tolerance. The specific linking role played by PGE2 is likely to be through its potent induction of the key regulatory molecules IL-10 and TGFβ.

7.11 Perspectives on the future

These substantial recent findings from the basic science arena promise (some allergists might say threaten) to rewrite the textbooks and tenets of food allergy, with a shift in emphasis from the downstream effector mechanisms of IgE response towards a broader consideration of mucosal tolerance. Does a genetic tendency to high IgE response simply mean that adverse immune reactions are more noticeable? Certainly doctors are happier to have specific tests to use, and non-IgE-mediated allergy is thus an uncomfortable area for many. The absence of specific tests can also lead to over-diagnosis, as a few minutes on the internet will testify.

However, a time when paradigms are shifting is also an immensely exciting time with major opportunities for real advance. The whole area of basic research, now seen to involve both intestinal inflammation and allergy because of shared tolerance mechanisms, begins to explain many of the important demographic shifts in allergy. We can say with some justification that a lack of appropriate early immune infectious priming may specifically hinder the development of normal gut tolerance. Such events may be occurring right at the start of life, and infant handling at the time of initial colonization may have impact on allergic sensitization. One study which shows potentially huge promise is the recent placebo-controlled trial by Isolauri's group in which neonatal administration of a probiotic organism (*Lactobacillus rhamnosus*) led to a 50% reduction in the later development of eczema (Kalliomaki *et al.*, 2001).

In only a hundred years there has been unprecedented alteration in the initial colonization of the intestine of human infants in the developed world. We now have evidence that this was important. Further studies focusing more specifically on food allergy are almost certain, and while prediction is always a hazardous business, it is likely that future therapeutic approaches towards food allergy will be as strongly based on stimulation of innate immune responses in early life as on antigen exclusion.

References and further reading

American Academy of Pediatrics, Committee on Nutrition. Hypoallergenic infant formulas. *Pediatrics* 2000; 106: 346–349.

Barth B, Furuta GT. These FADS are here to stay – clinicopathological patterns of food allergic diseases. *Gastroenterology* 2004; 126: 1481–1482.

Carroccio A, Montalto G, Custro N *et al.* Evidence of very delayed clinical reactions to cow's milk in cow's milk-intolerant patients. *Allergy* 2000; 55: 574-579.

Catassi C, Ratsch IM, Fabiani E *et al.* Coeliac disease in the year 2000: exploring the iceberg. *Lancet* 1994; 343: 200–203.

ESPGHAN (European Society for Paediatric Gastroenterology and Nutrition Group for the Diagnostic Criteria for Food Allergy) Diagnostic criteria for food allergy with predominantly intestinal symptoms. *J Pediatr Gastroenterol Nutr* 1992; 14: 108–112.

Gell PGH, Coombs RRA. Classification of allergic reactions responsible for hypersensitivity and disease. In: *Clinical Aspects of Immunology* (PGH Gell, RRA Coombs, eds), p. 575. Oxford: Blackwells, 1968.

Hepatology and Nutrition (ESPGHAN) Committee on Nutrition. Dietary products used in infants for treatment and prevention of food allergy. *Arch Dis Child* 1999; 81: 80–84.

Hill DJ, Hosking CS, Heine RG. Clinical spectrum of food allergy in children in Australia and South-East Asia: identification and targets for treatment. *Ann Med* 1999; 31: 272–281.

Hogan SP, Mishra A, Brandt EB, Foster PS, Rothenberg ME. A critical role for eotaxin in experimental oral antigen-induced eosinophilic gastrointestinal allergy. *Proc Natl Acad Sci USA* 2000; 97: 6681–6686.

Iacono G, Cavataio F, Montalto G *et al.* Intolerance of cow's milk and chronic constipation in children. *New Engl J Med* 1998; 339: 1100–1104.

Kalliomaki M, Salminen S, Arvilommi H, Kero P, Koskinen P, Isolauri E. Probiotics in primary prevention of atopic disease: a randomised placebo-controlled trial. *Lancet* 2001; 357: 1076–1079.

Latcham F, Merino F, Lang A *et al.* A consistent pattern of minor immunodeficiency and subtle enteropathy in children with multiple food allergy. *J Pediatr* 2003; 143: 39–47.

Matricardi PM, Rosmini F, Riondino S *et al.* Exposure to foodborne and orofecal microbes versus airborne viruses in relation to atopy and allergic asthma. *BMJ* 2000; 320: 412–417.

Newberry RD, Stenson WF, Lorenz RG. Cycloxygenase-2-dependent arachidonic acid metabolites are essential modulators of the immune response to dietary antigen. *Nature Medicine* 1999; 5: 900–906.

Rook GAW, Stanford JL. Give us this day our daily germs. *Immunology Today* 1998; 19: 113–116.

Sampson HA, Sichere SH, Bimbaum AH. AGA technical review on the evaluation of food allergy in gastrointestinal disorders. American Gastroenterological Association. *Gastroenterology* 2001; 120: 1026–1040.

von Mutius E, Weiland SK, Fritzsch C, Duhme H, Keil U. Increasing prevalence of hay fever and atopy among children in Leipzig, East Germany. *Lancet* 1998; 351: 862–866.

8
Nutritional Support

Karin Barndregt and Peter Soeters

Key messages

- Disease-related malnutrition is a frequent clinical finding in hospital populations.
- Improvement in nutritional intake can be achieved with food fortification and dietary counseling, oral nutritional supplements, enteral feeding, parenteral nutrition, or a combination of these approaches.

- Nutritional support can effectively contribute to improved functional and clinical outcomes, not only in hospitals, but also in the community setting.
- Evidence-based practice means combining the best available clinical evidence from research with clinical expertise within available resources.

8.1 Introduction

Nutritional support refers to the provision of adequate nutrients to meet the nutritional requirements of patients at risk of developing malnutrition. This can be in the form of oral diet, diet and nutritional supplements, or artificial nutritional support such as enteral or parenteral feeding. Identifying people at risk from undernutrition is the first step in the management of these patients. Many studies have shown that a substantial proportion of hospitalized patients are at risk of developing malnutrition. This proportion may increase in certain population groups. Assessing nutritional status and assessing nutritional requirements is necessary before optimal nutritional support can be instigated. Causes and consequences of malnutrition and the process of assessing nutritional status are discussed in Chapter 2. Specific guidelines for disease groups are discussed in the chapters specific to those conditions within this textbook. Ethical issues should always be considered before considering nutritional support and these are covered very comprehensively in Chapter 9. This chapter aims to outline general considerations in providing nutritional support and the methods and products available to do so.

8.2 Meeting nutritional needs

Energy, macronutrients, minerals, vitamins, trace elements, fluid, and electrolytes are all necessary for optimal body function. Without sufficient energy, fat and protein stores will be mobilized and these fuels will be oxidized in order to meet energy needs. Since the loss of protein stores directly affects body function, it is important to administer sufficient amounts of energy and protein. Protein synthesis and protein degradation occur simultaneously in all body tissues and the difference between these two processes determines whether the body is anabolic or catabolic. Whereas in the diseased patient protein synthesis can be stimulated by feeding, protein intake cannot influence whole body protein breakdown that occurs during inflammation. In severely ill patients an increased protein intake of 1.5–1.7 g/kg body weight per day (normally 0.8 g/kg body weight/day) optimally stimulates protein synthesis, resulting in the least negative nitrogen balance.

Carbohydrates are not essential nutrients because they can be produced from amino acids and glycerol. However, carbohydrates yield energy, and delivering carbohydrates in food prevents unnecessary stimulation of gluconeogenesis, and thus slows down the rate of protein breakdown.

Fat is an excellent energy source that yields, on a weight basis, more than twice as much energy as carbohydrates. Dietary fat is also a source of essential fatty acids that cannot be synthesized by the body. Essential fatty acids maintain biomembrane structure, influence coagulation characteristics and are precursors for leukotrienes and prostaglandins.

During disease, fluid and electrolyte balances can become disturbed. Overloading of fluids and electrolytes may impair gastric motility and delay the use of the enteral route for feeding. Fluid retention will also affect body weight, and if not accounted for can lead to inaccuracies in assessing nutritional requirements. Therefore, water and electrolyte balance should be carefully monitored and intake should be adapted accordingly (see Chapter 24).

In the past, hyperalimentation (the delivery of energy in excess of requirements) was thought to be efficient in improving nutritional status. However, hyperalimentation has been shown to induced severe metabolic abnormalities such as hyperglycemia, hyperlipidemia, and increased carbon dioxide production. Patients receiving nutritional support should be fed to their requirements. In clinical practice, basal energy expenditure is often calculated using empirical formulas which are often regression equations computed on the basis of energy expenditure and some anthropometric variables. Selected methods for estimating energy requirements are shown in Box 8.1. The Schofield equation is another frequently used formula and is used in Chapter 25 (Table 25.1). A frequently used simple guideline for estimating the daily energy needs of a patient is 25–35 kcal/kg body weight.

Energy requirements are strongly dependent on body composition. The body can be divided into fat mass and fat-free mass. Of the fat-free mass the body cell mass is metabolically the most active and consumes, on a weight basis, more energy than the fat mass. Patients with a higher body cell mass have higher energy needs than patients with a lower body cell mass. For example, young adult men who are tall and heavy need more energy compared with women or elderly and small or slim people. This can be explained by the fact that men have a higher body cell mass than women and need more energy even if they are of the same age, height, and weight. Women have 10% more fat mass than men. During aging, both men and women lose body cell mass which is replaced by fat mass, leading to a decrease in overall energy expenditure. Obese people

---

Box 8.1 Selected methods for estimating energy requirements

Harris–Benedict equation (estimates basal energy expenditure)
Male: $13.75W = 5H - 6.76A + 66.47$
Female: $9.56W + 1.85H - 4.68A + 655.1$

where W is weight in kilograms; H is height in centimeters; A is age in years.
   To predict total energy expenditure (TEE), add an injury/activity factor of 1.2–1.8 depending on the severity and nature of illness.

Ireton–Jones energy expenditure equations
   Obesity
   $IEE = 606S + 9W + 12A + 400V + 1444$

   Spontaneously breathing patients
   $EEE_s = 629 - 11A + 25W - 609O$

   Ventilator-dependent patients
   $EEE_v = 1925 - 10A + 5W + 281S + 292T + 851B$

   EEE is in kcal/day; subscript V indicates ventilator dependent; subscript S indicates spontaneously breathing.

   S: sex (male = 1, female = 0)
   V: ventilator support (present = 1, absent = 0)
   T: diagnosis of trauma (present = 1, absent = 0)
   B: diagnosis of burn (present = 1, absent = 0)
   O: obesity > 30% above ideal body weight from 1959 Metropolitan Life Insurance tables (present = 1, absent = 0)

---

have considerable amounts of fat mass but their body cell mass is also increased, resulting in a higher energy requirement than they would have if they were a normal body weight. Energy requirements in obesity should be calculated based on an adjusted body weight to compensate for the fact that adipose tissue is less metabolically active than lean body mass. Cutts ME *et al.*, 1997, have suggested the following formula to adjust body weight where obesity is present:

$$\text{Obesity-adjusted weight} = \text{IBW} + \frac{(\text{ABW} - \text{IBW})}{4}$$

where ABW is actual body weight and IBW is ideal body weight.

Basal energy expenditure, together with additional factors such as physical activity levels, have to be assessed to calculate total energy expenditure. In the clinical situation, additional disease-associated factors should be taken into account during the calculation of the required energy needs. These include disease stress factor, activity factor, and temperature factor. Fever raises basal energy expenditure approximately 10% per degree above normal. Energy and nutrient losses from malabsorption should be taken into account when present.

In view of differences in the nutritional needs between patients it is always important to assess needs on an individual basis.

8.3 Oral feeding and oral nutritional supplements

Nutritional screening is an effective way of identifying patients at nutritional risk. Once these patients are identified, a decision can be made with regard to oral feeding and nutritional supplements.

Regular hospital food should contain sufficient energy and nutrients for the vast majority of people and this should be the first option of feeding wherever possible. If a patient can be fed orally and is malnourished or at risk of developing malnutrition, oral intake must be optimized. The purpose of this diet is to increase energy and protein intake in order to meet the increased nutritional needs. Consumption of food rich in protein and fat should be encouraged due to the high energy density of fat, and the fact that illness is often accompanied with an increased energy and protein need. The energy and protein intake can be improved by the supply of additional appetizing and nourishing normal foods and snacks, supply of modular products and alteration of food consistency or sip feeding. In Figure 8.1 the different options for oral feeding are shown. Nutritional intake should be assessed by a dietitian/clinical nutritionist at regular intervals to adjust nutritional support if necessary.

If the addition of normal foods does not improve nutritional intake, commercially available modular products can be used. Modular products are single macronutrients and are used to augment oral feeding. They exist as glucose polymers, protein powders, and fat emulsions. Typically modular products do not provide a source of micronutrients.

If sufficient energy intake cannot be achieved with fortified foods, many nutritional supplements are available which can be taken in addition to the diet to provide extra macro- and micronutrients. Most of these oral nutritional supplements (ONS) are supplied in the form of a drink and are nutritionally complete, providing protein, carbohydrate, fat, vitamins, and minerals. These drinks can be sipped during the day in between meals and have been shown to have beneficial effects on nutritional status and outcome. The majority of ONS formulas are commercially available either over the counter in supermarkets or pharmacies, or on prescription. Homemade liquidized supplements have the advantage of being more palatable, but the disadvantage of being of unknown nutritional composition.

ONS drinks have been demonstrated to increase energy intake in a variety of patient groups. In most studies they have had little suppressive effect on food intake and in some patients groups they have been shown to actually stimulate appetite and food intake. Although ONS drinks can promote weight gain, changes in body composition have been infrequently assessed. Functional changes such as muscle strength, activity levels as well as physical and mental well-being, have been shown to improve with supplementation. Although the impact of supplements may be limited in patients with severe end stage disease, mortality rates are sig-

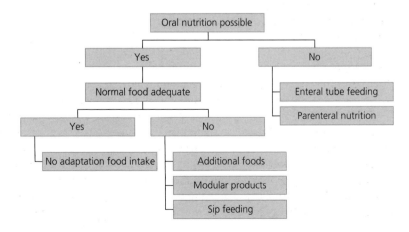

Figure 8.1 Oral feeding options.

nificantly lower in other patients receiving ONS compared with those not receiving supplements. Complication rates are also lower and length of hospital stay is reduced, resulting in considerable cost savings with the appropriate use of ONS. They have also been shown to have a beneficial role in the community setting with improved intake and weight as well as improved functional and clinical outcomes.

8.4 Enteral tube feeding

If oral intake is insufficient to meet nutritional requirements, or if it is contraindicated due to dysphagia, obstruction, or lack of consciousness, enteral tube feeding (ETF) should be considered (Figure 8.2). In both hospitals and the community, tube feeding is used in a variety of clinical conditions and ages and over varying periods of time, from weeks to years. It can be used as a sole source of nutrition, or as a supplementary source of nutrition. ETF has been shown to increase nutritional intake, attenuate loss of body weight and lean tissue, and improve functional and clinical outcomes (see Table 8.1). Patients with a functional gastrointestinal (GI) tract who will not, cannot, or should not eat, and are candidates for nutritional support, should be fed enterally.

Enteral tube feeding is contraindicated in patients with intestinal obstruction distal to the tube, high output fistulas, GI bleeding, or bowel ischemia. A mechanical obstruction distal to the tube results in accumulation of enteral feeding proximal to the obstruction. This can lead to severe bowel extension, abdominal pain, and even bowel rupture. Enteral feeding is also contraindicated in patients with paralytic ileus due to the lack of peristalsis. Enteral feeding in patients with a high output fistula or enterostomy stimulates the production of GI juices. Losses of water and electrolytes through the fistula can be replaced, but stimulation of the gut by enteral feeding can lead to a high fistula output, resulting in considerable losses of fluids and electrolytes through the fistula or enterostomy. These patients should be limited in their enteral intake in order to reduce electrolyte and fluid losses.

During bowel ischemia there should be no enteral provocation because the feed cannot be absorbed and may increase ischemia. Enteral nutrition should be avoided in patients with active GI bleeding and nutri-

tional support should only commence once a patient is hemodynamically stable.

Feeding routes

Access routes for enteral feeding vary according to the individual patient. In deciding which route to use, the anticipated length of feeding and the presence of delayed gastric emptying are two major considerations. Access to the GI tract via the nasal route such as nasogastric (into the stomach), nasoduodenal (into the duodenum), or nasojejunal (into the jejunum) tubes are usually short term (less than 6–8 weeks). During tube placement patients are asked to swallow the tube after advancing the tube through the nose. The nasoenteral tubes are usually placed into the stomach, but may migrate through the pylorus to the small bowel. Nasogastric tubes are usually placed at the bedside. Naso small bowel tubes can be placed in the endoscopy unit or under fluoroscopic guidance in the X-ray department, but some units have success in placing small bowel feeding tubes at the bedside with the aid of a motility agent such as erythromycin or maxolon.

Feeding tubes can increase the incidence of gastroesophageal aspiration as the cardiac sphincter at the top of the stomach cannot fully close. Sitting the patient at an angle of 45 degrees can reduce the incidence of aspiration. With ongoing problems a motility agent can be given, or the tube placed post-pylorically.

When enteral feeding is anticipated for a longer period of time an enterostomy tube should be considered. This is a more invasive category of enteral feeding where the tube accesses the GI tract through the abdominal wall. This procedure can be carried out in an endoscopy unit, radiology department or in theatre. Access can be to the stomach or small bowel. Complications associated with these procedures are infrequent, but include reaction to anesthesia, perforation of adjacent organs, bleeding, and infection. Special precautions should be taken when feeding into the small bowel due to the lack of gastric volume or acidity. Contraindications for enterostomy access are summarized in Box 8.2 (page 121).

Physical characteristics of enteral feeding tubes

A working knowledge of the physical characteristics of enteral access devices including tubes, connectors,

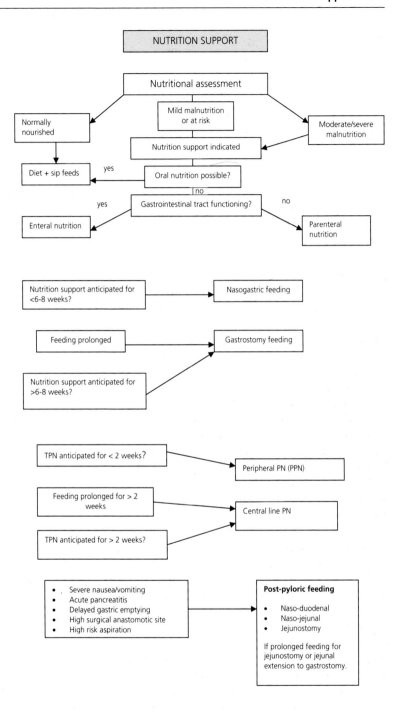

Figure 8.2 Decision tree for deciding on optimal route for nutrition support.

giving sets, and feeding pumps will be needed by the clinical nutritionist/dietitian to best suit the needs of a patient. Nasoenteric tubes for adults are available in lengths from 94 cm (36 in) (enteral) to 156 cm (60 in) (small bowel). Gastrostomy tubes are shorter, and recently very short gastrostomy skin level devices called 'buttons' have become available. These are very useful for GI access in patients who are young, aware of the cosmetic appearance of the tube, or in agitated, confused patients who are at risk of pulling out the tube.

Feeding tubes have variable diameters, measured in French size (the higher the French size the wider the

Table 8.1 Summary of improved functional and clinical outcomes according to disease group following enteral tube feeding in hospital and community

Disease/patient group	Functional/clinical outcome
Burns	Shorter hospital stays
	Fewer wound infections
COPD	Frequency and duration of hospital stays reduced
	Improved maximal inspiratory pressure and sustained inspiratory pressure (endurance)
	Improved maximal inspiratory and expiratory pressures, hamstring strength and endurance
	Less breathlessness
Critical illness/injury	**Lower number of infective complications**
	Lower mortality
	Prevention of increases in intestinal permeability seen in those not given enteral tube feeding
	Improved immune function
	Better neurological outcome
Cystic fibrosis	Lower mortality and hospital admissions
	Fewer episodes of pneumonia
	Improved well-being
	Less deterioration or improvements in pulmonary function
	Improved clinical scores
	Improved forced expiratory
	Increased daily activity
Elderly	**Reduction in pressure ulcer surface area**
	Shorter length of hospital stay
	Improved immune function
Gastrointestinal disease	**Lower rate of reoperations**
	Lower rate of other complications
	Lower mortality
	Reduced medication use
	Earlier return of GI function
	Reduction in Crohn's disease activity[a]
	Improved clinical scores
	Improvements in Crohn's disease activity/inflammatory markers
	Improved vitamin status
General medical	Lower mortality rate with earlier introduction of enteral tube feeding
	Improved quality of life
	Improved immunological parameters
	Improved intestinal absorption and GI function
HIV/AIDS	Improved quality of life
	Immunological benefits
Liver disease	**Lower mortality**
	Lower complication rate, including viral complications
	Improved liver function
Malignancy	Lower mortality
	Improved physical and emotional functioning and dyspnea symptoms
	Improved quality of life
	Immunological improvements
Orthopedics	**Shorter rehabilitation**
	Shorter length of hospital stay[b]
	Lower mortality
Pediatrics	Shorter length of hospital stay
	Reduced parenteral nutrition use
Renal disease	Reduced number of days in hospital
Surgery	**Lower rate of postoperative complications, including infective complications**
	Shorter length of hospital stay
	Slightly lower mortality
	Earlier return of bowel function
	Significant attenuation of increase in gut permeability
	Greater wound healing rate
	Immunological benefits
	Less parenteral nutrition use after enteral tube feeding and shorter requirement for intravenous catheter

Significant changes from randomized controlled trials in **bold**, others are non-significant trends and non-randomized data.
[a]Significant in pediatrics only.
[b]Very thin patients only.

Box 8.2 Contraindications for gastrostomy tube placement

- Disturbed coagulation
- Neoplasms in the stomach
- Morbid obesity
- Gastric varices

tube). Wider bore tubes should be used in postoperative or critical care situations where the tube is aspirated to monitor gastric emptying when enteral feeding is being established. Feeding solutions with a high viscosity may require a larger diameter tube to prevent blockages. When enteral feeding is administered with a pump, tube occlusions occur less frequently and a smaller diameter can be used. Finer bore tubes are more comfortable.

Enteral feeding tubes are made from a variety of materials, including silicone, polyvinylchloride (PVC), latex, or polyurethane (PUR). PVC and latex tubes are stiff and often uncomfortable for long-term use. PUR and silicone tubes are more comfortable and can be used over a longer period of time.

The advantages and disadvantages of different feeding routes are shown in Table 8.2.

Enteral feeding solutions

The selection of an enteral feed should depend upon the nutritional needs of the individual patient, taking into account fluid and energy requirements and renal function as well as the absorptive capacity of the patient. Figure 8.3 shows the decision tree for using specialized enteral formulas. Attention should also be paid to the osmolarity of the solution. Administration of a high osmolar solution directly into the bowel lumen leads to an increased fluid secretion of the bowel in order to dilute this high osmolar solution. This can lead to diarrhea and dizziness and other symptoms of dumping syndrome.

The rationale for the use of other disease-specific formulas is discussed in a useful review of the topic (ASPEN Board of Directors, 2002). The micronutrient profile of feeds is usually in line with recommended levels. These levels may be adjusted in some disease-specific formulas in line with recommendations for specific disease states.

Feeding rate

The time over which enteral feeding is given depends on the patient's needs and tolerance as well as local practices. If a patient requires full nutritional support it is usual to feed over about 20 h with a 4-h rest period to allow the gastric acidity to return to normal. It can also give a slot in the day for washing, physiotherapy, and X-ray when a patient is not connected to the feed. If the patient is given antacids, the feeding can continue over 24 h if required as the gastric acidity is already altered.

If the patient is tolerating enteral feeding, the length of time that they are fed can be reduced. The key factor to remember in this situation is that as the time reduces so the rate must increase to make sure all requirements are met. In situations where adult patients are well established on feeding, feeds can be administered at a rate of up to 200 ml/h by pump or bolus. This can facilitate a mobile patient to be disconnected from the feed for several hours at a time. Patients requiring supplementary nutrition can receive feeds overnight. This allows them to maximize their oral intake during the day.

Monitoring and complications of enteral nutrition

Monitoring patients on enteral tube feeding should be carried out by professionals with knowledge of nutritional requirements, feeding routes, feeding devices, enteral solutions, as well as the associated risks and complications of enteral feeding. Clinical, anthropometric, and biochemical parameters should be monitored before the start and throughout the period of feeding (see Chapter 2).

Complications associated with enteral tube feeding may be of mechanical, gastrointestinal, or metabolic nature. The most common complications of enteral feeding and advice about how to minimize them are shown in Table 8.3 (page 124). Severe complications such as bowel necrosis or GI perforation occur rarely.

8.5 Drugs and enteral feeding

If a patient cannot take medications orally they will need to be administered through the feeding tube.

Table 8.2 Advantages and disadvantages of different enteral feeding routes

Feeding route	Advantages	Disadvantages
Through nose: Nasogastric tube Nasoenteral tube	Not invasive Quick Cheap Feeding can be initiated immediately after tube placement and confirmation of tube location	Oropharyngeal and esophageal irritation Increased risk for sinusitis, esophagitis, nasopharyngitis Swallowing may be painful and difficult Increased risk for reflux Coughing, vomiting or sneezing may result in migration of the tube into the esophagus or pharynx, with an increased risk of aspiration Abnormalities in nose, neck, or esophagus area may prevent tube placement Tube can be placed in the trachea The tube can easily be removed as a result of coughing, vomiting, sneezing, improper tube taping, or by disoriented patients Stigmatizing Tubes should be replaced at a regular basis Location of the nasoenteral tubes often requires an endoscopic approach and X-ray confirmation
Through abdominal wall: Percutaneous endoscopic gastrostomy Gastrostomies Enterostomies Jejunostomy catheters	Less stigmatizing Better psychosocial acceptance Less migration of tube Less tube removal Less reflux or aspiration No oropharyngeal and esophageal irritation Surgical options can be performed when disorders in nose, neck or esophagus are present No difficulties with swallowing No replacement of tubes	Invasive access method with increased risks for postoperative complications Sedation and antibiotics may be necessary Placement may be time consuming Skin around tube can be irritated Leakage of nutrients or intestinal juices into the abdomen Translocation of the bowel around the jejunostomy catheter Occlusion of bowel caused by hematomas Jejunostomy catheter can dislocate and clog Jejunostomy catheter requires X-ray confirmation Abnormalities in the oropharyngeal-esophageal area may prevent percutaneous endoscopic gastrostomy placement

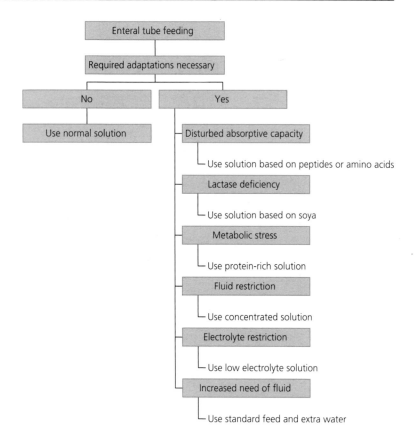

Figure 8.3 Enteral tube feeding options.

The following section outlines considerations for the administration of drugs through a feeding tube. The dietitian or health professional should liaise with a pharmacist to decide on the most appropriate method of drug administration.

Drugs that are liable to cause gastric irritation, or those that are better absorbed with food, should ideally be given while the patient is being fed. Drugs which should be given on an empty stomach are ideally given during the feeding break.

If patients can swallow tablets and capsules, then they should be encouraged to take these orally. If the patient cannot swallow, a liquid formulation of the drug should be tried. Viscous liquids should be diluted with water for injection to aid passage through the tube. The enteral feed should be stopped and the tube cleared by flushing with 15–30 ml of water for injection before and after drug administration.

Dispersible tablets and effervescent granules do not need to be crushed and are least likely to cause obstruction. They are more cost effective than liquid formulations.

Many drugs are only available as tablets or capsules. For optimum drug absorption, and to minimize tube occlusion, a mortar and pestle is recommended for crushing. A tablet crusher or serrated syringe may also be used. Most tablets if left in tepid water for 10–15 min, may soften sufficiently to allow them to be mixed to a slurry using a mortar and pestle. This method reduces the risk of powder inhalation while crushing the tablet. Alternatively a compressed tablet may be crushed to a fine powder and mixed to a suspension with water. The coating of sugar-coated or film-coated tablets will dissolve if crushed finely. Small compressed tablets may be difficult to crush in a serrated crushing syringe but a mortar and pestle may be used.

Drugs formulated as hard gelatin capsules containing a fine powder may be twisted open and the contents mixed in 10–15 ml of water for injection. There is no need to crush the contents. One exception to this is phenytoin. Mixing the contents of phenytoin capsules with water may cause clumping and obstruction of the tube so the suspension form of the drug should be used.

Table 8.3 Possible complications of enteral tube feeding

Complication	Probable causes	Actions/advice
Mechanical complications:		
Tube clogging	Displacement or kink in tube	Check tube for displacements or kinks, change tube if necessary
	Administration of medications	Advise to flush the tube with water when medication is administered
	Diameter is too small	Advise a larger diameter when highly viscous formulas are used
	Nutritional residue adhering to tube	Advise to flush the tube frequently, every 4 h with water
Tube displacement	Coughing, sneezing, vomiting	Reposition of tube
	Migration of tube	Replace tube and consider placement of a tube with a larger diameter
	Dislodgement by patient	Replace tube, if necessary restrain patient
	Inadequate taping of tube	Consider other feeding route. Replace tube and fasten tube properly
Irritations of nose, throat and esophagus	Tube diameter is too large	Advise a tube with a smaller diameter
	Tube is stiff	Advise a flexible tube
	Improper positioning of tube	Reposition the tube properly. Replace tube through other nostril
	Tube is placed too long	Consider other feeding routes
	Inadequate taping of tube	Tape tube properly. The tube should be able to move during swallowing
Gastrointestinal complications:		
Problems in the oral cavity	Decreased or no stimulation of salivary glands	Advise to rinse the mouth regularly or sip fluids if possible. Advise to chew on sugar-free gum or peppermints if allowed
	Dry mouth	Advise proper mouth care and regular rinsing of the mouth
	Time period of tube placing is too long	Replace tube or consider other feeding route
Nausea or vomiting	Formula is too cold	Advise only to administer enteral formulas at room temperature
	Rate of infusion is too high	Decrease rate of infusion
	Volume is too high	Decrease volume, consider a more concentrated formula
	Formula is too concentrated	Decrease concentration of formula
	Disturbed gastric emptying	Check gastric residuals. Monitor for diseases or drugs that may influence gastric motility. Advise prokinetics if possible. Consider nasoenteral feeding
	No bowel movements	Advise to exclude an ileus. If indicated, advise to stimulate bowel movements with a clysma
	Ileus	Immediately stop enteral feeding. If indicated advise parenteral nutrition
	Dislocation of tube	Replace tube and confirm position
	Possible lactose intolerance	Switch to lactose-free formula
	Infectious origin	Check performance of infection control protocol
Aspiration	Delayed gastric emptying	Check gastric residuals. Monitor for diseases or drugs that may influence motility. Advise prokinetics if possible
	Patient only in lying position	Elevate head of bed with 30 degrees
	Administration of bolus feeding	Alter bolus to continue feeding or decrease bolus volume
	High infusion rate	Decrease infusion rate. Consider concentrated solutions
	Displaced feeding tube.	Replace tube. Consider nasoenteral feeding
Constipation	Inadequate fluid intake	Monitor fluid balance, if necessary increase fluid administration
	Medication	Check medication use which can cause a decrease in bowel motility
	Inactivity	Advise more physical activity if possible
	Inadequate fiber intake	Consider formula rich in dietary fiber
Diarrhea	Formula too cold	Advise only to administer formula at room temperature
	Infusion rate too fast	Decrease infusion rate
	Hyperosmolar formula	Change to isotonic formula
	Bolus feeding	Decrease bolus volume or change to continuous feeding
	Infectious origin	Evaluate tube feeding handling and infection control strategies
	Malabsorption	Monitor malabsorption, change to elemental formula if indicated
	Lactose intolerance	Switch to lactose-free formula
	Increased bowel motility	Review possible effects of medication or diseases on bowel motility. If possible advise to start with medications that slow bowel motility
	Extremely low albumin levels	Since adequate enteral feeding is difficult to achieve, advise parenteral nutrition. If possible, a small amount of enteral tube feeding can be administered
	Medications	Monitor medications which may induce diarrhea such as antibiotics

Complication	Probable causes	Actions/advice
Metabolic complications (see also refeeding and overfeeding):		
Dehydration	Inadequate water supply	Monitor fluid balance with special interest in kidney function, serum values of electrolytes, urea, and creatinine. Check changes in body weight. If indicated increase volume
Hyper-/hypoglycemia	Feeding and insulin therapy incompatible	Adjust feeding or insulin therapy. Considerations about bolus or continuous feeding depends on insulin therapy. Monitor blood sugar frequently. If necessary stop nutrition
Serum electrolyte and mineral disturbances	Disease related	Adjust enteral formula to abnormalities, if indicated
Deficiencies of essential nutrients	Insufficient supply of nutrients	Administer the recommended daily allowances of all essential nutrients. If indicated, advise to supply
	Losses of nutrients	Monitor nutrient losses. Check serum values and advise supplementation if necessary
	Disease-related deficiencies	Check deficiencies when they can be expected and advise to supply them if indicated

Drugs formulated as soft gelatin capsules may be delivered by piercing a hole at one end of the capsule, squeezing out the contents and mixing with water for injection. If this is not possible, it is advisable to dissolve the capsule in a glass of warm water, taking care to avoid administration of the undissolved gelatin, which may clog the tube.

The purpose of an enteric coating is to bypass dissolution of the drug in the stomach so that the active compound is released into the small intestine. If the enteric coated tablet is crushed, it loses this property and it may cause undesirable side effects (e.g. gastric irritation with aspirin) or decreased effectiveness of the drug if it is degraded by stomach acid. However, if the drug is only available as an enteric coated formulation, crushing it may be unavoidable.

Controlled release products

Controlled release products are described by a variety of names including long-acting (LA), retard, modified release (MR), and sustained release (SR). These formulations are designed to release the active ingredient over an extended period of time. Tablets, hard gelatin capsules containing granules, and sachets may contain drugs in a controlled release formulation. Crushing SR products to facilitate passage through the enteral tube will alter the drug absorption profile and pharmacokinetics. The pharmacist should be contacted for advice in these situations.

Cytotoxic drugs

Crushing cytotoxic drugs is hazardous due to the risk of powder inhalation and skin contact. These should be administered parenterally. Some cytotoxic drugs should not be opened for enteral administration.

Hormonal drugs

Hormonal drugs should be crushed using a closed system. To avoid powder inhalation, a tablet crusher or a serrated crushing syringe is recommended. They may also be wet crushed.

Alternative routes of delivery

In some instances, alternative routes of drug delivery for the enterally fed patient may be worth considering. These include the topical, rectal, transdermal, buccal, or sublingual, nebulized or parenteral routes.

Adding drugs to the feed

Drugs should not be added to the enteral feed. There is a potential risk of microbiological contamination of the feed and difficulties in predicting the effect medication may have on the physical characteristics of the enteral feed. This may lead to problems, including tube obstruction.

Phenytoin

Enteral nutrition formulas may interact with the absorption or the action of certain drugs. When given concurrently with enteral feed there may be up to 70–80% reduction in serum phenytoin levels. Phenytoin is formulated as a powder in hard gelatin capsules but this tends to clump when dispersed in water. Therefore, the suspension is recommended for enteral administration. In order to maximize phenytoin bioavailability to the enterally fed patient it should be given as a single daily dose in the middle of the tube feeding break, which lasts 4 h or more.

It is important to remember that the bioavailability of phenytoin syrup is greater than that of the capsule.

Warfarin

Several reports have shown that there may be an increase in warfarin resistance in enterally fed patients. Close monitoring of the patient's international normalized ratio (INR) and prothrombin time is recommended, especially when enteral nutrition is started and discontinued.

The hospital pharmacist should be consulted for advice on any drugs whose absorption or bioavailability may be affected by enteral feed. When enteral feeding is stopped, notify the pharmacist so that the patient's medications can be reviewed. It is particularly important to restabilize the blood levels of drugs with a narrow therapeutic index. Other items, which may have been held during enteral nutrition, may need to be restarted.

8.6 Parenteral nutrition

Parenteral nutrition (PN) is used to provide nutrition support when the oral or enteral route cannot be used (Figure 8.2). Indications for parenteral feeding are listed in Box 8.3. Parenteral nutrition consists of a hypertonic solution with glucose, amino acids, fat, electrolytes, vitamins, trace elements, and minerals. It should be administered to patients who are already depleted or are at risk of developing depletion and who are not candidates for enteral feeding. An indication for parenteral nutrition can be short bowel syndrome. The most

---

Box 8.3 Indications for parenteral nutrition

- Mucositis following chemotherapy
- A minority of patients with inflammatory bowel disease where enteral nutrition has failed to prevent or reverse malnutrition (i.e. severe malabsorption)
- Patients with multiorgan failure where nutritional requirements cannot be met by the enteral route alone
- Intestinal atresia
- Radiation enteritis
- Motiliy disorders such as scleroderma or chronic idiopathic intestinal pseudoobstruction syndromes
- Extreme short bowel syndrome of any etiology

---

important feature of this syndrome is insufficient absorption of nutrients, indicating the need for parenteral nutritional support. Malabsorption can be due to massive bowel resection or caused by severe inflammation of the bowel. In the latter case we speak of a functional short bowel, since there is only loss of function. Multiple organ failure, often caused by sepsis, is a condition in which several organs malfunction or do not function at all. The bowel is often involved and does not tolerate full enteral nutrition. In this situation complete or supplementary parenteral nutrition is indicated.

Another indication for parenteral support consists of entero-cutaneous fistulas, especially high output fistulas, which are often located proximally in the small bowel. The proximal location of such fistulas (the jejunum, for example) does not allow adequate absorption of nutrients. An adynamic ileus, another indication for parenteral support, is characterized by lack of peristalsis and passage. Enteral nutrition can therefore not be administered and parenteral nutrition is indicated.

Patients with chronic bowel obstruction also require parenteral nutrition, since enteral nutrition may cause severe bowel distension or even bowel rupture. Since delivery of parenteral nutrition requires a catheter in a central vein, parenteral nutrition is contraindicated in patients with hemodynamic instability, since they have an increased risk of pneumothorax (see the section about complications). Percutaneous puncture of a central line is also contraindicated in patients with clotting abnormalities since they have an increased risk of bleeding. Hyperglycemia can be easily managed with insulin.

It is especially important with parenteral nutrition not to exceed the body's metabolic handling capacity of glucose (4–5 mg/kg per min) or fat (50 mg/kg per min).

Catheter access

In general, parenteral delivery of nutrients can be executed via peripheral or central access. Peripheral parenteral nutrition provides partial or total nutritional support in patients who have an inadequate intake and in whom central vein access is not possible. Peripheral access can only be used for short periods as hypertonic parenteral solutions irritate small veins with a low blood flow, causing phlebitis or thrombosis of the vein. The basilic vein is mostly used for peripheral access. Parenteral nutrition via a central vein with a larger blood flow resulting in a quick dilution of the solution is more successful and can be maintained for longer periods even at home. The most commonly used central vein is the subclavian vein. Other suitable veins are the internal and external jugular veins.

In rare instances when upper veins are not available, the femoral vein is used, which has great impact on the mobility of the patient. An indwelling catheter is another option for patients with poor venous access or for those who require parenteral nutrition for longer periods of time. This device is placed under the skin, in the upper part of the chest. It has a small reservoir that is connected to a major vein inside the chest. This device facilitates the administration of parenteral nutrition into the venous system. Rarely, arteriovenous shunts are employed, but these are only suitable for long-term parenteral nutrition.

Aseptic techniques employed in the cleaning and maintenance of sites is imperative for successful feeding.

Parenteral nutrition solutions

Parenteral nutrition solutions are complex formulas including macronutrients and micronutrients (glucose, amino acids, triglycerides, electrolytes, vitamins, and trace elements). There have been reports of serious harm and even death caused by instability and contamination of parenteral solutions. The stability and compatibility of parenteral formulas can be influenced by the chemistry of lipid emulsions, emulsion stabilization, electrostatic forces, and the effects of single components.

Some hospitals provide homemade parenteral nutrition solutions. These should only be provided to patients with the involvement of a pharmacist with understanding of this complex pharmaceutical chemistry. In 1998 the American Society for Parenteral and Enteral Nutrition (ASPEN) developed guidelines for safe practices for parenteral nutrition formulations. During the preparation of a parenteral solution several aspects should be taken into account. To control bacterial and fungal contamination trained personnel should produce intravenous nutrition in an aseptic work area, using aseptic techniques under laminar flow conditions. Routine microbiological testing of the prepared solution should also be performed. The majority of hospitals using parenteral nutrition use commercially prepared solutions.

The vitamin and mineral requirements for parenteral nutrition are described elsewhere (American Medical Association, 1979; Federal Register, 2000). It should be noted that not all essential nutrients (e.g. iron) can be mixed in a parenteral solution. Serum values of these nutrients should be monitored frequently and supplied via other routes when necessary.

Monitoring and complications of parenteral nutrition

Given the risks and complications associated with parenteral nutrition and the fact that these patients are often critically ill and immunosuppressed, patients receiving parenteral feeding should be carefully monitored. Fluid balance, biochemical parameters, and anthropometric measurements should be performed frequently. In Table 8.4 parameters that should be evaluated and frequency of measurement are listed. (For more detailed information the reader is referred to ASPEN, 2002).

Complications associated with parenteral nutrition can be mechanical, metabolic, or infectious. The most frequent infectious complication of parenteral nutrition is catheter-related sepsis. The incidence varies from 12% to 25%. The catheter hub is the most common site of origin of organisms who cause catheter tip infection and bacteremia. Catheter care is one of the most important factors that influence the incidence of catheter sepsis. Performed strictly according to protocol, catheter care achieves a significant decrease in infectious complications. Subcutaneous tunneling, a

Table 8.4 Parameters that should be evaluated during parenteral nutrition

Parameter	Daily	1–2 per week	Once every two weeks
Fluid balance	✓		
Anthropometry		✓	
Biochemical parameters:			
Hemoglobin		✓	
Leukocytes		✓	
Thrombocytes		✓	
Sodium		✓	
Potassium		✓	
HCO$_3$		✓	
Chloride		✓	
Calcium		✓	
Magnesium		✓	
Phosphate		✓	
Urea		✓	
Creatinine		✓	
Alkaline phosphatase		✓	
Gammaglutamyl transpeptidase		✓	
Bilirubin		✓	
Triglycerides		✓	
Albumin		✓	
Glucose	✓	✓	
Zinc			✓
Copper			✓
Folate			✓
Hydroxycobalamin			✓
Iron			✓

technique to increase the distance between the insertion site of the catheter to the bloodstream in order to prevent migration, has not proven to be effective.

Possible differences in infectious risk between single or multilumen catheters remain controversial. Other factors that can contribute to catheter sepsis are catheter insertion, production and delivery of the parenteral solution, and thrombogenic properties of the catheter, related to the texture of the catheter and the tendency of platelets to adhere to it.

It is important that patients are not fed in excess of their requirements parenterally as this can lead to a variety of metabolic problems such as:

- disorders in fat metabolism (hypertriglyceridemia),
- glucose metabolism (hyperglycemia),
- electrolyte (sodium, potassium) disorders and mineral imbalances (magnesium, phosphate), and
- hepatic disorders.

8.7 Special considerations with nutritional support

There is now good evidence to demonstrate that perioperative nutritional support is of benefit, particularly for patients with severe malnutrition (see Chapter 19). Enteral feeding is usually considered to be the preferred route of feeding as it is more physiological as well as being cheaper and safer. However, it is increasingly recognized that enteral nutrition often fails to achieve targeted caloric requirements, especially in critically ill patients, as a consequence of poor tolerance of feeding manifested by large gastric aspirates. The increased use of invasive methods of post-pyloric feeding and enterostomies have seen a rise in complications such as tube dislodgement, peritonitis, and infection at insertion sites.

Maintaining gut barrier function is often quoted as a reason for enteral feeding. The gut barrier is not a single entity, but instead a number of factors including mechanical defenses, intestinal microflora, immunological defenses, bile salts, and gastric acids, all working to prevent the movement of bacteria and endotoxins from the lumen of the gut through the intestinal lumen to extraintestinal sites. In humans, the evidence to support the theory of bacterial translocation has been extensively discussed and it now seems that bacterial translocation can occur in humans and is associated with an increase in septic morbidity.

There is little or no evidence supporting the theory that short-term parenteral nutrition results in mucosal atrophy or that intestinal permeability is a valid measurement of barrier function. Although enteral tube feeding is always preferred when the GI route is functional, one should consider that disease alters GI function. During critical illness such as sepsis patients are often hemodynamically unstable and blood supply to the GI intestinal tract can be insufficient. Enterocyte integrity and function may be compromised by the response to sepsis induced by cytokines and other modulators. Decreased pancreatic function, fat malabsorption, glucose and lactose malabsorption, delayed gastric emptying, decreased hydrogen ion production, and prolonged colonic transit time have all been described during sepsis. Administration of enteral nutrition to patients with disturbed GI function may cause bowel distension, delayed gastric emptying, paralytic ileus, and diarrhea.

The mode of nutritional support should be decided based on intestinal tolerance. In many instances, a combination of enteral and parenteral feeding may be necessary to meet nutritional requirements.

Post-pyloric feeding

Dumping syndrome results from the administration of a high osmolar solution directly into the small bowel. This leads to an increased fluid secretion from the bowel in order to dilute this high osmolar solution. Dumping syndrome may cause diarrhea, dizziness, and an exaggerated insulin response and ensuing hypoglycemia. This situation is worsened when the administration rate is increased too quickly. It is generally recommended that the infusion rate of small bowel feeding in adults should not exceed 125 ml/h.

Refeeding syndrome

Feeding the undernourished patient warrants particular caution (see Chapter 4). Refeeding syndrome is defined as severe fluid and electrolyte shifts in malnourished patients precipitated by the introduction of nutrition. In starvation, the secretion of insulin is decreased in response to a reduced intake of carbohydrates. Instead fat and protein stores are catabolized to produce energy. This results in an intracellular loss of electrolytes, in particular phosphate. When these patients start to feed, a sudden shift from fat to carbohydrate metabolism occurs and secretion of insulin increases. This stimulates the cellular uptake of phosphate, potassium, and magnesium and concentrations in plasma can fall dramatically and must be supplemented.

Phosphate is directly related to intermediates in energy metabolism such as ATP. Potassium, one of the most important intracellular minerals, is an important component of cellular metabolism. Magnesium, also a relevant intracellular mineral, is a cofactor in many enzyme systems. Decreased levels of such important minerals may lead to serious disorders such as altered myocardial function, cardiac arrhythmia, hemolytic anemia, liver dysfunction, neuromuscular abnormalities, acute ventilatory failure, GI disturbances, renal disorders, and even death.

Identifying patients at risk of refeeding syndrome helps to prevent the syndrome. Patients at greatest risk are those with chronic alcoholism, oncology patients

---

Box 8.4 Practical guidelines to help prevent refeeding syndrome

- Patients identified as requiring nutritional support should start feeding as soon as possible; however, electrolyte disturbances should be corrected before nutritional support is commenced
- Electrolyte levels should be monitored daily during first week of refeeding and twice weekly thereafter
- Food and fluid intake and output should be monitored
- Feeding should be introduced slowly (e.g. 20 kcal/kg for the first 24 h)

---

on chemotherapy, chronic diuretic users, chronic antacid users, those with chronic malnutrition (elderly patients and anorexia nervosa patients), and patients unfed for 7–10 days with evidence of stress and depletion. Postoperative patients have an incidence of severe hypophosphatemia at least twice that of other groups of patients.

Guidelines for preventing refeeding syndrome are summarized in Box 8.4.

Nutrition support team

Since parenteral nutrition is an invasive method of feeding associated with severe complications, a specialized team is necessary to support these patients. A nutrition support team should be a consulting service with knowledge in the field of nutritional and metabolic support of patients. To achieve such expertise an interdisciplinary approach (including a medical doctor, dietitian, pharmacist, and a nurse) is preferable if not essential. The primary goals of a nutrition support team should be the identification of patients who have nutrition-related problems, the performance of nutritional assessment, and the provision of effective nutritional support under continuous guidance. It has been shown that a nutrition support team encourages nutritional support in depleted patients, prevents not-indicated or short-term parenteral nutrition, reduces metabolic and mechanical complications, and decreases the incidence of catheter sepsis.

Swallowing difficulties

Many patients experience problems with swallowing which can cause aspiration pneumonia. It is very important to identify these as soon as possible to minimize the risk. Patient groups at risk include those with head and neck cancer, those with a tracheostomy, stroke, and neurological disease such as motor neurone disease and multiple sclerosis. A swallow assessment should be carried out by qualified personnel (ideally a speech and language therapist) and consistency of the diet altered as necessary. It was former practice to check for possible aspiration by adding blue food dye to feeds. This has been shown to be ineffective as a clinical tool and potentially life threatening and should not be used (http://vm.cfsan.fda.gov/~dms/col-ltr2.html).

Diarrhea and constipation

Since the advent of ready-to-use feeding systems the bacterial contamination of feeds is rarely seen, especially where clean techniques are used by staff. Some feeds may need to be decanted or reconstituted prior to feeding, and in these instances the incidence of bacterial contamination of feeds is greatly increased. The manufacturer's guidelines on feed hanging times should be referred to in all cases. Usually, giving sets should be used over 24 h, but they may be required to be changed more frequently in critically ill or immunocompromised patients.

Diarrhea in the enterally fed patient is most likely to be drug related, due to *Clostridium difficile*, or disease related. The offending cause should be removed if possible. The key medications causing diarrhea include antibiotics, sorbitol-containing medications often present in syrups, and magnesium-containing medications. Treating with fluid and electrolyte replacement must be first-line therapy. If *C. difficile* infection is suspected then a stool should be sent for analysis and the patient started on treatment as required.

Constipation may be caused by many drugs. If possible, the offending agent should be discontinued. Factors that can be used to reduce constipation include:
- increased water intake,
- the use of a high fiber feed to increase fecal bulk, or
- laxatives and stool softeners.

Nausea and vomiting

This should be assessed medically. Patients who have an impaired swallow are at risk of aspiration if they vomit. It is important to confirm placement of the feeding tube. The patient may just need a couple of hours with the feed disconnected, but long periods of discontinu-ation of the feed should be avoided. Antiemetic agents can be used and in extreme cases post-pyloric feeding or parenteral nutrition may be required.

8.8 Future directions

In this section some aspects of nutritional support which may be of importance in the future will be discussed. All clinicans working in the field of nutrition support should keep updated as to current evidence-based practice in the area.

Immunonutrition

In the last decade, the use of immunonutrition to different patient groups in the form of oral nutritional supplements, enteral nutrition, or parenteral nutrition has been extensively researched and discussed. Immunonutrients can be in the form of vitamins, minerals, fatty acids, or amino acids and have been suggested to accelerate recovery or to positively alter metabolic responses to illness. The most important nutrients and their related functions will be briefly discussed. An excellent review of the topic was published in 2001 (Kudsk *et al.*, 2001).

Glutamine

Glutamine is a non-essential amino acid. It is also the most abundant free amino acid in the body. Glutamine is a precursor of nucleotides, proteins, and glutathione (involved in the antioxidant defense system), serves as fuel for enterocytes and lymphocytes, and plays a role in the regulation of the acid–base balance. It is hypothesized that under certain circumstances such as severe nutritional depletion or stress, glutamine is insufficiently produced, making it a conditionally essential amino acid. Organ systems that require glutamine, such as the immune system or the gut, may lack glutamine, resulting in more complications in these severely depleted patients. Some, but not all, clinical studies have shown beneficial clinical outcome with better survival rates and less complications when glutamine-enriched nutritional support is administered. More research is necessary before definitive conclusions can be drawn, regarding the beneficial effects of glutamine.

Arginine

Arginine, also a non-essential amino acid, is produced by the kidneys and stimulates the secretion of several hormones such as growth hormone, glucagon, and insulin. Arginine supplementation is associated with positive effects on nitrogen balance and immune response. However, the clinical relevance of arginine supplementation has not been fully elucidated and there is some evidence that the use of arginine in critically ill patients may do more harm than good.

n-3 fatty acids

It is hypothesized that n-3 fatty acids (present in fish oil) positively influence the inflammatory response, resulting in a less severe inflammation and the production of anti-inflammatory cytokines. In general, although research which focused on the effects of the supplementation of specific nutrients showed some positive trends, no unequivocal conclusions can be drawn and more thorough confirmation is necessary. Therefore, the recommended daily allowances, designed for healthy individuals, are also generally applied in disease states.

Intradialytic parenteral nutrition

A new group of patients who might benefit from parenteral nutrition are the dialysis patients. Recent studies showed that administration of intradialytic parenteral nutrition in malnourished hemodialysis patients might improve their nutritional state.

Peripherally inserted central catheters

Recently, the use of another central venous access device, the peripherally inserted central catheter (PICC), has become increasingly popular. These catheters are inserted in a peripheral vein such as the basilic vein and are moved carefully to a central vein such as the subclavian vein. It is reported that PICCs are not associated with increased line sepsis or thrombosis but have an increased incidence of leaking catheters, phlebitis, and malposition. However, this technique is associated with fewer complications due to the catheter access.

References and further reading

American Medical Association. Department of Foods and Nutrition. Guidelines for essential trace element preparations for parenteral use. A statement by an expert panel. *JAMA* 1979; 241: 2051–2054.

ASPEN Board of Directors and the Clinical Guidelines Task Force. Guidelines for the use of parenteral and enteral nutrition in adult and pediatric patients *JPEN J Parenter Enteral Nutr* 2002; 26(Suppl).

Cutts ME, Dowdy RP, Ellersieck MR, Edes TE. Predicting energy needs in ventilator dependent critically ill patients. Effect of adjusting weight for oedema and adiposity. *Am J Clin Nutr* 1997; 66: 1250–1256.

Federal Register. Parenteral multivitamins products; drugs for human use; drug efficacy study implementation; amendment (21CFR 5.70). *Federal Register* 2000; 65: 21200–21201.

Fein BI, Holt PR. Hepatobiliary complications of total parenteral nutrition. *J Clin Gastroenterol* 1994; 18: 62–66.

Heyland DK, and the Canadian Critical Care Clinical Practice Guidelines Committee. Canadian clinical practice guidelines for nutrition support in mechanically ventilated, critically ill adult patients. *JPEN J Parenter Enteral Nutr* 2003; 27: 355–373.

Klein CJ, Stanek GS, Wiles CE. Overfeeding macronutrients to critically ill adults: metabolic complications. *J Am Diet Assoc* 1998: 98: 795–806.

Klein S, Kinney J, Jeejeebhoy K *et al*. Nutrition support in clinical practice: review of published data and recommendations for future research directions. *JPEN J Parenter Enteral Nutr* 1997; 21: 133–156.

Proceedings from Summit on Immune-Enhancing Enteral Therapy. May 25–26, 2000, San Diego, California, USA. *JPEN J Parenter Enteral Nutr* 2001; 25(Suppl): S1–63.

McClave SA, DeMeo MT, DeLegge MH *et al*. North American Summit on Aspiration in the Critically Ill Patient: consensus statement. *JPEN J Parenter Enteral Nutr* 2002; 26(Suppl): S80–S85.

National Advisory Group on Standards and Practice Guidelines for Parenteral Nutrition. Safe practices for parenteral nutrition formulations. *JPEN J Parenter Enteral Nutr* 1998: 22: 49–66.

Solomon SM, Kirby DF. The refeeding syndrome: a review. *JPEN J Parenter Enteral Nutr* 1990; 14: 90–97.

Useful websites

www.ajcn.org
www.arborcom.com/frame/clin_4
www.bapen.org.uk
www.clinical-nutrition.com
www.criticalcarenutrition.org
www.espen.org
www.faseb.org/ascn
www.harcourt-international.com/journals/clnu/
www.nutrition.org.uk
www.nutritioncare.org (ASPEN)
www.stockton-press.co.uk/ejcn/

9
Ethics and Nutrition

John MacFie

Life is short; and the art long; and the right time an instant; and treatment precarious; and the crisis grievous. It is necessary for the physician not only to provide the needed treatment but to provide for the patient himself, and for those beside him, and to provide for his outside affairs.

Attributed to Hippocrates circa 400BC
(translation by Dickinson Richards)

Man is an animal with primary instincts of survival. Consequently, his ingenuity has developed first and his soul afterwards. Thus, the progress of science is far ahead of man's ethical behaviour.

Sir Charles Spencer Chaplin (1899–1977)

Let the doctors work out the ethical implications: let them face the problems in the context of ethics, I think the courts have given the medical profession the opportunity to get their ethical house in order, If they do, then common law will follow the guidance of the ethical solutions reached.

Lord Scarman, 1984

9.1 Introduction

Medicine is inherently a moral enterprise; the very practice of medicine involves making decisions between good and bad, right and wrong. This has been part of the practice of medicine for centuries. Nonetheless, it is only in relatively recent years that the principles of ethics applied to medicine have come to dominate contemporary practice. Traditionally, doctors are seen as experts in addressing the 'can we?' questions which are technical questions, but the ethics questions, the 'should we?' questions, are comparatively new to clinical practice.

The term 'bioethics' was coined in the early 1970s to denote a new, rapidly expanding discipline in medicine. There were many reasons for this growth, the most important of which can be summarized as follows:

- *The explosion of medical technology.* As patients, researchers, and technicians discover newer and improved methods of treatment then each development is matched by an extension of the ethical dilemmas that surround each new innovation. Gradually the ethical issues are focused, they evolve and, occasionally, they may be resolved.
- *The changing doctor–patient relationship.* Traditionally, the paternalistic physician unilaterally made decisions about what was appropriate for a particular patient. Paternalism, however, has been seen to be flawed and current case law in most countries of the world recognizes the essential principle of autonomy and the fact that the competent patient is empowered to participate in medical decisions.
- *Concerns about cost containment.* Medical decisions used to be made by one physician who would provide the professional service almost irrespective of cost. This inevitably resulted in dramatic increases in utilization of new medical technologies. As third party payers (insurance companies, governments, health authorities) became alarmed about increasing costs they demanded not only accountability, but also some voice in decisions about the use of expensive technology. In addressing this dilemma about costs there are two different perspectives. There is the medical practice perspective, which attempts to maximize the good of the individual patient. This perspective looks at personal concerns on a case-by-case basis, and is particularly concerned about the ethical principles of beneficence (doing good for the patient) and autonomy (the patient's right to self-determination). In contrast, there is the health policy perspective, which seeks to maximize the good of society rather than the individual. This

perspective reflects the importance of the ethical principles of utilitarianism and justice.

The issue of nutritional support in clinical practice exemplifies these changing attitudes to ethical dilemmas. The administration of artificial nutrition and hydration was originally intended as a temporary bridge to the restoration of a patient's normal digestive functioning. It is now, however, often given to patients who have irretrievably lost all higher brain function. It is a strange paradox that society and many members of the medical profession frequently recommend nutritional support in those with severe neurological disease or terminal illness but at the same time fail to recognize or treat malnutrition in hospitalized patients.

An analysis of the ethical issues surrounding malnutrition and nutritional support serves to emphasize not only the changing face of bioethics but also demonstrates how the ethical issues themselves have influenced the clinical application of nutritional support techniques.

9.2 A brief history of medical ethics

Hippocrates is considered the father of medical ethics. He is thought to have been born around 460BC, but little is known of his life and there may, in fact, have been several men of this name. Whether Hippocrates was one man or several, the works attributed to him mark the stage in western medicine where disease was coming to be regarded as a natural rather than a supernatural phenomenon and doctors were encouraged to look for physical causes of illness. Hippocrates laid much stress on diet in the treatment of disease and the use of few drugs. He emphasized the importance of the natural history of disease, recognizing the futility of treatment in many instances. Perhaps his greatest legacy was the charter of medical conduct embodied in the so-called Hippocratic oath, which has been adopted as a pattern for physicians throughout the ages. Although not strictly an oath it was rather an ethical code or ideal, an appeal for right conduct. In one or other of its many versions it has guided the practice of medicine for more than 2000 years.

The fundamental tenets of the Hippocratic tradition were to do away with suffering, to lessen the violence of disease and to refuse to treat those who were overwhelmed by their disease in the realization that in such cases medicine or treatment was powerless. Nontreatment was not considered to violate the concept of doing no harm because these physicians accepted a limit to their abilities. Provision of food and water was not deemed 'necessary' in the face of overwhelming disease. The Hippocratic concepts of beneficence, the providing of benefit, and non-maleficence, the avoidance of harm, remain fundamental to contemporary medical ethics.

This Hippocratic tradition remained largely unchallenged for the best part of the next two millennia. Comparatively little was written on the subject of ethics until the fifteenth and sixteenth centuries, when contemporary theologians recorded their thoughts for posterity. Sixteenth-century theologian Bonez, for example, was the first to expound the theory of ordinary versus extraordinary treatment in prolonging life. It is important to emphasize here that extraordinary does not refer to the techniques employed but rather to the condition of the patient. Historically even the most simple remedy was deemed extraordinary if it offered no hope to the patient. Such remedies were, therefore, morally optional. Even food and water were considered to be extraordinary therapies and, therefore, as in the Hippocratic tradition, morally optional.

British physician Thomas Percival was arguably the first to formulate a doctrine of medical ethics. In 1803 he published a treatise entitled, 'Code of institutes and precepts adapted to the professional conduct of physicians and surgeons'. This treatise was to be the most influential document on ethics on both sides of the Atlantic for over 100 years. His work served as a prototype for the American Medical Association's first code of ethics in 1847. Percival believed that the welfare of the patient was governed by the good and virtuous behavior of doctors. He believed in the assets of a strong interprofessional relationship achieved through the propriety and dignity of the conduct of a doctor. His was the philosophy of the doctor–doctor relationship – the doctor knows best. This philosophical approach to medical care is termed 'paternalism.'

While there are many different aspects to paternalism, the fundamental principle of this philosophy is the presumption that the doctor is in the best position to make decisions on behalf of the patient. Percival argued that non-maleficence and beneficence fix the physician's primary obligations and triumph over the patient's preferences and rights in any circumstance of serious conflict. It was accepted that doctors determined by themselves, or in conjunction with colleagues, the most appropriate care for their patients. This rendered unnecessary the inconvenience of discussing with either the patient or their surrogates the relative merits or demerits of any given therapy. Percival failed to foresee the power of the principles of autonomy and distributive justice that in the twentieth century became ubiquitous in discussions of biomedical ethics.

One catalyst to the dramatic shift away from paternalism towards acceptance of the critical importance of autonomy was the publication of the Nuremberg Code, which followed the unpleasant discovery of human experiments performed during World War II. The doctor–doctor relationship was seen to be flawed and the Nuremberg Code established the importance of the doctor–patient relationship. Implicit in this is the recognition of a patient's right to self-determination; the right to know, the right to choose, and the right to be informed.

Another important principle in contemporary ethical debate relates to justice. Common to all theories of justice is a minimal requirement that equals are treated equally, a concept originally attributed to Aristotle. These days the principle of distributive justice refers to fair, equitable, and appropriate distribution in society determined by justified norms that structure the terms of social cooperation. Most governments of the day and certainly all democracies would claim to support the principles inherent in distributive justice.

9.3 Medical ethics: the 'four-principles' approach

From the foregoing discussion it can be seen that four principles underpin present approaches to medical ethics (Box 9.1).

- *Autonomy* is the principle of self-determination and is a recognition of patient rights. This is now the pre-eminent theme in law in most democratic states.
- *Non-maleficence* is the deliberate avoidance of harm.
- *Beneficence* is the concept that the patient is provided with some kind of benefit.
- *Justice* is the fair and equitable provision of available medical resources to all.

Application of these four principles offers a systematic and relatively objective way to approach ethical dilemmas. The advocates of this 'four-principles' approach to biomedical ethics stress that these principles should be seen not as specific precise action guides that will inform doctors of appropriate action for any circum-

> **Box 9.1** The four principles of medical ethics
>
> - Beneficence
> - Non-maleficence
> - Justice
> - Autonomy

stance, but rather as a framework of virtues or values that are relevant to ethical debate. It is important to note that there are alternative ethical approaches including virtue-based theories, the ethics of caring, casuistry, narrative ethics, and others. These are outwith the scope of this chapter and the interested reader is referred to standard texts on ethical theory and moral philosophy.

Analysis of ethical dilemmas employing principalism as outlined above results in three common themes that distinguish different individuals' perspectives on ethical debate:

- The *duty-based moralist* is concerned predominantly with the intrinsic merits or otherwise of a medical decision rather than its consequences. A wholly committed duty-based moralist would support the sanctity of life at all costs.
- The *utilitarian or goal-based moralist* requires the doctor to judge the general aggregate of good according to the consequences of an action rather than the act itself. Thus, this doctor would stand by the principles of a controlled clinical trial thereby justifying the morbidity and even mortality of a few patients for the potential benefit to be gained by a majority of patients.
- The *rights-based moralist* is, as already pointed out, the dominant contemporary theme and is now the fundamental principle of medical law. This doctor would condemn an action if it wronged someone or if it violates the rights of a patient to determine their own destiny.

Application of these themes to the issue of nutritional support gives very different recommendations for treatment. The duty-based moralist would always feed the patient whatever the anticipated outcome, on the basis that this was the right and responsibility of the doctor. The goal-based or utilitarian doctor would feed when appropriate in their health care setting and if the results of such intervention were justified on the basis of scientific evidence. The rights-based moralist would argue that the patient should always be offered nutritional support and, if requested by the patient on the basis of information given, then the moral responsibility must be to provide nutritional support. Equally, if the patient or their surrogate refuses nutritional support then the patient's wishes must be respected.

Obviously there is some conflict between these three themes, as well as with the four principles of autonomy, beneficence, non-maleficence, and justice. These conflicts serve to emphasize that ethics is a process of reasoning whereby a morally respectable and defensible position can be reached, which protects the best interests of the patient. There are no absolutely satisfactory resolutions of ethical dilemmas and the most that one can hope to achieve is a balance between the conflicting interests and goals of different individuals involved in patient care. While this is a very simplistic approach to a complex area it is hoped that the foregoing discussion will have provided the reader with an insight into how these ethical principles have evolved and provided some feeling for their relative importance.

9.4 Definitions and ethical terms

The definitions and terms described here are adopted from the British Medical Association's publication *Withholding and Withdrawing Life-prolonging Medical Treatment*. This text is highly recommended.

Oral nutrition and hydration: 'basic care'

The provision of food or water by mouth, whether simply moistening a patient's mouth for comfort, or by the use of cup, spoon, or other assistance is deemed part of basic care. Basic care means those procedures deemed essential to keep a patient comfortable. It is a health professional's duty to ensure the provision of basic care to all patients unless actively resisted by the patient. Food and water should therefore always be offered unless the process of feeding produces an unacceptable burden to the patient.

Many patients, such as babies, young children, and people with disability, may require assistance with feeding but retain the ability to swallow if the food is placed in their mouths; this forms part of basic care. Evidence suggests that when patients are close to death, however, they seldom want nutrition or hydration and its provision may exacerbate discomfort and suffering. Good practice should include moistening the mouth as necessary to keep the patient comfortable.

Artificial nutrition and hydration

The term artificial nutrition should be used specifically for those techniques for providing nutrition that are used to bypass a pathology in the swallowing mechanism. All parenteral and the majority of enteral feeding techniques (except perhaps sip feeding using oral supplements) are forms of provision of artificial nutrition. In America and in most European countries artificial nutrition is now considered a medical treatment as opposed to simply an aspect of basic care and therefore subject to same ethical constraints in their instigation or withdrawal as any other life-prolonging therapies.

Some people continue to argue that tube feeding should be regarded as part of basic care and others have made a distinction between the insertion of a feeding tube, which is classed as treatment, and the administration of fluid or nutrients through a tube, which they consider basic care. If this view were generally accepted then decisions not to insert a feeding tube or not to reinsert it if it became dislodged would be legitimate medical decisions, whereas a decision to stop providing nutrition through an existing tube would not. This distinction is not generally accepted.

Competence

Assessing competence is critical. Failure to do so denies the patient's right to autonomy. Hard and fast rules for appraising competence do not exist. In the UK, guidelines have been advocated as indicating a patient's competence to consent to treatment or to non-treatment. These are summarized in Box 9.2. Each of these abilities must be present over a sustained period for competence to be firmly established.

In contrast to the assessment of competence, it is important to also consider that there are an increasing number of conditions in which a consensus of medical opinion is such that non-treatment is regarded as

Box 9.2 Competence guidelines

A patient is considered to be competent if able to:
- Understand a simple explanation of their condition, prognosis, and proposed treatment or non-treatment
- Reason consistently about specific goals linked to their personal beliefs
- Choose to act on the basis of such reasoning
- Communicate the substance of their choice and the reasons for that choice
- Understand the practical consequences of their choice

Box 9.3 Conditions for non-treatment of incompetent patients

- Imminent and irreversible closeness to death
- Extensive neurological damage leading to the permanent destruction of both self-awareness and intentional action
- Little self-awareness accompanied by such severe motor disability that sustained independent and intentional action becomes impossible
- Destruction of both long- and short-term memory to such a degree that the person that used to exist no longer does and no other person can evolve instead
- Severely limited understanding by patient of distressing and marginally effective life-saving treatment that leads to a demonstrably awful life

being legally justified. Conditions for non-treatment of incompetent patients are summarized in Box 9.3.

'Time limited trials' of treatment

Considerable anxiety is produced by reports of mistaken diagnosis or a belief that had treatment been provided the patient may have recovered to a level that would have been acceptable to that individual. One of the difficulties for health professionals is that it is often not possible to predict with certainty how any individual will respond to a particular treatment or, in the final stages of an illness, how long the dying process will take. Doctors have an ethical obligation to keep their skills up to date and to keep abreast of new developments in their speciality and to base their decisions on a reasonable assessment of the facts available. There will, however, always remain some areas of uncertainty and empirical judgments are necessarily based on probability rather than certainty.

Wider consultation including a second opinion should be sought where the treating doctor has doubt about the proposed decision. In emergency medicine procedures may be instituted that appear unjustified when more information is available. Where there is genuine doubt about the ability of a particular treatment to benefit the patient that treatment should be provided but may be withdrawn if, on subsequent review, it is found to be inappropriate or not beneficial. This uncertainty about outcomes of disease often leads to reticence to commence therapy such that dilemmas on stopping such treatment are avoided. In these cases it is worth considering time-limited trials of therapy. In these, specific goals are agreed, often between rela-

tives and staff, and progress carefully monitored over previously specified periods of time.

Many studies have demonstrated that ethical problems can be pre-empted if they have been discussed with the patient, where possible, the family, and the health care team at the outset.

Time-limited trials recognize that the beneficial effects of treatment often cannot be foreseen, making it inappropriate to withhold treatment. Treatment is therefore initiated in order to ascertain potential benefit even though it may subsequently be stopped when more information becomes available. Time-limited trials also permit wider consultation of complex problems, which can help to diminish uncertainty in medical treatment. When there is genuine doubt about possible benefit, treatment should be given but may be withdrawn if on subsequent review it is found to be inappropriate or not beneficial. End points, for example, are objective signs of recovery or deterioration in multiorgan failure or neurological status. It would be reasonable to assess these on a weekly basis. Ideally, clinicians should determine the goals of therapy or response to illness after discussion with colleagues as well as with relatives. In the case of nutritional support it would seem sensible to involve a nutrition team.

Advance directives/proxies

Advance directives enable patients to express in advance their individual preferences in respect of medical treatment should they subsequently become incompetent. Advance directives may express refusal of any therapy or procedure that would require consent of the patient if competent. The British Medical Association has published a code of practice on advance directives. It should be noted that there is no statute on advance directives in English law although a number of cases have established legal precedent. In the US, California was the first state to enact a law (The Natural Death Act) in 1976 and many other states have since followed suit. It is now generally accepted that artificial nutrition may be considered as being one of the treatments that might be included in an advance refusal of treatment. Clinical dilemmas may arise if patients establish advance directives in which advance refusals of basic care including the offer of oral nutrition and hydration are included. It can be argued that it should never be binding on health professionals to deny a patient basic care. The importance of distinguishing between basic care and artificial nutritional support is self-evident.

In most western countries advance refusals have the same legal authority as contemporaneous refusals of treatment and legal action can be taken against a doctor who provides treatment in the face of a valid refusal. Advance directives are usually presented as formal written documents but it is not necessary for the refusal to be in writing for it to be valid. If prior discussions with a health professional have been clearly recorded in a patient's notes then this may constitute a valid advance directive. In the UK, relatives, friends, or other interested parties have no authority to overrule an advance directive. In this regard it is interesting to note that recently the UK government announced its intention to legislate to allow adults to appoint friends or relatives to take health care decisions for them if they later become too incapacitated to decide for themselves. Under these plans any competent adult will be able to draw up continuing power of attorney authorizing the chosen proxy to consent or refuse treatment. However, a general authority to take health care decisions will not allow the proxy to authorize the withdrawal of artificial nutrition unless this was specifically stated. Legal appointment of proxies already exists in some American states and European countries.

Futility and the concept of net patient benefit

There are many aspects to medical futility and many definitions. In considering the principle of futility it is important to differentiate between effect and benefit. In patients with persistent vegetative states nutritional therapy will maintain organ function and keep the patient alive. However, nutritional therapy is unlikely to restore the patient to a conscious and sapient life. It is arguable, therefore, that nutritional therapy, in these instances, is futile. This is certainly the view accepted by British and European Courts of Justice. The British Medical Association has defined benefit for patients as treatment conferring a net gain or advantage. It does not necessarily equate with simply achieving certain physiological goals. The same principles might apply to the perioperative patient with multiorgan failure being sustained on long-term hemodialysis and artificial ventilation. It is worthy of emphasis, with regard to assessment of futility in clinical practice, that the courts in the UK have made clear on a number of occa-

sions that doctors are not obliged to provide treatment contrary to their clinical judgment.

9.5 Some common ethical dilemmas

Withdrawing and withholding nutritional support: persistent vegetative states

Landmark 'right to die' cases, all diagnosed as being in a persistent vegetative state, both in this country and elsewhere have generated much ethical debate and established important legal precedent. In the UK, the Bland case was the first of these judgments. Tony Bland was a 21-year-old man who suffered anoxic brain damage when a soccer stadium collapsed. He was subsequently confirmed as being in a persistent vegetative state. Nutrition and hydration were maintained by tube feeding. After some months in this condition his attending physicians approached the courts to enquire as to the legality of withdrawing nutritional support. They were informed that this would constitute judicial murder. The case was ultimately heard in the House of Lords, which constitutes the highest court in the UK, and they authorized the removal of the feeding tube. Tony Bland died 11 days later.

This case clarified the law relating to withholding and withdrawing life-prolonging treatments and highlighted several important legal points:

- medical decisions for a mentally incapable patient should be made in the best interests of the patient;
- if a decision to withdraw or withhold treatment was in the best interests of the patient then it is lawful;
- there is no legal difference between withdrawing or withholding treatment;
- artificial nutrition and hydration constitute medical treatments and can be withdrawn if it is in the best interests of the patient to do so.

The situation in the USA and the UK is now similar to that which already exists in many European countries in that there is no legal or ethical restraint on the discontinuation of feeding in a patient with an established persistent vegetative state if this can be shown to accord with the patient's wishes and if no doubt exists as to the diagnosis of persistent vegetative state. These patients were unable to express a view and, therefore, the weight of evidence in all these court cases has revolved around a discussion with relatives, proxies, or surrogates. On each occasion the courts have taken the view that the weight of evidence must show clearly that a decision to discontinue feeding would accord with the patient's wishes were they able to express them. In other words, the principle of patient autonomy, that is the right to self-determination, is pre-eminent in any ethical debate as this applies to the withholding or withdrawing of any medical therapy.

A recent report by the British Medical Association on the subject of withholding and withdrawing medical treatment provides a comprehensive overview of all the issues involved and the current legal position. It emphasizes that treatments must bring about net benefits to the patient (not simply the achievement of physiological goals) and that decisions should be made on the basis of what is right for the individual patient. The important consideration is whether any proposed measure can restore the patient to a way of living that he or she would have considered acceptable. Legally, doctors are bound by a patient's right to refuse treatment.

In clinical practice, at least in the UK, there is now the paradox that there is clear legal precedent for withdrawal of artificial nutrition in patients confirmed as being in a persistent vegetative state but not for the many other patients with severe neurological illness who are not designated as being in a vegetative state. For those in a persistent vegetative state a declaration to the courts must be sought to authorize discontinuation of feeding but for other patients whose death is not imminent and for whom it is deemed that their best interests are served by cessation of nutritional therapy there is currently no requirement for court review. It is clearly important for these patients that additional safeguards should be implemented including the use of a routine second opinion and the establishment of systems to record and monitor decisions and progress.

9.6 Can we afford it? The principle of justice

Resources for health care are not infinite. As medical technology becomes sophisticated and therefore more expensive, difficult and at times controversial decisions must be made about priorities. This is particularly apposite to the question of adjuvant nutritional support. A report on medical ethics to the UK government in 1994 stated that health care teams should not be put in a position of having to make resource decisions in the course of their day-to-day clinical practice. Their

concern must be for the welfare of the individual patient. Decisions about treatments should be made on the basis that such treatments as society does wish to fund must be available equally to all who might benefit from them.

With regard to nutritional support it is noteworthy that recent guidelines on parenteral and enteral nutritional support, published by the American Society of Parenteral and Enteral Nutrition in 1995, stated that 'healthcare providers should not make unilateral decisions to provide, withhold or withdraw nutritional support on the basis of limiting costs or of rationing scarce resources for the benefit of society unless required by the law. No such laws exist at this time'.

There is an ethical requirement for doctors to consider the broader issue of resource availability. Doctors are in a unique position to influence economic reality. Permitting largesse in prescribing drugs or the use of modern technology can no longer be justified. Physicians can ethically participate in cost containment so that the health care system on the whole is morally just. This requires the physician to critically appraise treatment and is a good advertisement for evidence-based medicine. Collective research and reflection on optimal resource use is morally, medically, and economically preferable to individual cost cutting. The moral question is no longer whether to participate in cost containment but how to do so in a morally creditable way. Although economic constraints may force physicians to weigh more carefully the cost of each benefit, they do not require that the physician appraise the value of the individual patient or weigh his or her benefit to society. The physician can still be the patient's best advocate even if he or she is not obliged to provide benefits without limit.

The application of the ethical principle of justice as this applies to the treatment of malnutrition or the provision of nutritional support necessitates that physicians carefully appraise treatments for each and every individual. Physicians can help control costs by choosing the most economic way of delivering optimal care. Why use parenteral nutrition if enteral nutrition will do? Why use percutaneous endoscopic gastrostomy (PEG) if short-term enteral nutrition or sip-feeding will suffice? Doctors should also be aware of evidence from studies which specifically address cost benefit. One obvious example in the field of nutrition is the use of nutrition teams. Much evidence exists to show that the creation of a nutrition team provides substantial savings in the costs of nutritional support. Despite this, only 30% of UK hospitals had a properly established nutrition team in 1995.

9.7 Force-feeding

It is well established in law and ethics that competent adults have the right to refuse any medical treatment even if that refusal results in their death. This includes artificial nutrition and hydration. There are guidelines for assessing competence in adult patients (see above). In the UK, most of Europe, and the US there is no acceptance of the principle of 'retroactive consent' whereby a patient gives consent after receiving a therapy which was initially refused. In Israel, however, the patients' rights law does permit competent patients to be treated against their will on the basis that there is reason to believe that they would change their mind after treatment. This has led, for example, to enforced force-feeding of prisoners on hunger strike. Some authorities have reported this as an example of a severe breech of individual patient autonomy. Force-feeding hunger strikers or any other competent individual in most countries would constitute assault.

There is an ethical dilemma in the management of confused, semi-conscious, or demented patients who remove or dislodge feeding tubes or lines. The use of restraint may be seen as violating patient freedom and therefore their autonomy. Clinicians must exercise judgment, compassion, and commonsense in dealing with these scenarios.

The Mental Health Act in the UK permits the compulsory detention in hospital of patients with recognized mental disorders. This includes eating disorders such as anorexia nervosa. The law permits under certain circumstances the use of artificial nutritional support in these patients against their will on the basis that feeding is an integral part of their treatment. This might also apply to other patients deemed incompetent.

9.8 Conflict between relatives, friends or proxies, and carers

The views of people close to an adult patient carry no legal weight, although those with parental responsibility have the legal authority to make most decisions for children. Of course the opinions of relatives and others close to a patient may assist in the process of determining what is in the best interests of a patient if they are deemed incompetent. Studies have shown, however, that a relative's perceptions of a patient's likely views often differ substantially from the patient's own wishes.

It should be noted that clinicians are not obliged to offer useless interventions and these do not need to be discussed with patients. In the situation whereby a relative demands artificial nutrition against medical advice then, legally, the clinician is not obliged to accede to such requests. Such cases have already come to the courts in America. Clearly, the clinician must act in what he or she considers the best interests of the patient and where possible decisions should be evidence-based.

Many authors have referred to this potential conflict between relatives and carers. Most now agree that doctors have little to fear in the legal arena when withholding therapy if the clinical judgment is made in the best interests of the patient. The Canadian Law Report examined three options for ensuring consent and protection of patients. These included a judicial model, a family or guardian consent model, and the medical model. The Law Commission comprised of leading Canadian lawyers embraced the last placing primary responsibility for prescribing on the physician. It was emphasized however that medical decisions should be made after consultation with those close to the patient. This view has been echoed in the UK and by the American Medical Association. It would appear therefore that there is a consensus that doctors remain the final arbiters of treatment decisions. Against this, it must be recognized that the massive increase in medical litigation worldwide may reflect a growing public opinion that challenges the appropriateness of doctors taking decisions in isolation. There is undoubted pressure on the medical establishment to involve patients, their carers, or patient interest groups in difficult or controversial treatment decisions.

Conflicts might also arise because of strongly held cultural or religious beliefs. When religious principle conflicts with medical opinion, legal judgments have ruled that personal conviction cannot override public policy. Thus a doctor cannot be forced to treat against the dictates of his or her professional conscience, especially when acting according to a widely held professional view.

9.9 Application of ethical principles to artificial nutritional support: clinical scenarios

Stroke

Cerebrovascular accidents are common. Many are minor and the effects transitory. However, in some the effects are devastating. Up to a third of patients may have dysphagia with inevitable problems with oral intake. There is evidence to show that the nutritional status of these patients deteriorates during admission and this, together with dysphagia, is associated with poorer outcomes. There would seem to be, therefore, a strong case to be made for artificial feeding in these patients and indeed many clinicians recommend early instigation of feeding, although the evidence in favor of this practice is limited. A number of studies have reported their experiences with feeding, usually with nasogastric tubes or percutaneous gastrostomies. A recent review of this topic concluded that there was no evidence to suggest that tube feeding improves outcomes such as aspiration pneumonia, survival, risk of pressure sores, infections, or function. Further, there is conflicting evidence regarding the optimum time for instigation of therapy. Some studies have reported high mortalities soon after PEG insertion, with most deaths occurring as a consequence of the stroke or other concurrent disease.

Against this background of uncertainty over the benefits of nutritional support in patients with stroke disease, how should the clinician approach the problem of deteriorating nutritional status in these patients? A number of factors are important: first it must be recognized that the poor results so far reported in the literature may well reflect the inappropriate feeding of patients with pre-existing poor prognosis. Second, it is imperative to carefully assess patients for a few days after admission. Several studies indicate that the patient's condition on admission is the best indicator of prognosis. The most significant determinant factors are dysphagia, anthropometric measures, and albumin. Mortality in stroke patients is more than 50% at one month and outcomes are worse in those with deteriorating nutritional status. Dysphagia is present in up to 40% of patients on admission and this will reduce to about 16% at one week. A powerful case can be made therefore for delaying the instigation of feeding for one week after admission. Not only will this policy prevent ongoing malnutrition in those patients with

an expectation of satisfactory outcome, but in addition it permits time for full assessment of the patient, including discussions with medical staff, speech therapists, dietitians, and relatives.

More importantly, delay for a week may permit recovery from aphasia or dysarthria such that the patient's views can be carefully considered. Where reasonable doubt exists over outcomes then time-limited trials of therapy should be considered. Most authorities would agree that feeding in these patients should in the first instance be through a fine-bore nasogastric tube. These are associated with minimal morbidity and feeding is easily discontinued if ability to swallow returns. Several published studies advocate the use of a percutaneous gastrostomy if long-term feeding is required, either because of persistent dysphagia or inadequate intake. Most recommend that these invasive methods of feeding should only be considered 2–4 weeks after the initial stroke.

Considering the principles of beneficence and nonmaleficence in these patients there is no doubt harm will result from inadequate intakes and that some will benefit from some form of nutritional support. The duty of the doctor is to employ those feeding techniques that are most effective and impose least burden on the patient. The concept of justice necessitates the attending physician to make a judgment of outcome. Allocation of resources is justified if recovery is anticipated, particularly if a good quality of life is expected. The problem for the ethicist arises if recovery is uncertain. This raises the question of medical futility. In practice it is often impossible to know what progress the patient may or may not make. In these circumstances there is much to recommend the instigation of time-limited trials of therapy. The implementation of time-limited trials of therapy facilitate decision-making by emphasizing that clinical situations evolve. Thus, whereas nutritional support may be justified early in the course of the disease, after some weeks without tangible progress or actual deterioration then the clinician is ethically justified to discontinue therapy on the basis of medical futility.

Recognition of the principle of autonomy in any unconscious patient necessitates the clinician making an assessment of what the patient would have wanted had they been in a position to express a view. All efforts must be made to ensure the patients right to self-determination. In some instances patients may have expressed their views in an advance directive which has to be accepted.

Dementia

One consequence of the aging of the population has been a dramatic rise in the incidence of Alzheimer's disease. It has been estimated that there are currently four million cases in the United States. Patients with advanced dementia frequently have difficulties with swallowing and lose interest in eating. In these, the decision is often made to insert a feeding tube. A number of factors need to be considered before embarking upon artificial feeding in these patients; first, it should be recognized that feeding tubes often fail to provide adequate nutrition because of problems with diarrhea, clogging, and the tendency of patients with dementia to pull out the tubes. Secondly, tubes are sometimes employed on the basis that they interrupt the cycle of eating, predisposing to aspiration with consequent pneumonia. There is now good evidence to show that feeding tubes do not prevent aspiration. Some authorities recommend the use of gastrostomies or jejunostomies but the evidence that these reduce aspiration is tenuous and on any account they are themselves associated with considerable morbidity. Thirdly, there is little evidence that tube feeding prolongs life. One reason for this which is important in the assessment of patients with dementia is that difficulty with eating is a marker of severe dementia. Its occurrence probably indicates that patients have entered the terminal phase of their disease. Finally, patients with dementia do not have the cognitive capacity to understand the purpose of feeding tubes, whether nasogastric or transabdominal, with the result that they require restraining to prevent them from pulling them out.

There is increasing support for the view, eloquently argued by Gillick (2000), that artificial feeding techniques should not be used in patients with advanced dementia. It is recognized that there will always be exceptions and uncertainties such as the patient with vascular disease in whom improvements in cognitive function may occur. This emphasizes the importance of careful neurological assessment in confirming diagnoses. It is noteworthy that a consideration of patient autonomy supports these views. In a prospective study of 421 randomly selected and competent nursing home residents only a third would favor a feeding tube if they were unable to eat because of permanent brain damage. Furthermore 25% of respondents who initially favored feeding changed their minds when informed that physical restraint might be necessary. It is interesting to speculate that even more patients would

have opposed feeding if they were fully informed as to outcome data for feeding in patients with dementia.

Clearly, there will be many occasions when relatives and friends will place considerable pressure on medical staff to instigate feeding in the belief that not to do so is commensurate with starving their loved one to death. These understandable anxieties need to be discussed in full. It needs to be emphasized that the balance of benefits and burdens is rarely in support of feeding in these patients and there is evidence to suggest that these patients will not experience hunger or thirst. Where conflict or uncertainty prevail, time-limited trials using therapies with minimal morbidity may be justified.

Wasting disorders: cancer, AIDS, and terminal illness

These conditions are characterized by involuntary loss of body weight and lean tissue in the setting of chronic illness. There is a direct relationship between mortality and loss of either body weight or lean body mass. Furthermore, starvation-induced malnutrition has numerous deleterious effects on physiological and cognitive function which impair daily activities and quality of life. The association between wasting and death has led to the assumption that prevention or reversal of wasting might delay or prevent death and be associated with improved quality of life. Regrettably there is little evidence to support this view.

These patients are frequently cachectic and their appearance is distressing to those around them. It is understandable that the view is often taken that correction of malnutrition is justified as correction of obvious malnutrition or dehydration must bring about improved quality of life. These assumptions are difficult to substantiate but are fundamental to the ethical debate that surrounds the withholding or withdrawing of artificial nutrition from terminally ill patients. In essence, the critical question is whether or not the absence of feeding leads to or causes a cruel and painful demise. There is little in the literature that addresses this question but existing documentation suggests that death accompanied by starvation and dehydration is in fact painless and humane. For example, studies in the hospice movement have shown that terminally ill patients do not experience more than transient hunger and that any thirst can be easily offset by mouthcare.

The paucity of evidence for benefit for nutritional support in these patients and the fact that any nutritional intervention can itself be associated with harm does not mean that nutritional support is never indicated. Basic care in the form of offered oral nutrients should never be withdrawn and there will often be cases where the clinician feels that the patient has not entered the terminal phase of their illness where nutritional support might be indicated to achieve specific short-term goals. This merely serves to emphasize that patients need to be assessed on an individual basis. Decisions over nutritional therapy must be discussed with the patient and relatives in the context of available evidence. The responsibility of clinicians is to avoid interventions that they know to be futile.

Clinical judgment must decide whether the patient's inability to eat is irreversible and a consequence of overwhelming disease. If so, then nutritional support can at best delay the dying process and at worst result in discomfort or morbidity with no benefits in terms of quality or quantity of life. Inappropriate feeding has resource implications, but more importantly is unfair on the individual patient, who is given unrealistic expectations of therapy.

Malnutrition in the hospitalized patient

Many patients in hospital suffer malnutrition. These include the preoperative patient, the postoperative patient, the cancer patient, and the chronically ill. In all of these groups starvation and subsequent malnutrition may occur as a complicating factor during the course of the patient's illness. Considering the principles of beneficence and non-maleficence one is immediately confronted with the dilemma that no consensus exists as to the benefit of nutritional support therapy in many patient groups. This probably reflects the use of inappropriate outcome measures in many studies. Nutritional therapy, like ventilatory or renal support, is not a disease-specific treatment and assessment of benefit should be based primarily on the correction or otherwise of nutritional abnormality. In other words it is important in assessing any potential benefit as opposed to the burden of nutritional therapy to separate the benefits of treating any underlying disease from allaying the effects of starvation.

There is no doubt that starvation is harmful; death from protein–energy malnutrition occurs within 60–70 days of total starvation in normal adults. Functional metabolic deficits occur after some 10–15 days semi-starvation in previously healthy adults and shorter periods in those already compromised by disease. The consequences of starvation are well known and, apart from weight loss, include impairment of the immune response, alterations in organ function, malaise, lethargy, and changes in cognitive function. Against this background of information on the causes and consequences of malnutrition, it is a relatively simple matter to make recommendations for treatment. For instance, the American Society of Parenteral and Enteral Nutrition recently published guidelines for the use of parenteral and enteral nutritional support and recommends that a maximum period of seven days of a severely limited nutrient intake is the empirical absolute most investigators set for hospitalized patients (Allison, 1992). Most would add that a weight loss of 10–15% recalled pre-illness weight was also an indication for nutritional support.

What then is the ethical situation in those patients who have already or who are anticipated to be subjected to inadequate intakes of seven days or more? Taking the four principles previously outlined:

- *Beneficence*: There can be no doubt that nutritional deprivation does harm and that nutritional repletion by whatever means will prevent this, and presumably therefore, it is reasonable to assume that the nutritional support therapy provides benefit.
- *Non-maleficence*: There is no doubt that certain techniques of nutritional support, such as total parenteral nutrition (TPN) in inappropriate patients, can be harmful. The small percentage of complications arising from tube or PEG feeding, some of which can be serious or fatal, must be considered within the clinical background of each patient. This emphasizes the importance of the clinician tailoring the method of nutritional support that for a given patient will provide maximal benefit for minimal morbidity. The expected clinical benefit of feeding must always outweigh the significant risks and suffering caused to the patient.
- *Justice*: If it is accepted that some form of nutritional support should be considered in all patients with significant weight loss or in those who have sustained seven or more days of inadequate oral intake, then the resource implications are clearly enormous. Recent evidence suggests that up to one-fifth of all hospital admissions may be malnourished and up to one-half of all hospital patients have one or more abnormal parameters of nutritional status. Application of the ethical principle of justice requires that health professionals assess cost benefit of their treatments

and that these are based on sound evidence. It is very significant, therefore, that it is well established that malnourished patients have longer hospital stays and a greater incidence of morbidity and death than well-nourished individuals. The hospital cost associated with the treatment of a malnourished patient is significantly greater than that of a well-nourished patient without complications. Clinical trials have demonstrated that nutritional intervention improves clinical outcome, enhances wound healing, facilitates return of normal physiological function, and reduces hospital stay. It is worth reiterating that there is no precedent, legal or ethical, that justifies the absence of resources as a reason not to treat. The inability of clinicians to provide nutritional support either because of personal beliefs or institutional policy will necessitate the clinician making reasonable efforts to arrange for the prompt transfer of the patient's care to a practitioner or facility willing to implement appropriate treatment. This does not, however, permit the clinician to abrogate his or her responsibilities to ensuring that every effort is made to provide cost-effective nutritional support.

- *Autonomy*: If patients are made aware of the deleterious consequences of short-term starvation then it would seem reasonable to conclude that, if informed, they would request active measures to prevent harm. Unlike sophisticated medical therapies, patients understand the principles of nutritional support. The provision of food and water to the sick has a symbolic and an emotional role that transcends cultural, ethnic, and socioeconomic barriers. Patients already ask about antimicrobial therapy and other well-publicized treatments and will surely do the same with regards to nutrition therapy when there is a greater public awareness of the dangers of malnutrition as well as an appreciation of the options for nutritional support. There may be patients who specifically object to artificial means of nutritional support and in these cases the wishes of the patients will have to be respected.

9.10 Clinical guidelines in ethical care

The decision-making process surrounding the provision or withdrawal of artificial nutrition can be difficult. A clear understanding of the clinical goals of therapy, together with an appreciation of the ethical issues involved facilitates resolution of dilemmas. Ap-

plication of the four principles of autonomy, beneficence, non-maleficence, and justice is one approach and is recommended. Figure 9.1 illustrates how these principles may be used to assist the clinician in the decision as to whether to feed or not to feed. Contemporary thinking, both ethical and legal, places most emphasis on the patient's right to self-determination, autonomy, which is reflected here.

The first question that must be asked is whether or not the patient is eating normally. Clearly, if so, then he or she must be encouraged to maintain adequate intakes and ideally these should be monitored by the health care team. If uncertainty exists, formal assessment of intakes is appropriate. In these situations no ethical dilemmas occur. If the patient is not eating adequately, then the next question must be to involve the patient. Is the patient competent? If so, then the pros and cons of feeding must be discussed with clear expositions as to possible outcomes and potential morbidity. The patient has the right to refuse therapy. If he or she does so, then respect for the patient's wishes is paramount. If appropriate, all palliative care must be offered together with unforced offers of oral hydration or nutrients. The patient should have the opportunity to change his or her mind at any point. Doctors here have a responsibility to outline the futility of treatments if this is relevant to a given situation.

If the patient is deemed incompetent, then the next enquiry should be towards establishing whether or not the patient has an advance directive. Note that this does not have to be a formalized witnessed written document. Contemporaneous records in a patient's notes, such as a general practitioner's, may suffice. If there is an advance directive and this specifically refers to life-prolonging therapy then the wishes of the patient must be observed. Not to do so renders the attending doctor liable to the charge of assault. In the absence of a valid advance directive then the doctor must make a decision as to whether or not treatment is futile. This necessitates a clear decision as to the objectives of therapy. Does the patient fulfil any of the justifiable conditions for non-treatment, would treatment not be in the best interests of the patient. Doctors are not obliged to instigate therapies which they perceive will do no good for the patient.

Genuine uncertainty over the futility of treatment necessitates discussions with other members of the health care team, possible second opinions, and involvement of the relatives. All endeavors must be made to attempt to establish what the patient might have

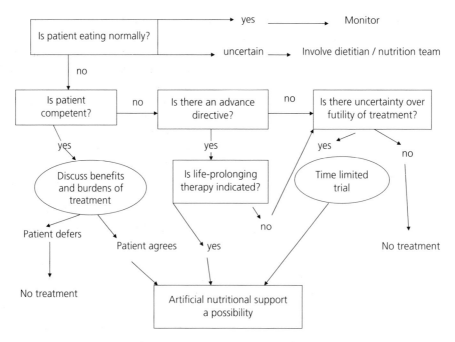

Figure 9.1 How the four principles of autonomy, beneficence, non-maleficence, and justice may be used to assist the clinician in the decision as to whether to feed or not to feed. Consider:
- Is swallowing normal? – sip feeding, nasogastric feeding, PEG
- Is the gut functioning? – sip/enteral feeding versus parenteral
- Specific nutrient requirements – vitamin B$_{12}$, thiamine, trace elements
- Have outcomes been decided?
- Has it been written in the notes?
- Has it been discussed with colleagues? (nutrition team/relatives, second opinion)
- Is it hospital or community?

wanted were they in a position to express a view. The overriding factor must be to do what is in the best interests of the patient. Continuing uncertainty is a good reason for commencement of a time-limited trial of therapy. The goals and timespan of such trials must be clearly recorded and frank and open discussions with relatives and other carers are essential.

When a decision is made to consider artificial nutrition support, whether indefinitely or as a time-limited trial, then the following questions must be asked: is swallowing normal, is the gut functioning, are there specific nutrient requirements, have outcomes been decided, has it been recorded in the notes, are the relatives and other members of the team involved, and is the intention hospital or community care? In this way optimal nutritional support appropriate to an individual patient ensuring minimal morbidity is more certain.

Throughout this process patients should be encouraged to state their preferences and, if this is not possi-

ble, then the views of the patient's surrogates, relatives, friends, or medical or legal representative should be sought. The most important factor is the best interests of the patient. In some circumstances there will be disagreement between members of the health care team or patient surrogates as to what is in the best interests of the patient. This might reflect conflicts in religious, ethnic, or other value systems. These must be discussed openly before the instigation or withdrawal of therapy, particularly if disagreements have been identified. Clinicians must be seen to be transparently honest in their discussions with all concerned. They must avoid the temptation to arbitrarily impose their value systems or preferred biases in feeding modality in the absence of evidence. It is not for the individual clinician to make recommendations for treatment or its withdrawal on the basis of resource considerations. When doubt persists as to the validity of treatments it is the patient's preferences, when fully informed, or their presumed preferences based on discussions with others that take precedence over health care systems or an individual doctor's opinions, providing this serves the patient's best interests.

9.11 Perspectives on the future

The implications of recognizing nutritional support as a medical therapy and of assessing its provision on the basis of accepted ethical principles are far reaching. First, there would seem to be a sound philosophical argument that dictates that all patients who have inadequate intakes for seven days or more should at least be offered advice on nutritional care. A documented dietetic referral may suffice. Secondly, failure to appraise and document nutritional status may, in the future, have medico-legal consequences. Thirdly, there is an urgent need to raise the awareness of nutritional problems and their treatment in both medical and nursing professions. Finally, the financial implications of these recommendations are enormous. While dietetic advice, sip feeding, and certain techniques of enteral nutrition are not in themselves expensive, the inevitable consequence of an increased awareness of nutritional problems will be an increase in the use of expensive nutritional support techniques.

The giving of artificial nutrition, where indicated, is not sufficient in itself. It must also be done well and conducted according to nationally accepted standards and guidelines. Failure to do this or to provide resources and expert staff to carry this out may be construed as unethical and may leave doctors and hospitals, in the future, open to legal action in the courts.

Clinical decision-making, including the provision of nutritional support, is increasingly informed by ethical and legal, as well as clinical considerations. Doctors must practice on the basis of evidence concerning the efficacy of nutritional support and the means of providing it, moderated by compassion and consideration for the patient and their families. All clinicians involved in the provision of nutritional support should keep updated with legal amendments to the ever-changing landscape of medical ethics. New legal precedents are being created on a regular basis and clinicians involved with end-of-life decisions must keep abreast of these developments. For instance, there was extensive press coverage recently concerning a patient with spino-cerebellar ataxia. In the Court of Appeal it was ruled that not to provide nutritional support in the future for this patient might cause 'intolerable' suffering. The implication of this judgment was that, in future, doctors might be expected to provide artificial nutrition and other life-prolonging treatments for all legally incompetent patients, unless they had previously rejected it by signing valid advance directives. This has major implications and the decision is being appealed by the General Medical Council (Gillon, 2004). Another recent development is the argument that hospital nutrition should be considered a human right (Kondrup, 2004). If accepted this also has wide ranging clinical implications.

In conclusion, the application of simple ethical principles to the use of nutritional support is likely to have a significant impact on clinical practice, particularly in western society where the morality of different treatment strategies are increasingly being subjected to public scrutiny.

References and further reading

American Society of Parenteral and Enteral Nutrition. Guidelines for the use of parenteral and enteral nutrition in adult and pediatric patients. *JPEN J Parenter Enteral Nutr* 1993; 17: 1SA–52SA.

Allison SP. The uses and abuse of nutritional support. *Clin Nutr* 1992: 11; 319–330.

Arras JD, Steinbock B, eds. *Ethical Issues in Modern Medicine*, 4th edn. California: Mayfield Publishing, 1995.

Beauchamp TL, Childress JF, eds. *Principles of Biomedical Ethics*, 4th edn. Oxford, New York: Oxford University Press, 1994.

British Medical Association. *Withholding and Withdrawing Life-prolonging Medical Treatment*. London: BMA Books, 1999.

Gillick MR. Rethinking the role of tube feeding in patients with advanced dementia. *N Engl J Med* 2000; 342: 206–210.

Gillon R. Why the GMC is right to appeal over life prolonging treatment. *BMJ* 2004; 329: 810–811.

Gillon R, Lloyd A. *Principles of Health Care Ethics*. London: John Wiley and Sons, 1993.

Glick SM. Unlimited human autonomy – a cultural bias? *N Engl J Med* 1997; 336: 994–996.

Kondrup J. Proper hospital nutrition as a human right. *Clin Nutr* 2004:135–137.

Leaning J. War crimes and medical science. *BMJ* 1996; 313: 1413–1415.

Lipman T. Enteral nutrition and dying. Ethical issues in the termination of enteral nutrition in adults. In: *Enteral and Tube Feeding*, 3rd edn (J Rombeau, Rolando H Rolandelli, eds). Philadelphia: WB Saunders and Co, 1997.

10
The Gastrointestinal Tract

Miguel A Gassull and Eduard Cabré

Key messages

- Celiac disease is an intestinal mucosal disorder caused by hypersensitivity to gluten present in several cereal grains, such as wheat, barley, rye, and possibly oats. Symptoms range from severe malabsorption to oligosymptomatic cases, often with extradigestive symptoms (anemia, osteopenia), which are particularly frequent in adults.
- The only effective treatment for celiac disease is the absolute withdrawal of gluten from the diet for life. This is particularly important to minimize the risk of late complications, such as intestinal lymphoma or other gastrointestinal malignancies.
- Tropical enteropathy and tropical sprue are a group of disorders mainly affecting the small intestine of individuals living in, or visiting, the tropics. Correction of water and electrolyte imbalances and nutritional replacement are the

basis for the management of tropical sprue.
- Protein–energy malnutrition and other micronutrient deficiencies are frequent in patients with inflammatory bowel disease (IBD) and result from a combination of poor nutrient intake, increased metabolic demands, increased intestinal protein losses, and nutrient malabsorption.
- If patients with IBD are severely malnourished or suffering from severe inflammatory bouts of the disease, they will need to be treated with artificial nutrition.
- Many patients with irritable bowel syndrome believe that their symptoms are triggered by specific foods but this is difficult to prove scientifically. However, specific sugar malabsorptions should be investigated, by means of the hydrogen breath test, in those patients in whom diarrhea and/or bloating continue to occur.

10.1 Introduction

The majority of the diseases of the gastrointestinal (GI) tract are not fatal but are significant causes of poor health, responsible for significant proportions of patients attending hospital and local medical services. The major conditions associated with the GI tract are summarized in Box 10.1.

Infectious diseases of the GI tract are covered in Chapter 20, malignant disease of the GI tract is dealt with in Chapter 21, pancreatitis in Chapter 12, and liver disease in Chapter 11. Management of food allergy is covered in Chapter 7.

Dysphagia

Dysphagia (difficulty in swallowing) is a common consequence of many different types of illness or injury resulting in mechanical or neurological impairment of the swallowing process. Swallowing occurs in two phases

Box 10.1 The major conditions associated with the GI tract

- Diarrhea and vomiting
- Dyspepsia
- Peptic and duodenal ulcers
- Constipation, abdominal pain, and irritable bowel
- Hemorrhoids and anal fissure
- Dysphagia
- Hernia
- Gallstones
- Appendicitis
- Malabsorption syndromes
- Ulcerative colitis and Crohn's disease
- Diverticular disease of the colon
- Pancreatitis
- Liver disease
- Food intolerance

– oropharyngeal and esophageal. In the oropharyngeal phase, food in transferred from the mouth via the pharynx to the upper esophagus. The esophageal phase carries

Table 10.1 The most common causes of dysphagia

Type of dysphagia	Causes
Oropharyngeal	
Neuromuscular	Stroke
	Head injury
	Muscular disorders
	Motor neuron disease
	Parkinson's disease
Physical obstruction	Pharyngeal pouch
	Goiter
Physiological	Globus hystericus
Infections	Tonsillitus
Oesophageal	
Neural	Achalasia
	Multiple sclerosis
	Diffuse esophageal spasm
Muscular	Scleroderma
	Dystrophia myotonica
Physical obstruction	Stricture
	Cancer
	Chronic esophagitis
	Diverticulum
	External compression (aortic aneurysm)
	Postoperative
Infections	*Candida*

food from the pharynx to the stomach. Some of the most common causes of dysphagia are listed in Table 10.1.

Attempting to swallow foods or liquids without the ability to do so carries a high risk of aspiration pneumonia and is potentially fatal. It is very important that if dysphagia is suspected that the patient's swallow is assessed by a health professional qualified to do so. Dysphagia is almost always accompanied by a reduced food intake leading to significant weight loss, compromised immune function, and a high risk of dehydration. The primary aims of management of dysphagia are listed in Box 10.2.

Box 10.2 The primary aims of management of dysphagia

- Assess the nature of the swallowing problem
- Determine a safe and adequate feeding route
- Determine the appropriate texture and consistency of food and fluids
- Meet nutritional needs
- Ensure adequate hydration status
- Educate patient and/or carers
- Monitor progress and ensure continuity of care

Box 10.3 Causes of gastroesophageal reflux disease

- Esophageal sphincter weakness
- Increased pressure within the stomach
- High pressure from the abdominal area (obesity or pregnancy)
- Hiatus hernia

Gastroesophageal reflux disease

Gastroesophageal reflux occurs as a normal event and clinical features only occur when antireflux mechanisms fail enough to allow gastric contents to make prolonged contact with the lower esophageal mucosa. The presence of acid and enzymes irritates the mucosa, causes pain, and repeated attackes may cause mucosal damage and inflammation (esophagitis). This in turn increases the risk of adenocarcinoma. Causes of gastroesophageal reflux disease are listed in Box 10.3.

About 50% of patients can be treated successfully with simple antacids, loss of weight, and raising the head of the bed at night. Dietary changes that may help to manage gastroesophageal reflux disease include:

- Eating smaller meals more frequently
- Avoiding eating late at night
- Avoiding bending, lifting, or lying down after meals
- Reducing weight if overweight
- Avoiding excessive consumption of caffeine-containing drinks and alcohol
- Avoiding highly spiced foods or those foods known to exacerbate symptoms.

Cancer of the esophagus and stomach

Surgical treatment of cancer of the esophagus may be partial or total esophagectomy, esophagogastrectomy, or partial or total gastrectomy, depending on the site and extent of the cancer. Since many of these patients may be severely nutritionally compromised, preoperative and early postoperative nutritional support is often necessary (see Chapter 8). Weight loss, iron deficiency anemia, vitamin B_{12} deficiency, and osteomalacia may all occur after gastric surgery and must be identified and managed.

Short bowel syndrome

Short bowel syndrome occurs after small bowel resection where less than 1 m of the bowel remains. The management of these patients depends on the amount of bowel resection, the site of the section and the presence or absence of the ileocecal valve. Intestinal adaptation can occur postoperatively, leading to hypertrophy of the mucosal surface and lengthening of the villi, leading to a substantial increase of the absorptive surface.

The fact that GI tract disease is a major cause of malnutrition for patients both in hospital and the community is not surprising, given its pivotal role in digestion and absorption. In some conditions, such as celiac disease and some food allergies, the illness is caused by the intolerance of some nutrient, and treatment is based on the withdrawal of the offending foodstuff. In other situations, such as GI tract infections and tropical enteropathy, the causative agent is not dietary, but consequences of the illness are nutritional and metabolic in nature and need to be managed.

In other conditions, such as IBD (ulcerative colitis and Crohn's disease), where the etiology is unknown, nutritional support may not only provide macro- and micronutrients, but certain elements may play a pharmacological role in the management of the disease itself. Finally, in functional intestinal diseases, dietary management may play a role in alleviating or reducing symptoms.

This chapter will focus on the nutritional consequences and management of some non-neoplastic diseases of the small bowel and the colon. These include:

- celiac disease,
- tropical enteropathy and tropical sprue,
- IBD, and
- irritable bowel syndrome and diverticular disease.

10.2 Celiac disease

Celiac disease – also termed celiac sprue or gluten-sensitive enteropathy – is a disease of the small bowel characterized by:

- malabsorption of nutrients by the damaged portion of the small intestine,
- a characteristic, although unspecific, lesion of the intestinal mucosa, and
- prompt clinical and histological improvement after withdrawal of gluten from the diet.

Epidemiology

The true prevalence of celiac disease is probably unknown since many patients have mild or no symptoms, and in these cases the disease often remains undiagnosed. In most European countries, the prevalence of the disease ranges from 0.05% to 0.2%. Some studies report an increased incidence of celiac disease in the last 20 years. This must be due, at least in part, to an increasing awareness of the disease and the recognition of oligosymptomatic patients. Classically, celiac disease seemed to be less frequent in the USA. However, recent studies of serological screening in blood donors suggest that the frequency is the same as in Europe.

Although some ethnic groups – including Scandinavians, Italians, Irish, British, Spaniards, Jews, and Palestinians – are particularly at risk, celiac disease is considered worldwide. However, it is rare in Africa, the Far East, and the Caribbean.

Pathogenesis

Celiac disease is a hereditary illness. Its development is strongly associated (90–95% of cases) with the HLA haplotype DQw2 on chromosome 6. However, environmental factors also play a role in the development of the disease.

The most important environmental factor for developing celiac disease in susceptible individuals is gluten, a protein component of several cereal grains. Some alcohol-soluble fractions of gluten, termed prolamines, are particularly harmful. These are α, β, γ, and Ω gliadins (from wheat), hordeins (from barley), secalins (from rye), and possibly avidins (from oats). In contrast, rice and corn are not harmful to the intestinal mucosa.

Some factors may play a role in precipitating symptoms. These include GI surgery, pregnancy, high-dose or early gluten challenge, and viral infection. Breast-feeding seems to delay the age of onset of celiac disease, but there is no clear evidence that it reduces the lifetime risk for developing the disease.

There is now evidence that celiac disease is an intestinal immunological disease. In brief, selected prolamin peptides are presented by distinctive surface HLA heterodimers to specific T cells. T cell activation then results in a cascade of proinflammatory cytokines. At the same time, B cells and plasma cells produce antibodies which stimulate the release of other noxious mediators, possibly causing cell-mediated cytotoxicity. As a result of this process the intestinal mucosa becomes damaged.

Celiac disease may occur in association with other immune-based diseases (Box 10.4). Individuals suffering from these conditions should be screened for celiac disease. Amongst these associated diseases, dermatitis herpetiformis deserves special mention. This is a itchy bullous skin rash that involves the extensor surfaces of the limbs, trunk, and scalp, characterized histologically by the deposition of immunoglobulin A (IgA) granules in the dermal–epidermal junction. The disease is accompanied by intestinal damage, sometimes asymptomatic, but indistinguishable from that seen in celiac disease. In fact, both the intestinal and cutaneous lesions regress with dietary gluten withdrawal. Thus, dermatitis herpetiformis is at present considered as part of the spectrum of gluten-sensitivity rather than a condition merely associated with celiac disease.

Magnitude of the problem: The spectrum of gluten-sensitivity

Celiac disease involves the mucosa of the small bowel, whereas the submucosa, muscularis, and serosa are usually unaffected. Proximal segments of the bowel (duodenum and jejunum) are more often damaged, while ileal involvement is less frequent. The mucosal damage in celiac disease varies from almost normal morphology (latent celiac disease) to the classical picture of villous atrophy and 'flattened mucosa.'

Traditionally, celiac disease has been considered a pediatric disease, but it is also frequently diagnosed in adult life. Classical symptoms in children include diarrhea, vomiting, anorexia, irritability or apathy, and failure to thrive. In adults, the 'complete' celiac syndrome consists of chronic diarrhea, weight loss, malabsorption, and iron-deficiency anemia. In most severe cases, the so-called 'celiac crisis' would ensue if left untreated – with tetany, hemorrhagic diathesis, and edema – constituting a true GI emergency.

In the last decade it has become evident that celiac disease may present with only scarce and/or mild symptoms. This is particularly true in the adult, so that the diagnosis of the disease could be delayed. Digestive symptoms can be recurrent abdominal pain in children, as well as complaints of indigestion and bloating in adults. A number of patients have only extradigestive symptoms. Some of the most frequent manifestations, which may occur (alone or in combination) in absence of the classic malabsorptive syndrome in celiac disease, are listed in Box 10.5. Celiac disease may remain clinically silent for years despite the existence of histological lesions. This situation has been reported to occur in first-degree relatives of celiac patients and other risk groups.

Diagnosis and screening

The diagnosis of celiac disease is based on the demonstration of the characteristic histological findings in a well-oriented jejunal biopsy specimen, followed by clinical remission when the patient is put on a gluten-free diet. In 1990, the European Society of Paediatric Gastroenterology and Nutrition (ESPGAN) revised its diagnostic criteria, stating that a single jejunal biopsy could be enough for the diagnosis of celiac disease. The old ESPGAN criteria required a second biopsy after withdrawing gluten from the diet (which must be normal), followed by a third one after gluten challenge (where histological lesion must reappear). These two additional biopsies are no longer necessary except for:

- children younger than two years, when celiac disease can be difficult to distinguish from cow's milk protein intolerance, and
- patients who are asymptomatic at diagnosis, or those with minimal clinical response to a gluten-free diet.

Serologic tests, based on the detection of circulating antibodies to gliadin or connective tissues (endomysium, reticulin), are at present available for screening of celiac disease. These tests differ in their sensitivity and specificity (Table 10.2). Low-titers of antigliadin antibodies are often detectable in the general population, whereas anti-endomysium antibodies are usually negative in healthy subjects. Antigliadin antibodies have a lower specificity in younger children. Anti-endomysium and antireticulin antibody assays are much more specific, although antigliadin antibodies have been reported to be more sensitive in some studies. Thus, combinations of both antigliadin and anti-endomysium probably maximize the negative predictive value.

Serologic screening should be made in patients with clinical suspicion of celiac disease, in first-degree relatives of celiac patients, or in individuals suffering from any of the conditions associated with the disease (see Box 10.4). However, it must be stressed that serologic tests do not replace intestinal biopsy in the diagnosis of celiac disease. Moreover, patients with malabsorptive symptoms or signs must undergo jejunal biopsy irrespective of the results of the serological tests, in order to rule out an enteropathy other than celiac disease.

Negativization of antibodies can be used as monitoring test for compliance to the gluten-free diet.

Treatment

Celiac disease is perhaps the only disease above all other GI disorders where diet is the key to management. Patients with celiac disease and/or dermatitis herpetiformis must adhere to a strictly gluten-free diet for life. Cutaneous manifestations of dermatitis herpetiformis usually respond to treatment with sulfones (dapsone), but such a therapy fails to reverse the intestinal disease. A major reason for recommending absolute removal of gluten from the diet is prevention of late development of malignancies. Celiac patients have been found to have increased risk for malignancy – particularly T cell lymphoma of the small bowel, esophageal cancer, and cancer of the oropharynx – compared with the general population. A strict gluten-free diet for life decreases such a risk, although unfortunately this is not fully eliminated in the case of lymphoma.

Avoiding gluten is easier to say than to do. Follow-up studies indicate that only 50–70% of celiac patients maintain a strict gluten-free diet later in life. Non-compliance is more frequent in children and, particularly, in teenagers. Removal of obvious sources of the offending grains (wheat, rye, barley, and oats) such as bread, breakfast cereals, pasta, cakes, and pastry is relative easy. However, hidden sources of gluten are frequent as wheat flour is added in many manufactured food products. Adequate food labeling is very important in this setting. Lists of foods obviously containing gluten (and, then, forbidden), positively gluten-free (and, then, permitted), or possible surreptitious sources of gluten (to be considered with caution) are provided in Boxes 10.6 to 10.8.

Table 10.2 Serologic tests for celiac disease

Antibody class	Antigen	Method	Sensitivity (%)	Specificity (%)
IgG	Gliadin	ELISA	46–100	67–100
IgA	Gliadin	ELISA	31–100	85–100
IgA	Endomysium	IIF	57–100	95–100
IgA	Reticulin	IIF	29–100	95–100

ELISA, enzyme-linked immunosorbent assay; IIF, indirect immunofluorescence.

Box 10.6 Foods forbidden for celiac patients (obviously containing gluten)

- Bread and flour from wheat, rye, barley and oats (note: some patients can probably tolerate certain amounts of oats without risk)
- Cakes, pastry, biscuits, pies, and other baked goods made with these flours
- Italian pasta (spaghetti, macaroni, etc.), wheat semolina
- Manufactured products with the above flours (flans, custard, ice-creams, jelly, etc.)
- Malted foods (e.g. malted milk)
- Drinks containing cereals (beer, ale)

Box 10.7 Foods permitted for celiac patients (obviously gluten-free)

- Milk and other dairy products
- Any kind of fresh meat, fish, or other seafood
- Eggs
- Rice, corn, millet, buckwheat, sorghum, and any foodstuff made with flour from these cereals
- Tapioca, soybean
- Fruits, vegetables, potatoes
- Butter, margarine, oils and other fats
- Salt, pepper, vinegar
- Sugar, honey
- Coffee made with ground coffee beans, tea and other herbal infusions
- Homemade cakes and pastry without the offending flours

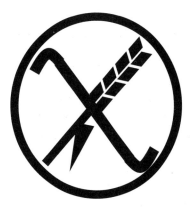

Figure 10.1 The international logo to identify gluten-free foodstuffs.

Box 10.8 Surreptitious presence of gluten in foods (not to be eaten by celiac patients, unless explicitly labeled as gluten-free by the manufacturer)

- Manufactured foodstuffs which might contain cereal flours as additive, thickening or flavoring agents
- Sausages, patés, luncheon meats, canned meats and poultry
- Meat sauces (soy, Worcestershire, etc.)
- Cheese spreads
- Salad dressings, mustard, catsup, tomato sauce, etc.
- Instant and canned soups, bouillon cubes
- Instant coffee and tea
- Candy bars, chocolate mixes
- As a rule, *any canned food*
- Contamination with flour of gluten-free products during harvesting, packaging, storage, or in the kitchen
- Residual gluten in 'gluten-free' wheat starch used in baked products
- Non-food items with trace amounts of gluten
- Excipients of some medications (either prescriptions or over-the-counter)
- Communion wafers
- Grain-derived alcoholic drinks (whisky, vodka, etc.)
- Misleadingly labeled foods

The institution of an effective gluten-free diet requires extensive education of the patient by his or her physician, as well as the advice of an experienced professional dietitian. Recipe books are also available in some countries. In addition, patients should be encouraged to contact and join the Celiac Societies or other support groups existing in many countries, which produce up-to-date lists of brands of gluten-free foods.

Commercially available brands of gluten-free foods (e.g. pasta, biscuits, bread) help to diversify the diet of celiac patients. These brands are internationally identified with a special logo (Figure 10.1). The Codex Alimentar-ius defines a food as gluten-free when 'the total nitrogen content of the gluten containing cereal grains used in the product does not exceed 0.05 g/100 g of these grain on a dry matter basis.' It is important to note that this norm does not refer to the minimal amount of gluten tolerated by a celiac patient. In some particularly susceptible patients, even this small amount could induce insidious symptoms. In addition, gluten-free brands are expensive. Therefore, they should be used merely as a complement of the celiac diet, which must be essentially based on naturally occurring gluten-free foods.

In the last 10 years, there is increasing evidence which suggests that some celiac patients can tolerate moderate amounts of oats. The source of oats must be free of gluten contamination (in harvesting, storing, or packaging) to be safe, and it is uncertain whether larger and long-term oats challenges would be harmless in these patients. Thus, if a celiac patient is going to consume oats, a pure source should be used, and continued monitoring for relapse should be maintained.

Besides avoiding gluten, celiac patients must eat an otherwise balanced diet, with normal amounts of nitrogen, fat, and carbohydrates. In most symptomatic cases the administration of iron, folate, fat-soluble vitamins (parenterally), and oral medium-chain triglycerides (as a caloric supplement) at the beginning of the therapy is useful. Epithelial damage leads to the loss of brush border enzymes and then to hypolactasia. In this setting, transient withdrawal of milk and its derivatives from the diet may be advisable. Patients with 'celiac crisis' would need intravenous fluid and electrolyte replacement, as well as calcium and magnesium administration to prevent tetany. Severely malnourished cases would benefit from enteral nutrition. These formulas may accelerate the recovery since most of them are absolutely free of both gluten and lactose.

Therapeutic failure

The great majority of celiac patients will recover both clinically and histologically on a strict gluten-free diet. Clinical improvement is usually apparent after only one or two weeks on the diet, although complete recovery may take several months.

A minority of patients (about 15%) do not improve with the diet, or their symptoms relapse after a variable period of time. The most important cause of therapeutic failure is incomplete removal of gluten from the diet. In many cases, the patient is unaware of this circumstance and an in-depth dietary interview is required to reveal it. As mentioned before, anti-endomysium antibodies usually become negative with total gluten withdrawal and are a useful tool for monitoring dietary compliance.

Recent studies indicate that a number of patients with celiac disease and persistent diarrhea suffer from another coexisting disease including exocrine pancreatic insufficiency, microscopic colitis, lactose or fructose malabsorption, intestinal bacterial overgrowth, and irritable bowel syndrome. This fact should be taken into account in assessing unresponsive celiac patients.

Another cause of therapeutic unresponsiveness in celiac disease is the development of an associated intestinal malignancy (mostly T cell lymphoma), particularly if the patient has low-grade fever. The risk for this neoplasm is increased in celiac patients despite a complete adherence to a gluten-free diet.

In a minority of celiac patients with therapeutic failure (either *de novo* or after initial response), none of the above circumstances can be demonstrated. This situation is arbitrarily termed refractory sprue. Some, but not all, of these patients will respond to steroids or other immunosuppressors.

10.3 Tropical enteropathy and tropical sprue

Concept and epidemiology

Aside from infectious intestinal diseases with known etiology, there is a group of GI disorders mainly affecting the small intestine of individuals predominantly living in – and less often visiting or returning from – developing countries, usually in the tropics. These disorders range from asymptomatic or oligosymptomatic structural and/or functional abnormalities of the intestinal mucosa (tropical enteropathy) to a fully symptomatic condition with malabsorption of nutrients, nutritional deficiencies, and a 'celiac-like' appearance of the intestinal mucosa (tropical sprue). It has been suggested that tropical enteropathy and tropical sprue may be the two ends of the same clinical and pathological spectrum, but this is far from been proven.

Epidemiological distribution of both conditions is one of the arguments against this view. Tropical enteropathy has been detected in most tropical regions of Asia, Africa, the Middle East, the Caribbean, and Central and South America. Tropical sprue, however, has a much more restricted geographical distribution, occurring in southern Asia, South-East Asia, the Caribbean and, to a much lesser extent, Central and South America. It almost never occurs in Africa.

Pathology, and clinical relevance

Tropical enteropathy is characterized by some reduction in intestinal villi height, often associated with hyperplasia of the intestinal crypts. This results in a reduction of the absorptive surface, cellular infiltration of the lamina propria, as well as cytological changes in the enterocytes. The clinical repercussion of tropical enteropathy is usually mild, so that it has been argued that this would be the 'normal state' for individuals living in these tropical developing areas.

In contrast to tropical enteropathy, tropical sprue is a much better defined clinical entity. Tropical sprue is a syndrome of chronic diarrhea often associated with steatorrhea, anorexia, abdominal cramps and bloating, weight loss, megaloblastic anemia, and edema. It may occur in epidemics in which the illness begins as an acute attack of watery diarrhea with fever and malaise which precede the chronic phase. When the situation has been maintained for months or even years, the clinical picture is dominated by nutritional deficiencies, sometimes in the absence of diarrhea.

Histopathologic changes in tropical sprue vary in intensity depending on the duration and severity of the illness. In well-established cases, the small intestinal histology mostly resembles that of celiac disease. In fact, celiac disease was formerly known as non-tropical sprue. Severe cases may also cause chronic atrophic gastritis (leading to vitamin B_{12} malabsorption due to the lack of intrinsic factor), and changes in the colonic mucosa similar to those of the small bowel, which lead to impaired absorption of water and sodium.

Pathogenesis

Tropical enteropathy is an acquired condition since newborns in developing countries have intestinal villi as high as those of newborns in western countries. The intestinal abnormalities begin to appear between the ages of four and six months, and could be due to a relatively hostile postweaning environment for the small intestine. The most plausible environmental factors are either an intestinal infection and/or bacterial overgrowth, or a nutritional deficiency. However, studies in British Indian and Afro-Caribbean people living for more than 30 years in the UK revealed the persistence of intestinal abnormalities, suggesting that a genetic predisposition to develop this disease may play a role.

As in tropical enteropathy, the cause of tropical sprue has not been clearly defined, but nutritional and infectious mechanisms seem to be involved. An important role has been proposed for bacterial colonization of the small bowel by both aerobic and anaerobic bacteria, but protozoal infection by agents such as *Cryptosporidium parvum*, *Isospora belli*, *Blastocystis hominis*, and *Cyclospora cayetanensis* may also be involved. Initial infectious damage would induce hormonal and functional abnormalities in the gut which would lead to active secretion of water and electrolytes and impaired intestinal motility, thus perpetuating the disease.

Treatment

Correction of water and electrolyte imbalance and nutritional replacement are the mainstay of the early management of cases of tropical sprue. In fact, nutritional intervention alone is responsible for the dramatic decrease in mortality of epidemic bouts of tropical sprue in southern India. Oral supplements of folic acid and iron and parenteral vitamin B_{12} should be promptly administered, leading to a rapid recovery of anemia and a marked appetite gain.

There is no specific pharmacological treatment for tropical sprue, but the long-term use of broad-spectrum antibiotic (such as tetracycline 250 mg four times daily from four weeks to several months) is recommended. However, subclinical malabsorption remains in a significant proportion of patients many years after being apparently cured with tetracyclines.

10.4 Inflammatory bowel disease

Definition

The term inflammatory bowel disease (IBD) includes ulcerative colitis and Crohn's disease. In both entities there is inflammation of the bowel mucosa with different patterns and degrees of severity. In ulcerative colitis the inflammatory phenomena only occur in the mucosa and submucosa of the colon, whereas the whole thickness of the bowel wall, from mucosa to serosa, is involved in Crohn's disease. In contrast to ulcerative colitis, which involves only the colon, Crohn's disease may affect any portion of the GI tract from the mouth to the anus, often in a segmentary pattern, although involvement of the terminal ileum and the right colon is the most frequent. In some cases of IBD involving only the colon, features of both ulcerative colitis and Crohn's disease are observed, so that a clear-cut diagnosis cannot be established. For these cases, the term indeterminate colitis is used.

Epidemiology

Incidence rates range between 2 and 12 per 100 000 population for ulcerative colitis, and 0.1 and 7 per 100 000 population for Crohn's disease. Both diseases are more frequent in northern countries (e.g. UK, Scandinavia, USA) than in southern countries (e.g. Mediterranean countries, South Africa, Australia), but in recent years these differences are decreasing. The incidence of ulcerative colitis remains stable, the occurrence of Crohn's disease appears to be increasing.

White populations are more often affected than non-white populations, and in some ethnic groups (e.g. Askenazi Jews) the frequency of the disease is particularly high. In most studies the incidence of IBD peaks in subjects between 15 and 30 years of age. A second smaller peak in incidence has been observed between 60 and 80 years, particularly for Crohn's disease.

Pathogenesis

The etiology of IBD is unknown. In both diseases there is a pattern of family aggregation suggesting a genetic basis which is not fully elucidated. It is thought that the pathogenesis of IBD may be the result of a combination of

- an exaggerated intestinal immune response to GI antigens or normal bacterial flora,
- a normal immunological response to noxious and as yet unknown stimuli, and
- autoimmune involvement.

All of these will trigger the release of inflammatory mediators (cytokines, eicosanoids, etc.), which will be responsible for the clinical and histological manifestations of the disease.

Clinical features and diagnosis

A detailed description of the clinical features of IBD is beyond the scope of this chapter. Both diseases typically have a chronic relapsing course. Bloody diarrhea is the main symptom of ulcerative colitis, whereas patients with Crohn's disease may present with different combinations of diarrhea, weight loss, abdominal pain, fever, and other digestive complaints. Fistulas between the intestinal loops, or between the gut and the skin or any hollow viscus in its vicinity, as well as perianal disease (abscess, fistulas) often occur in Crohn's disease. Moreover, both diseases may be associated with extraintestinal complaints including rheumatologic, ophthalmologic, cutaneous, and hepatobiliary diseases.

IBD is diagnosed by a set of clinical, endoscopic, and histologic characteristics. In ulcerative colitis, only the colon is involved and colectomy, either with permanent ileostomy or with an ileo-anal pouch anastomosis, is considered to be curative. In contrast, Crohn's disease may involve any part of the GI tract, often two or more segments at the same time. Moreover, after the surgical removal of the involved segment, the disease may recur at any level of the GI tract. Thus, although necessary in some cases, surgery cannot be envisaged as a curative therapeutic approach for Crohn's disease.

The chronic relapsing character of IBD, its predominance in young people, and the fact that the disease has no cure (except for colectomy in ulcerative colitis) contribute to a very negative socioeconomic impact of the disease, as well to a poor quality of life of these patients.

Treatment

As there is not a curative medical therapy for IBD, standard therapy, both in ulcerative colitis and Crohn's disease, relies on corticosteroids or amino-salicylates, depending on the severity and extent of the attack. A number of patients become resistant to these therapies or require long-term steroid therapy to remain asymptomatic. For these patients, a number of therapeutic strategies have been developed in the last two decades, including immunosuppressors (azathioprine, 6-mercaptopurine, cyclosporine, methotrexate), antibiotics (metronidazole, ciprofloxacin), or, more recently, the so-called modifiers of the biological response (monoclonal anti-tumor necrosis factor alpha (TNFα) antibodies, rh-IL-10).

Malnutrition in inflammatory bowel disease

Nutritional deficits are frequently observed in IBD, especially in Crohn's disease patients with extensive involvement of the small bowel. Malnutrition may manifest as weight loss, growth retardation, and delayed sexual maturation, anemia, asthenia, osteopenia, diarrhea, edema, muscle cramps, impaired cellular immunity, or poor wound healing.

The prevalence of protein–energy malnutrition in IBD ranges from 20% to 85%. This wide range is due to the fact that most studies put together ulcerative colitis and Crohn's disease, as well as hospitalized and ambulatory patients. This results in a marked heterogeneity of disease extension, inflammatory activity, and organ involvement (small or/and large bowel). It is considered that irrespective of steroid use, around 20–30% of children will become adults with abnormally short stature.

Two factors, seldom mentioned, may be relevant regarding the severity and type of malnutrition in IBD: (a) the time elapsed since the onset of the disease, which is usually longer in Crohn's disease, and (b) the acuteness of the attack, which is usually greater in ulcerative colitis. These factors are related to the type of protein–energy malnutrition developed, which is predominantly marasmatic or mixed in Crohn's disease, and hypoalbuminemic (kwashiorkor-like) in ulcerative colitis.

Pathogenic mechanisms for malnutrition in inflammatory bowel disease

- Poor nutrient intake
- Anorexia
- Upper GI tract involvement[a]
- Drug-induced dyspepsia
- Intestinal obstruction[a]
- Inadequate or restrictive diet
- 'Therapeutic' fasting
- Increased metabolism
- Increased energy expenditure
- Increased protein turnover (mainly breakdown)
- Increased intestinal protein losses
- Mucosal inflammation and ulceration
- Enteric fistulas[a]
- Impaired intestinal lymph drainage (mesenteric involvement)[a]
- Malabsorption
- Extensive small bowel involvement[a]
- Multiple intestinal resections (short bowel)[a]
- Intestinal bacterial overgrowth[a]
- Bile salt malabsorption (ileal dysfunction or resection)[a]
- Impaired intestinal lymph drainage (mesenteric involvement)[a]

[a]Only in Crohn's disease.

Pathogenesis of malnutrition in inflammatory bowel disease

Several factors are involved in the development of malnutrition in IBD (Box 10.9). The most important factors are poor nutrient intake, increased metabolism, increased intestinal protein losses, and nutrient malabsorption.

Poor nutrient intake

Inadequate intake of nutrients is common in IBD. Anorexia, nausea and vomiting, abdominal pain or discomfort, and/or medical restrictions on some foods are frequent in acute attacks of ulcerative colitis and Crohn's disease. In addition, in almost one-third of patients with Crohn's disease the upper GI tract (esophagus, stomach, and duodenum) may be involved, and approximately the same proportion will suffer from one or more episodes of intestinal obstruction during the course of their disease. In addition, some drugs used in the treatment of active disease may induce gastric upset (sulphasalazine, metronidazole, 5-ASA). All these factors negatively impact on food intake.

The possibility that alimentary antigens might act as triggering factors for the inflammatory response in IBD, and the fact that diarrhea is the most prominent symptom of these patients, led to the use of fasting as part of the treatment of acute attacks of both ulcerative colitis and Crohn's disease, in order to achieve 'bowel rest.' The consequence of this therapeutic approach was the deterioration of nutritional status and this treatment should no longer be advocated. Decreased food intake is still sometimes erroneously reinforced by attendants' and physicians' advice: in almost one-third of the patients a reduction in food intake could be related to an inadequate restricted diet, which prescribed a reduction of fat- and fiber-rich foods. Adequate dietary assessment may be crucial in preventing malnutrition in these patients. This may be achieved by offering palatable energy- and protein-rich foods which do not exacerbate the disease or symptoms of obstruction.

Increased metabolism

Reports on energy metabolism in patients with IBD have been contradictory. Energy expenditure has been reported to be either increased or reduced in these patients as compared with healthy subjects. This may be partly due to the fact that patients with different disease extension, inflammatory activity, and nutritional status were put together in the studies. However, when adjusted for body composition, an increase in resting energy expenditure is generally disclosed.

Protein turnover is also enhanced in IBD. Increase in both synthesis and breakdown of protein account for accelerated turnover. However, protein breakdown usually exceeds synthesis, the result being protein depletion.

Increased intestinal protein losses

Increased blood and protein losses through the inflamed intestinal mucosa is another contributing factor in the development of malnutrition in IBD. Protein losses parallel the degree of inflammation of the intestinal mucosa and the quantification of this phenomenon has been used as an index of disease activity. Moreover, the possible existence of intestinal bacterial overgrowth, abnormalities in the intercellular tight junctions of the mucosal epithelium, and the difficulties in the lymphatic drainage of the intestine may contribute to the protein-losing enteropathy associated with IBD.

Nutrient malabsorption

When Crohn's disease involves the small intestine, malabsorption of various nutrients may occur. This may be an important contributing factor for the development of protein–energy malnutrition in these patients. However, the inflamed mucosa itself is seldom the primary cause of gross nutrient malabsorption in Crohn's disease, except when the disease involves a very extensive area of the small intestine, or successive surgical resections have led to a short bowel syndrome. Nutrient malabsorption is more often secondary to bile acid malabsorption or intestinal bacterial overgrowth. Bile salt malabsorption often occurs when the terminal ileum is extensively diseased or has been resected. In such a situation, spill over of bile salts through the colon produces diarrhea, and decreases the bile salt pool leading to abnormal micellar solubilization and fat malabsorption. Intestinal bacterial overgrowth occurs in 30% of Crohn's disease patients, as a result of strictures in the small bowel or to the resection of the ileo-cecal valve. In addition to an increased consumption of vitamin B_{12}, small intestine bacterial overgrowth deranges carbohydrate and protein absorption and bile salt metabolism.

Micronutrient deficiencies in inflammatory bowel disease

Deficiencies of micronutrients in IBD, as well as their possible role in its pathogenesis, have been scarcely documented in the literature. The main problems in interpreting the reported results are:

- the absence of reference values in healthy individuals from the same geographical area,
- the lack of agreement about the type of sample to be analyzed for a particular micronutrient (whole blood, plasma, urine, or other tissue), and
- the concept of subclinical deficiency or inadequacy for a given element.

This concept may be of importance in IBD, since clinically apparent vitamin or trace element deficiencies seldom do appear (except for iron and folate). However, micronutrient inadequacies might play an important role in metabolic pathways relevant for the pathogenesis of the disease.

Vitamins

It is well known that patients on sulphasalazine can develop folate deficiency. Also, vitamin B_{12} malabsorption may occur in Crohn's disease patients with ileal involvement or resection, or intestinal bacterial over-

growth. Deficiencies of individual vitamins have been reported in IBD patients. In many cases low plasma vitamin levels are not accompanied by clinical signs of vitamin deficiency. The pathophysiological and clinical implications of suboptimal vitamin status found in active IBD are unknown. However, some vitamin-dependent enzyme systems are presumably altered in these patients. Low folate levels were associated to epithelial dysplasia in ulcerative colitis. Inappropriate levels of antioxidant vitamins (beta-carotene, vitamins A, E, and C) as well as biotin and vitamin B_2, involved in the scavenging of reactive oxygen metabolites and in the polyunsaturated fatty acid biosynthesis, may prove to be of pathobiological importance in the future.

Minerals and trace elements

Iron-deficiency anemia because of acute or chronic blood loss is frequent in patients with IBD. Deficiency of many other minerals and trace elements, including magnesium, zinc, selenium, copper, chromium, manganese, and molybdenum have been also described in these patients. Of these, zinc and selenium status deserve especial mention.

The clinical interest in evaluating zinc status in IBD relates to its role in growth retardation and because overt zinc deficiency associated with total parenteral nutrition can occur. Low serum zinc levels have been found in active and inactive Crohn's disease, and in active ulcerative colitis.

Serum selenium is low in patients with severe attacks of IBD, associated malnutrition, and/or long-standing disease. Glutathione peroxidase is a selenium-dependent enzyme with antioxidant functions, activity of which has been found to be decreased in plasma of patients with both ulcerative colitis and Crohn's disease. However, overt symptoms of deficiency, which include myopathy and cardiomyopathy, are rare.

Consequences of impaired nutrition in inflammatory bowel disease

General consequences of malnutrition in IBD (Box 10.10) do not differ from those in other disease states. Malnutrition is the second most common cause of secondary immunodeficiency (the first one is AIDS). Thus malnutrition renders patients with ulcerative colitis and Crohn's disease immunodepressed and hence more susceptible to infectious complications. A well-demonstrated effect of malnutrition in children with IBD is growth retardation and delayed sexual maturation. In both children and adults malnutrition contributes to the osteopenia associated with Crohn's disease. Additional consequences of malnutrition include delayed fistula healing, increased surgical risk and impaired healing of wounds, deficient transport of drugs by plasma proteins, and hypoplasia of the intestinal epithelium, which contributes to autoperpetuate the nutritional derangement. In recent years, there are growing evidences that some specific nutritional derangements may even play a role in the pathogenesis of abnormal immune response of IBD patients.

Nutritional support in inflammatory bowel disease

In previous sections, the rationale for nutritionally supporting patients with active IBD has been provided. Patients with mild to moderate attacks could be managed with an oral conventional diet. No major dietary restrictions should be prescribed in active disease except for avoiding coarse fiber (particularly in patients with ulcerative colitis, and in the presence of bowel strictures in Crohn's disease). Milk and its derivatives should not be restricted unless overt intolerance (e.g. increase in diarrhea) is observed.

Patients with inactive disease must eat a normal well-balanced diet. Coarse fiber has to be restricted in those patients with persistent intestinal strictures. The use of exclusion diets to maintain remission in Crohn's disease has been advocated by some authors but, with few exceptions, do not seem to be effective.

A significant number of patients with either ulcerative colitis or Crohn's disease will need to be nutri-

tionally supported with artificial nutrition at any time during the course of their illness. This is a major issue that will be discussed in more detail in the following paragraphs.

Artificial nutrition as adjuvant therapy in inflammatory bowel disease

As in other disease states, total parenteral nutrition (TPN) was the first modality of artificial nutrition to be used in patients with acute attacks of IBD. The rationale for this was the concept that 'bowel rest' was a cornerstone for the treatment of these patients. However, current available data indicate that 'bowel rest' is by no means necessary to induce remission both in Crohn's disease and ulcerative colitis. Randomized controlled trials in patients with both Crohn's disease and ulcerative colitis treated with steroids indicated that the remission rate was the same when patients received either TPN, or total enteral nutrition (TEN). Moreover, the frequency of side effects related to artificial nutrition is usually lower with TEN than with TPN. Interestingly enough, in those ulcerative colitis patients unresponsive to steroids who required to be colectomized, the rate of postoperative complications was also lower in those who had received TEN.

In the light of these data, TEN should be preferred to TPN in patients with IBD in whom artificial nutrition is indicated. In fact, enteral feeding has physiological advantages as it contributes to maintain intestinal trophism, and it is cheaper and safer than TPN. However, TPN must be used in patients who do not tolerate enteral feeding or in those situations where this is contraindicated, such as those with toxic megacolon, intestinal perforation, complete intestinal occlusion, massive GI bleeding, or fistulas arising in the mid-jejunum where the enteral diet could not be infused far enough (either proximally or distally) from the origin of the fistula.

Short-term enteral nutrition should be used in patients with active IBD (both ulcerative colitis and Crohn's disease) who are malnourished or at risk of become rapidly malnourished (e.g. those with severe attacks). In these cases, diet infusion through a fine nasoenteric tube with the aid of a peristaltic pump improves tolerance. Long-term enteral feeding (either nocturnal or cyclic) is a well-established treatment for preventing or reversing growth retardation in children and adolescents with Crohn's disease. Patients with complicated Crohn's disease may need long-term home enteral nutrition to maintain their nutritional status. In these circumstances, the insertion of a percutaneous endoscopic gastrostomy has to be considered. Prior to performing these procedures a careful endoscopic and histological study must be performed in order to rule out the possibility of gastric involvement by the disease, since a permanent fistulous tract may be favored if percutaneous gastrostomy is carried out on a previously diseased gastric wall.

Repeated or extensive intestinal resections may lead some patients with Crohn's disease to a status of intestinal insufficiency termed short bowel syndrome. In the early phases of the short bowel syndrome, protein and energy requirement should be provided with TPN, but small amounts of enteral feeding should also be administered to favor intestinal adaptation. In most patients, progressive weaning from TPN will be possible. A minority, however, will become dependent on home TPN for life. Factors influencing the adaptation of short bowel syndrome to enterally administered foods include the extent and site of the resected segment, as well as the presence of residual disease in the remnant bowel.

Enteral nutrition as primary treatment in Crohn's disease

Since the early 1980s, the possibility that enteral feeding could be used as primary treatment (i.e. could be able, *per se*, to induce remission) in this disease has been a matter of debate.

Meta-analyses of the published randomized controlled trials comparing TEN versus steroids in the treatment of active Crohn's disease have concluded that steroids are better than any type of enteral feeding. In spite of that, the overall remission rate with TEN is about 60%, a figure which is substantially higher than the 20–30% placebo response obtained in placebo-controlled therapeutic trials in Crohn's disease. This suggests that enteral nutrition would indeed have a role as primary treatment in active Crohn's disease. In addition, enteral feeding has been shown to be useful in preventing relapse in inactive Crohn's disease, particularly in children.

On the other hand, meta-analysis of the randomized trials comparing elemental (e.g. amino acid-based) and non-elemental (e.g. peptide- or whole protein-based) diets, as primary therapy in Crohn's disease, showed that both types of diets were equally effective. In other words, the primary therapeutic effect of TEN does not appear to depend on the type of nitrogen source.

The remission rates of 26 studies (both controlled and uncontrolled), including 673 compliant adult patients with active Crohn's disease treated with enteral diets for at least two weeks ranged from 36% to 100%, with a mean value of 75%. This wide range of remission indicates that not every enteral diet is equally effective. It has been hypothesized that differences in the amount or type of fat may partly account for these differences, but this is far from proven. Hence, identifying the nutrient (or nutrients) responsible for the therapeutic effect of enteral diets in Crohn's disease will be a hard task for the future. On the other hand, it could well be that some patients were more susceptible than others to the effect of enteral diet. Reliable assessment of disease-related predictive factors of response to enteral feeding will require the performance of large-scale trials. While such studies were not available, TEN should be tried as primary therapy for active Crohn's disease in those patients in whom steroids are especially harmful (i.e. children and adolescents, as well as in osteopenic elder patients or postmenopausic women). In any case, TEN should be kept in mind as a possible therapeutic alternative for steroid-resistant and, particularly, steroid-dependent Crohn's disease patients.

10.5 Irritable bowel syndrome and diverticular disease

Definition of irritable bowel syndrome

Irritable bowel syndrome – also referred to as irritable or spastic colon – is one or the commonest disorders seen at gastrenterology clinics (20–50% of referrals). Irritable bowel syndrome is a combination of chronic or recurrent GI symptoms not explained by structural or biochemical abnormalities. Although irritable bowel syndrome is a disorder of the whole bowel, colonic symptoms usually predominate. Thus, two general subsyndromes are recognized:

- abdominal pain plus constipation (often alternating with diarrheic episodes), which is more usual, and
- a less frequent picture of painless diarrhea.

Other symptoms include bloating, excess of flatus, passage of mucus in the stools, a sensation of incomplete rectal emptying, and proctalgia fugax (fleeting rectal pain).

At least three months of continuous or recurrent symptoms consisting of:

- Abdominal pain which is
- Relieved by defecation or
- Associated with a change in stool consistency or
- Associated with a change in stool frequency

With two or more of the following (at least on 1/4 of occasions or days):

- Altered stool frequency (>3 times/day or <3 times/week)
- Altered stool form (lumpy/hard or loose/watery)
- Altered stool passage (straining, urgency, or feeling of incomplete evacuation)
- Passage of mucus
- Bloating or abdominal distension

The absence of pathognomonic features makes irritable bowel syndrome a diagnosis of exclusion. Keeping this is mind, and to reduce the need for expensive and unnecessary investigations, attempts have been made for a positive diagnosis of irritable bowel syndrome. At present, the most widely accepted definition of irritable bowel syndrome are the so-called 'Rome criteria' which were reached by consensus of a panel of international experts who met in Rome in 1989 and 1992 (Box 10.11).

In addition of symptom assessment by means of the Rome criteria, a limited screening for organic disease seems mandatory. This includes complete physical examination, hematology counts and routine biochemistry analysis (including erythrocyte sedimentation rate and, probably, serum thyroid hormones), a search for ova and parasites in the stool, and a flexible sigmoidoscopy plus barium enema (or total colonoscopy in patients older than 50). Additional tests may be necessary according to the syndromic subtype or the particular characteristics of the patient.

Epidemiology of irritable bowel syndrome

As mentioned, irritable bowel syndrome is one of the most frequent causes of referral to the gastroenterologist. However, many patients do not seek for medical care. Thus, the true prevalence of irritable bowel syndrome must be estimated by symptom questionnaire in population surveys. A recent review of the published studies indicate that, in Britain and the USA, irritable bowel syndrome affects 14–24% of women and 5–19%

of men. In general, irritable bowel syndrome is more frequent in females. In studies that stratified groups by age there is a decrease in frequency among older subjects. The prevalence seems to be equal in white and black people, but may be lower in Hispanics. However, data on racial prevalence of irritable bowel syndrome are confounded by cultural influences. There are few epidemiological studies in non-western countries. The available data suggest that irritable bowel syndrome is rare in the sub-Saharian Africa, but would be common in Japan, China, the Indian subcontinent, and South America.

Pathogenesis of irritable bowel syndrome

A detailed description of the pathogenic mechanisms thought to be involved in the development of irritable bowel syndrome exceeds the purpose and scope of a textbook devoted to clinical nutrition. A neurobiological pathophysiological model for irritable bowel syndrome, which includes alterations in autonomic, neuroendocrine, and pain modulatory mechanisms, is currently being developed. Altered viscerosomatic sensitivity (the so-called 'visceral hyperalgesia') seems to play a key role in these models, leading to the development of symptoms of irritable bowel. Psychological stress and/or specific psychological disturbances (anxiety/depression) contribute to exacerbate symptoms. Intestinal infections have also been incriminated as a triggering factor. The role of dietary components in this pathogenic network will be discussed in the next section.

Food intolerance and irritable bowel syndrome

Many patients with irritable bowel syndrome believe that their symptoms are triggered by specific foods but this causative relationship is difficult to prove. Many studies have investigated the role of a variety of foodstuffs in the development of symptoms of irritable bowel with controversial results. Positive response to an elimination diet ranges from 15% to 71%, and double-blind placebo-controlled challenges identify problem foods in 6–58% of cases. Milk, wheat, and eggs, as well as foods high in salicylates (coffee, nuts, corn, wine, tomato, etc.) or amines (chocolate, bananas, wine, tomato, etc.) are most often identified as causing symptom exacerbation. However, studies had major limitations in their design, so that it is unclear whether adverse reactions to foods are a key factor in exacerbating symptoms or whether dietary manipulation is a valid therapeutic option.

The role of individual sugar (i.e. lactose, fructose, sorbitol) malabsorption in the development of symptoms of irritable bowel deserves particular comment. Lactose malabsorption has been reported to occur in about 25% of patients with irritable bowel syndrome in the USA and Northern Europe, whereas the prevalence may be as high as 52–68% in Mediterranean countries. In addition to geographical influences, patient selection may account for these differences. Lactose malabsorption can cause osmotic diarrhea and bloating, and hence may be more frequent in the subset of patients in whom these symptoms predominate. In a series of unselected Finnish patients, there was a poor relationship between lactose malabsorption, lactose intolerance, and symptoms of irritable bowel. In the light of these data, routine investigation of lactose malabsorption in every patient with irritable bowel syndrome does not seem advisable. However, lactose malabsorption should be investigated, by means of a hydrogen breath test after an oral load of lactose, in those patients in whom diarrhea and/or bloating predominate, particularly in countries where lactase deficiency is highly prevalent.

Fructose and sorbitol malabsorption also occur among patients with irritable bowel syndrome. The prevalence of malabsorption is particularly when both sugars are administered together (31–92%). Although these figures do not differ from those found in healthy controls, the intensity of symptoms after the ingestion of these sugars is significantly higher in irritable bowel syndrome patients. Such a difference does not appear to be due to intestinal dysmotility and hypersensitivity to distension, but to an increased fermentative capacity in patients with irritable bowel syndrome. As in the case of lactose, hydrogen breath tests using fructose, sorbitol and fructose + sorbitol mixtures as substrate should be performed in irritable bowel syndrome patients with predominating diarrhea and/or bloating symptoms.

Nutritional consequences of irritable bowel syndrome

Fortunately, malnutrition is not particularly prevalent among irritable bowel syndrome patients. In fact, the diagnosis of irritable bowel syndrome must be questioned in the presence of marked nutritional deficiencies or weight loss. In this setting, the diagnostic work-up for organic disease must be expanded with specific imaging and laboratory tests to rule-out IBD, celiac disease, GI neoplasm, chronic pancreatitis, pancreatic cancer, etc.

Despite the rarity of malnutrition in irritable bowel syndrome, some patients tend to attribute all their symptoms to the 'last meal they ate.' Thus, they sometimes eat an increasingly restrictive and imbalanced diet which can lead to protein–energy malnutrition or micronutrient deficiencies.

Dietary management of irritable bowel syndrome

The treatment of irritable bowel syndrome should be based on the nature and severity of the symptoms, the degree of physiological disturbance and functional impairment, and the presence of psychosocial disturbance affecting the course of the illness. Patients with mild symptoms respond to education and reassurance, whereas antispasmodic (anticholinergic) drugs or low-dose antidepressant agents (either tricyclic or serotonin reuptake inhibitors) are recommended in more symptomatic patients. However, it should be kept in mind that 40–70% respond to placebo alone.

In this setting, it is important to avoid restrictive and monotonous diets since, as mentioned, many patients tend to exclude from their diet a great number of foodstuffs without a firm reason to do that. After an accurate dietary interview, most patients will realize that a given foodstuff which apparently caused symptoms on one occasion was well tolerated in many other instances. Therefore, in general, most patients with irritable bowel syndrome could (and should) eat a balanced diet without restrictions. However, in some patients in whom symptoms are repeatedly triggered by eating, an exclusion diet may be of benefit. Also, a substantial percentage of patients with associated sugar malabsorption will improve after excluding the offending sugar from the diet.

For years, high-fiber diets and/or the addition of bulking agents (i.e. bran) have been accepted as effective therapeutic measures for irritable bowel syndrome patients. In fact, such a recommendation still appears in the more recent editions of authoritative gastroenterology textbooks. However, several randomized cross-over trials have shown that the administration of 12–15 g of bran or 20 g of corn fiber per day was not better that placebo in improving symptoms of irritable bowel. In fact, more than a half of patients from a large uncontrolled series felt that they get worse after bran supplementation. High-fiber diets might, at least in part, aggravate symptoms through an increase in gas production because, as mentioned before, patients with irritable bowel syndrome appear to have an increased fermentative capacity.

In spite of these considerations, high-fiber diets or fiber supplements should not be totally withdrawn from the therapeutic armamentarium for irritable bowel syndrome. Fiber supplements would be particularly useful in those patients with constipation. Hydrophilic colloids such as psyllium derivatives and methyl-cellulose tend to produce less gas (or at an slower rate). In addition, because of their hydrophilic properties, these agents bind water and prevent both excessive stool dehydration and excess liquidity. Thus, they may be equally effective for patients in whom either constipation or diarrhea predominate.

Diverticular disease

Definition and epidemiology
Although diverticula (i.e. pouches protruding outwards the wall of the bowel) may occur anywhere in the gut, the term 'diverticular disease' usually denotes the presence of diverticula in the large intestine, particularly in the sigmoid colon. In fact 95% of cases of colonic diverticular involve this segment, and it is exclusively affected in 65% of patients.

Diverticular disease is very common, particularly in industrialized countries. The prevalence of this condition increases with the age, being rare in individuals younger than 40, whereas it occurs in more than one-third of subjects over 65. Diverticular disease is rare in people who live in developing countries. However, the risk rapidly increases when these people migrate to western societies.

About 80% of patients with diverticular disease never have any symptoms. When symptomatic, patients complain from pain in the left lower quadrant of the abdomen, usually colic, and changes in bowel habit. In fact, these symptoms mostly resemble those of irritable bowel syndrome. Complications occurs in about 5% of cases and mainly consist of infection of a diverticulum (diverticulitis) which may lead to bowel perforation or abscess formation. Gastrointestinal bleeding may also occur, particularly from diverticula arising in the right colon.

Dietary fiber and diverticular disease
Colonic hypersegmentation resulting in intraluminal hypertension has been incriminated as the primary cause of diverticular disease. Increased intraluminal pressure (myochosis) would result in mucosal herniation and diverticula production, but these motility disturbances are not present in all patients with diverticula.

In spite of the fact that there is no direct evidence to prove it, there are a number of data suggesting that diverticular disease could be caused by a fiber-deficient diet. In fact, it occurs more often in omnivores than in vegetarians, and individuals consuming a high-meat, low-fiber diet are particularly at risk. The essential pathology in diverticular disease is colonic muscular hypertrophy. It is thought to be due to the need to propel hard fecal contents. Once the muscular thickening occurs the bowel lumen becomes narrowed, forming small chamber with high pressure leading to diverticula formation.

Treatment of uncomplicated diverticular disease relies on the use of a high-fiber diet. Bran supplements had proven to be effective both in uncontrolled and controlled trials. Bran appears to be more effective than other sources of non-starch polysaccharides or bulk-forming agents. As in irritable bowel syndrome, however, fiber supplements may increase flatus production and bloating. Thus a high-fiber diet alone should always be tried first.

10.6 Perspectives on the future

Future research on the role of nutrition and nutrients in the GI tract is likely to focus on the effects of individual nutrients on gene expression. Over the past years, the hypothesis has emerged that digestive end products and/or their metabolic derivatives may regulate pancreatic gene expression directly and independently of hormone stimulation. The role of fatty acids in the control of gene expression is now at an early stage of understanding and, whether or not this mechanism is related to pancreatic adaptation to dietary fat is unknown and will have to be defined by additional research.

Current information on developmental gene expression in the intestine as well as the dietary regulation of genes expressed in the developing intestinal epithelium is limited to only a handful of genes, which are primarily highly expressed genes involved in differentiated cellular functions (see chapter 10 in *Nutrition and Metabolism*). The carbohydrate structure and amounts in many foods and ingredients can be manipulated to achieve specific physiochemical properties of benefit for food structure and to produce a diverse range of physiological effects. It can be expected that many functional foods of the future will contain such specially selected or modified carbohydrates, but the metabolic and health consequences of these carbohydrates should be examined in more detail before health claims can be justified (see chapter 5 in *Nutrition and Metabolism*).

The area of probiotics is another area of ongoing research, and manipulation of colonic microflora has real potential for therapeutic management of GI disease.

More knowledge in all of these areas will lead to a better understanding of the mechanisms through which nutrients affect GI health.

References and further reading

Drossman DA, Whitehead WE, Camilleri M. Irritable bowel syndrome: A technical review for practice guideline development. *Gastroenterology* 1997; 112: 2120–2137.

Farthing MJG. Tropical malabsorption and tropical diarrhea. In: *Selisenger & Fordtran's Gastrointestinal and Liver Disease* 6th edn (M Feldman, BF Scharschmidt, MH Sleisenger, eds), pp. 1574–1584. Philadelphia: W.B. Saunders, 1998.

Fernández Bañares F, Cabré E, Esteve Comas M, Gassull MA. How effective is enteral nutrition in inducing clinical remission in active Crohn's disease? A meta-analysis of the randomized clinical trials. *JPEN J Parenter Enteral Nutr* 1995; 19: 356–364.

Fine KD, Meyer RL, Lee EL. The prevalence and causes of chronic diarrhea in patients with celiac sprue treated with a gluten-free diet. *Gastroenterology* 1997; 112: 1830–1838.

Francis CY, Whorwell PJ. Bran and irritable bowel syndrome: Time for reappraisal. *Lancet* 1994; 344: 39–40.

Gassull MA, Cabré E. The role of nutrition in the pathogenesis of inflammatory bowel disease. In: *Falk Symposium 106: Advances in Inflammatory Bowel Disease* (P Rutgeerts, J-F Colombel, S Hanauer, J Schölmerich, GN Tytgat, A Van Gossum, eds), pp. 80–88. London: Kluwer Academic, 1999.

Gassull MA, Fernández Bañares F, Cabré E, Esteve Comas M. Enteral nutrition in inflammatory bowel disease. In: *Clinical Nutrition. Enteral and Tube Feeding*, 3rd edn (JL Rombeau, RH Rolandelli, eds), pp. 403–416. Philadelphia: W.B. Saunders, 1997.

Gassull MA, Fernández Bañares F. Nutrition in inflammatory bowel disease. In: *Artificial Nutrition Support in Clinical Practice*, 2nd edn. (J Payne-James, G Grimble, DBA Silk, eds), pp. 553–573. London: Greenwich Medical Media, 2001.

Gray GM. Persistence of diarrhea in treated celiac sprue: refractory disease or another organ's malfunction? *Gastroenterology* 1997; 112: 2146–2147.

Jewell DP. Ulcerative colitis. In: *Selisenger & Fordtran's Gastrointestinal and Liver Disease*, 6th edn (M Feldman, BF Scharschmidt, MH Sleisenger, eds), pp. 1735–1761. Philadelphia: W.B. Saunders, 1998.

Mäki M, Collin P. Coeliac disease. *Lancet* 1997; 349: 1755–1759.

Murray JA. The widening spectrum of celiac disease. *Am J Clin Nutr* 1999; 69: 354–365.

Ramsey DJ, Smithard DG. Assessment and management of dysphagia. *Hosp Med* 2004; 65: 274–279.

Simmang CL, Shires GT. Diverticular disease of the colon. In: *Sleisenger & Fordtran's Gastrointestinal and Liver Disease*, 6th edn (M Feldman, BF Scharschmidt, MH Sleisenger, eds), pp. 1788–1798. Philadelphia: W.B. Saunders, 1998.

Somers SC, Lembo A. Irritable bowel syndrome: evaluation and treatment. *Gastroenterol Clin North Am* 2003; 32: 507–529.

Ukleja A, Scolapio JS, Buchman AL. Nutritional management of short bowel syndrome. *Semin Gastrointest Dis* 2002; 13: 161–168.

Wilmore DW. Indications for specific therapy in the rehabilitation of patients with the short-bowel syndrome. *Best Pract Res Clin Gastroenterol* 2003; 17: 895–906.

11
Nutrition in Liver Disease

Marietjie G Herselman, Demetre Labadarios, Christo J Van Rensburg, and Aref A Haffejee

Key messages

- The liver is intimately involved in the metabolism and storage of nutrients, as well as the homeostasis of water and sodium, and impaired hepatic function is bound to result in a wide range of nutritional abnormalities.
- Patients with liver disease are often undernourished and need sufficient protein, energy, and micronutrients to meet their requirements and to promote regeneration of hepatocytes. Dietary excess may, however, be a risk factor for liver pathology itself (e.g. excessive amounts of vitamins A and energy).

- Protein should be included in the diet as needed, since elimination of protein from the diet will not only contribute to protein–energy malnutrition (PEM), but can in fact worsen hepatic encephalopathy.
- The long-term benefits of nutrition support in liver disease, the best route of feeding, and the best sources of protein remain to be confirmed by larger and better controlled studies.

11.1 Introduction

Anatomy

The liver is the largest organ in the body and is located in the right upper quadrant of the abdomen. There are two anatomical lobes, with the right lobe being approximately six times the size of the left. It has a double blood supply, with the portal vein carrying venous blood from the intestines and spleen, and the hepatic artery supplying the liver with arterial blood. These blood vessels enter the liver through the porta hepatis, where they divide into branches to the left and right lobes of the liver. The hepatic vein returns blood from the liver to the heart. The liver is covered almost completely with peritoneum and is kept in place by peritoneal ligaments.

Functions

The liver plays a central role in the metabolism of protein, carbohydrate, fat, and drugs. Other functions include the storage of vitamins and trace elements, conversion of beta-carotene, folate, and vitamin D to their biologically active forms, bile formation and excretion, and sodium and water homeostasis. Impaired liver function, therefore, is associated with a number of metabolic disturbances, some of which have profound consequences on the nutritional status of such patients (Table 11.1). Further to this, it should be noted that catabolic conditions, such as trauma and sepsis, are associated with many metabolic interrelationships between the liver, muscle, and other organs. Depending on the degree of catabolism, it is accompanied by adaptive responses in the liver, most notably the synthesis of acute phase proteins, a decrease in the rate of albumin synthesis, an increase in glycogenolysis or gluconeogenesis, increased urea production, and impaired ketogenesis.

Anabolic functions

Control of blood glucose
The healthy liver is intimately involved in the control of blood glucose via the processes of glycogenesis, glycogenolysis, glycolysis, and gluconeogenesis. In advanced liver disease, these processes are impaired due to increased levels of glucagon, insulin resistance, increases in tumor necrosis factor (TNF) and interleukin 1 (IL-1), decreased levels of insulin-like growth

Table 11.1 Summary of the functions of the healthy liver and abnormalities associated with impaired liver function

Function	Common effects of impaired liver function
Anabolic	
Carbohydrate metabolism and control of blood glucose	Blood glucose levels may be normal, increased, or decreased
Protein synthesis	Hypoalbuminemia and edema or ascites
	Impaired transport functions
	Bleeding tendency due to impaired synthesis of clotting factors
	Abnormal BCAA : AAA ratio
Lipid metabolism	Malabsorption of fat
Synthesis of bile salts	Cholesterol may be increased (cholestasis), decreased (malnutrition), or normal (cirrhosis)
Synthesis of LCAT	
Conversion of vitamin D to its active form	Low levels of active vitamin D
Catabolic	
Oxidation of fatty acids	Triglycerides may be increased
Detoxification	Low urea levels
	Hyperammonemia
	Prolonged action of medication
Phagocytosis	Inflammatory response
Conjugation and excretion of bilirubin	Jaundice
Inactivates and excretes aldosterone, glucocorticoids and sex hormones	Hyperaldosteronism and hypokalemia
	Altered estrogen and androgen metabolism
Storing	
Fat-soluble vitamins	Deficiency of vitamin K with bleeding tendency
	Elevated levels of vitamin K with necrotic hepatocytes, hepatitis, active cirrhosis, primary liver cancer
	Vitamin D deficiency with bone disorders
Vitamin B_{12}	Low vitamin B_{12} and folate stores
Folate	
Trace elements	
Homeostatic	
Water and sodium	Sodium and water retention with ascites and edema, due to hyperaldosteronism

Adapted from Sherlock and Dooley (1993), Morgan (1999) and Stolz (2002).
LCAT, lecithin cholesterol acyl transferase; BCAA, branched-chain amino acids; AAA, aromatic amino acids.

factor (IGF-1), and a reduced storage capacity due to hepatic fibrosis. In the presence of mild liver impairment, blood glucose concentration is usually maintained within the normal range. In advanced chronic liver disease, however, impaired glucose tolerance has been reported in about 36% of patients with cirrhosis with 37% of these being diagnosed as diabetics. In acute and terminal cases of liver disease, hypoglycemia may occur due to a decrease in gluconeogenesis and glycogen synthesis. Hypoglycemia, due to decreased conversion of pyruvate to glucose, may also occur in alcoholic liver disease.

Protein and amino acid metabolism
The liver is responsible for the synthesis of a number of proteins including albumin, transferrin, prealbumin, retinol-binding protein, alpha-fetoproteins, acute phase proteins, complement, ceruloplasmin, and proteins involved in coagulation. With impaired liver function, the serum concentration of these proteins may be abnormal due to increased levels of glucagon and cytokines, and decreases in their concentration may be associated with hypoalbuminemia, impaired transport of nutrients, and a bleeding tendency. The liver also plays a role in maintaining a normal amino acid profile through the process of transamination, deamination, and decarboxylation. Impaired liver function is usually associated with an increase in the aromatic amino acids (phenylalanine, tyrosine, and tryptophan) and methionine, and a decrease in the branched-chain amino acids (valine, leucine, and isoleucine).

Lipid metabolism

The liver plays an important role in the synthesis of triacylglycerols, lipoproteins, cholesterol, lecithin cholesterol acyl transferase (LCAT – involved in the reverse cholesterol transport pathway), and bile acids. In the presence of liver disease, there is an increase in lipolysis, enhanced oxidation of non-esterified fatty acids, and normal or increased ketogenesis. Serum cholesterol is elevated in cholestasis, and is thought to be the result of increased hepatic synthesis, reduced LCAT activity, and regurgitation of biliary cholesterol into the circulation. Increased serum cholesterol concentrations may also be seen during recovery from virus hepatitis, in fatty infiltration of the liver, and in some patients with gallstones. In cirrhosis, serum cholesterol is usually normal, and low levels may indicate the presence of protein–energy malnutrition or hepatic decompensation. Triacylglycerol levels may be normal or moderately increased in hepatocellular disease and obstructive jaundice, with the excess being found in low-density lipoprotein (LDL) cholesterol. Failure of hepatic apoprotein synthesis may lead to fatty infiltration of the liver due to impaired export of triacylglycerols from the liver in the form of very low density lipoproteins (VLDL), and a reduction in the bile acid pool may lead to steatorrhea.

Catabolic functions

The liver also has some catabolic functions, which include the following:

- the oxidation of fatty acids for use as an energy source,
- detoxification of ammonia and drugs,
- phagocytosis of bacteria and endotoxin from the gastrointestinal tract,
- conjugation and excretion of bilirubin, and
- catabolism of aldosterone.

The liver plays a crucially important role in ammonia homeostasis. The majority of ammonia is derived from the small intestine by the degradation of glutamine to glutamate in the mucosal cells, and from the large intestine where ammonia is formed as a product of protein and urea breakdown by intestinal flora. Ammonia is, however, also synthesized to a smaller extent in the skeletal muscle and the kidneys, and an increase in ammonia synthesis is known to occur during diuretic treatment and in hypokalemia. In the liver itself, large amounts of ammonia are formed as a product of protein breakdown, but it is utilized in the synthesis of urea and glutamine. In the presence of normal liver function there is hardly any ammonia released from the liver. With impaired liver function, however, the conversion of ammonia to urea may be reduced by up to 80%, a reduction that is associated with an increase in the blood concentration of ammonia and a decrease in blood levels of urea.

Liver dysfunction may further lead to a prolonged half-life and action of medication (which may require dose reduction), and the development of jaundice due to impaired conjugation and/or excretion of bilirubin. The phagocytic function of the Kupfer cells is also impaired in the presence of liver dysfunction, and may lead to an inflammatory response that adversely affects metabolism and tissue function. Finally, a decrease in the metabolism of aldosterone results in increased aldosterone levels, which in turn is associated with sodium and water retention, potassium loss in the urine, and the development of hypokalemia, which is thought to contribute to the precipitation of hepatic encephalopathy.

Nutrient storage

The liver is the storage site for glucose in the form of glycogen, which amounts to approximately 90 g.

The liver also has the capacity to store large amounts of fat-soluble vitamins, vitamin B_{12}, magnesium, and metals such as zinc, iron, and copper. It is also responsible for the conversion of carotene to vitamin A, of folate to 5-methyltetrahydrofolate, pyridoxine to pyridoxal-5-phosphate, and of vitamin D to 25-hydroxy-vitamin D. Abnormalities found in liver disorders include a bleeding tendency due to vitamin K deficiency, and decreased hydroxylation of vitamin D.

Homeostatic function

The liver plays an important role in water and sodium homeostasis as well as the maintenance of normal plasma volume. The renin–angiotensin–aldosterone system is activated in patients with hepatic cirrhosis and ascites. The result is a decrease in the clearance of free water, and an increase in sodium absorption, which may lead to an increase in plasma volume.

Table 11.2 Classification of acute viral hepatitis

	HAV	HBV	HCV	HDV	HEV
Transfer	Fecal-orally	Parenteral	IV drug users	Parenteral	Fecal-orally
	Sexual	Blood	Blood	Blood	Perinatal
		Sexual	Sexual, rare	Sexual, rare	
		Saliva	Saliva		
		Perinatal	Perinatal		
Genome	RNA	DNA	RNA	RNA	RNA
Incubation period	15–50 days	28–180 days	14–160 days	30–180 days	15–60 days
Prevalence	High	High	Moderate	Low, regional	Regional
Hepatic necrosis	Seldom	Seldom	Yes	Seldom	Yes
Chronic hepatitis	No	Yes	Yes	Yes	No
Hepatocellular carcinoma	No	Yes	Yes	Yes	No
Carrier	No	Yes	Yes	Yes	No
Therapy	No	Interferon	Interferon	Interferon	No
		Nucleoside	Ribavirin		
Prophylaxis	Hygiene	Recombinant HBsAg	Routine testing of donor blood	Recombinant HBsAg	Hygiene
	Inoculation	Behavior modification			

Adapted from Sherlock and Dooley (1993), Berenguer and Wright (2002), Gerlich and Thomssen (1999), Ryder and Beckingham (2001).
HAV, hepatitis A virus; HBV, hepatitis B virus; HCV, hepatitis C virus; HDV, hepatitis D virus; HEV, hepatitis E virus; HBsAg, hepatitis B surface antigen.

11.2 Diseases of the liver

Acute viral hepatitis

Acute hepatitis can be caused by viruses A, B, C, D, or E. Their mode of transmission, genome, and clinical characteristics differ, as do the treatment and prophylactic measures for preventing infection (Table 11.2).

Hepatitis A is highly contagious but usually resolves within weeks and does not become chronic. In children, about 80% of cases remain asymptomatic. Hepatitis A is more likely to produce symptoms in adults, with about one-third of cases developing jaundice. Management is conservative and patients are monitored carefully to identify the small number of patients who may develop fulminant liver failure.

Infection with hepatitis B virus (HBV) is usually asymptomatic, with 70% of subjects having a subclinical infection and 20–25% presenting with acute hepatitis. Most patients will clear up, but approximately 10% of patients progress to chronic hepatitis, with 1% of patients with acute hepatitis dying from hepatic encephalopathy (Figure 11.1). Patients chronically infected with hepatitis B can be further subdivided into those who are carriers and who do not need treatment, and those with chronic hepatitis B that may progress to cirrhosis and liver failure. All cases with hepatitis B infection must be notified and close contacts must be screened and vaccinated.

Infection with hepatitis C virus (HCV) is a major cause of chronic hepatitis and 20% of patients eventually develop cirrhosis. Although early identification of cases of acute hepatitis C is difficult, it is desirable as early treatment with interferon alpha may reduce the risk of chronic infection. Approximately 80% of untreated patients develop chronic hepatitis C compared with less than 50% of those treated with interferon. The delta virus is an incomplete RNA virus that requires HBV for replication. Delta virus infection (HDV) can affect all risk groups for HBV infection, and can become chronic. Vaccination against HBV infection also

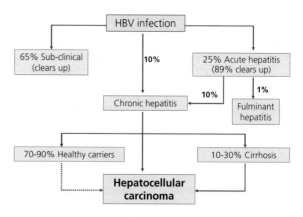

Figure 11.1 The course of acute hepatitis B infection. Adapted from Sherlock and Dooley (1993) and Dusheiko (1999).

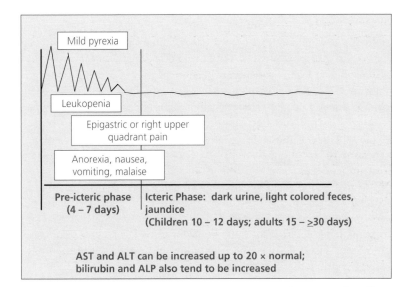

Figure 11.2 Signs and symptoms of acute viral hepatitis. From Sherlock and Dooley 1993; Hasse *et al.* (2000); Popper (1964).

protects against HDV. Hepatitis E virus (HEV) infection may cause epidemics of acute, self-limiting hepatitis with a course similar to that of hepatitis A.

Common signs and symptoms of acute viral hepatitis include anorexia, nausea, and vomiting during the pre-icteric phase (4–7 days), abdominal tenderness, and jaundice which can last up to 30 days or more (Figure 11.2). Aspartate and alanine transaminase (AST and ALT) may be increased up to 20-fold, and bilirubin and alkaline phosphatase (ALP) are usually also increased. Leukopenia is also common. Other symptoms include fatigue and malaise, changes in smell or taste sensation, headache, photophobia, and diarrhea. A large percentage of cases, however, remain asymptomatic.

During acute illness protein and energy requirements will depend on the degree of catabolism. Due to anorexia and vomiting, patients may prefer smaller meals given more frequently throughout the day. The enteral or parenteral route should be considered if adequate intake via the oral route is not possible, and fluid balance needs to be monitored carefully, as patients with severe hepatitis may not be able to excrete a water load.

Chronic hepatitis

Chronic hepatitis is defined as the persistence of liver injury, without improvement, for longer than six months. It can be viral (HBV, HCV, or HDV), autoimmune or, drug-induced in origin and carries the risk of cirrhosis, liver cancer, and liver failure. All types of chronic hepatitis have the same clinical, biochemical, and histological features. Patients may be asymptomatic, with portal hypertension complicated by bleeding from esophageal varices being late features. Biochemical abnormalities may include elevated bilirubin, hepatocellular enzymes, and gamma-globulin levels. Weight loss is a common feature of chronic hepatitis C, and may be related to an increase in energy expenditure. Resting energy expenditure (REE) has been reported to be markedly elevated in 47 patients with chronic hepatitis C (patients were not cirrhotic), and REE/fat-free mass (FFM) was significantly higher in patients than in healthy controls. REE was also correlated with the viral load but not with histological status or hepatocellular function, suggesting that hypermetabolism is the direct result of HCV replication rather than the consequence of hepatic inflammation. Interferon treatment significantly reduced the degree of hypermetabolism in responders, with a dramatic decline in both virus load and REE/FFM.

Acute liver failure

Acute liver failure is often caused, amongst others, by drug toxicity or viral hepatitis, and is characterized by massive liver cell necrosis, which is rapidly followed by cardiopulmonary dysfunction, marked coagulation disorders, renal failure, and cerebral edema. Fulminant hepatic failure is reserved for the clinical setting in which patients with previously existing liver disease suddenly develop rapidly progressive liver failure with hepatic encephalopathy within eight weeks of the onset of acute illness. Even if patients are in good nutritional status at the onset of fulminant hepatic failure, they tend to develop protein–energy malnutrition (PEM) within 7–10 days. Nutrition support in these very unstable patients can be a challenge due to problems with venous access, coagulopathy, sepsis, deteriorating renal function, and rapid hemodynamic changes. Prokinetic agents may be indicated in patients with delayed gastric emptying in order to provide optimal nutrition.

In patients who require hemodialysis for the treatment of renal failure, care must be taken to replace amino acid losses. This is especially important in the case of continuous renal replacement therapy where such losses can be high. Once the patient has recovered, the focus should be on restoring nutritional status using basic healthy eating principles. Although this clinical setting carries a high mortality rate, the prognosis has lately been improved due to better intensive care. Patients with fulminant hepatic failure are susceptible to a wide variety of complications in addition to encephalopathy (which is part of the definition of the disorder). These include cerebral edema, renal failure, hypoglycemia, metabolic acidosis, sepsis, coagulopathy, and hemodynamic collapse. All patients with fulminant hepatic failure should be managed in an intensive care unit at a facility capable of performing liver transplantation. The only proven therapy that improves patient outcome in fulminant hepatic failure is orthotopic liver transplantation, which is associated with one-year survival rates of greater than 80%. The provision of optimal nutrition in these patients is of vital importance in order to facilitate regeneration of hepatocytes.

Alcoholic liver disease

Alcoholic liver disease can be classified into fatty infiltration of the liver or steatosis (80% of heavy drinkers), alcoholic hepatitis (10–35%), and fibrosis and/or cirrhosis (10%). Alcoholic hepatitis is potentially reversible in its early stages, but can progress to cirrhosis. However, it might be fatal even in the absence of cirrhosis. The risk of developing cirrhosis depends on both the amount and duration of alcohol intake. The amount of alcohol necessary to cause alcoholic liver disease is controversial, but has been associated with the daily consumption of more than 40 g absolute al-

cohol over many years. The Royal College of Physicians in the UK advises a weekly limit of 21 units of alcohol for men and 14 units for women. Women absorb about 30% more alcohol than men for the same amount of alcohol consumed. They are also more susceptible to hepatic damage, more likely to relapse after treatment, and are more likely to progress to cirrhosis even if they stop drinking. The pattern of alcohol consumption is also important, as it has been shown that alcoholic liver damage is increased in those drinking on an empty stomach and those who drink multiple different alcoholic beverages. Absorption of alcohol is also lower when drinking low-concentration beverages such as beer, compared with beverages with a high concentration of alcohol.

Pathogenesis and complications of alcoholic liver disease

There are several putative mechanisms involved in the development of alcoholic liver disease, including the effects of acetaldehyde, redox alteration, oxidant stress, and hypoxia.

Acetaldehyde

The main metabolic pathway in ethanol metabolism is its conversion to acetaldehyde via the alcohol dehydrogenase (ADH) system (Figure 11.3).

The microsomal ethanol oxidation system (MEOS) pathway, which is stimulated in chronic ethanol abuse, also generates acetaldehyde. Acetaldehyde is an extremely reactive and toxic metabolite, and its possible hepatotoxic effects include the following:

- Free radical production at high concentrations of acetaldehyde, with an increase in lipid peroxidation
- Adduct formation with protein (antigenic), which may promote hepatic collagen synthesis
- Increased expression of proinflammatory cytokines (TNFα, transforming growth factor alpha (TGFα), IL-1β, and IL-6), which stimulate collagen-producing stellate cells
- Binding to phospholipids
- Interference with mitochondrial electron transport
- Inhibition of nuclear repair
- Interference with microtubule function

Redox alteration

ADH-mediated ethanol oxidation is accompanied by the conversion of reduced nicotinamide adenine dinu-

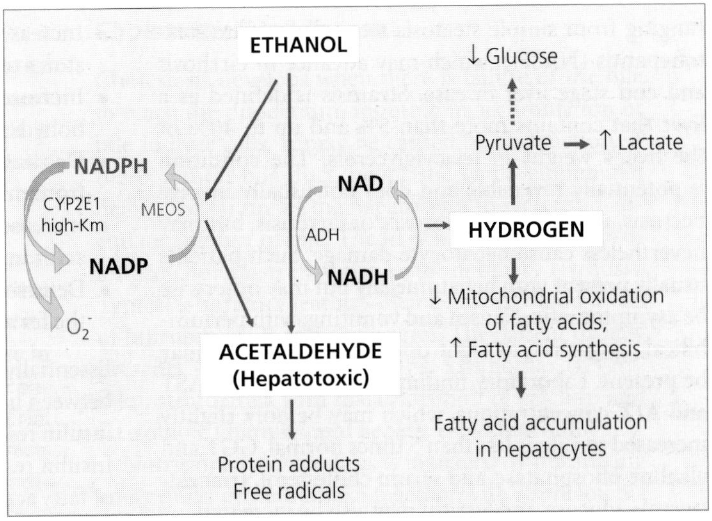

Figure 11.3 Pathogenesis and complications of alcoholic liver disease. Excess NADH shifts the redox state of hepatocytes, which in turn affects other NAD-dependent processes such as lipid and carbohydrate metabolism (e.g. steatosis) and gluconeogenesis (can lead to profound hypoglycemia). These changes are reversible with abstinence, but with chronic ethanol consumption, the redox state can become prolonged. Adapted from Sherlock and Dooley (1993); Maher (2002).

cleotide phosphate (NADH) to nicotinamide adenine dinucleotide (NAD), which shifts the redox state of hepatocytes (Figure 11.3). The latter is associated with the development of hepatic steatosis due to an increase in the synthesis of fatty acids and inhibition of mitochondrial beta-oxidation of fatty acids. This leads to accumulation of fatty acids in hepatocytes where they are esterified and stored as triacylglycerols. There is also a decrease in the conversion of pyruvate to glucose (which may lead to hypoglycemia), and an increased conversion to lactate and therefore an increased risk to develop acidosis.

Oxidant stress

Ethanol oxidation is associated with the formation of several free radical species which can cause oxidative damage to the liver. Free radicals are thought to result from ethanol oxidation by cytochrome P-4502E1 (CYP2E1) (Figure 11.3), but more importantly, they may derive from Kupfer cells. Other factors that may contribute to free radical formation include mobilization of iron from ferritin due to excess NADH generation, recruited leukocytes, and neutrophils. Free radicals have been associated with direct injury to hepatocytes by lipid peroxidation. These effects may be amplified if chronic ethanol consumption leads to a depletion of antioxidants such as vitamins E and A and glutathione.

Hypoxia

Ethanol consumption has been associated with a hyper-

metabolic state in the liver with increased oxygen consumption by hepatocytes. This leaves the pericentral hepatocytes in a state of relative hypoxia, leading to depletion of adenosine triphosphate (ATP) and liver damage. However, the increase in hepatic oxygen consumption is believed to be offset by concomitant increases in splanchnic blood flow, so that hypoxia may only occur during periods of abstinence or withdrawal.

Alcoholic hepatitis, which may eventually progress to cirrhosis, is characterized by degeneration of the liver parenchyma and alcoholic fibrosis, which like the hepatitis lesion, first appears in the pericentral zone and then progresses to panlobular fibrosis in those who continue to drink. Common biochemical abnormalities include raised serum transaminases (with the ratio of AST/ALT > 2), and gamma-glutamyl transferase (GGT), hypokalemia due to poor dietary intake, low plasma zinc levels, normal or decreased levels of serum albumin, an increased mean corpuscular volume (MCV) and white cell count, and anemia. Other abnormalities that may be present include elevated alkaline phosphatase (ALP), hyperbilirubinemia, impaired platelet function, a raised temperature, anorexia, nausea, vomiting, diarrhea, hyperaldosteronism, and clinical signs of liver disease. The most important treatment for alcoholic liver disease is to ensure total and immediate abstinence from alcohol.

Non-alcoholic fatty liver disease (NAFLD)

NAFLD refers to a wide spectrum of liver damage

crease in serum levels of copper and ceruloplasmin, and Kayser–Fleisch rings. Complications include liver damage with cirrhosis, neurological, and psychiatric disturbances, hemolysis, renal tubular damage, and demineralization of bone. Treatment options include D-penicillamine (chelates copper), trientene (if sensitive to D-penicillamine), zinc (sequestrates copper in the gut), or liver transplantation. Dietary treatment is of limited value, but a diet low in copper (1.5 mg/day) may be of some value. Sources high in dietary copper include shellfish, dried fruit, chocolate, nuts, broccoli, liver, mushrooms, and legumes. With early and effective treatment patients can live a normal life.

Hemochromatosis

Hemochromatosis is a autosomal recessive metabolic defect with an increase in the intestinal absorption of iron, leading to excessive iron deposition in the liver, pancreas, spleen, heart, kidneys, gastrointestinal mucosa, skin, and testis. Hepatic complications include liver fibrosis, cirrhosis, and hepatocellular carcinoma. Diabetes has been estimated to occur in about two-thirds of patients with hemochromatosis, but its frequency has now decreased due to earlier diagnosis of the condition, and it is usually not seen in the absence of cirrhosis. If present, it may be controlled by diet and/or oral medication, but in some patients treatment may be difficult even with large doses of insulin. The brain and central nervous system is not affected. Iron can damage the liver via lipid peroxidation, deposition of hemosiderin in lysosomes, and increased collagen synthesis. In the initial stages of the disease, there is only

increased iron absorption, and later in the course of the disease, it is followed by a decrease in serum transferrin, an increase in serum iron, hepatic iron, total body iron, progressive tissue damage, and finally cirrhosis at the age of about 40–50 years (Figure 11.5).

Characteristics of the disease include abdominal pain, hepatomegaly, splenomegaly, a fibrotic pancreas, testicular atrophy, skin pigmentation, increased serum iron, ferritin, transferrin saturation, and an increase in the hepatic iron index. In the absence of anemia, treatment includes venesection (500 ml once or twice a week until the hematocrit value drops below 37%), which removes about 250 mg iron at a time. This is followed by maintenance phlebotomy of 1 unit of whole blood every 2–3 months (folate supplementation is essential). If anemia is present, however, chelating agents may be used. Dietary restriction of iron is not very effective, but a reduction in heme iron, vitamin C, and alcohol has been advocated. Food should also not be cooked in iron pots. If treatment is initiated before the onset of cirrhosis, patients will have a normal life expectancy.

Liver cirrhosis

Liver cirrhosis is the end stage of a number of different chronic liver diseases. It may develop as a result of chronic alcohol abuse, viral hepatitis, drugs, toxic substances, prolonged cholestasis, vascular, autonomic and metabolic disorders, intestinal bypass surgery, or it may be cryptogenic in nature. It is characterized by hepatocellular damage with necrosis of hepatocytes,

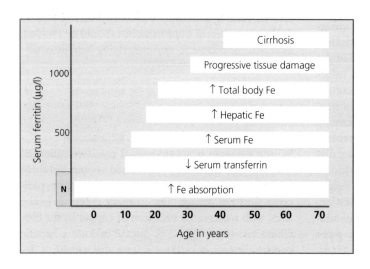

Figure 11.5 The clinical course and iron status in hemochromatosis. Sherlock and Dooley (1993). N, normal range.

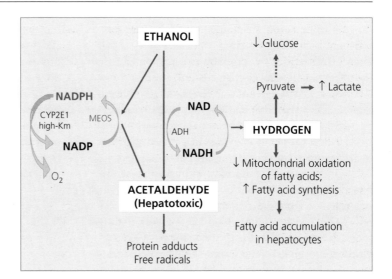

Figure 11.3 Pathogenesis and complications of alcoholic liver disease. Excess NADH shifts the redox state of hepatocytes, which in turn affects other NAD-dependent processes such as lipid and carbohydrate metabolism (e.g. steatosis) and gluconeogenesis (can lead to profound hypoglycemia). These changes are reversible with abstinence, but with chronic ethanol consumption, the redox state can become prolonged. Adapted from Sherlock and Dooley (1993); Maher (2002).

cleotide phosphate (NADH) to nicotinamide adenine dinucleotide (NAD), which shifts the redox state of hepatocytes (Figure 11.3). The latter is associated with the development of hepatic steatosis due to an increase in the synthesis of fatty acids and inhibition of mitochondrial beta-oxidation of fatty acids. This leads to accumulation of fatty acids in hepatocytes where they are esterified and stored as triacylglycerols. There is also a decrease in the conversion of pyruvate to glucose (which may lead to hypoglycemia), and an increased conversion to lactate and therefore an increased risk to develop acidosis.

Oxidant stress
Ethanol oxidation is associated with the formation of several free radical species which can cause oxidative damage to the liver. Free radicals are thought to result from ethanol oxidation by cytochrome P-4502E1 (CYP2E1) (Figure 11.3), but more importantly, they may derive from Kupfer cells. Other factors that may contribute to free radical formation include mobilization of iron from ferritin due to excess NADH generation, recruited leukocytes, and neutrophils. Free radicals have been associated with direct injury to hepatocytes by lipid peroxidation. These effects may be amplified if chronic ethanol consumption leads to a depletion of antioxidants such as vitamins E and A and glutathione.

Hypoxia
Ethanol consumption has been associated with a hyper-

metabolic state in the liver with increased oxygen consumption by hepatocytes. This leaves the pericentral hepatocytes in a state of relative hypoxia, leading to depletion of adenosine triphosphate (ATP) and liver damage. However, the increase in hepatic oxygen consumption is believed to be offset by concomitant increases in splanchnic blood flow, so that hypoxia may only occur during periods of abstinence or withdrawal.

Alcoholic hepatitis, which may eventually progress to cirrhosis, is characterized by degeneration of the liver parenchyma and alcoholic fibrosis, which like the hepatitis lesion, first appears in the pericentral zone and then progresses to panlobular fibrosis in those who continue to drink. Common biochemical abnormalities include raised serum transaminases (with the ratio of AST/ALT > 2), and gamma-glutamyl transferase (GGT), hypokalemia due to poor dietary intake, low plasma zinc levels, normal or decreased levels of serum albumin, an increased mean corpuscular volume (MCV) and white cell count, and anemia. Other abnormalities that may be present include elevated alkaline phosphatase (ALP), hyperbilirubinemia, impaired platelet function, a raised temperature, anorexia, nausea, vomiting, diarrhea, hyperaldosteronism, and clinical signs of liver disease. The most important treatment for alcoholic liver disease is to ensure total and immediate abstinence from alcohol.

Non-alcoholic fatty liver disease (NAFLD)
NAFLD refers to a wide spectrum of liver damage

ranging from simple steatosis to non-alcoholic stea-tohepatitis (NASH), which may advance to cirrhosis and end stage liver disease. Steatosis is defined as a liver that contains more than 5% and up to 40% of the liver's weight in triacylglycerols. The condition is potentially reversible and does not usually involve necrosis, inflammation, fibrosis, or cirrhosis, but may nevertheless cause hepatocyte damage. Such patients usually present with hepatomegaly but may otherwise be asymptomatic. Nausea and vomiting, with perium-bilical, epigastric, or right upper quadrant pain may be present. Laboratory findings include elevated AST and ALT concentrations, which may be only slightly increased to values less than 5 times normal. GGT and alkaline phosphatase, and serum cholesterol, triacylg-lycerols, glucose, and ferritin may also be increased.

NASH is a syndrome of liver pathology resembling alcoholic hepatitis, but it is not the result of alcohol, drugs, or any other single identifiable cause. It is almost invariably associated with the insulin resistance (meta-bolic) syndrome. It is very common, usually relatively mild and overlapping with steatosis, but it can progress to end stage liver disease. Prevention and treatment is aimed at the correction of insulin resistance, correc-tion of central obesity, treatment of dyslipidemia, and physical activity.

The pathogenesis of NAFLD remains speculative, but retention of triacylglycerols within hepatocytes is a prerequisite for its development. In view of the crucial role of the liver in fatty acid metabolism (Figure 11.4), steatosis is thought to occur when there is:

- Increased delivery of free fatty acids from the fat stores to the liver
- Increased hepatic synthesis of fatty acids from car-bohydrates via acetyl-CoA
- Decreased oxidation of free fatty acids resulting from mitochondrial damage
- Increased triacylglycerol production from fatty acids in the liver
- Defective triacylglycerol removal from the liver in the form of VLDL.

Essentially, NAFLD occurs when there is an imbalance between lipogenic and lipotrophic factors, and in this, insulin resistance is thought to play an important role. Insulin resistance is associated with the accumulation of fatty acids in hepatocytes due to an increase in lipol-ysis (which increases circulating levels of fatty acids) and hyperinsulinemia (which increases glycolysis and favors triacylglycerol accumulation in hepatocytes due to a decreased production of apolipoprotein B-100).

Increased levels of fatty acids in hepatocytes may further lead to an increase in cytochrome P-450, which may result in the production of free radicals and lipid peroxidation of hepatocytes membranes, and the pro-gression from simple steatosis to NASH and cirrhosis.

Conditions associated with the development of NAFLD include kwashiorkor, obesity, non-insulin-dependent diabetes mellitus, hypertriglyceridemia, jejeno-ileal bypass, and total parenteral nutrition. Steatosis in kwashiorkor is due to a shortage of lipo-trophic factors, and it resolves rapidly with protein feeding. It does not usually progress to cirrhosis, but

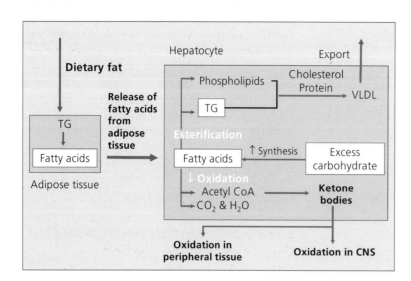

Figure 11.4 Role of the liver in fatty acid metabolism. Adapted from Sherlock and Dooley (1993); Angulo (2002).

hepatic fibrosis may develop. Morbid obesity (>70% overweight) is associated with fatty infiltration of the liver due to increased lipolysis from the fat depots and an increased flow of free fatty acids to the liver. It is present in about 60–90% of obese subjects, and although it is usually reversible with weight loss, it has been associated with NASH (a progressive fibrotic form of NAFLD) in 20–40% of subjects.

With jejeno-ileal bypass steatosis is already present preoperatively due to obesity, but it has been reported to be exacerbated postoperatively due to a decrease in lipotrophic factors, an increase in lipolysis due to energy shortage, and the hepatotoxic effect of bacterial overgrowth. Between 1% and 17% of such subjects may develop cirrhosis and liver failure, but the condition may resolve partially upon repair of the bypass.

Total parenteral nutrition (TPN) is sometimes associated with cholestasis and fatty infiltration of the liver, with an increase in AST, ALT, ALP, and bilirubin concentrations after two weeks on TPN. It usually normalizes when TPN is stopped, but patients who are on TPN for long periods of time may develop hepatitis, cirrhosis, and cholelithiasis. The mechanisms are thought to include an increase in free fatty acid (FFA) synthesis and a decrease in fatty acid oxidation and lipoproteins. Fatty infiltration of the liver is thought to be less likely with the administration of a balanced carbohydrate–lipid source of energy, and it has been suggested that carbohydrate should not exceed 4 mg/kg per min, with fat contributing 30–40% of total energy. The ratio of energy to nitrogen should be approximately 150 cal:1 g N. It is further recommended that the gallbladder should be stimulated during TPN in order to prevent bacterial overgrowth and cholestasis.

Other causes of fatty liver disease include drugs (corticosteroids, carbon tetrachloride, tetracycline, valproate, and others), hepatotoxins, metabolic or genetic factors, human immunodeficiency virus infection, inflammatory bowel disease, and diverticulosis with bacterial overgrowth. Treatment of fatty infiltration is aimed at eliminating the causative underlying condition (abstinence from alcohol, adequate protein intake, moderate weight reduction in the obese, discontinuation of TPN, and control of serum glucose and lipid levels). It is worth noting that rapid weight loss in obese subjects may lead to necroinflammation, portal fibrosis, and bile stasis. Current recommendations are that weight loss should not exceed 500 g per week in children, or 1600 g per week in adults.

Cholestatic liver disease

Cholestasis develops when there is failure of the bile to reach the duodenum, resulting in accumulation of bile in liver cells. It may be caused by obstruction of the common bile duct, neoplastic or developmental defects, or failure of the hepatocytes to secrete an adequate amount of bile. The liver is enlarged, and prolonged cholestasis may also result in biliary cirrhosis. Typical laboratory features include raised blood levels of bilirubin, ALP, and cholesterol. The patient usually presents with jaundice, pruritis, xanthomas (reversible), steatorrhea with malabsorption of calcium and fat-soluble vitamins, and hepatic osteodystrophy.

Nutritionally, cholestasis is managed by optimizing energy and protein intake together with supplements of fat-soluble vitamins, and a low-fat diet (<40 g/day) supplemented with medium-chain triacylglycerols (up to 40 g per day). In the presence of bone changes, vitamin D_2 (100 000 units) is given intramuscularly every four weeks, adapting the dose according to serum levels. The active form of vitamin D is preferred in cases with symptomatic osteomalacia. Calcium gluconate (6 g) should be given in cases with prolonged cholestasis, and phosphate supplements should be given if serum levels are low. The latter should be given on alternate days with the calcium to avoid the formation of complexes in the gut. With severe bone pain, intravenous calcium (15 mg calcium/kg as calcium gluconate in 500 ml 5% dextrose) can be given over 4 h daily for about 7 days, with close monitoring of blood levels. Cholestyramine is useful in the treatment of pruritis as it binds with bile salts in the gastrointestinal tract. However, it should be kept in mind that cholestyramine also binds calcium and fat-soluble vitamins. Glucocorticoids are helpful in the management of pruritis, but should be avoided, as it will contribute to any underlying hepatic osteodystrophy.

Inherited disorders

Wilson's disease

Wilson's disease is an autosomal recessive inherited disorder characterized by increased copper accumulation in the liver, brain, kidneys, heart, muscle, pancreas, and the cornea. The primary defect is in the liver, with a decreased excretion of copper in the bile. Characteristics of Wilson's disease include a hepatic copper content of >200–250 µg/g dry weight, a decrease in serum levels of copper and ceruloplasmin, and Kayser–Fleisch rings. Complications include liver damage with cirrhosis, neurological, and psychiatric disturbances, hemolysis, renal tubular damage, and demineralization of bone. Treatment options include D-penicillamine (chelates copper), trientene (if sensitive to D-penicillamine), zinc (sequestrates copper in the gut), or liver transplantation. Dietary treatment is of limited value, but a diet low in copper (1.5 mg/day) may be of some value. Sources high in dietary copper include shellfish, dried fruit, chocolate, nuts, broccoli, liver, mushrooms, and legumes. With early and effective treatment patients can live a normal life.

Hemochromatosis

Hemochromatosis is a autosomal recessive metabolic defect with an increase in the intestinal absorption of iron, leading to excessive iron deposition in the liver, pancreas, spleen, heart, kidneys, gastrointestinal mucosa, skin, and testis. Hepatic complications include liver fibrosis, cirrhosis, and hepatocellular carcinoma. Diabetes has been estimated to occur in about two-thirds of patients with hemochromatosis, but its frequency has now decreased due to earlier diagnosis of the condition, and it is usually not seen in the absence of cirrhosis. If present, it may be controlled by diet and/or oral medication, but in some patients treatment may be difficult even with large doses of insulin. The brain and central nervous system is not affected. Iron can damage the liver via lipid peroxidation, deposition of hemosiderin in lysosomes, and increased collagen synthesis. In the initial stages of the disease, there is only increased iron absorption, and later in the course of the disease, it is followed by a decrease in serum transferrin, an increase in serum iron, hepatic iron, total body iron, progressive tissue damage, and finally cirrhosis at the age of about 40–50 years (Figure 11.5).

Characteristics of the disease include abdominal pain, hepatomegaly, splenomegaly, a fibrotic pancreas, testicular atrophy, skin pigmentation, increased serum iron, ferritin, transferrin saturation, and an increase in the hepatic iron index. In the absence of anemia, treatment includes venesection (500 ml once or twice a week until the hematocrit value drops below 37%), which removes about 250 mg iron at a time. This is followed by maintenance phlebotomy of 1 unit of whole blood every 2–3 months (folate supplementation is essential). If anemia is present, however, chelating agents may be used. Dietary restriction of iron is not very effective, but a reduction in heme iron, vitamin C, and alcohol has been advocated. Food should also not be cooked in iron pots. If treatment is initiated before the onset of cirrhosis, patients will have a normal life expectancy.

Liver cirrhosis

Liver cirrhosis is the end stage of a number of different chronic liver diseases. It may develop as a result of chronic alcohol abuse, viral hepatitis, drugs, toxic substances, prolonged cholestasis, vascular, autonomic and metabolic disorders, intestinal bypass surgery, or it may be cryptogenic in nature. It is characterized by hepatocellular damage with necrosis of hepatocytes,

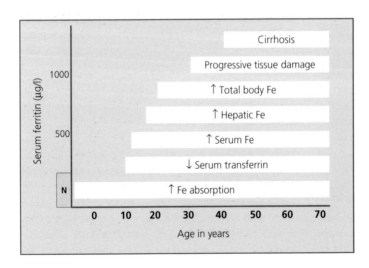

Figure 11.5 The clinical course and iron status in hemochromatosis. Sherlock and Dooley (1993). N, normal range.

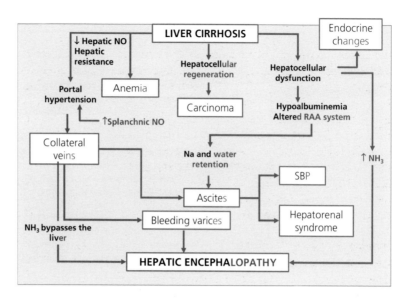

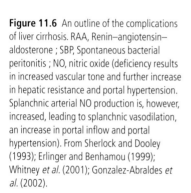

Figure 11.6 An outline of the complications of liver cirrhosis. RAA, Renin–angiotensin–aldosterone ; SBP, Spontaneous bacterial peritonitis ; NO, nitric oxide (deficiency results in increased vascular tone and further increase in hepatic resistance and portal hypertension. Splanchnic arterial NO production is, however, increased, leading to splanchnic vasodilation, an increase in portal inflow and portal hypertension). From Sherlock and Dooley (1993); Erlinger and Benhamou (1999); Whitney *et al.* (2001); Gonzalez-Abraldes *et al.* (2002).

collapse of reticulin, nodular regeneration, and fibrosis, and it may predispose to the development of hepatocellular carcinoma. The early stage of liver cirrhosis may be asymptomatic, or the patient may present with clinical evidence of cirrhosis, which implies a dramatic decline in the functional reserve of the liver. With the development of complications (Figure 11.6) such as ascites, encephalopathy, and variceal bleeding, the prognosis deteriorates, with a mean survival period of 1–5 years. Severe complications such as spontaneous bacterial peritonitis or refractory ascites are associated with a lifespan of about one year.

Increased intestinal protein losses have been reported in liver cirrhosis, which is thought to be caused by an increased splanchnic lymph flow, and is associated with venous, portal, and lymphatic hypertension. Posthepatic venous obstruction in patients with liver cirrhosis has been shown to increase the formation of protein-rich hepatic and thoracic duct lymph, which 'weeps' into the peritoneal cavity to initiate ascites. The treatment aspects of the latter are discussed elsewhere in this chapter.

11.3 Laboratory assessment of liver function

Tests of liver function are required for diagnostic purposes, to estimate severity of the disease, to assess prognosis, and to evaluate the response to therapy (Table 11.3). These tests can be divided into three categories according to the underlying mechanisms of hepatic disease:

- hepatocyte damage characterized by the release of hepatocellular enzymes with an accompanying rise in their plasma concentration(s),
- cholestasis characterized by retention of conjugated bilirubin and alkaline phosphatase, and
- reduced mass of functioning hepatocytes characterized by alterations in protein synthesis/degradation, for instance reduction in the synthesis of albumin and prothrombin.

11.4 Manifestations and complications of cirrhosis

Clinical signs of liver disease

The clinical signs of liver disease can be grouped into those caused by impaired liver function and those caused by portal hypertension (Table 11.4).

The Child–Turcotte–Pugh score (Table 11.5) can be used to predict the prognosis of patients with liver disease who has undergone surgery. The mortality rate has been estimated at 10% for class A, 30% for class B, and 82% for class C patients. The score has also been associated with postoperative complications like renal failure, ascites, encephalopathy, infections, and worsening of liver function.

Table 11.3 Summary of biochemical parameters used in the assessment of liver disease

	Parameter	Comments
Plasma protein	Albumin	Decreased in advanced liver disease; assess severity
		Decreased with the acute phase response
		Decreased with increased plasma volume
		Usually normal with biliary obstruction and acute hepatitis due to short half-life
	Prealbumin	Decreased in liver disease
	Globulin	High immunoglobulin A and G (chronic hepatitis and cirrhosis)
		High immunoglobulin M (primary biliary cirrhosis)
	Ceruloplasmin	Decreased activity in Wilson's disease
		Decreased in liver failure
		Increased with the acute phase response
		Increased with obstructive jaundice
	Ferritin	Increased with hemochromatosis and hepatocellular damage
		Increased with the acute phase response
Bilirubin	Conjugated	Increased with dysfunction of liver parenchyme or bile ducts
		Increased with obstruction of the bile ducts
	Unconjugated	Increased with hemolysis
		Increased with abnormal bilirubin metabolism
Tests indicating hepatocellular damage	AST	Early diagnosis of hepatocellular disease; follow progress
		AST/ALT usually >2 in alcoholic liver damage, with the value of each <300 U
	ALT	Increased with liver damage – may be 100 times normal. More specific for liver cell damage than AST
	LD	More indicative of myocardial infarction and hemolysis
		May be markedly increased with neoplasms, especially with hepatic involvement
Tests indicating cholestasis	ALP	Derived from the liver, bone, kidneys, gut, tumors and placenta and excreted via the bile
		Serum activity rises with intrahepatic cholestasis or extrahepatic obstruction
		Modest elevation in many types of liver disease
		Markedly elevated in cholestases
	GGT	Derived from the liver, kidneys, pancreas, gut, spleen, heart, lung, brain, prostate, bile
		Suggests alcoholic liver disease if GGT/ALP > 2.5
		Increased in acute cholesistitis, cholestasis or obstruction, diabetes and acute pancreatitis, and may also be induced by drugs
Other	Prothrombin time	Prolonged with parenchymal liver dysfunction
		Prolonged secondary to vitamin K deficiency (fat malabsorption)
		Increased with advanced liver disease; assess severity
	Ammonia	Elevation has been implicated as a risk factor for hepatic encephalopathy
		Increased during fits, inborn errors of metabolism
	Urea	Decreased with advanced liver disease

Adapted from Sherlock and Dooley (1993), Ryder and Beckingham (2001), Leevy *et al.* (1994), Davern and Scharshmidt (2002) and Beckingham and Ryder (2001).
AST, aspartate transaminase; ALT, alanine transaminase; LD, lactate dehydrogenase; ALP, alkaline phosphatase; GGT, gamma-glutamyl transferase.

Portal hypertension

The portal venous system drains the stomach, gut, pancreas, and spleen, and carries a large volume of blood. There are also communications with the systemic circulation, which are not usually in use (natural 'collateral veins'). Portal hypertension develops as a result of obstruction to blood flow, as the large volume of blood cannot pulse easily through the scarred tissue of a cirrhotic liver. Under these conditions, the collateral veins dilate to allow the portal venous blood to return to the systemic circulation (Figure 11.6). In the process, the liver may also be bypassed so that gut-derived toxins and microbes reach the systemic circulation.

The increase in pressure leads to the enlargement of the collateral veins and the formation of varices. The esophageal varices, especially, are prone to rupture and massive bleeding which carries a 20–30% risk of death per bleeding episode. Also, patients who have once bled from esophageal varices carry a 70% risk to bleed again. It has further been shown that even a moderate amount of oral alcohol consumption worsens the portal hypertensive syndrome, and that it may increase the risk of variceal bleeding in patients with

Table 11.4 Summary of the clinical signs found in advanced liver disease

Effect of liver disease	Asterixis	Flapping tremor of the dorsiflexed hand with the arm outstretched
	Ascites and edema	Caused by hypoalbuminemia, portal hypertension, and sodium and fluid retention
	Bleeding tendency	Rupture of varices
		Impaired synthesis of clotting factors
	Fetor hepaticus	Sweetish, slightly fecal smell of breath
		Correlates with severity of disease
		Might be derived from sulfur compounds like methionine.
		Often precedes coma.
	Gynecomastia/testicular atrophy	Due to altered estrogen and androgen metabolism
		Alcoholic liver disease is the commonest association
	Jaundice	Yellow discoloration of body tissues due to increased blood levels of bilirubin (> 34μmol/l)
	Palmar erythema	Hands are warm and palms bright red, flushing synchronously with the pulse rate
		Most prominent on the hypothenar and thenar eminences and the fingertips
		Feet may also be affected
		Due to altered estrogen and androgen metabolism
		May be familial
	Pruritis	Unknown cause
		Found in biliary obstruction
	Xanthomas/xanthelasma	Increased serum cholesterol
		Found in biliary obstruction/cholestasis
	Spider nevi	Consists of central arteriole, radiating from which are numerous small blood vessels resembling a spider's legs (3–15 mm)
		Blanch when skin is compressed or stretched
		Commonly found in necklace area, face, back, forearms, dorsum of the hand
		Common with cirrhosis, especially in alcoholics; also found in pregnancy
		May disappear with improving hepatic function
		Due to altered estrogen and androgen metabolism
	Paper money skin	Usually found on the upper arms and face
		Numerous small vessels scattered in random fashion through the skin, resembling the silk threads in United State's dollar bills
	White spots	Found on the arms and buttocks on cooling of the skin
		Centre of the spot represents the beginnings of a spider
	White nail	Opacity of the nail bed.
		A pink zone is seen at the tip of the nail
		Bilateral, especially involving the thumb and index finger
Effect of portal hypertension	Esophageal varices	Caused by portal hypertension, due to obstruction of the blood flow
	Caput medusae	Enlarged veins around the umbilicus
	Edema and ascites	Caused by hypoalbuminemia, portal hypertension, and sodium and fluid retention
	Decreased red cells, white cells, and platelets	Caused by hypersplenism

Sherlock and Dooley (1993); Leevy *et al.* (1994).

Table 11.5 Child–Turcotte–Pugh scoring system to assess the severity of liver disease

Clinical and laboratory measurements	Points scored for increasing abnormality		
	1	2	3
Encephalopathy (grade)	None	1–2	3–4
Ascites	None	Mild or controlled by diuretics	At least moderate despite diuretic treatment
Prothrombin time (seconds prolonged) or	<4	4–6	>6
International normalized ratio (INR)	< 1.7	1.7–2.3	>2.3
Albumin (g/dl)	> 3.5	2.8–3.5	< 2.8
Bilirubin (mg/dl)	< 2	2–3	> 3

Grade A: 5–6; Grade B: 7–9; Grade C: 10–15.
From Davern and Scharschmidt (2002)

alcohol-induced cirrhosis. The same effect could not be demonstrated in a placebo-controlled study where a 10% solution of ethanol in 5% dextrose was given intravenously to raise blood alcohol levels to 100 mg/dl over 30 min. Larger intravenous doses (1 g alcohol/kg body weight), however, have been shown to increase portal hypertension significantly. Acute bleeding from varices needs to be controlled in order to prevent encephalopathy and death, and rebleeding must be prevented. Options for long-term management include sclerotherapy, endoscopic ligation or balloon tube tamponade, beta-blockers, surgical shunt, and liver transplantation. Patients who are treated with sclerotherapy may experience dysphagia due to stricture formation, and may require a soft diet.

Pharmacologic management with vasoactive drugs is the treatment of choice for esophageal varices that have not yet bled. Spironolactone, an aldosterone antagonist, and sodium restriction is effective in reducing plasma volume and portal pressure, but sodium-restricted diets are often unpalatable and may contribute to poor intake and the development of malnutrition. The effect of spironolactone administration given concomitantly with an unrestricted sodium diet to 18 patients with compensated cirrhosis and portal hypertension, was investigated in a placebo-controlled study (6 patients in placebo and 12 in control group). None of the patients had encephalopathy, edema, or ascites. Spironolactone was associated with a significant reduction in hepatic venous pressure gradient, cardiac output, wedged hepatic venous pressure, and plasma volume at eight weeks, but no significant change in heart rate, mean arterial pressure, free hepatic venous pressure, hepatic blood flow, or hepatic vascular resistance. Ascites and edema were not clinically apparent and weight did not increase, indicating that sodium balance was maintained by increased sodium output. However, it was also evident in this study that spironolactone with an unrestricted sodium diet decreased portal pressure only in Pugh–Child's A, but not in Pugh–Child's B grade patients. Spironolactone together with sodium restriction may therefore well be necessary in the treatment of portal hypertension in Pugh–Child's grade B patients.

Ascites

The development of edema and ascites in liver cirrhosis results from the alterations in the balance of albumin

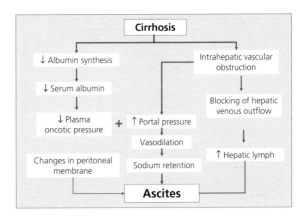

Figure 11.7 The pathogenesis of ascites. Adapted from Sherlock and Dooley (1993); Arroyo *et al.* (1999); Runyon (2002).

synthesis/degradation by the liver, which in turn leads to a reduction in serum albumin and plasma oncotic pressure. This, together with portal hypertension, results in the extravasation of plasma into the abdominal cavity, causing ascites (Figure 11.7). There may also be an accumulation of hepatic lymph due to blockage of the hepatic venous outflow, and permeability changes in the peritoneal membrane may further contribute to the development of ascites. As fluid accumulates in the abdomen, there is a reduction in blood volume and a decrease in blood flow to the kidneys. The latter increases the synthesis of aldosterone and antidiuretic hormone, leading to sodium and water retention. In the presence of hepatic impairment aldosterone levels remain high, thus enhancing sodium and water retention. Early stages of cirrhosis thus appear to be characterized by sodium retention and extracellular volume expansion even with low sodium diets of 100 mEq/day.

The complications of ascites include tense ascites, pleural effusions, spontaneous bacterial peritonitis, increase in portal pressure, early satiety and anorexia, herniation of the abdominal wall, gut edema, and the hepatorenal syndrome. Spontaneous bacterial peritonitis is the most common infection in cirrhotic patients with ascites and is thought to be associated with poor nutritional status and, possibly, bacterial translocation. Ascites has also been associated with an increase in energy expenditure, and removal of ascitic fluid via paracentesis has been reported to decrease REE parallel to the weight loss achieved.

Ascites is best treated with bed rest, diuretics, and sodium restriction (see section on Nutritional management in liver disease). Treatment with diuretics may result in intravascular volume depletion, electrolyte imbalance, and renal impairment. Low doses of albumin infusion have been reported to reduce the recurrence of ascites in cirrhotic patients treated with diuretics. Large volume paracentesis (removal of >5 liters of ascitic fluid at once) has been used successfully in tense ascites in decompensated liver cirrhosis, with the administration of albumin or other plasma expanders usually being recommended to prevent complications like hyponatremia and renal insufficiency. Paracentesis is reported to be associated with amino acid losses, which amounted to no more than 3 g of amino acids. However, the protein content of ascitic fluid is known to vary widely and is expected to directly influence the loss of amino acids induced by paracentesis.

Jaundice

Jaundice is one of the most common symptoms of liver disease, and it can be clinically detected when the sclera, skin, and mucous membranes become yellow, usually at a blood bilirubin concentration of about 40 µmol/l. Jaundice is classified as prehepatic (unconjugated bilirubinemia), hepatic (parenchymal disorder), or posthepatic (obstructive), depending upon the underlying cause. With prehepatic jaundice, bilirubin is produced at a faster rate than the liver can conjugate it for excretion, as with hemolysis. The most common causes of hepatic jaundice include viral hepatitis, alcoholic cirrhosis, primary biliary cirrhosis, drug-induced jaundice, and alcoholic hepatitis. Posthepatic jaundice most often results from biliary obstruction by stones or carcinoma. With hepatic parenchymal disorders, both conjugated and unconjugated levels of bilirubin are increased, and stools and urine are typically normal in color.

Jaundice due to prehepatic causes is characterized by unconjugated hyperbilirubinemia, whereas jaundice due to posthepatic causes (both intrahepatic cholestases and extrahepatic obstruction) is characterized by increased levels of conjugated bilirubin. Conjugated bilirubin is water-soluble and is excreted in the urine, giving it a typically dark color, whereas the absence of bilirubin in the stools imparts a 'putty' color to it. Stool color on its own is, however not a very reliable indicator of the underlying disorder. Jaundice *per se* does not usually require dietary restriction of fat, unless it is accompanied by nausea and vomiting.

Steatorrhea

Steatorrhea (resulting from fat malabsorption) may develop as a result of decreased secretion of bile acids by the failing liver, and may be present in about 50% of patients with chronic liver disease. It is accompanied by malabsorption of fat-soluble vitamins and calcium, and may lead to the development of hepatic osteodystrophy. The dietary management of steatorrhea is discussed elsewhere in this chapter.

Hepatic encephalopathy

Hepatic encephalopathy describes the spectrum of potentially reversible neuropsychiatric abnormalities seen in patients with liver dysfunction after exclusion of unrelated neurologic and/or metabolic abnormalities. The term implies that altered brain function is due to metabolic abnormalities, which occur as consequence of liver failure. The symptoms may range from subclinical to coma, with neuropsychiatric symptoms being present to varying degrees. Encephalopathy can be present in both acute and chronic liver failure, and the neuropsychiatric manifestations are potentially reversible. The acute form of hepatic encephalopathy carries a high mortality risk, and is associated with fulminant liver failure, which quickly progresses to profound coma, seizures, and a decerebrate state. Death is usually due to cerebral herniation and hypoxia. The chronic form of encephalopathy is characterized by persistence of neuropsychiatric symptoms despite adequate medical treatment. It may be associated with irreversible brain damage but the survival rate is relatively high.

Classification of hepatic encephalopathy
Hepatic encephalopathy can be divided into five different clinical stages on the basis of elicited symptoms and signs as well as special investigations (Table 11.6).

The Glasgow Coma Scale (Table 11.7) is widely used in the assessment of structural and metabolic disorders of brain function, and may also be applied in acute and chronic liver disease to determine the level of consciousness.

Precipitating factors for hepatic encephalopathy
The exact causes of hepatic encephalopathy remain unclear, but it is postulated that nitrogenous substances derived from the gut adversely affect brain

Table 11.6 Classification of hepatic encephalopathy

Stage	Consciousness	Intellect	Neurologic	Tremor	Behavior	EEG
Subclinical	Normal	Action IQ ↓	Abnormal psychometric tests	Absent	Normal	Normal
Stage 1	Sleeping disorder Absent minded Lack of awareness	Calculation ↓	Impaired handwriting (asterixis)	Slight finger tremor	Accentuation of normal behavior Euphoria or depression	Slightly ↓ (7–8/s)
Stage 2	Drowsy Lethargic	Time orientation ↓	Asterixis Ataxia Slurred speech	Flapping tremor easily provoked	Disinhibition Apathy	Slow (6–7/s)
Stage 3	Sleeps most of the time but can be woken	Spatial orientation ↓	Asterixis Increased reflexes Positive Babinski	Flapping tremor present most of the time	Delusion Aggression	Slow (3–5/s)
Stage 4	Comatose	Comatose	Pupil dilation Decerebral condition Opistotonus	Absent	–	Very slow (2–3/s)

Adapted from Gerber and Schomerus (2000); Abou-Assi and Vlahcevic (2001); Blei *et al.* (2001).
IQ, intelligence quotient; EEG, Electroencephalogram

Table 11.7 Level of consciousness with the Glasgow Coma Scale

Eyes open		Best motor response		Best verbal response	
Spontaneously	4	Obeys verbal orders	6	Oriented, conversant	5
To command	3	Localises painful stimuli	5	Disoriented, conversant	4
To pain	2	Painful stimulus, flexion	3	Inappropriate words	3
No response	1	Painful stimulus, extension	2	Inappropriate sounds	2
		No response	1	No response	1

From Blei *et al.* (2001). [Add permissions]
To obtain the score, the best ocular, verbal, and motor responses are summed. The best score is 15 and the worst 3. Severe encephalopathy is defined as a score of <12

function, due to failure of the liver to metabolize these substances and other toxins. These reach the systemic circulation as a result of impaired liver function and portal-systemic shunts, which bypass the liver (Figure 11.8). They then cross the blood–brain barrier, and alter neurotransmission in the brain that may affect consciousness and behavior.

Potential precipitating factors for hepatic encephalopathy are listed in Table 11.8.

Ammonia

The gut is an important source of nitrogen-containing substances since colonic bacteria produce ammonia by the deamination of glutamine to glutamate. It has been estimated that approximately 40% of ammonia in the gut is derived from the ingestion and metabolism of nitrogenous substances, with the remaining 60% being derived from the conversion of glutamine to glutamate,

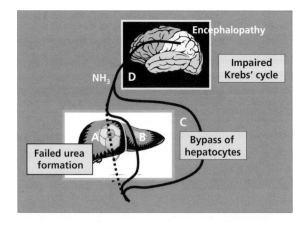

Figure 11.8 Liver cell bypass/damage in patients with impaired hepatic function. (A) Decreased conversion of ammonia to urea due to liver cell damage. (B and C) Failure in the hepatic conversion of ammonia to urea due to liver cell bypass (intrahepatic (B) and extrahepatic (C) shunts due to cirrhosis). (D) Impaired Krebs' cycle (due to excess ammonia) contributes to the development of hepatic encephalopathy.

Table 11.8 Precipitating factors in the pathogenesis of hepatic encephalopathy

Mechanism	Precipitating factors
Increased ammonia production	High protein intake
	Constipation (longer contact time with the gut and hence increased time for ammonia absorption)
	Fluid restriction
	Gastrointestinal bleeding
	Infection (increased protein catabolism)
	Blood transfusion
	Alkalosis (increased renal production of ammonia)
	Surgery
Ammonia diffusion across blood–brain barrier	Alkalosis
Decreased ammonia detoxification	Skeletal muscle wasting (reduces the ability to metabolize ammonia)
Decreased urea formation	Acidosis
Decreased metabolism of toxins due to hypoxia	Dehydration
	Arterial hypotension
	Hypovolemia
	Hypoxia
	Anemia
	Fever
Central nervous system depression and binding with GABA receptors	Medication (antidepressants, morphine)
Decreased hepatic metabolism	Portosystemic shunts
Increased susceptibility to infections and hepatic dysfunction	Alcohol

Adapted from Sherlock and Dooley (1993); Gerber and Schomerus (2000).
GABA, gamma-aminobutyric acid.

as well as the deamination and transamination of other amino acids. In the liver, ammonia is normally metabolized to urea, which is then excreted in the urine. Another means of detoxifying ammonia is via formation of glutamine from glutamate in the muscle, liver, and brain. Elevated ammonia levels usually result from impaired hepatic function together with excessive protein intake, constipation, malnutrition, gastrointestinal bleeding, infections, and metabolic alkalosis. When ammonia reaches the brain, it crosses the blood–brain barrier by simple diffusion. Since there is no urea cycle in the brain, ammonia combines with glutamate (an excitatory neurotransmitter) to form glutamine in the perineural astrocytes under the influence of glutamine synthetase, in order to prevent excitotoxicity. Ammonia also appears to enhance the transfer of tryptophan across the blood–brain barrier by an unknown mechanism, thus stimulating seretonin metabolism.

Hyperammonemia has a neurotoxic effect and has been associated with the development of hepatic encephalopathy. The mechanism for this neurotoxicity is not clear but may include a direct as well as an indirect effect. A direct effect is suggested by ammonia's ability to block extrusion of chloride ions and to decrease excitatory transmission by postsynaptic action. The degree of ammonia elevation does, however, not correlate with the severity of encephalopathy, and some patients with encephalopathy may even have normal blood levels of ammonia. A possible explanation for this finding is that blood levels do not always correlate very well with brain concentrations of ammonia, and that arterial levels of ammonia seem to correlate better with hepatic encephalopathy than venous levels. It has further been shown that blood ammonia levels correlate better with encephalopathy when determined in patients with impending or established coma upon admission and before institution of therapeutic procedures such as antibiotics, which may rapidly reduce ammonia levels. Permeability of the blood–brain barrier is increased in patients with hepatic encephalopathy, and, therefore, blood levels would be expected to correlate weakly with ammonia levels in the brain. Recent studies, however, suggested that this correlation can be improved by correcting ammonia levels to blood pH.

The indirect effect of ammonia in hepatic encephalopathy may be mediated by stimulation of glutamine synthesis. Glutamate is an excitatory neurotransmitter released from presynaptic neurons, and it has been suggested that increased glutamine synthesis may deplete brain glutamate levels, thereby promoting encephalopathy. Also, high rates of astrocytic glutamine synthesis have been shown to disrupt neurotransmitter uptake. This hypothesis has, however, been questioned since it has been shown that extracellular glutamate levels in the brains of rats with acute liver failure or hyperammonemia were increased despite decreased levels of total brain glutamate. It has also been speculated that glutamine synthesis is associated with the development of cerebral edema which may eventually lead to increased intracranial pressure and tissue hypoxia, and that glutamate promotes the uptake of aromatic amino acids by the blood–brain barrier.

False neurotransmitters

The neurotransmitter theory can be divided into the amino acid–neurotransmitter theory and the gamma-aminobutyric acid (GABA) theory. The existence of an abnormal amino acid ratio (an increase in serum aromatic amino acids (AAA) and a decrease in branched-chain amino acids (BCAA)) in patients with severe liver failure and hepatic encephalopathy is well known. In liver failure, the metabolism of AAAs and methionine is decreased due to failure of hepatic deamination, leading to increased blood levels. BCAAs, on the other hand, are catabolized at an accelerated rate by muscle, resulting in lower blood levels. A decrease in the BCAA : AAA ratio from 3.5 : 1 to 1 : 1 is proposed to lead to an increase in the uptake of AAAs by the brain. The increase in AAAs in the central nervous system is thought to interfere with physiologic neurotransmission by competitively inhibiting normal neurotransmitters such as dopamine and norepinephrine, and the attendant synthesis of false neurotransmitters such as octopamine.

GABA is derived from bacterial flora in the gut, and is the principal inhibitory neurotransmitter in the brain. It passes through the blood–brain barrier and induces its own receptors in the brain. It has been postulated that hepatic encephalopathy is associated with increased numbers of binding sites for GABA. It has also been suggested that elevated ammonia levels may enhance GABA-ergic neurotransmission, but other studies failed to confirm a pathogenic role of GABA in chronic liver disease. Elevated plasma GABA concentrations have, however, been associated with acute liver disease.

Mercaptans

The proposed theory, which needs to be confirmed, on the role of mercaptans in hepatic encephalopathy is based on the reported increase in serum mercaptans, which are formed from methionine by colonic bacteria in patients with cirrhosis. High concentrations of serum mercaptans is associated with the typical fetor hepaticus odor in patients with encephalopathy. Theoretically, these products may have a neurotoxic effect by their reported inhibition of Na^+/K^+-ATPases, with subsequent accumulation of sodium intracellularly, and brain edema.

Short-chain fatty acids

The mode of action of short-chain fatty acids in hepatic encephalopathy is thought to be based on the inhibition of Na^+/K^+-ATPase and urea synthesis in the liver. Free fatty acids may also increase tryptophan uptake by the brain by decreasing the affinity of albumin for tryptophan resulting in increased cerebral formation of seretonin, a decrease in the density of seretonin receptors but with an increase in affinity. The latter may explain the altered sleep–wake rhythm in hepatic encephalopathy.

Zinc and manganese

A more recent hypothesis associates zinc deficiency and manganese deposition (due to portal-systemic shunting and from impaired hepatobiliary elimination) in the basal ganglia of the brain, with hepatic encephalopathy. However, short-term oral zinc supplementation failed to improve hepatic encephalopathy.

Alkalosis

Patients with hepatic encephalopathy are often alkalotic, due to toxic stimulation of the respiratory center by ammonia, the administration of alkali, or hypokalemia. The latter has been associated with clinical deterioration and increased ammonia levels in the blood, irrespective of the rate of alimentary synthesis of ammonia.

Alcohol

Alcohol is not only known to be injurious to the liver, but it is also thought to precipitate hepatic encephalopathy because of its neurodepressant properties. Alcoholics also have an increased susceptibility to infections due to underlying malnutrition, which may indirectly contribute to encephalopathy.

Helicobacter pylori

The relationship between infection with *Helicobacter pylori* (a urease-containing organism) and hyperammonemia as a precipitating factor for hepatic encephalopathy is not clear, and remains speculative. Therefore, eradication of *H. pylori* cannot be recommended as a therapeutic strategy at this stage.

In conclusion, a variety of metabolites/substances have been evoked to explain the mechanism(s) of hepatic encephalopathy, but all remain mostly speculative. In addition, interactions between the various factors seem likely, and it is also possible that reported 'abnormalities' may indeed be the effect rather than the cause of hepatic encephalopathy.

Treatment of hepatic encephalopathy

In patients with chronic end stage liver disease, orthotopic liver transplantation, when possible, remains the treatment of choice. When transplantation is not feasible, the recommended treatment goals are as follows:

Provision of supportive care

Adequate supportive care, including nutrition support, is critical during all stages of hepatic encephalopathy.

Identification and removal of precipitating factors

Treatment of precipitating factors such as gastrointestinal bleeding, infections, electrolyte disturbances, constipation, excessive protein intake, sedatives, and diuretics, which may contribute to the precipitation and/or exacerbation of hepatic encephalopathy in up to 80% of patients, is of crucial importance.

Cleansing of the gut

Intestinal cleansing is a standard therapeutic measure to remove nitrogen-containing precursors of ammonia, and is especially important in patients with gastrointestinal bleeding and constipation. Methods used to cleanse the gut include lactulose (β-galactosidofructose) and lactilol (β-galactosido-sorbitol). Both are non-absorbable disaccharides, which are metabolized by colonic flora to acetic acid, lactate, and propionic acid. Their metabolism leads to a decrease in the colonic pH, assimilation of ammonia as a nitrogen source by bacteria, a decrease in portal blood ammonia and as a result, a reduction in the peripheral levels and total body pool of ammonia. There may also be a decrease in ammonia absorption due to fecal acidity,

and a decrease in ammonia-producing bacteria. Additionally, their acid metabolites lead to an increase in the osmotic pressure in the intestinal lumen, which has a laxative effect and decreases the intestinal transit time. Lactulose is usually given orally at a dosage of 30–60 g (30–45 g lactilol), sufficient to produce 2–3 soft stools per day. Side effects of lactulose include flatulence, diarrhea (which must be avoided as it can cause hypertonic dehydration and electrolyte imbalances which may aggravate the patient's mental state), and abdominal cramping. Lactilol, on the other hand, has fewer side effects and it is more palatable.

Antibacterial drugs such as aminoglycosides (neomycin) can be used to limit the growth of gut bacteria, and are as effective as disaccharides, but they are associated with nephro- and ototoxicity. Neomycin also impairs the activity of glutaminase of the intestinal villi, leading to a decrease in ammonia production from glutamine. The nephro- and ototoxicity of aminoglycosides is reported to be a cumulative effect and usually irreversible, and these antibiotics should therefore not be used for longer than one month. Metronidazole is a useful alternative to neomycin, affecting a different bacterial population. It is neurotoxic, especially in patients with severe liver disease, which impairs the clearance of the drug.

Promotion of optimal nutritional status

See section on Nutritional management in liver disease.

Stimulation of ammonia metabolism

The predominant ammonia detoxification mechanisms are the urea cycle in the liver and the conversion of glutamate to glutamine. Both glutamate and α-ketoglutarate promote glutamine production. Ornithine is a substrate for the urea cycle and supplementation of ≥20 g of ornithine aspartate has been shown to increase the conversion of ammonia to urea. Aspartate is also a substrate for the synthesis of glutamine via transamination to glutamate. Preliminary evidence with these amino acids in prospective, randomized, placebo-controlled, double-blind trials have documented improvements in mental state.

Other options for the treatment of hepatic encephalopathy with questionable outcomes include sodium benzoate (decreases ammonia via excretion in the urine), antipsychotic drugs, liver transplantation, and colectomy or colon bypass (carries a high mortality risk and is rarely performed in non-transplant candidates) and modification of gut flora by *Lactobacillus acidophilus* and *Enterococcus fecium*.

11.5 Nutritional management in liver disease

Patients with cirrhosis of the liver have presented with nutritional problems since the condition was first recognized around 400BC. Hippocrates stressed the importance of nutrition in the treatment of this disease and believed the main problem could be attributed to poor digestion. Despite the major advances made in the field of clinical nutrition, our knowledge of the influence of a malfunctioning liver on the nutritional state of the body is surprisingly small, as is our ability to effectively use nutritional intervention in the treatment of some of the consequences of liver disease.

In acute liver failure malnutrition is rarely a problem. However, in patients with chronic liver disease, mixed protein–energy malnutrition is common and is associated with a poor prognosis. It is important to separate the effect of malnutrition from the effect of the liver disease itself when one considers prognosis. As a result of these gray areas, nutritional support is still under debate in patients with liver cirrhosis, despite several studies showing positive effects on liver function and prognosis.

Assessment of nutritional status

The assessment of nutritional status in liver disease is complicated by the effect of impaired liver function on nutrient metabolism and the effect of the disease itself as well as ascites and water retention on anthropometric measurements. Assessment of nutritional status should focus on dietary intake and history of weight loss, detection of edema and ascites, assessment of somatic protein reserves and body fat, and manifestations of micronutrient deficiencies. Serum proteins are used for assessment of the visceral protein compartment, but may correlate better with the degree of liver failure and level of stress than with nutritional status. The use of creatinine-height index will be limited in patients with renal failure, bioelectrical impedance will have limited value in the presence of ascites and edema, and urea nitrogen appearance may provide unreliable data on nitrogen balance due to the decrease in urea synthesis in liver disease.

Newer techniques of measuring body composition include dual-energy X-ray absorptiometry (DXA) and bioelectrical impedance analysis (BIA). The latter is a more convenient method of assessing body composition but its accuracy in liver disease is poor due to varying states of hydration. The validity of DXA in assessing body composition in patients with end stage liver disease and fluid retention has also not been determined.

Nevertheless, the use of some such parameters (Table 11.9) have been useful in the assessment of nutritional status of patients with severe alcoholic liver disease.

Prevalence and causes of malnutrition

The prevalence of malnutrition in chronic liver disease ranges widely from 0% to 100%. Much of this variation results from the difficulties in assessment due to the lack of a standardized diagnosis and classification of malnutrition in patients with liver cirrhosis. Malnutrition is also common in patients with other liver disorders, with reports of anergy to skin hypersensitivity tests in 60%, weight loss greater than 20% of the predicted value in 14% and deficiencies in fat-soluble vitamins occurring in 40% of patients. It is therefore not surprising that protein–energy malnutrition is considered by some to be the most common complication in chronic liver disease.

Since combined kwashiorkor-like malnutrition and marasmus coexist in liver disease, it has been recommended that malnutrition in liver disease be defined as protein–energy malnutrition (PEM). However, protein malnutrition has often been a more frequent finding than energy malnutrition. In hospitalized patients with moderately severe disease, evidence of protein malnutrition has been reported in 30–40% of patients. Furthermore, moderate and severe malnutrition has been reported in 48% of patients, with the most severe deficits being observed in visceral proteins with short half-life such as prealbumin and retinol-binding protein. Smaller deficits were seen in midarm muscle area and skinfold thicknesses. In liver cirrhosis, PEM is a common complication with patients frequently presenting with a low body mass index <18.5 kg/m^2, low albumin and immunoincompetence with abnormal response to skin tests. In alcoholic liver cirrhosis, ascites, and hepatic encephalopathy are significantly more frequent compared with patients with non-alcoholic liver cirrhosis. Other studies have reported that nu-

Table 11.9 Parameters for assessment of nutrition status in patients with liver disease

Parameters of nutritional status	Invalidation
Body weight corrected for edema and ascites	Edema, ascites, diuretic therapy
Skinfold thickness and fat stores	Edema, interobserver variability
Triceps	
Biceps	
Subscapular	
Iliac	
Midarm muscle area	
Creatinine-height index	Renal insufficiency
Visceral proteins	Impaired liver function
Albumin	
Transferrin	
Prealbumin	
Retinol-binding protein	
Urea nitrogen appearance	Decreased urea synthesis
Skin test responsiveness to a battery of antigens	Non-nutritional impairment
DXA	Not validated in end–stage liver disease

Wicks (2001); Mendenhall *et al.* (1995); Pomposelli and Burns (2002).

tritional abnormalities are present in all patients with moderate or severe alcoholic hepatitis, and that mean values for creatinine-height index, hemoglobin, cholesterol, and complement C4 are significantly lower in severe liver failure only in patients with alcoholic cirrhosis. In liver transplant recipients, malnutrition occurs in between 18% and 65% of patients.

The etiology of malnutrition in liver disease is multifactorial in nature (Tables 11.10 and 11.11) and is thought to be due to decreased dietary intake, increased nutrient losses, and alterations in substrate utilization and energy expenditure. Irrespective of its cause(s), the European Society for Clinical Nutrition and Metabolism (ESPEN) summarized the effects of PEM on the course of liver cirrhosis as follows:

- Nutritional status is correlated to mortality in the total group of patients with liver cirrhosis and in Child A and B patients if analyzed separately.
- Malnutrition is an independent predictor for the first bleeding episode and survival in patients with esophageal varices.
- Malnutrition is associated with the presence of refractory ascites.
- Preoperative nutritional status is related to postoperative complications and mortality.

Table 11.10 Possible causes of wasting in patients with liver disease

Reduced nutrient intake	Excessive nutrient losses	Increased requirements
Abdominal pain	Blood loss via GI bleeding	Ascites (increased metabolic rate)
Anorexia	Purgation and diarrhea	Infections
Gastroparesis	Malabsorption	Cytokines
Early satiety	Drugs	Malnutrition
Esophageal varices	Steatorrhea	Drugs
Drugs	Vomiting	Energy cost of alcohol metabolism
Nausea	Large volume paracentesis	
Restrictive/unpalatable diet		
Vomiting		
Refractory ascites		
Hepatic encephalopathy		
Zinc deficiency		
Hyperglycemia		
Leptin (anorexia)		
Increased TNF-α, IL-1, IL-6		

Lochs and Plauth (1999); Whitney *et al.* (2001); Wicks (2001); Scolapio *et al.* (2002).

Table 11.11 Nutritional related side effects of drugs used commonly in patients with liver disease

Medication	Indication for use	Side effects
Antidiabetic drugs	Hyperglycemia	Hypoglycemia
		Decreased serum folate and vitamin B_{12}
		Nausea, vomiting, flatulence
		Diarrhea or constipation
Antihypertensives	Portal hypertension	Pyridoxine depletion
		Hyperkalemia
		Diarrhea
		Dry mouth, nausea, and vomiting
Neomycin	Cleansing of the gut	May require vitamin K
		Nephrotoxicity
		Anemia and fatigue
Antilipemics	Hyperlipidemia	Nausea, dyspepsia, altered taste
		Constipation
		Decreased absorption of fat, fat-soluble vitamins, folate, calcium, iron, zinc, and magnesium
Megestrol acetate	Appetite stimulant	Nausea, vomiting
Dronibanol		Diarrhea
Spironolactone	Potassium-sparing diuretic	Elevated blood levels of potassium, magnesium, glucose
		Nausea, vomiting, diarrhea
Azathioprine	Liver transplantation	Macrocytic anemia
		Mouth sores, sore throat
		Nausea, vomiting, anorexia
		Decreased taste acuity
		Diarrhea
Cyclosporine	Immunosuppression	Sodium retention
		Hyperkalemia
		Hyperlipidemia
		Hyperglycemia
		Hypomagnesemia
		Nausea, vomiting
Tacrolimus	Immunosuppression	Hypertension
		Hyperglycemia
		Hyperkalemia
		Diarrhea/constipation
		Nausea, vomiting
Sirolimus	Immunosuppression	Possible hyperlipidemia
		Possible hyperglycemia
		Possible gastrointestinal symptoms
Glucocorticoids	Immunosuppression	Sodium retention
		Hyperlipidemia
		Hyperglycemia
		False hunger
		Protein wasting
		Decreased absorption of calcium and phosphorus
Interferon		Nausea, vomiting
		Weight loss
		Fever
		Fatigue
		Depression
Lactulose	Cleansing of the gut	Belching and cramps, flatulence
		Diarrhea
Penicillamine	Wilson's disease	Altered taste
		Anorexia, nausea and vomiting
		Diarrhea
		Vitamin B_6 deficiency
		Iron deficiency
		Proteinuria

Hasse and Matarese (2000); Whitney *et al.* (1998); Mahan and Escott-Stump (2000).

Table 11.12 Dietary recommendations for patients with liver disease

Clinical condition	NPE (kcal/kg per day)	Protein (g/kg per day)	Other
Compensated liver disease	25–35 or REE × 1.3	1.0–1.2	*Alcohol* Stop for 6–12 months in case of acute hepatitis *Fat* 40–50% NPE (25–40% TE) 35–50% NPE (TPN) low fat diet plus MCT (15 ml 3–4 times per day) in cases with steatorrhea *Carbohydrate* 60–50% NPE Hypoglycemic (small frequent meals) Hyperglycemia (as for diabetics) *Sodium* Restrict only as necessary to control ascites (usually not <2 g/day) *Water* 1–1.5 l/day with ascites (if serum sodium <120 mmol/l) *K, Mg, Ca, Zn, P* According to individual needs Supplementation may be indicated Ca supplementation (cholestasis, steatorrhea) *Zinc* Zinc acetate (220 mg b.i.d. in deficient patients) *Vitamin supplements* PEM and alcoholic liver disease (B-complex vitamins, folate, thiamin, vitamin B_6, B_{12}, and C) Cholestasis and bleeding (vitamin K) Steatorrhea (fat-soluble vitamins) *Meal frequency* 6–7 Small frequent meals including a late night snack rich in carbohydrate is effective in increasing food intake and improving N-balance
Complications			
Inadequate intake Malnutrition Ascites Hypercatabolic	35–40 or REE × 1.5	1.5	
Encephalopathy (grade 1–2)	25–35 or REE × 1.3	Transiently 0.5 then 1–1.5 Increase by 0.25–0.5 g/kg every 2nd to 3rd day or 10 g/day every 2nd to 3rd day If protein-tolerant, use plant protein or BCAA supplement (0.25 g/kg) Increase protein in combination with non-absorbable disaccharides	
Encephalopathy (grade 3–4)	25–35 or REE × 1.3	0.5–1.2 BCAA-enriched amino acid solution Increase as for grade 1 or 2	

Adapted from Whitney *et al.* (2001); Blei *et al.* (2001); Lochs and Plauth (1999); Scolapio *et al.* (2002); Pomposelli and Burns (2002).
NPE, non-protein energy; TE, total energy; REE, resting energy expenditure; TPN, total parenteral nutrition; BCAA, branched-chain amino acid; PEM, protein–energy malnutrition.
Use actual dry weight for calculations.
Correct body weight for ascites and edema.
Ascites: minimal 2.2 kg; moderate 6 kg; severe 14 kg.
Peripheral edema: mild 1 kg; moderate 5 kg; severe 10 kg.

Nutritional recommendations for patients with liver disease

Energy

Adequate energy intake is essential for hepatic regeneration and to prevent protein catabolism. Energy requirements are increased with ascites, malabsorption, and infections. An increased REE has been observed in patients with viral hepatitis and cirrhosis, but whether increased REE is increased in all cirrhotic patients remains controversial. In one study, significant variations were found in patients with liver disease, with 18% being hypermetabolic and 31% being hypometabolic, with hypermetabolism being correlated more to extrahepatic factors. The use of stress factors and energy equations to determine energy requirements are, therefore, not very helpful, and a more accurate method to determine energy requirements is by using indirect calorimetry. For use in a clinical situation, this is unfortunately not practical, and ESPEN recommended the use of energy intake ranges based on body weight (Table 11.12). The patient's desirable or preferably dry weight should be used as the basis for calculating energy requirements. It should be pointed out that overfeeding of the malnourished metabolically stressed liver failure patient should be avoided, as it may lead to hyperglycemia, lipogenesis, increased carbon dioxide production, and septic complications.

Protein

The estimated protein intake to maintain nitrogen balance in liver cirrhosis is estimated at 1.0–1.2 g/kg per day. In a study on 271 patients with severe alcoholic liver disease, an intake of 1.2 g/kg of protein was associated with a positive nitrogen balance in all patients. This amount of protein was well tolerated despite the severity of liver disease. Although encephalopathy was observed in 20% of these patients, it was not correlated with protein intake. In another study on 345 patients with severe alcoholic liver disease (115 test subjects and 230 controls), it was reported that a diet high in protein (140 g/day) and supplemented with B vitamins was associated with a significant improvement in survival (65% versus 39% survival in the test and control subjects respectively at one year). Although this was not a randomized study, a number of other smaller scale studies are supportive of the concept that patients do tolerate a relatively high protein intake. In patients with liver disease who do not show any signs of im-

pending coma, protein restriction is therefore not recommended as it may contribute to increased protein catabolism, resulting in increased ammonia production and an increased susceptibility to infections. In addition, the accompanying muscle breakdown seen with low protein intakes is associated with a reduction in the extrahepatic ammonia detoxification potential.

It has been recommended that patients with hepatic encephalopathy should be aggressively treated with standard measures such as lactulose before consideration of protein restriction. In patients who do not tolerate protein, intake should be restricted initially to 0.5–0.6 g/kg per day and advanced by 0.25–0.5 g/kg per day until the target level is reached or progression of encephalopathy occurs (Table 11.12). The ESPEN recommendation for protein intake in patients with hepatic encephalopathy is the maximum that can be tolerated, usually aiming at 1.2 g/kg per day with a range of 1–1.5 g/kg per day, the higher levels being reserved for more catabolic patients.

The quality of protein is also thought to be important in the precipitation and management of encephalopathy. In this regard, increased intake of vegetable protein may be considered in patients who are unable to tolerate protein intakes greater than 1 g/kg per day, since in such patients vegetable protein appears to be better tolerated than animal protein. In a randomized cross-over study on eight patients with cirrhosis and chronic encephalopathy, nitrogen balance was significantly better on the vegetable protein diet compared with an isonitrogenous and isocaloric animal protein diet due to a reduced urinary nitrogen excretion. Clinical grading of encephalopathy and psychometric tests, although it remained abnormal, also improved on the vegetable protein diet. The beneficial effect of vegetable proteins has been ascribed to:

- a higher fiber intake (which accelerates gastrointestinal transit time),
- a more favorable composition of amino acids with lower AAA and methionine content,
- a reduction in pH of the intestinal lumen similar to non-absorbable disaccharides via promoting fermentation by intestinal bacteria, and
- a higher energy-to-nitrogen ratio.

Diets containing more than 50 g/day of vegetable protein may, however, be poorly tolerated in some individuals due to their reported side effects such as bloating, early satiety, and flatulence.

In patients with protein intolerance BCAAs may be administered orally at a dosage of 0.25 g/kg per day to promote nitrogen balance. BCAAs have been reported to be superior to isonitrogenous casein infusions, and associated with improved nitrogen balance without inducing encephalopathy. The use of BCAA- and casein-based supplementation of the diet was investigated in a double-blind randomized controlled study on 64 patients with cirrhosis and chronic hepatic encephalopathy. Thirty patients received the BCAAs and 34 the isonitrogenous casein-based supplementation. After three months of treatment, encephalopathy significantly improved in patients receiving the BCAA supplementation but not in the casein group. It was further found that casein-treated patients who were given BCAA improved rapidly, with the changes in neuropsychological function being associated with an improvement in nitrogen balance.

In addition, a meta-analysis of five randomized controlled trials using parenteral solutions high in BCAAs has shown a highly significant improvement in mental recovery of patients with cirrhosis and hepatic encephalopathy. Although the available evidence regarding the possible benefits of BCAAs in the management of encephalopathy appear promising, it does not support the unqualified recommendation of BCAA solutions, because the safety and efficacy of such a practice has never been determined. Furthermore, the impact of such a practice on mortality has been reported to vary considerably and follow-up periods have been too short. Although the clinical relevance of BCAAs in the management of encephalopathy remains to be defined, BCAA use may be beneficial in patients who are protein intolerant.

Carbohydrate and fat

Lipids are the preferred oxidative fuel in the postabsorptive state, and this is most pronounced in patients with advanced cirrhosis. However, these changes depend on substrate availability and are soon reverted after nutrition support. Therefore, no specific recommendations for the different amounts of substrate are required. Carbohydrate should generally provide 50–60% of energy intake or less than 5 mg/kg per min, and a bedtime snack may help to prevent breakdown of protein during overnight fasting. Small, frequent meals should be given to patients presenting with hypoglycemia, and patients with insulin resistance or diabetes mellitus should follow the dietary guidelines for diabetics.

Fat is an important energy source and also helps to make food more appetizing, therefore it should only be restricted in patients with steatorrhea. Medium-chain triacylglycerols can safely replace some of the fat in these cases, even in patients with hepatic encephalopathy. In patients with compensated liver cirrhosis clearance of intravenous triacylglycerols is impaired, but moderate amounts of fat may be removed from the bloodstream at a normal rate. In the case of TPN, non-protein energy may be given in the ratio of 50–60% carbohydrate and 50–35% fat. Intravenous fat should not exceed 1 g/kg per day, however, and should be given over 24 h to prevent hypertriglyceridemia and immunosuppression, as it has previously been shown that intravenous lipid in humans inhibited chemotaxis of neutrophils. When using 3-in-1 TPN admixtures, the minimum dose of lipid should be 20 g/l or 2% final concentration, as more dilute lipid formulas are unstable in the presence of hypertonic dextrose and amino acids. Triacylglycerol levels should be monitored throughout in patients receiving TPN.

Sodium and fluid

Dietary treatment of ascites entails sodium restriction to 500–2000 mg/day, depending on its severity. Very low sodium diets are, however, impractical and unpalatable and should be avoided if possible. Fluid restriction only becomes necessary if serum levels of sodium fall to below 120 mmol/l and if weight continues to rise as a result of fluid retention. It is important that treatment of ascites is not too vigorous (about 0.5 kg/day diuresis) as it may predispose the patient to the development of encephalopathy and the hepatorenal syndrome.

Vitamins

Micronutrient deficiencies occur in about 50% of cirrhotic patients, and are more common in alcoholic liver disease. Vitamin supplementation may be required in many patients with advanced liver disease, as deficiency of thiamin, folate, vitamin B_6, and riboflavin are common. In a recent case–control study, vitamin status (specifically thiamin and riboflavin) was strongly correlated with brain metabolic changes as assessed by proton magnetic resonance spectroscopy. An important consideration in hypoglycemic alcoholic patients is that thiamin should be administered before giving a glucose load, as the latter may deplete already borderline thiamin stores and precipitate Wernicke's encephalopathy. Fat-soluble vitamin deficiency in the presence of steatorrhea has been reported, and vitamin K deficiency is associated with increased bleeding time, with the subsequent increase in the risk of gastrointestinal bleeding. In addition, the liver's ability to convert vitamin D into its more active form ($25\text{-}OH\text{-}D_3$) is also impaired and may contribute to hepatic osteodystrophy, which generally does not respond well to vitamin D supplementation.

Minerals

Deficiencies of minerals are known to occur in patients with liver disease due to steatorrhea (calcium), alcohol abuse, increased levels of aldosterone (potassium), and the use of diuretics (potassium, calcium, magnesium, zinc). Severe hypophosphatemia (<0.32 mmol/L) has been reported following major liver resection and in patients with fulminant liver failure, and may result in respiratory, cardiac, immunologic, neurologic, hematologic, and muscular alterations. Zinc stores may also become depleted due to liver damage. Zinc deficiency may lead to a decrease in the activity of urea cycle enzymes as two of the five enzymes in the urea cycle are zinc dependent.

Zinc supplementation has previously been shown to cause an increase in urea synthesis, and improvement in glucose tolerance. In a study on 15 patients with advanced cirrhosis before and after oral supplementation (200 mg zinc sulfate 3 times daily) for 2–3 months, zinc levels returned to normal and liver function also improved significantly. There was also an improvement in serum albumin, prealbumin, retinol-binding protein, and IGF-1, although levels remained below normal. Changes in IGF-1 were correlated with improvement in glucose tolerance after an intravenous glucose load and it was concluded that IGF-1 increased glucose disposal. These results are, however, uncontrolled and need to be confirmed. Although the optimum dosage and duration for treatment with zinc supplements remains to be determined, it is currently recommended that oral zinc supplementation (220 mg zinc acetate twice daily) be given to patients with documented zinc deficiency.

Anabolic agents

There has recently been an interest in the use of anabolic agents combined with nutritional therapy to improve nutritional status of patients with liver disease. The use of oxandrolone was investigated in a study on 273 male patients with severe alcoholic hepatitis and some degree of protein–energy malnutrition. Patients with moderate malnutrition who received oxandrolone had a mortality rate of 9.4% compared with 20.9% of control patients, with a significant improvement in the severity of liver injury and malnutrition. In patients with severe malnutrition, however, there was no significant improvement, and oxandrolone did not have an effect in the presence of inadequate energy intake.

Nutritional support

Enteral nutrition

The oral route is usually the preferred choice for nutrition support, but nausea, vomiting, early satiety, and encephalopathy may prevent sufficient intake. In patients who are fed orally, it may be helpful to give frequent small meals in order to increase feeding tolerance, since patients with liver cirrhosis may have reduced gastric emptying, a slow transit time, as well as reduced gastric accommodation and relaxation. Patients who cannot eat enough to meet their increased nutritional requirements must be considered for enteral supplementation, total or partial enteral nutrition, and total or partial parenteral nutrition. Patients without PEM will usually tolerate 5–7 days of *nil per os* before nutrition support is initiated. However, those patients who will predictably not eat before 7 days, and those with PEM or >15% weight loss should be started on nutrition support as soon as possible to prevent nitrogen losses. Contraindications to enteral feeding include significant gastrointestinal bleeding, intestinal obstruction and pancreatitis, and patients with tense ascites who may not be able to tolerate the required volume of enteral feeds to meet nutrient requirements.

Coagulopathy or esophageal varices are not an absolute contraindication to prolonged placement of nasogastric tubes. However, performing percutaneous endoscopic gastrostomy in cirrhotic patients is difficult and dangerous because of ascites and portal hypertension. It is usually accepted that patients without large esophageal varices should generally be able to tolerate soft small-bore feeding tubes. Patients who bleed from esophageal varices may be unable to consume food by mouth and are often given intravenous fluid and electrolytes.

The effect of early enteral nutrition in this clinical setting was investigated in a randomized controlled trial on 22 patients with cirrhosis with bleeding esophageal varices. In this study, all patients admitted for acute variceal bleeding underwent emergency sclerotherapy or banding ligation and continuous infusion of octreotide, and were randomized into two groups to either receive discontinuous polymeric enteral nutrition via nasogastric tube, or were kept nil per mouth. On day 4 of the study, all patients received an oral diet. Recurrence of bleeding occurred in 33% of patients who were fed by nasogastric tube, compared with only 10% of the patients who were kept nil per mouth. Furthermore, early enteral feeding had no beneficial effect either on nutritional status or liver function. On the basis of the available evidence, therefore, this practice cannot be recommended in such patients.

Total parenteral nutrition (TPN)

This mode of nutrition support is reserved for patients with a non-functional gastrointestinal tract or those who cannot be fed adequately by the oral or enteral route. In the majority of patients standard amino acid solutions are recommended. BCAA solutions, if available, are usually reserved for patients with encephalopathy and those intolerant to protein because of their reported anticatabolic effects. Whether they are superior to standard solutions remains to be determined. Although the optimal amounts of carbohydrate and fat in the TPN admixtures for these patients have also not been evaluated systematically, their composition is usually aimed at maintaining euglycemia (glucose infusion of 2 g/kg per day) and serum triacylglycerol levels below 3 mmol/l. Patients who are fluid overloaded and those with hyponatremia should be treated with concentrated TPN solutions.

Nutrition in liver transplantation

Liver transplantation is the treatment of choice for end stage liver disease, with survival rates exceeding 85% at one year and 70% at five years post-transplantation. The majority of patients waiting for a transplant have chronic end stage liver disease with the likelihood of associated malnutrition. In contrast, patients with acute liver failure do not present with the wasting associated with chronic disease, but instead are severely catabolic and often septic with a rapidly deteriorating nutritional state.

The relationship between malnutrition and patient survival following liver transplantation was evaluated by Shaw and co-workers. They developed a malnutri-

tion score based on general assessment of nutritional status and found this to be one of six variables to be highly correlated with patient survival. A randomized prospective study by Reilly et al. evaluated the benefits of nutritional support in patients immediately after liver transplantation surgery. During the first 7 postoperative days, 28 patients were assigned to one of three parenteral regimens: intravenous glucose solution alone (400 kcal/day), TPN containing 35 kcal/kg per day non-protein calories and 1.5 g/kg per day standard amino acid formula, or the same TPN solution enriched with BCAAs. Both TPN subgroups had significantly better nitrogen balance and tended to have shorter lengths of stay in the intensive care unit. The BCAA formula was not superior to standard amino acids. This investigation suggests that early postoperative nutritional support facilitates patient recovery in the intensive care unit.

More recently, Wicks et al. demonstrated the safe use of enteral feeding in the early postoperative period, showing that in the majority of patients the parenteral route is not necessary.

The few controlled studies on nutritional interventions in patients undergoing liver transplantation have focused on the postoperative period. A study investigating the effect of pretransplant nutrition showed improved growth in terms of height and body weight when BCAA supplementation was administered. However, in adult patients, BCAA-enriched solutions in the postoperative period did not reduce time spent on a ventilator or in the intensive care unit when compared with conventional amino acid solutions.

According to the clinical experience of European Transplant Centres, nutritional status is assessed in transplant candidates without defined exclusion criteria. The centers agree about the indication for nutritional support after transplantation, and whenever possible, the enteral route is preferred. Most centers administer normocaloric nutrition, and the ratio of glucose : fat non-protein calories is similar to that of other surgical patients. At present, there is only limited experience with supplemented nutrition by new substrates such as glutamine, arginine, and omega-3 fatty acids. However, most immunosuppressive medications, including cyclosporine, corticosteroids, azathioprine, and tarcrolimus, have metabolic effects resulting in impaired nutrient utilization. More clinical trials are necessary to evaluate the interaction of these immunosuppressive agents and nutrient substrates.

Long-term metabolic problems following liver transplantation include obesity, hyperlipidemia, diabetes mellitus, osteoporosis, and renal dysfunction. Hence, transplant recipients require regular nutritional assessment to monitor and treat such complications as they arise. Hepatic veno-occlusive disease of the liver is a common complication following high-dose cytotoxic therapy for bone marrow transplantation. The major pathological changes are seen in centrilobular (zone 3) hepatocytes and adjacent endothelium. Glutathione becomes depleted following chemotherapy and experimental evidence suggests reduced levels predispose to centrilobular hepatocyte and endothelial cell injury. A recent study suggests that glutamine infusions during bone marrow transplantation preserves hepatic function.

11.6 Perspectives on the future

Several studies (Table 11.13) document an improvement in the nutritional status and prognosis of patients on nutrition support. Nevertheless, the benefits of nutrition support in liver disease remains controversial due to inadequately controlled studies, small numbers of patients, variations in nutritional status of patients included in such trials, differences in the methods used to evaluate efficacy of nutrition support, and lack of sufficient understanding of the pathophysiological processes involved. The long-term benefits of nutrition support in liver disease, the best route of feeding, and the best sources of protein remain to be confirmed by larger and better controlled studies.

References and further reading

Abou-Assi S, Vlahcevic ZR. Hepatic encephalopathy. Metabolic consequence of cirrhosis often is reversible. *Postgrad Med* 2001; 109(2): 52–60, 63.

Angulo P, Lindor KD. Non-alcoholic fatty liver disease. *J Gastroenterol Hepatol* 2002; 17 Suppl: S186–S190.

Arroyo V, Gines P, Planas R, Rodés. Pathogenesis, Diagnosis, and Treatment of Ascites in Cirrhosis. In: Bircher J, Benhamou J-P, McIntyre N, Rizetto M, Rodés J, editors. *Oxford Textbook of Clinical Hepatology*. Oxford: Oxford University Press, 1999.

Arteel G, Marsano L, Mendez C, Bentley F, McClain CJ. Advances in alcoholic liver disease. *Best Pract Res Clin Gastroenterol* 2003; 17: 625–647.

Beckingham IJ, Ryder SD. ABC of diseases of liver, pancreas, and biliary system. Investigation of liver and biliary disease. *BMJ* 2001; 322(7277): 33–36.

Berengeuer M, Wright TL. Viral Hepatitis. (Eds). In: Feldman M,

Friedman LS, Sleisenger MH, editors. *Sleisenger & Fordtran's Gastrointestinal and Liver Disease*. Pathophysiology/Diagnosis/Management. London: Saunders, 2002.

Blei AT. Infection, inflammation and hepatic encephalopathy, synergism redefined. *J Hepatol* 2004; 40: 327–330.

Blei AT, Cordoba J. The Practice Parameters Committee of the American College of Gastroenterology. Hepatic encephalopathy. Practice Guidelines. *Am J Gastroenterol* 2001; 96: 1968–1976.

Bonkovsky HL, Fiellin DA, Smith GS, Slaker DP, Simon D, Galambos JT. A randomized, controlled trial of treatment of alcoholic hepatitis with parenteral nutrition and oxandrolone. I. Short-term effects on liver function. *Am J Gastroenterol* 1991a; 86: 1200–1208.

Bonkovsky HL, Singh RH, Jafri IH *et al*. A randomized, controlled trial of treatment of alcoholic hepatitis with parenteral nutrition and oxandrolone. II. Short-term effects on nitrogen metabolism, metabolic balance, and nutrition. *Am J Gastroenterol* 1991b; 86: 1209–1218.

Butterworth RF. Pathogenesis of hepatic encephalopathy: new insights from neuroimaging and molecular studies. *J Hepatol* 2004; 39: 278–285.

Cabre E, Gonzalez-Huix F, Abad-Lacruz A *et al*. Effect of total enteral nutrition on the short-term outcome of severely malnourished cirrhotics. A randomized controlled trial. *Gastroenterology* 1990; 98: 715–720.

Davern TJ, Scharschmidt BF. Biochemical Liver Tests. In: Feldman M, Friedman LS, Sleisenger MH, editors. *Sleisenger & Fordtran's Gastrointestinal and Liver Disease*. Pathophysiology/Diagnosis/ Management. London: Saunders, 2002

Dusheiko G. Hepatitis B. In: Bircher J, Benhamou J-P, McIntyre N, Rizetto M, Rodes J, editors. *Oxford Textbook of Clinical Hepatology*. Oxford: Oxford University Press, 1999.

Erlinger S, Benhamou J-P. Cirrhosis: Clinical Aspects. In: Bircher J, Benhamou J-P, McIntyre N, Rizetto M, Rodes J, editors. *Oxford Textbook of Clinical Hepatology*. Oxford: Oxford University Press, 1999.

Farrell G. Non-alcoholic steatohepatitis: What is it, and why is it important in the Asia-Pacific region? *J Gastroenterol Hepatol* 2003; 18: 124–138.

Gerber T, Schomerus H. Hepatic encephalopathy in liver cirrhosis: pathogenesis, diagnosis and management. *Drugs* 2000; 60(6): 1353–1370.

Gerlich WH, Thomssen R. The Viruses of Hepatitis. In: Bircher J, Benhamou J-P, McIntyre N, Rizetto M, Rodes J, editors. *Oxford Textbook of Clinical Hepatology*. Oxford: Oxford University Press, 1999.

Gonzalez-Abraldes J, Garcia-Pagan JC, Bosch J. Nitric oxide and portal hypertension. *Metab Brain Dis* 2002; 17(4): 311–324.

Hasse JM, Matarese LE. Medical Nutrition Therapy for Liver, Biliary System, and Exocrine Pancreas Disorders. In: Mahan LK, Escott-Stump S, editors. *Krause's Food, Nutrition, & Diet Therapy*. London: WB Saunders Company, 2000.

Hirsch S, Bunout D, de la Maza P *et al*. Controlled trial on nutrition supplementation in outpatients with symptomatic alcoholic cirrhosis. *JPEN J Parenter Enteral Nutr* 1993; 17: 119–124.

Ichida T, Shibasaki K, Muto Y, Satoh S, Watanabe A, Ichida F. Clinical study of an enteral branched-chain amino acid solution in decompensated liver cirrhosis with hepatic encephalopathy. *Nutrition* 1995; 11(2 Suppl): 238–244.

Leevy CM, Sherlock S, Tygstruo N, Zetterman R. Diseases of the Liver, and Biliary Tract. New York: Raven Press, 1994.

Lochs H, Plauth M. Liver cirrhosis: rationale and modalities for nutritional support – the European Society of Parenteral and Enteral Nutrition consensus and beyond. *Curr Opin Clin Nutr Metab Care* 1999; 2: 345–349.

Table 11.13 Summary of studies on the effect of nutrition support in liver disease

Study	Subjects	Design	Intervention	Outcome
Ichida *et al.* 1995	96 Patients with grade II coma or history of encephalopathy	No controls	BCAA	Improvement in plasma amino acid profiles, serum albumin, coma, quality of life, and performance Adverse reactions in 17% (GI symptoms) Safety rate 90%
Tangkijvanich *et al.* 2000	Not clear	Controlled	BCAA	Improvement in liver function
Meng *et al.* 1999	Not clear	Controlled	BCAA	Improvement in liver function Shorter hospital stay
Cabre *et al.* 1990	35 Severely malnourished cirrhotic patients	RCT	Enteral nutrition (BCAA, MCT, maltodextrin) Standard oral diet (isocaloric, isonitrogenous)	Serum albumin improved in enterally fed group only Child's score improved in enterally fed group only Mortality lower in enterally fed group
Mezey *et al.* 1991	44 Patients with severe alcoholic hepatitis	RCT 1 Month Standard hospital diet	2 l dextrose + AA versus dextrose only	Significant increase in N-balance in the experimental group No difference in mortality, change in body weight, AMC, creatinine height index, and triceps
Hirsch *et al.* 1993	51 Patients with decompensated alcoholic cirrhosis	Controlled trial 1 Year	*Experimental group* Enteral supplement of 1000 cal and 34 g protein/day (Energy and protein intake was significantly higher in the experimental group) *Controls* Placebo capsule	Frequency of hospitalizations, but not total days, were significantly lower in experimental group Mortality was not different between groups Liver function improved in both groups
Bonkovsky *et al.* 1991	39 Patients with moderate to severe alcoholic hepatitis	RCT Metabolic ward 35 days	Standard therapy or standard therapy plus oxandrolone or standard therapy plus 2 l parenteral AA in dextrose or standard therapy plus oxandrolone plus parenteral AA in dextrose	Oxandrolone plus parenteral supplementation plus standard therapy was well tolerated, and resulted in more rapid improvement in serum albumin, transferrin, prothrombin time, and liver volume.
Bonkovsky *et al.* 1991	Patients with severe alcoholic hepatitis	RCT Metabolic ward 35 days	Standard therapy or standard therapy plus oxandrolone or standard therapy plus 2 l parenteral AA in dextrose or standard therapy plus oxandrolone plus parenteral AA in dextrose	Oxandrolone did not enhance appetite, food intake, or nitrogen balance Oxandrolone had a favorable effect on serum levels of pre-albumin and transferrin Intake of 125 g protein/day did not lead to hepatic encephalopathy or increased ammonia levels

BCAA, branched-chain amino acids; GI, gastrointestinal; RCT, randomized controlled trial; MCT, medium-chain triglycerides.

Mahan LK, Escott-Stump S. *Krause's Food, Nutrition, & Diet Therapy*. 10 edn. London: WB Saunders Company, 2000.

Maher JJ. Alcoholic Liver Disease. In: Feldman M, Friedman LS, Sleisenger MH, editors. *Sleisenger & Fordtran's Gastrointestinal and Liver Disease*. Pathophysiology/Diagnosis/Management. London: Saunders, 2002.

Mendenhall CL, Moritz TE, Roselle GA, Morgan TR, Nemchausky BA, Tamburro CH *et al*. Protein energy malnutrition in severe alcoholic hepatitis: diagnosis and response to treatment. The VA Cooperative Study Group #275. *JPEN J Parenter Enteral Nutr* 1995; 19(4): 258–265.

Meng WC, Leung KL, Ho RL, Leung TW, Lau WY. Prospective randomized control study on the effect of branched-chain amino acids in patients with liver resection for hepatocellular carcinoma. *Aust N Z J Surg* 1999; 69: 811–815.

Mezey E, Caballeria J, Mitchell MC, Pares A, Herlong HF, Rodes J. Effect of parenteral amino acid supplementation on short-term and long-term outcomes in severe alcoholic hepatitis: a randomized controlled trial. *Hepatology* 1991; 14(6): 1090–1096.

Morgan MY. Nutritional Aspects of Liver and Biliary Disease. In: Bircher J, Benhamon J-P, McIntyre N, Rizzetto M, Rodes J, editors. *Oxford Textbook of Clinical Hepatology*. Oxford: Oxford University Press, 1999.

Pomposelli JJ, Burns DL. Nutrition support in the liver transplant patient. *Nutr Clin Pract* 2002; 17: 341–349.

Popper H. Viral Hepatitis 1. Acute Form. In: Netter FH, editor. *The Ciba Collection of Medical Illustrations*. Part III. Liver, Biliary Tract and Pancreas. Cincinatti: The Hennegan Company, 1964.

Runyon BA. Ascites and Spontaneous Bacterial Peritonitis. In: Feldman M, Friedman LS, Sleisenger MH, editors. *Sleisenger & Fordtran's Gastrointestinal and Liver Disease*. Pathophysiology/Diagnosis/Management. London: Saunders, 2002.

Ryder SD, Beckingham IJ. ABC of diseases of liver, pancreas, and biliary system: Acute hepatitis. *BMJ* 2001; 322(7279): 151–153.

Reilly J, Mehta R, Teperman L, Cemaj S, Tzakis A, Yanaga K *et al*. Nutritional support after liver transplantation: a randomized prospective study. *JPEN J Parenter Enteral Nutr* 1990; 14(4):386–391.

Scolapio JS. Nutrition therapy in liver disease. *Nutr Clin Pract* 2002; 17: 331–340.

Scolapio JS, Ukleja A, McGreevy K, Burnett OL, O'Brien PC. Nutritional problems in end-stage liver disease: contribution of impaired gastric emptying and ascites. *J Clin Gastroenterol* 2002; 34(1): 89–93.

Sherlock S, Dooley J. Diseases of the Liver and Biliary System. 9th ed. Oxford: Blackwell Scientific, 1993.

Shaw BW, Jr., Wood RP, Gordon RD, Iwatsuki S, Gillquist WP, Starzl TE. Influence of selected patient variables and operative blood loss on six-month survival following liver transplantation. *Semin Liver Dis* 1985; 5(4):385–393.

Stolz A. Liver Physiology and Metabolic Function. In: Feldman M FLSM, editor. *Sleisenger & Fordtran's Gastrointestinal and Liver Disease*. Pathophysiology/Diagnosis/Management. London: Saunders, 2002.

Tangkijvanich P, Mahachai V, Wittayalertpanya S, Ariyawongsopon V, Isarasena S. Short-term effects of branched-chain amino acids on liver function tests in cirrhotic patients. *Southeast Asian J Trop Med Public Health* 2000; 31(1): 152–157.

Whitney EN, Cataldo C, DeBruyne LK, Rolfes SR. Nutrition for Health and Health Care. 2 edn. London: Wadsworth, 2001.

Wicks C, Bray G, Williams R. Nutritional assessment in primary biliary cirrhosis. The effect of disease progression. *Clin Nutr* 1995; 14: 29–34.

Wicks C. Nutrition and Liver Disease. In: Payne-James J, Grimble G, Silk D, editors. *Artificial Nutrition Support in Clinical Practice*. London: Greenwich Medical Media Limited, 2001.

12
Nutrition and the Pancreas

Jean-Fabien Zazzo

Key messages

- The pancreas is a dual function organ consisting of exocrine and endocrine cells. Ninety-eight per cent of the pancreas is made up of exocrine cells. Disease of the pancreas can result in diabetes, pancreatitis (acute or chronic), or both.
- The dietary management of diabetes has changed radically in the last century in response to the increased understanding of the pathophysiology of diabetes and the increased and improved range of available insulins.
- Pancreatitis represents a wide spectrum of clinical disease involving a diffuse inflammatory process of the pancreas with variable involvement of other regional tissues and/or remote organ systems.
- The metabolism of acute pancreatitis involves a stress state very similar to that seen in sepsis.

- Not all patients suffering from acute pancreatitis need nutritional support but in severe acute pancreatitis nutritional support is indicated to supply metabolic demands, to prevent wasting, to attempt to modulate the inflammatory response, to protect gut barrier function, and to prevent bacterial translocation.
- Total parenteral nutrition should only be considered in those patients with severe pancreatitis who are intolerant for enteral feedings or in whom enteral access cannot be obtained.
- There remains a need for larger randomized controlled trials in severe acute pancreatitis to study the effect of nutrition support on morbidity, and to define the optimal composition and timing of enteral nutrition support.

12.1 Introduction

The pancreas consists of endocrine and exocrine cells. The main pancreatic duct joins the common bile duct to enter the duodenum as a single duct at the ampulla of vater. The exocrine cells of the pancreas produce digestive enzymes, which are stored in secretory granules and released when stimulated to do so by several hormones, including vasoactive intestinal polypeptide (VIP), secretin, and cholecystekinin (CCK). Pancreatic exocrine function is controlled by both neural and hormonal mediators. CCK is produced by cells in the intestinal mucosa in response to the presence of fat, protein, and amino acids. It then stimulates (by nerve pathways) pancreatic secretion of enzymes and bicarbonate. The enzymes produced by the pancreas are listed in Box 12.1. Pancreatic polypeptide inhibits pancreatic secretion via the vagus nerve. Secretin is produced in response to the acidic chyme entering the duodenum. This stimulates pancreatic secretion of

bicarbonate which educes the acidity of the luminal contents.

Scattered throughout the pancreas are the islets of Langerhans. There are four main types of islet cell which have different secretory granules in their cytoplasm:

- β cells are the most common type – they produce insulin,
- α cells produce glucagon,
- D cells produce somatostatin, and
- PP cells produce pancreatic polypeptide.

> **Box 12.1** Enzymes produced by the pancreas
>
> - Amylase
> - Lipase
> - Co-lipase
> - Phospholipase
> - Trypsinogen
> - Chymotrypsinogen

12.2 Diabetes mellitus

Diabetes mellitus is a chronic disease caused by inherited and/or acquired deficiency in production of insulin by the pancreas, or by the ineffectiveness of the insulin produced. Such a deficiency results in increased concentrations of glucose in the blood, which in turn damage many of the body's systems, in particular the blood vessels and nerves.

There are two principal forms of diabetes:

- In type 1 diabetes (formerly known as insulin-dependent) the pancreas fails to produce the insulin which is essential for survival. This form develops most frequently in children and adolescents, but is being increasingly noted later in life.
- Type 2 diabetes (formerly named non-insulin-dependent) results from the body's inability to respond properly to the action of insulin produced by the pancreas. It is much more common than type 1 and accounts for around 90% of all diabetes cases worldwide. It occurs most frequently in adults, but is being noted increasingly in adolescents as well.

Certain genetic markers have been shown to increase the risk of developing type 1 diabetes. Type 2 diabetes is strongly familial, but it is only recently that some genes have been consistently associated with increased risk for type 2 diabetes in certain populations. Both types of diabetes are complex diseases caused by mutations in more than one gene, as well as by environmental factors. Diabetes in pregnancy may give rise to several adverse outcomes, including congenital malformations, increased birth weight, and an elevated risk of perinatal mortality. Strict metabolic control may reduce these risks to the level of those of non-diabetic expectant mothers.

As type 2 diabetes has been covered in Chapters 3 and 5, this chapter will only deal with type 1 diabetes.

Symptoms and diagnosis

The symptoms of diabetes may be pronounced, subdued, or even absent. In type 1 diabetes, the classic symptoms are excessive secretion of urine (polyuria), thirst (polydipsia), weight loss, and tiredness. The World Health Organization (WHO) has published recommendations on diagnostic values for blood glucose concentration. The diagnostic level of fasting blood glucose concentration was last modified in 1999.

Box 12.2 Methods and criteria for diagnosing diabetes mellitus (WHO, 2002)

(1) Diabetes symptoms (i.e. polyuria, polydipsia, and unexplained weight loss) plus a random venous plasma glucose concentration ≥11.1 mmol/l **or** a fasting plasma glucose concentration ≥7.0 mmol/l (whole blood ≥6.1 mmol/l) **or** 2-h plasma glucose concentration ≥11.1 mmol/l 2 h after 75 g anhydrous glucose in an oral glucose tolerance test (OGTT).

(2) With no symptoms, diagnosis should not be based on a single glucose determination but requires confirmatory plasma venous determination. At least one additional glucose test result on another day with a value in the diabetic range is essential, either fasting, from a random sample or from the 2-h post glucose load. If the fasting or random values are not diagnostic the 2-h value should be used.

Methods and criteria for diagnosing diabetes mellitus are shown in Box 12.2.

A diagnosis of diabetes has important legal and medical implications for the patient and it is therefore essential to be secure in the diagnosis. A diagnosis should never be made on the basis of glycosuria or a stick reading of a finger-prick blood glucose alone, although such tests may be useful for screening purposes. HbA1c measurement is also not currently recommended for the diagnosis of diabetes. Diabetes UK recommends that the diagnosis is confirmed by a glucose measurement performed in an accredited laboratory on a venous plasma sample, although the WHO do give values for whole blood as well. This should mean that there is less need to perform oral glucose tolerance testing on the majority of the population, although in the elderly and some ethnic groups the fasting glucose may not be a reliable indicator of diabetes. For this group, and in the absence of symptoms of diabetes, a glucose tolerance test is often recommended as the definitive second test.

Treatment

Insulin was isolated by Frederic Banting and Charles Best in 1921 in Canada. This revolutionized the treatment of diabetes and prevention of its complications, transforming type 1 diabetes from a fatal disease to one in which long-term survival became achievable. People with type 1 diabetes are usually totally dependent on daily insulin injections for survival. Insulin is unavailable and unaffordable in many poor countries, despite being listed by the WHO as an essential drug.

Access to insulin by those who require it is thus a subject of special concern to international health agencies and national health authorities.

Complications associated with diabetes mellitus

Diabetic retinopathy

Diabetic retinopathy is a leading cause of blindness and visual disability. Diabetes mellitus is associated with damage to the small blood vessels in the retina, resulting in loss of vision. Findings, consistent from study to study, make it possible to suggest that, after 15 years of diabetes, approximately 2% of people become blind, while about 10% develop severe visual handicap. Loss of vision due to certain types of glaucoma and cataract may also be more common in people with diabetes than in those without the disease. Good metabolic control can delay the onset and progression of diabetic retinopathy. Loss of vision and blindness in persons with diabetes can be prevented by early detection and treatment of vision-threatening retinopathy: regular eye examinations and timely intervention with laser treatment, or through surgery in cases of advanced retinopathy. There is evidence that, even in developed countries, a large proportion of those in need are not receiving such care due to lack of public and professional awareness, as well as an absence of treatment facilities. In developing countries, in many of which diabetes is now common, such care is inaccessible to the majority of the population.

Nephropathy

Diabetes is among the leading causes of renal failure, but its frequency varies between populations and is also related to the severity and duration of the disease. Several measures to slow down the progress of renal damage have been identified. They include control of high blood glucose, control of high blood pressure, intervention with medication in the early stage of renal damage, and restriction of dietary protein. Screening and early detection of diabetic renal disease are an important means of prevention.

Heart disease

Heart disease accounts for approximately 50% of all deaths among people with diabetes in industrialized countries. Risk factors for heart disease in people with diabetes include smoking, high blood pressure, high serum cholesterol, and obesity. Diabetes negates the protection from heart disease which premenopausal women without diabetes experience. Recognition and management of these conditions may delay or prevent heart disease in people with diabetes.

Diabetic neuropathy

Diabetic neuropathy is probably the most common complication of diabetes. Studies suggest that up to 50% of people with diabetes are affected to some degree. Major risk factors of this condition are the level and duration of elevated blood glucose. Neuropathy can lead to sensory loss and damage to the limbs. It is also a major cause of impotence in diabetic men.

Diabetic foot disease

Diabetic foot disease due to changes in blood vessels and nerves often leads to ulceration and subsequent limb amputation. It is one of the most costly complications of diabetes, especially in communities with inadequate footwear. It results from both vascular and neurological disease processes. Diabetes is the most common cause of non-traumatic amputation of the lower limb, which may be prevented by regular inspection and good care of the foot.

12.3 Nutritional management of type 1 diabetes

The dietary management of diabetes has changed radically in the last century in response to the increased understanding of the pathophysiology of diabetes and the increased and improved range of available insulins. There has been a move away from the prescriptive diets of the 1980s, when a strict carbohydrate and even fat exchange lists were in vogue. Management has now moved towards education and helping people to change behavior in a way which best maintains glucose and lipid levels while maximizing quality of life. The evidence base for current nutritional recommendations has been extensively reviewed by the European Association for the Study of Diabetes (EASD) and the American Diabetic Association (ADA) as well as Diabetes UK. The following is a brief synopsis of the current recommendations for people with diabetes. For further information on this topic go to the websites quoted at the end of the chapter.

Body weight

People with type 1 diabetes should be encouraged to maintain a healthy body weight with a body mass index in the range 18.5–25 kg/m². Waist circumference is a simple measure to determine whether fat deposition is central or visceral and ideally both should be measured at clinic visits (see Chapters 3 and 5 for more details on measuring waist circumference).

Physical activity

Regular physical activity improves insulin resistance and lipid profile (reduction in triacylglycerols and increase in total high-density lipoprotein (HDL) concentration), and lowers blood pressure in the long term. It has also been shown to reduce mortality in type 1 diabetes.

Most people with diabetes should be encouraged to take at least 20–30 min of physical activity on most days. The physical activity varies according to age and fitness.

The energy content of the diet must be sufficient to sustain growth in children, prevent or correct obesity in adults, and maintain body weight in those who are ill. Monounsaturated fat intake (MUFA) is promoted as the main source of dietary fat because of its lower susceptibility to lipid peroxidation and consequent lower athrogenic potential. There is also a further liberalization in the consumption of sucrose from the previous recommendations, plus an active promotion of carbohydrate foods with a low glycemic index.

Dietary education is an ongoing interactive process between patient and health professional and cannot be expected to be achieved in a single session.

Glycosylated hemoglobin (HbA1c) is an indicator of medium to long-term glycemic control and has been shown to improve after regular dietetic follow-up in an outpatient setting.

Glycemic index

Many factors affect the glycemic response to foods, including amount of carbohydrate consumed, composition of the carbohydrate (content of glucose, fructose, sucrose, resistant starch, etc.), and effects of cooking or processing.

The glycemic index is a useful tool in managing blood sugar levels; however, it is important to remember that the amount of carbohydrate in meals and snacks has a much greater influence on glycemia than source or type of carbohydrate.

The introduction of the new insulin systems such as the basal-bolus system using either conventional insulins or short-acting analogs, as well as the availability of insulin pumps and fast-acting glucometers, has allowed greater flexibility in the timing of meals and variation in intakes of carbohydrate. It is important to remember that the effective management of these adjustments depends on the individual's knowledge and motivation.

Alcohol

Advice on alcohol consumption within sensible drinking limits should be given to the general population. The major issues relating to alcohol use for the person with diabetes are:

- its ability to reduce blood sugar and cause unawareness of a hypoglycemic event,
- its energy content for those with excessive body weight, and
- its ability to cause or aggravate hypertriacylglycerolemia.

More detailed information on nutritional recommendations for people with diabetes can be found in the reading list at the end of this chapter.

12.4 Pancreatitis

Pancreatitis represents a wide spectrum of clinical disease involving a diffuse inflammatory process of the pancreas with variable involvement of other organ systems. Patients with mild pancreatitis account for 80% of hospital admissions for pancreatitis. These patients can usually be supported with intravenous fluid resuscitation and analgesia and rapidly return to oral diet. Severe pancreatitis is differentiated from mild cases by the presence of organ failure or evidence of necrosis on CT scan. This group accounts for 20% of hospital admissions for pancreatitis, has a higher mortality (about 5–10%), and is more likely to require nutritional support. Gallstones are the most common cause of acute pancreatitis worldwide. Other risk factors include alcohol, hyperlipidemia, hypercalcemia, endoscopic retrograde cholangiopancreatography (ERCP), and trauma. In 10–25% of the patients with acute pancreatitis no obvious risk factors are present.

12.5 Pathogenesis of acute pancreatitis

Mortality from acute pancreatitis has fallen over the last two decades from around 30–40% to 5–10%, but the mortality rate may approach 50% in patients with severe pancreatitis with more than 50% necrosis. The early deaths are related to the presence of comorbid conditions and to the development of a systemic inflammatory response syndrome (SIRS) and multiorgan failure (MOF) occurring mainly in the necrotizing forms of pancreatitis.

The first phase is characterized by SIRS, during which MOF and death may supervene (Figure 12.1).

In severe acute pancreatitis, shock induces intestinal ischemia, loss of gut barrier function, and then contributes to SIRS that ultimately leads to MOF. There is increasing evidence that intestinal injury can result in the gut becoming a cytokine-generating organ. Early increased permeability has also been demonstrated in patients suffering from acute pancreatitis. This increased permeability correlates with disease severity, being significantly greater in severe attacks. Similarly, significantly higher levels of endotoxemia were detected in patients who developed MOF or died. Unless this process is arrested and reversed by natural defenses or therapeutic intervention, the second phase ensues.

The second phase is characterized by local complications such as infected pancreatic necrosis, usually becoming apparent in the second week of the illness.

The bacterial flora related to the necrotic infection is dominated by enteric bacteria, indicating that the gut may play an important role in the pathogenesis of pancreatitis-related infection. In the early phase after induction of experimental pancreatitis, there is a persistent reduction in intestinal motility with bacterial overgrowth in the ileum and colon and bacterial translocation to mesenteric lymph nodes.

In acute pancreatitis, the gut may be the primary origin of the bacteria which are present in infected necrosis. Bacterial translocation has been proposed as a mechanism of sepsis in critically ill patients and especially in pancreatitis. A decrease in intestinal motility and transit causes an increased intraluminal count of bacteria. Intestinal motility may be worsened by morphine administration, often used to control pain in these patients. Experimental studies suggest that this is a cause of bacterial translocation. In rat models of acute pancreatitis, the gut is the primary source of infection. Enteric bacteria within the gut and in adjacent mesenteric lymph nodes increased as intestinal transit decreased.

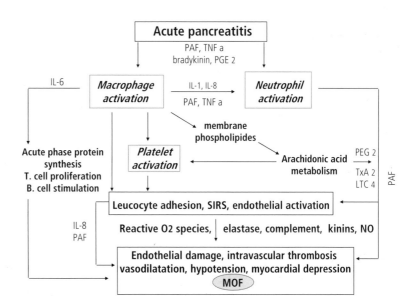

Figure 12.1 Pathways in acute pancreatitis leading to systemic inflammatory response syndrome (SIRS) and multiorgan failure (MOF). Adapted from Neoptolemos *et al.* (1998).

12.6 Severity scores

Acute pancreatitis may be a fatal disease with a reported mortality rate up to 20–25%. This mortality depends on the severity of the disease and the severity depends on whether or not pancreatic necrosis is present. Distinction must be made between mild and severe forms, necrotic and edematous lesions, since acute pancreatitis in its severe form requires urgent treatment in an intensive care unit.

At admission, clinical examination is unreliable in predicting severity of pancreatitis. Authors tried to develop a combination of criteria to predict severity. Three of them are used in literature: Ranson score (Table 12.1), Glasgow Score (Table 12.2), and Acute Physiology and Chronic Health Evaluation (APACHE) II. Monitoring of patients with severe pancreatitis must include a baseline contrast-enhanced CT scan repeated at least weekly or until improvement. The presence of necrosis increases the morbidity and mor-

tality. Most complications of acute pancreatitis occur in patients in whom the initial diagnosis is based upon peripancreatic fluid collections (grade D or E) and an excellent correlation has been established between the CT depiction of necrosis and the development of complications and death. Patients with pancreatic necrosis have been shown to have a morbidity of about 82% and a mortality of 23% whereas those without necrosis have a morbidity of 6% and a mortality of 0%.

12.7 Metabolic consequencies of acute pancreatitis

The metabolism of acute pancreatitis involves a stress state very similar to that seen in sepsis, characterized by hyperdynamic changes, hypermetabolism, and hypercatabolism. These changes are important in considering appropriate feeding.

Alterations in carbohydrate metabolism may result from increased cortisol and catecholamine secretion. Gluconeogenesis is increased while glucose oxidation is diminished. This and insulin resistance lead to a glucose intolerance which may necessitate insulin use even in the non-diabetic patient. Alterations in fat metabolism are less frequent. Lipolysis and lipid oxidation are usually increased but clearance from the blood can be reduced, resulting in hyperlipidemia and hypertriacylglycerolemia.

In acute pancreatitis, skeletal muscle proteolysis and amino acid release is associated with an increased consumption of circulating amino acids. This results in amino acid depletion, increased ureagenesis and nitrogen excretion that can reach more than 30 g per day. Total amino acid concentrations in the plasma of patients with acute pancreatitis have been shown to be lower than that of normal controls. Amino acids involved in gluconeogenesis such as alanine, threonine, and serine were particularly low. The concentration of glutamine may fall to levels of only 55% of normal. Depression in glutamine and alanine in plasma occurs despite an increased release of both amino acids from skeletal muscle. These important changes suggest that administration of amino acid solutions may be beneficial to prevent wasting by supplying amino acids exogenously.

The most common mineral abnormalities described in acute pancreatitis are hypocalcemia and hypomagnesemia, particularly occurring in alcoholic patients.

Table 12.1 Prognostic factors in acute pancreatitis by Ranson score

On admission	
Age	>55 years
White cell count	>16 000/mm^3
Glucose	>11 mmol/l
LDH	>700 UI or 1.5 N
ASAT	>250 IU/l or 6 N
Within 48 h of admission	
Hematocrit drop	>10%
Blood urea nitrogen increase	>5 mg/l or 1.8 mmol/l
Serum calcium	<8 mg/l or 2 mmol/l
Pa_{O_2}	<60 mmHg or 8 kPa
Base deficit	>4 mmol/l
Fluid sequestration	>6 l

Reproduced from Ranson et al. (1974) with permission of the *Journal of the American College of Surgeons*.

Table 12.2 Prognostic factors in acute pancreatitis by Glasgow Score

Age	>55 years
White blood cell count	>15 000/mm^3
Glucose	>10 mmol/l
Blood urea nitrogen increase	>16 mmol/l
Pa_{O_2}	<8 kpa
Serum calcium	<2 mmol/l
Serum albumin	<32 g/l
LDH	>1.5 N

Reproduced from Blamey et al. (1984) with permission of the BMJ Publishing Group.

Reactive oxygen species and related oxidative damage have been implicated in the initiation of acute pancreatitis. A significant correlation between disease severity and endogenous antioxidant status in patients with mild or severe pancreatitis has been shown. Markers of oxidative stress include antioxidant vitamins (alpha-tocopherol, ascorbic acid), lucigenin-amplified chemiluminescence, and thiobarbituric acid reactive substances.

12.8 Artificial nutrition

Not all patients suffering from acute pancreatitis need nutritional support. In mild pancreatitis, the majority of patients (80%) are likely to return to oral diet within 7 days. Early refeeding is usually well tolerated and leads to exacerbation of the disease process in only a small percentage of patients. Elevated serum lipase concentrations the day before refeeding has been shown to be associated with an increased risk of pain relapse.

In severe acute pancreatitis, as in other critical situations, nutritional support is indicated in order to supply metabolic demands, to prevent wasting, to modulate (if possible) the inflammatory response, to protect gut barrier function, and prevent bacterial translocation.

Recent experimental data suggest that the function of the gut as a barrier against sepsis may be impaired in pancreatitis. Nutritional therapy may influence this barrier function.

In a rat model of acute pancreatitis, jejunal administration of enteral nutrition maintains immune responsiveness and gut integrity, and reduces bacterial and/or endotoxin translocation when compared with total parenteral nutrition but without improving outcome. In animals, chow and complex enteral diet maintain a normal balance between immunoglobulin A (IgA)-stimulating and IgA-inhibiting cytokines while preserving normal antibacterial and antiviral immunity. These data are consistent with severely impaired mucosal immunity with intravenous total parenteral nutrition (TPN) and partial impairment with intragastric TPN and provide a cytokine-mediated explanation for reduction in diet-induced mucosal immunity. A few data suggest that maintaining gut barrier and local immune function by nutritional intervention could potentially improve outcome in pancreatitis, as has been suggested in other critical situations.

Parenteral nutrition

In some experimental studies, glucose given parenterally has been shown to suppress pancreatic function, whereas amino acid solutions do not. A series of controlled studies have refuted these early reports, demonstrating that parenteral infusion of fatty acids does not stimulate pancreatic exocrine secretion in humans.

In animal studies and some case reports in humans suffering from external pancreatic fistula, results suggest that intravenous infusion of amino acids, glucose, or fat emulsion alone or in combination does not stimulate exocrine pancreatic secretion and sometimes decreases pancreatic enzyme secretory capacity. Pancreatic secretion has never been prospectively studied in severe necrotic pancreatitis.

Clinical experience with parenteral nutrition

The only available randomized study included only mild acute pancreatitis. Patients were randomized within 24 h of admission to receive TPN or intravenous fluid (crystalloids or colloids). Compared with the control group, the patients receiving early TPN had a longer length of stay (16 versus 10 days). There was no difference in days to clear liquid diet, return of amylase to normal, or overall complications. All other studies were retrospective or case reports (Table 12.3). In the absence of properly conducted prospective, randomized clinical trials, it remains to be shown whether TPN has any clinical benefit on the outcome of the disease other than the ability to meet patients' nutritional needs in severe forms.

To meet increased metabolic demands and to 'rest' the pancreas, TPN through a central venous catheter was the first route used in patients with acute necrotizing pancreatitis.

Numerous clinical trials or reports have demonstrated the safety of administering intravenous lipids to patients with severe acute pancreatitis and in whom hypertriacylglycerolemia was not an etiologic factor (Table 12.3). Fat emulsion tolerance should be evaluated twice a week by measuring triacylglycerolemia 4 h after the infusion has been stopped. Plasma level must be under 2 g/l.

Enteral nutrition

The debate on the use of enteral feeds in pancreatitis has existed because of the potential risks of stimulating the inflamed pancreas. Bypassing the stomach is one

Table 12.3 Trials of intravenous nutrition with or without lipids in patients with acute pancreatitis

Study	Number of patients	Type of study	Severity	Type of nutrition	Observations
Hyde, 1984	21	PR	NA	Glucose or glucose + AA or glucose + AA + 10% lipid	WT, lipid safe
Durr, 1985	31	PR	Mild	IV lipids (1.5 g/kg/day) versus NPO	WT, lipid safe
Sax, 1987	54	PR	Mild	Glucose + AA + 10% lipid 2×/week	WT, lipid safe
Silberman, 1982	11	PNR	NA	Glucose + AA + Intralipid®	WT, lipid safe
Grant, 1984	73	PNR	38% RS > 3	Glucose + AA + 10% lipid	WT, lipid safe
Van Gossum, 1988	18	R	Mean RS = 5.6	30 kcal/kg/day non-protein energy-lipid = 55%	Triglyceride+glucose intolerance predicted poor outcome
Sitzmann, 1989	73	PNR	50% RS > 3	Glucose + lipid 2×/week or lipid daily or glucose	WR, lipid safe Mortality x 10 if negative N balance
Steininger, 1989	4	PNR	NA	Glucose + dipeptide + lipid	WT, lipid safe
Robin, 1990	156	R	29% RS > 3	Glucose + lipid 1×/week	WT, lipid safe
Kalfarentzos, 1991	67	PNR	Mean RS = 3.8	Glucose + AA + lipid (20–30% of calories as fat)	WT, lipid safe

PR, prospective, randomized; PNR, prospective non-randomized; R, retrospective; NPO, nothing per os; RS, Ranson score; TPN, total parenteral nutrition; IV, intravenous; WT, well tolerated; NA, not available; AA, amino acid.

way to prevent this from happening. There is a paucity of human studies on the effects of enteral nutrition on pancreatic secretion. In healthy volunteers fed either an elemental diet or a food homogenate via a nasojejunal tube, studies indicate that the latter has a greater stimulatory effect on the secretion of pancreatic lipase and chymotrypsin than the former. The osmolality of the infused solutions does not appear to be important. Infusion of a high caloric load into the jejunum has an inhibitory effect on pancreatic secretions. Nutrients entering the duodenum do not stop cycles of enzyme secretion. The limited number of randomized trials in this area suggest that there is no difference in the volume of pancreatic secretions or the content of bicarbonate, protein, or amylase between patients receiving either parenteral nutrition, or enteral nutrition via a needle catheter jejunostomy.

Clinical experience with enteral nutrition
The first report of enteral nutrition via a surgical jejunostomy goes back to 1967. Subsequent case studies suggest some benefit from early enteral nutrition, but only one small study has compared enteral nutrition ($n = 13$) versus no nutritional support ($n = 14$) in severe acute pancreatitis.

Early nutritional support
Clinical reports and the three randomized studies suggest that contrary to the conventional wisdom, early enteral feeding is both feasible and desirable in the management of patients with acute pancreatitis. The benefits relate primarily to reduced infectious and overall complication rates and to reduced costs. However, the benefit of early nutritional support (either parenteral or enteral nutrition) on severe pancreatitis outcome has not yet been established. The role of enteral nutrition deserves further prospective evaluation, particularly in the subgroup of patients with severe acute pancreatitis.

Enteral nutrition may not be feasible either because of gastrointestinal stasis, high gastric aspirates, or complications of pancreatitis. Enteral intakes are often lower than prescribed due to vomiting, diarrhea, interruption for procedures, or tube problems. In these cases, parenteral nutrition is indicated.

Even if TPN is required, it is probably useful to give a small amount of enteral feeding to prevent bacterial translocation and improve host immune function.

Substrates

Energy requirements
Patients with pancreatitis have a wide distribution of resting energy expenditure. It has been shown that 10% of patients are hypometabolic, 38% are normometabolic, and only 52% are hypermetabolic. The energy needs of patients with acute pancreatitis are variable due to the severity of the disease, the presence of infection, and treatment (pain control, sedation, myorelax-

ants). Although basal energy expenditure (BEE) is most often estimated by using the Harris–Benedict formula modified by stress factors to account for the severity of the disease, the most accurate way of assessing caloric requirements is by measuring the resting energy expenditure (REE) by indirect calorimetry. However, in a critically ill population, it has been demonstrated that the Harris–Benedict formula overestimated the energy needs when compared with REE measured by calorimetry. Since equipment for measuring indirect calorimetry is expensive and may not always be available, predictive formulas to calculate basal energy expenditure are more often used and help in preventing over- or underfeeding in this group of patients (see Chapter 8).

Glucose should provide 60–70% of the total non-protein caloric needs but never in excess of the maximal endogenous capacity to oxidize glucose (4–5 mg/kg per min). If the serum triacylglycerol is normal, 30% of non-protein energy can be provided as fat but never in excess of 1 g/kg per day to prevent cholestasis. In pancreatitis, all studies have been performed using long-chain triacylglycerol. The theoretical advantages of new emulsions (medium-chain triacylglycerol, structured lipids, olive oil, or n-3) have not be tested in pancreatitis.

Protein requirements
Protein needs are not different from the needs of critically ill patients. In parenteral studies, authors provided 0.25–0.30 g/kg per day nitrogen. In severe illnesses there may be a relative deficiency of glutamine, but the role of glutamine supplementation in human acute severe pancreatitis has yet to be confirmed.

Micronutrients
Multivitamin and trace elements solutions must be administered early when nutritional support is ordered. Recommended dietary allowances do not cover the needs during acute pancreatitis because of previous

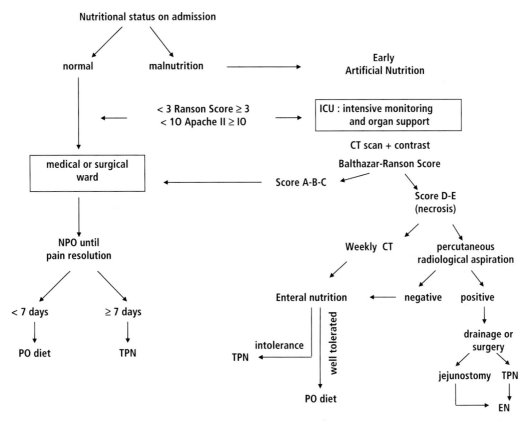

Figure 12.2 Guidelines for nutritional support.

to parenteral nutrition in severe acute pancreatitis: results of a randomized prospective trial. *Br J Surg* 1997; 84: 1665–1669.

Kalfarentzos FE, Karavias DD, Karatzas TM *et al.* Total parenteral nutrition in severe acute pancreatitis. *J Am Coll Nutr* 1991; 10: 156–162.

McClave SA, Greene LM, Snider HL *et al.* Comparison of the safety of early enteral versus parenteral nutrition in mild acute pancreatitis. *JPEN J Parenter Enteral Nutr* 1997; 21: 14–20.

Meier R, Beglinger C, Layer P *et al.* Consensus statement. ESPEN Guidelines on nutrition in acute pancreatitis. *Clin Nutr* 2002; 21: 173–183.

Nathens AB, Curtis JR, Beale RJ, *et al.* Management of the critically ill patient with severe acute pancreatitis. *Crit Care Med* 2004; 32: 2524–2536.

Neoptolemos JP, Raraty M, Finch M, Sutton R. Acute pancreatitis: the substantial human and financial costs. *Gut* 1998; 42: 886–891.

Ranson JH, Rifkind KM, Roses DF *et al.* Prognostic signs and the role of operative management in acute pancreatitis. *Surg Gynecol Obstet* 1974; 139: 69–81.

Robin AP, Campbell R, Palani CK. Total parenteral nutrition during acute pancreatitis: clinical experience with 156 patients. *World J Surg* 1990; 14: 572–579.

Sax HC, Warner BW, Talamini MA. Early total parenteral nutrition in acute pancreatitis: lack of beneficial effects. *Am J Surg* 1987; 153: 117–124.

Silberman H, Dixon NP, Eisenberg D. The safety and efficacy of a lipid-based system of parenteral nutrition in acute pancreatitis. *Am J Gastroenterol* 1982; 77: 494–497.

Sitzmann JV, Steinborn PA, Zinner MJ, Cameron JL. Total parenteral nutrition and alternate sustrates in treatment of severe acute pancreatitis. *Surg Gynecol Obstet* 1989; 168: 311–317.

Steininger R, Karner J, Roth E, Langer K. Infusion of dipeptides as nutritional substrates for glutamine, tyrosine, and branched-chain amino acids in patients with acute pancreatitis. *Metabolism* 1989; 38: 78–81.

Tesinsky P. Nutritional care of pancreatitis and its complications. *Curr Opin Clin Nutr Metab Care* 1999; 2: 395–398.

Van Gossum A, Lemoyne M, Greig PD, Jeejeebhoy KN. Lipid-associated total parenteral nutrition in patients with severe acute pancreatitis. *JPEN J Parenter Enteral Nutr* 1988; 12: 250–255.

Vidon N, Pfeiffer A, Franchisseur C *et al.* Effect of different caloric loads in human jejunum on meal-stimulated and non-stimulated biliopancreatic secretion. *Am J Clin Nutr* 1988; 47: 400–405.

WHO. *Laboratory Diagnosis and Monitoring of Diabetes Mellitus.* Geneva, Switzerland: World Health Organization, 2002.

Windsor AC, Kanwar S, Li AG *et al.* Compared with parenteral nutrition, enteral feeding attenuates the acute phase response and improves disease severity in acute pancreatitis. *Gut* 1998; 42: 431–435.

Websites

Diabetes UK. www.diabetes.org.uk/
American Diabetes Association. www.diabetes.org/home.jsp
European Association for the Study of Diabetes. www.easd.org/
European Society for Clinical Nutrition and Metabolism. www.espen.org/

13
The Kidney

Gianfranco Guarnieri, Roberta Situlin, and Gabriele Toigo

Key messages

- The functions of the kidney are to eliminate waste products, control body fluid volume and composition, produce erythropoietin, renin, and prostaglandins, and regulate the metabolism of vitamin D and small molecular weight proteins.
- In renal disease, these functions are impaired leading to the development of the uremic syndrome.
- Dietary therapy has an important role in renal disease to control the symptoms and metabolic consequences of renal dysfunction.
- Protein–energy malnutrition (PEM) is a common clinical finding in renal disease and has a negative bearing on quality of life, morbidity, mortality, and rate of progression of the disease.
- PEM can also have negative effects on renal function, which in turn exacerbates existing malnutrition.

13.1 Introduction

Medical nutrition therapy (MNT) plays an essential role in the management of renal disease. To appreciate the interaction between nutritional and renal dysfunction it is important to have an understanding of the normal physiology of the kidney. The kidney is essentially an excretory organ but it is also involved in the regulation of the volume and composition of body fluids, as well as having specific endocrine and metabolic functions. The functioning unit is the nephron, of which there are approximately 1 million in each kidney. The function and action of a nephron are shown in Figure 13.1.

A large volume of blood – about 1.3 liters – passes through the nephrons every minute. The rate of ultrafiltration is referred to as the glomerular filtration rate (GFR) and is approximately 125 ml/min. This value varies with age and sex. The filtrate formed in the glomerulus passes first into the proximal convoluted tubule, then into the loop of Henle and through the distal convoluted tubule to the collecting ducts. During this process, the filtrate is modified according to the needs of the body by re-absorption and secretion by the tubules (Figure 13.1b).

If as a result of renal disease, excretions are not optimal, serum levels of urea and electrolytes can become elevated and patients may become symptomatic. Dietary intervention has an important role by regulating protein, fluid, sodium, potassium, and phosphate intake. Plasma urea and electrolyte levels can be maintained within acceptable limits. The nutritional status of the patient must be considered and adequate energy, protein, macro- and micronutrients supplied, especially in children, to maximize growth, and to prevent malnutrition, commonly seen in this group of patients.

This chapter will be organized according to the type of renal disease as the role of nutritional management in each situation is quite different (Box 13.1).

13.2 Acute renal failure

Acute renal failure (ARF) is a clinical syndrome, characterized by a rapid loss of renal function (decreased glomerular and tubular function), with accumulation of metabolic end-products normally excreted by the kidneys. Increased levels of plasma urea, creatinine, hydrogen ions, potassium, and uric acid are some of the metabolic consequences of ARF.

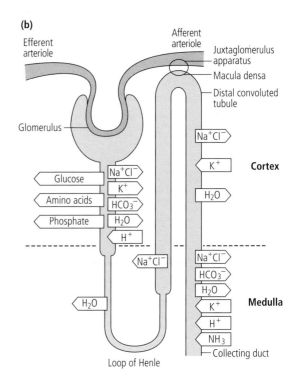

Figure 13.1 (a) The principal parts of the nephron. (b) Sites of removal or addition of electrolytes from, or into, tubular fluid. Redrawn from Kumar and Clark (1998) with permission from Elsevier.

Box 13.1 Types of renal disease

- Acute renal failure (ARF) – the onset of renal failure is rapid
- Chronic renal failure (CRF) – the onset of renal failure has developed over a longer period of time
- The nephrotic syndrome – a specific syndrome in which patients lose excessive amounts of protein in their urine
- End stage renal failure (ESRF) – the patient requires some form of renal replacement therapy (RRT) or transplantation

---

The prevalence of ARF has been estimated as 5% of all patients in the hospital setting, with the incidence being as high as 25% in the intensive care setting. The overall mortality is about 40–60%, despite many recent improvements in treatment and renal replacement therapy. Patients with shock or sepsis have the worst prognosis (up to 90% mortality), while medical and trauma patients have a better prognosis (30% and 50% respectively). Obstetric acute renal failure is rare today, but the group of patients showing increasing frequency of ARF are the elderly. Mortality has also been related to systolic blood pressure, assisted ventilation, congestive heart failure, sepsis, and gastrointesti-

nal dysfunction. Other determinants of outcome are the presence and degree of hypercatabolism, the need for dialysis (especially continuous treatment), and the degree of biocompatibility of dialysis membranes.

Metabolic changes

Protein catabolism
Severe catabolism with a highly negative nitrogen balance is characteristic of ARF. Hypercatabolism in ARF has been defined on the basis of daily increases in blood urea nitrogen (>11 mmol/l), blood urea nitrogen to creatinine ratio (>10), or of urea nitrogen appearance, UNA (>10 or >15 g/day) (Box 13.2). Box 13.3 lists the main causes of hypercatabolism in ARF patients.

Hypercatabolism causes severe negative nitrogen balance, with nitrogen losses as high as 150–200 g/day. Increased gluconeogenesis (insensitive to exogenous glucose infusion) and ureagenesis occur in response to this protein hypercatabolism. Endocrine abnormalities (Box 13.3) are characteristic of severe ARF and may be partly responsible for the increased gluconeogenesis, proteolysis, and accelerated protein turnover. There is

Box 13.2 Equations used to calculate urea nitrogen appearance and change in body urea nitrogen

The urea nitrogen appearance (UNA) can be calculated from the following formula:

UNA (g/day) = urinary urea nitrogen (g/day) + change in body urea nitrogen (g/day)

Change in body urea nitrogen (g/day) is calculated with the following formula:

$$\text{Change} = (\text{SUN}_f - \text{SUN}_i,\ \text{g/l/day}) \times 0.60 \times \text{BW}_i\ (\text{kg}) + (\text{BW}_f - \text{BW}_i,\ \text{kg/day}) \times \text{SUN}_f\ (\text{g/l})$$

where SUN is serum urea nitrogen (g/l), BW is body weight (kg), subscripts i and f indicate initial and final values for the period of measurement, and 0.60 is the estimate of the fraction of body weight that is body water.

Box 13.3 Factors responsible for hypercatabolism in acute renal failure

- Endocrine abnormalities
  - Raised glucagon
  - Raised cortisol
  - Raised catecholamines
  - Raised parathormone
  - Insulin resistance
- Immobilization
- Acidemia
- Uremic toxins
- Loss of nutrients
- Bleeding
- Associated events (SIRS, burns, shock, etc.)
- Increased proteases activity
- Increased cytokine activity
- Reduced nutrient intake
- Resistance to growth factors
- Renal replacement therapy

an increased secretion of counterregulatory hormones such as catecholamines, glucagon, and cortisol, leading to insulin resistance. Hyperparathyroidism can also be present in ARF.

As with chronically uremic patients, metabolic acidosis may be responsible for impaired insulin activity, protein breakdown, increased cortisol secretion, and low albumin plasma levels. Replacement therapy is often necessary in patients with ARF, although dialysis itself is considered a strong catabolic stimulus, due to loss of nutrients (amino acids, peptides, and vitamins) during the dialytic procedure and due to the production and release of cytokines and proteases from monocytes during the blood contact with the dialysis membranes. In some cases blood–membrane interactions can exert a catabolic stimulus, producing an increased release of amino acid from muscle. This loss can be lessened by using more biocompatible membranes.

Protein metabolism

Metabolic abnormalities, decreased renal function, or loss of the amino acids through the dialysis membranes may mean that amino acids that are considered non-essential in healthy subjects (e.g. histidine, arginine, tyrosine, serine, and cysteine) become conditionally essential in ARF patients.

Imbalances of plasma and intracellular amino acids have been described in ARF. The rate of elimination of amino acids from plasma is altered in acutely uremic patients and some amino acids, such as phenylalanine and methionine, may accumulate. Non-essential amino acids involved in the urea cycle (e.g. arginine and ornithine) may need to be supplemented in patients with ARF treated with artificial nutrition.

Lipid metabolism

Lipid metabolism is severely affected by ARF. Plasma lipid levels and clearances are altered. Plasma concentrations of triglyceride, very low-density lipoproteins (VLDL) and low-density lipoproteins (LDL) are usually elevated in renal patients, while cholesterol and high-density lipoprotein (HDL) levels are usually low. Impaired lipolysis is the main reason for this as the activities of the key enzymes of lipid metabolism (post-heparinic lipoprotein lipase, hepatic triglyceride lipase, and peripheral lipoprotein lipase) are altered both at peripheral and hepatic levels. Because a decreased ability to utilize exogenous lipids has been described, the amount of lipids given to ARF patients should be lower than that for non-uremic patients.

Nutritional treatment in acute renal failure

It is yet to be clearly demonstrated that nutritional intervention can improve outcome in ARF. This may be due to the fact that the patients have a widely varying etiology, severity, and treatment, making it difficult to carry out randomized prospective trials. In addition, the optimal composition of formulas for parenteral and enteral nutrition has not been clearly established. However, clinical experience indicates that treatments may have important clinical benefits even when it is difficult to demonstrate such benefits scientifically. The markedly negative nitrogen balance often seen in the most severe patients and their poor prognosis suggest the importance of a well-planned nutritional treatment, with an optimal amount of energy, nitrogen, and of other nutrients.

Energy requirements

ARF itself does not cause increased energy demand. On the contrary, patients with uncomplicated ARF may have a lower energy expenditure than healthy controls. The coexisting disease (e.g. sepsis, surgery, or trauma) determines the energy needs of these patients. Some authors have demonstrated that hypercatabolic patients receiving a moderate quantity of energy (26 kcal/kg per day) had a better outcome than patients with higher energy intakes (35 kcal/kg per day). Measuring or calculating energy expenditure on the basis of estimated dry weight is useful to avoid overfeeding. An amount of energy not exceeding 1.3 times the basal metabolic rate (i.e. 25–35 kcal/kg per day) is generally recommended in these patients, the higher amount being reserved for hypercatabolic patients with higher urea plasma levels and very negative nitrogen balance. Amounts of energy in excess of 35 kcal/kg per day are seldom needed.

In some conditions, replacement therapy is responsible for a heat loss that should be taken in account when calculating energy requirements. Glycemia must be carefully monitored because of the risk of hyperglycemia due to insulin resistance, increased gluconeogenesis, and acidosis. Due to the impaired ability to metabolize exogenous lipids, their intake should be limited to 20–25% of total energy and the serum triglycerides should be monitored frequently.

Nitrogen requirements

The nitrogen requirements of patients with ARF are determined by many factors including:

- the degree of renal impairment,
- the prognosis of renal failure,
- the underlying disease,
- the need for replacement therapy, and
- nutritional status.

Dialysis makes it possible to give amounts of protein or amino acids while maintaining low blood urea nitrogen values. However, the replacement therapy can itself be a cause of increased catabolism. Patients with ARF derived from primary renal involvement (most often drug or contrast media-induced) show a low degree of catabolism (UNA <6 g/day) and have a short expected duration of renal insufficiency: they can usually eat spontaneously 'per os,' and they can initially be treated with a low protein diet (0.6 g/kg per day); this amount can be progressively increased to 0.8–1.0 g/kg per day, maintaining blood urea nitrogen lower than 100 mg/dl (~36 mmol/l). In acutely ill patients with ARF, nitrogen requirements are higher: 1.0–1.5 g/kg per day of protein is generally suggested, depending on the degree of protein catabolism. Higher nitrogen intake may not promote a better nitrogen balance but may result in higher urea levels. However higher amounts are needed in highly catabolic patients treated with continuous renal replacement therapy.

Where possible, patients with ARF should be given an oral diet with, or without, nutritional supplements. In situations where this is not possible and the patients are not able to achieve full nutritional requirements orally within 5–7 days, nutritional support will be necessary. If the nutritional status of the patient is severely compromised and/or hypercatabolism is present, nutritional support should be started sooner. Enteral nutrition is preferable to parenteral nutrition, but not always possible, especially in some of the sicker patients.

Vitamin requirements

Large vitamin A molecules are not filtered, therefore over time their blood concentration can increase. For this reason, vitamin A supplementation should be avoided. Vitamin C should not exceed 30–50 mg/day. There has been much interest recently concerning the role of the antioxidant nutrients. Requirements for vitamins K, E, D, B_6, and folate are increased in ARF, and supplements are needed.

13.3 Chronic renal failure

Rationale and goals of nutritional therapy

The goals of MNT in chronic renal failure (CRF) are: the prevention of malnutrition, the slowing of the renal disease progression, the control of secondary hyperparathyroidism, of cardiovascular disease risk factors, and of uremia symptoms.

Delay the progression of kidney disease

Chronic kidney disease is characterized by a progressive nature which leads to a relentless loss of renal function even when the pathogenetic factors causing the original damage have been successfully treated. This is at first the consequence of adaptive mechanisms. The remaining functional nephrons (remnant nephrons) become hypertrophic with an increased glomerular plasma flow and transcapillary glomerular hydraulic pressure. These hemodynamic changes allow the total kidney GFR to increase in spite of a reduced kidney mass. In the long term, however, the glomeruli become sclerotic and renal function progressively declines.

In CRF much effort has been put into identifying the best interventions, both nutritional and non-nutritional, to control the factors involved in the progression of the kidney disease and delay the need for renal replacement treatment.

Protein intake
Proteins induce hemodynamic and structural changes in the kidney that are mediated by a number of mechanisms, including increased secretion of hormones (glucagon, growth hormone, corticosteroids, insulin-like growth factor), increased synthesis of angiotensin II, prostaglandins, and nitric oxide, activation of growth factors and complement fractions, induction of cytokines, and higher production of reactive oxygen species.

The effectiveness of a low-protein diet from the early stages of CRF in slowing the progression of kidney disease was shown at first in animal models and then extensively investigated in CRF patients. The level of protein restriction used in the clinical trials varied, in relation to the CRF stage, from low-protein diets (LPD) of about 0.6 g/kg ideal body weight per day to very low-protein diets (VLPD) of about 0.3 g/kg per day, supplemented with essential amino acids or their ketoanalogs. Low-protein diets are also phosphorus restricted, since the two nutrients are associated in the same types of food.

However, it remains uncertain whether protein and phosphate restriction can slow the rate of loss of renal function in progressive renal failure (Box 13.4). Some randomized studies, the largest and most sophisticated being the Modification of Diet in Renal Disease Study (MDRD), suggest that protein and phosphorus restriction is able to slow the worsening of progressive renal disease towards end stage renal disease and report a small or moderate beneficial effect on GFR in patients with advanced renal failure. In patients with early renal failure treated with an LPD a 28% reduction of GFR

Box 13.4 Reasons why it remains uncertain whether protein and phosphorus restriction can slow the rate of loss of renal function in progressive renal failure

Study design
- Heterogeneous populations
- Different rates of renal disease progression
- Different end points

Methodological approach
- Difficulties in measuring loss of renal function
- Difficulties in measuring dietary compliance

Interfering factors
- Other factors responsible for progression
- Whole diet composition
- Drug interference

worsening was found, in comparison with patients maintained on a normal protein diet. In a subsequent examination of the data, the supplemented VLPD showed a beneficial effect on renal failure in advanced renal failure (GFR lower than 25 ml/min). The amount of proteinuria was the main determinant of the blood pressure control on progression of renal failure.

Despite these positive analyses, unequivocal demonstration of the beneficial effect of a low protein–low phosphorus diet is still lacking. This is mainly due to the fact that in the first four months on the diet, patients treated with an LPD showed a more rapid decrease of GFR. This was suggested by the authors to be probably the result of hemodynamic adjustments rather than of renal structural injury. The effect was however large enough to confound the results of the trials.

Vegetable soy protein has shown to be more effective in slowing the progression of kidney disease than casein from milk.

Phosphate intake
Phosphate intake is also considered responsible for kidney damage, independently from protein, most likely through parenchymal deposition of calcium phosphate precipitates in the presence of hyperphosphatemia, and changes in intracellular calcium metabolism which may modify renal hemodynamics and mesangial growth factors. A low daily phosphate intake also allows an improvement in divalent ion metabolism, parathyroid hormone (PTH) functions, and hyperparathyroidism.

Dietary fat

Dietary fat may also have a role in the progression of kidney failure. Hypercholesterolemia may cause excessive activation of monocytes and macrophages. Both hyperlipemia and the intramesangial oxidative modification of LDL might be responsible for the glomerular damage. The combination of hypertension and hyperlipemia may have a very negative prognostic relevance. Quality of dietary fat may also have a role by its influence on production of eicosanoids involved in the inflammatory processes. Diets supplemented with polyunsaturated *n*-3 fatty acids in experimental conditions showed beneficial effects on renal functions, proteinuria, progression of renal failure, and survival. The data from clinical trials were inconsistent, however, with the exception of immunoglobulin A (IgA) nephropathy.

Proteinuria

Proteinuria favors the deposition of excess filtered proteins into the mesangium, causing tubular cell injury and interstitial fibrosis. Proteinuria has been defined as an independent risk factor for the progression of CRF.

Hyperglycemia

In diabetic patients dietary goals include the maintenance of a strict glucose control, since hyperglycemia is associated with an accelerated rate of renal failure.

Hypertension

The role of hypertension in determining the rate of progression of CRF is well established. Therefore a good control of blood pressure needs to be associated with the dietary modifications.

Type of nephropathy

The decrease in GFR is faster in patients with autosomal dominant polycystic kidney disease and chronic glomerulonephritis.

Avoid malnutrition

Besides the efficacy of LPDs and VLPDs on the progression of renal failure, it is also important to consider the safety and feasibility of such regimens. Many authors have confirmed that LPDs and supplemented VLPDs can maintain good nutritional status. However concerns exist regarding protein–phosphorus restricted diets in the genesis of PEM in chronically uremic patients from the observation of abnormalities of nutritional status (reduced nutrient intake, decline

of body weight, percentage body fat, arm muscle area, and serum protein levels) and of muscle metabolism after long-term treatment.

Control of uremia symptoms

Symptoms are the consequence of the accumulation of nitrogenous waste products, including urea and creatinine and other uremic toxins, and of the hormonal changes (increased levels of PTH, lack of vitamin D, or erythropoietin). In the more advanced stages, patients develop more severe symptoms of uremia which can be improved in the short run by a further restriction of protein and phosphate intake; however, renal replacement therapy (RRT) generally needs to be started in the short term.

In conclusion, present guidelines about MNT for chronic renal failure suggest protein and phosphate restriction and strongly recommend a strict and continuous surveillance of the risk of PEM.

Protein–energy malnutrition (PEM)

Nutritional status influences both quality of life and patient outcome. PEM is a negative prognostic predictor in CRF. The summary of studies measuring the prevalence of PEM in patients with chronic renal failure in Table 13.1 shows that PEM is a frequent clinical finding.

In CRF, PEM is generally evident when the GFR is less than 10–20 ml/min, even though biochemical and tissue abnormalities are present at earlier phases of renal damage. The finding of PEM in patients who start dialysis is often the result of inadequate nutritional status during the predialytic phase.

Causes of malnutrition

The causes of malnutrition are multifactorial and are illustrated in Figure 13.2.

Reduced food intake

One of the most relevant and common causes of PEM is an inadequate dietary intake. Energy intake is particularly low in CRF patients and it has been considered one of the most important reasons for the wasting syndrome of uremia.

Anorexia is a common feature in patients with a GFR below 60 ml/min. Some of the causes of anorexia are listed in Box 13.5. Recently, high levels of plasma leptin have been found in CRF both in predialysis and

Table 13.1 Prevalence of protein–energy malnutrition in patients with chronic renal failure

Study	Number and patient groups studies	Percentages of patients with values below references or score
Guarnieri et al., 1989a	CRF (18); HD (19); CAPD (19)	TST (64); AMC (36); Alb (87); Transf (40)
Guarnieri et al., 1989b	CRF on LPD from 5 (12) and 10 (9) years	TST (10); AMC (22); Alb (0); Transf (14)
		TST (12); AMC (0); Alb (71); Transf 14)
Young et al., 1991	CAPD (224)	SGA (41):
		Mod PEM = 33; S PEM = 8
Cianciaruso et al., 1995	CAPD (224)	SGA, 18–64 years: M–Mod PEM = 65; S PEM = 5
		>65 years: M–Mod PEM = 36; S PEM = 11
		SGA, 18–64 years M–Mod PEM = 30.3; S PEM = 3
		>65y: M-Mod PEM=43; S PEM=8
Qureshi et al., 1998	HD (128)	SGA (<65 years, 46; >65 years, 68), (M PEM = 51; Mod–S
		PEM = 13)
Heimburger et al., 2000	Advanced CRF (115)	SGA (48)

Figures in brackets are percentages of patients with values below references or scores.
CRF, chronic renal failure; HD, hemodialysis; CAPD, continuous ambulatory peritoneal dialysis; LPD, low-protein diet; TST, tricep skinfold thickness; AMC, arm muscle circumference; Transf, transferrin; Alb, albumin; PEM, protein–energy malnutrition; M, mild; Mod, moderate; S, severe; SGA, Subjective Global Assessment.

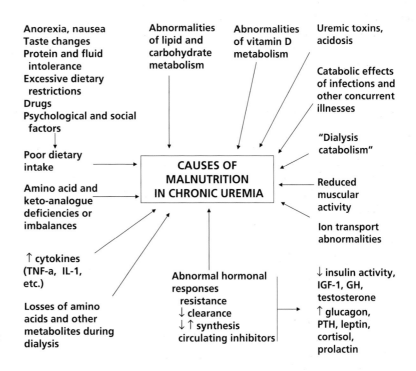

Figure 13.2 Causes of malnutrition in chronic uremia.

hemodialysis patients and even more in those on peritoneal dialysis. This high leptin level might be related to reduced renal clearance of the polypeptide, to the hyperinsulinemia, or to chronic inflammation. In particular it is noteworthy that the ratio leptin/body fat is inversely related to the protein intake in patients on

peritoneal dialysis, and may therefore be directly involved in the genesis of anorexia.

Metabolic acidosis
Metabolic acidosis (MA) plays a very important causal role in PEM. It acts as an uremic toxin: it directly fa-

vors protein catabolism by increasing branched chain amino acid oxidation, stimulating cortisol secretion, and promoting proteolytic enzyme activity and muscle mRNA for ubiquitin and proteasome synthesis. The normal adaptive metabolic mechanisms are inhibited by MA, which has an independent negative effect on plasma albumin levels. The net effects of MA associated with a reduced protein intake are a negative nitrogen balance and muscle wasting. Correction of acidosis can decrease the rates of whole body protein turnover and improve nitrogen balance, insulin sensitivity, and PTH response.

Changes in nutrient metabolism

- *Carbohydrate metabolism* Hyperinsulinemia and insulin resistance have been well documented in patients with renal insufficiency, and they may be involved in the genesis of accelerated atherosclerosis in uremia. Many other causes may be responsible, including metabolic acidosis, secondary hyperparathyroidism, as well as general uremic toxins. Increased plasma concentrations of glucagon and PTH promote gluconeogenesis and protein catabolism. The negative effect of CRF on glucose metabolism is demonstrated by the finding of high free glucose concentration at the intracellular level, while the glycogen concentration is low. The activity of phosphofructokinase is low in skeletal muscle, and its activity is inhibited by the ultrafiltrate of uremic sera. The acetate and pyruvate metabolic tolerance is impaired.

- *Lipid metabolism* The most frequent type of dyslipidemia in CRF in the predialysis phase and during the dialysis period is hypertriglyceridemia, with high levels of ApoB-rich VLDL and IDL. The causes of dyslipidemia are also multiple, and defects of the enzymes involved in lipid metabolism (LCAT, lipoprotein lipase, and hepatic lipase) have been described. Dietary recommendations to have a high carbohydrate intake may exacerbate high triglyceride serum levels, particularly if the soluble fiber intake is low.

- *Protein metabolism* Severe derangement of plasma and intracellular concentrations of amino acids has been found in uremic patients. The ratio of essential to non-essential amino acids in plasma is lower than in normal individuals. The concentration of the branched chain amino acids, especially valine, and of tyrosine, threonine, and lysine is reduced. In contrast, plasma levels of glycine, cystine, methionine, aspartate, and citrulline are increased. In muscle, normal levels of leucine and isoleucine were found, while valine, threonine, taurine, lysine, and histidine were low. Histidine and thyrosine are considered essential in chronic uremia owing to the specific metabolic impairment.

The protein depletion and muscle wasting that are characteristic of uremic patients can be a consequence of increased muscle degradation or decreased protein synthesis, with an imbalance between the two processes. Both muscle RNA : DNA and alkali-soluble protein : DNA ratios (respectively expressions of the cell capacity to synthesize protein and of the cell size) are reduced in chronically uremic patients. Experimental and clinical studies on total body and on skeletal muscle protein turnover have generally shown a reduced protein synthesis, while protein degradation has been found to be normal or reduced.

Both the uremic syndrome and malnutrition might be responsible for these adaptive mechanisms. Indeed, the adaptive mechanisms of normal individuals to a reduced dietary protein intake are preserved in the short and in the long term in uremic patients on LPD.

A regulatory effect of the degree of renal failure on the total body protein turnover is suggested by the finding of a direct correlation between plasma creatinine and leucine rate of appearance. Furthermore, a direct stimulatory effect of acidosis on protein catabolism has been recently demonstrated. Acidosis increases branched chain amino acids oxidation, enhances secretion of cortisol, and promotes proteolytic enzyme synthesis.

Role of inflammation

Inflammation may influence energy expenditure, nutrient intake, and metabolism. High levels of tumor necrosis factor alpha (TNFα) and interleukin 1 (IL-1) have been found in the plasma of patients with CRF. From our personal observations, CRF patients have increased secretion of TNFα which is associated with higher circulating levels of soluble TNFα receptors, directly related to serum creatinine.

The risk of developing atherosclerosis in CRF may be linked to the interaction between PEM, inflammation, and oxidative stress.

Effects of malnutrition on renal function

Not only does renal disease impact on the nutritional status of a patient, but low protein intake and PEM can also have negative effects on renal function, which in turn may exacerbate existing malnutrition. These effects include the following:

- Changes in urine concentration capacity can be the result of higher levels of prostaglandin E2 (PGE2). Furthermore, a low protein intake decreases the levels of urea in the kidney medulla necessary to create an adequate osmotic gradient and may impair antidiuretic hormone (ADH) activity.
- Acidosis from a lower ability to acidify urine. A low protein intake may reduce the activities of enzymes involved in the process while a low phosphate intake lowers the excretion of acid loads.
- Increased frequency of nosocomial urinary tract infections.

Assessment of nutritional status

Nutritional assessment should be performed regularly in patients with CRF in order to identify patients at risk of malnutrition. This should include anthropometry, biochemical determinations, clinical assessment, and dietary compliance (see Chapter 2).

Signs of PEM usually appear with a GFR around 60 ml/min. At this stage nutritional assessment should be conducted every 6–12 months. With further decline of GFR below 30 ml/min follow-up is better done at 1–3 month intervals (National Kidney Foundation, 2001). Standardization of screening method policies may help early recognition of nutritional risks. Multiple methods of assessment should be used to obtain more reliable data.

Subjective methods

Subjective methods of nutritional screening and assessment should include a nutrition-oriented medical history to obtain information on past and present illnesses, drug, vitamin and mineral supplement intake, weight, appetite and taste changes, and socioeconomical and psychological factors which may interfere with adequate nutrition. The Subjective Global Assessment (SGA) of nutritional status integrates history with physical examination data and has been validated in patients with CRF.

Assessment of nutrient intake

The assessment of dietary intake in CRF is important since many patients have difficulties in following long-term restrictive regimens. Dietary interviews by well-trained dietitians are recommended. Food diaries may also be useful to assess eating habits and to monitor the patient dietary compliance.

Anthropometric measurements

Anthropometric measurements include body weight, body mass index (BMI), subcutaneous skinfold thickness, and arm or leg circumferences. They are all easy and safe to perform, and most of them require simple and readily available equipment. Water retention in the end stages of renal failure may limit the reliability of anthropometric indices. The fluid balance state should therefore be always taken into account when performing these measurements.

Biochemical indices
Serum protein concentration

The concentration of serum proteins is an index of the status of visceral proteins, mainly synthesized by the liver. Albumin is a protein with a long half-life of 21 days, which is a marker of PEM. Its serum levels are influenced, however, by a number of factors including:

- massive extracorporeal losses (nephrotic syndrome, burns),
- inflammation-associated changes in vascular permeability with shift of albumin from the intra- to the extravascular space,
- fluid overload,

- protein hypercatabolism, and
- liver dysfunction.

In CRF low serum albumin level is associated with a bad prognosis. Determination of albumin is now considered a means to assess outcome rather than an index of nutritional status. Serum transferrin has a shorter half-life of 9 days, which makes it a more sensitive index of malnutrition; however, it is important to note that its concentration is also sensitive to iron status and to infectious and inflammatory diseases. Prealbumin has a very short half-life and may therefore detect short-term changes in visceral protein status. In predialysis patients, however, its assessment is not useful. The serum concentration of the protein is influenced by the level of renal functions and rises in CRF independently from nutritional status. Insulin-like growth factor 1 (IGF-1) has also been recently proposed as a sensitive index of PEM.

Plasma amino acid concentrations
In chronically uremic patients the pattern of free amino acids in plasma and skeletal muscle shows peculiar abnormalities that might be caused by uremia itself or by malnutrition. The value of plasma amino acid concentrations as reliable and sensitive markers of nutritional state, however, is low. In contrast, the finding of specific changes of intracellular amino acid in skeletal muscle has been helpful in treating uremia by tailored nutritional solutions for enteral or parenteral nutrition.

Blood urea nitrogen and nitrogen balance
In stable chronically uremic patients, the blood urea nitrogen (BUN) correlates with protein intake. However, it should always be considered that BUN values are also influenced by a worsening of renal failure (in predialysis patients), by the adequacy of the dialysis treatment in dialyzed patients, or by the degree of protein catabolism.

The urea nitrogen appearance (UNA) is a measure of protein intake in clinically stable patients. It can be calculated from the formula shown in Box 13.2. Changes in BUN (g/day) can be calculated with the formula shown in Box 13.2 and nitrogen balance can be derived from the difference between nitrogen intake and UNA.

Nitrogen balance studies with direct measurement of most nitrogen losses can give more precise measure of changes in body nitrogen/protein content and they are often used for research purposes. Bias may be introduced, however, by inaccurate sample collections.

A neutral nitrogen balance does not necessarily indicate an ideal nutritional state or therapy but rather shows a steady state of body nitrogen: a neutral balance is attained, but at the expense of reduced visceral and muscular protein pools. If severe malnutrition is present, a neutral nitrogen balance can be attained with lower protein intake. In addition, the nitrogen balance is also sensitive to an adequate intake of other nutrients such as energy or some micronutrients.

Immunological indices
Total lymphocyte count and complement fractions are frequently low in malnourished CRF patients. However, they can also be influenced by uremic toxicity and immune-mediated renal disease. Many effects of uremia on immunological function have been described but the relative importance of uremia and malnutrition is not clear. Cellular immunity and T cell subsets are altered in chronic uremia, and the number and function of T cells are predictive of prognosis. Higher levels of cytokines have been associated with malnutrition and mortality in hemodialysis patients. Leukocyte metabolism and function are also impaired in uremia. Immune depression is partially responsible for the close relationship between malnutrition and infections in chronic renal patients.

Body composition measurements
Several techniques have been developed to measure body composition with different levels of precision, accuracy, safety, and costs. These are discussed at greater length in chapter 2 of *Introduction to Human Nutrition* in this series.

Medical nutritional therapy

Medical nutrition therapy (Table 13.2) of CRF involves multiple goals and may therefore be difficult to understand and follow by many patients. Education and motivation of the patients and their families are therefore key factors in fostering dietary compliance. Furthermore the need for long-term follow-up to avoid malnutrition requires specific knowledge, commitment, cooperation, and adequate resources.

Table 13.2 Guidelines for dietary treatment of patients with chronic renal failure on conservative therapy

	ESPEN (Toigo *et al.*, 2000)	K/DOQI Guidelines, 2000	Kopple *et al.*, 2004
Protein, g/kg body weight[a] per day			
GFR >70 ml/min	0.8–1.0	–	As for GFR of 25–70 ml/min, only in patients with evidence of continuing GFR decline
Early/moderate renal failure (GFR 25–70 ml/min)	0.55–0.6 (75% HBV)	–	0.55–0.6 to 0.75 (at least 50% HBV)[b]
Advanced renal failure (GFR <25 ml/min)	0.55–0.6 (75% HBV) or VLPD[c]	0.55–0.6 to 0.75 (at least 50% HBV)[b]	0.55–0.6 to 0.75 (at least 50% HBV)[b]
Energy, kcal/kg body weight per day[a]	35 (±25% in obese or malnourished patients)	35	35
		30–35 (if age>60 years) (with GFR <25 ml/m)	30–35 (if age >60 years) unless weight >120% of relative weight or patient is gaining unwanted weight

[a]Body weight. ESPEN = ideal body weight, according to the Metropolitan Life Insurance tables; Kopple = relative weight as determined from NHANES II values, 1984.
[b]0.75 g/kg body weight/day of proteins if the patient is not compliant to the more restrictive diets or unable to maintain an adequate energy intake.
[c]Very low protein diet is 0.28 g/kg/day + essential amino acid (EAA) supplements or ketoanalogs of amino acids and EAA supplements. These supplements are not available worldwide. VLPD can be prescribed only in highly selected patients, with lower GFR (10–20 ml/min), highest compliance to an adequate energy intake, and under strict nutritional monitoring.
HBV, high biological value; VLPD, very low protein diet.

Protein intake

The prescription of a reduced protein diet requires the selection of:

- the patient who might benefit from protein restricted regimens,
- the time to start the diet, and
- the quantity and the quality of proteins.

There is no general consensus about the best time to start a protein-restricted diet. The following guidelines are those published by the European Society for Clinical Nutrition and Metabolism (ESPEN) in 2000 (www.espen.org). Generally, if the patient is being diagnosed a nephropathy but the GFR is >70 ml/min (i.e. there is no kidney insufficiency) there should be nutritional counseling to limit protein intake to the level recommended for normal subjects (0.8–1 g/kg per day). With a worsening of renal functioning (GFR between 25 and 70 ml/min) the protein intake should be reduced to 0.55–0.6 g/kg ideal body weight per day (75% of animal origin, high biological value protein, HBV).

This is the amount of protein needed to maintain the nitrogen balance in normal subjects when HBV proteins are used. HBV proteins allow the supply of the best quantity and proportion of essential amino acids needed for protein synthesis. Diets with lower protein intake should therefore include at least 75% of HBV proteins while assuring an adequate energy intake in order to avoid a negative nitrogen balance.

The acceptance of these type of diets depends also on the patient's food habits. When vegetable proteins are an important part of the usual diet (for example, pasta, bread, pizza, rice, pulses) the compliance to the low protein diet can be poorer. Aproteic vegetable food products are available but their taste and texture is not always accepted by patients.

When the renal function further deteriorates to a GFR <20–25 ml/min the same LPD can be continued. However, such a regimen might be inadequate to control uremic symptoms. At this point two options are available: (a) adopt a stricter reduction of protein intake, or (b) start dialysis treatment. The second option is mandatory if the patient shows signs of malnutrition since this condition has a negative prognosis on short-term survival. Furthermore, anorexia is a common finding with advanced uremia. The first option, which usually can be adopted in selected patients only for short periods of time, is a VLPD (0.28 g/kg per day), with no limitation about quality, supplemented with essential amino acids or their ketoanalogs. This regimen allows a nitrogen balance to be maintained, provided that the energy intake is adequate. Amino acid supplements are not available, however, in all countries.

A patient on any level of protein restriction will require careful monitoring to ensure that there is no deterioration in the nutritional status.

The National Institute of Diabetes and Digestive and Kidney Disease (NIDDK) have published in 1994 guidelines (www.niddk.nih.gov) that are somewhat less restrictive. The indications for protein intake are of 0.8 g/kg per day (60% HBV) with GFR above 55 ml/min and of 0.6 g/kg per day (60% HBV) with a GFR between 55 and 25 ml/min. In 2000 the National Kidney Foundation (NKF) Kidney Dialysis Outcome Quality Initiative (KDOQI) (http://www.kidney.org/professionals/kdoqi/guidelines.cfm) gave indications to reduce protein intake to 0.6 g/kg per day (50% HBV) only in patients with GFR lower than 25 ml/min who have not yet started dialysis and whose daily energy intake reached 35 kcal/kg. Otherwise and if the patient is not able to maintain the 0.6 g/kg per day diet, 0.75 g protein/kg per day are recommended.

For higher GFR levels no specific indications are given. Kopple *et al.* (2004) advise to keep protein intake at 0.6 g/kg per day (at least 50% HBV) or at 0.75 g/kg per day in non-compliant patients, starting from GFR levels <70 ml/min, and to follow the same indications of the KDOQI in patients with a GFR < 30 ml/min.

A schematic representation of different levels of dietary protein prescription during the clinical course of a patient with chronic renal failure is shown in Figure 13.3.

Energy intake

According to ESPEN Guidelines the maintenance of a nitrogen balance requires an energy intake around 35 kcal/kg per day in normal weight patients. This amount should be adapted by 25% in underweight and obese patients. The NKF K/DOQI Nutrition Guidelines suggest an intake of 35 kcal/kg per day with GFR <25 ml/min on low protein diet, since nitrogen utilization is enhanced by higher energy intake. This amount can be a little lower in elderly and more sedentary subjects (aged ≥60 years) or in subjects who are overweight or afraid to gain unwanted weight. Energy intake has been shown to be difficult to achieve with a low protein regimen.

Education of patients in selecting appropriate foods to achieve a low protein intake together with an adequate energy intake is of paramount importance. Dietary fat should be 30% of the total energy intake or 35% in subjects with hypertriglyceridemia. The indications from the Third Report of the National Cholesterol Education Program (NCEP) Expert Panel (http://www.nhlbi.nih.gov/guidelines/cholesterol/index.htm) may need to be applied to control the increased cardiovascular risk.

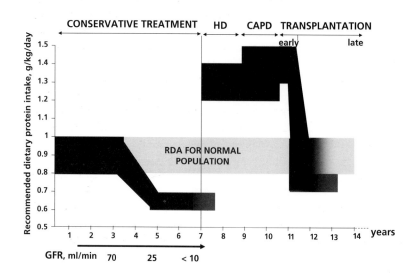

Figure 13.3 Schematic representation of different levels of dietary protein prescription during the clinical course of a patient with chronic renal failure. The sharp modifications of the protein intake recommendations may not be followed by metabolic adaptation or by adequate patient compliance. CAPD, continuous ambulatory peritoneal dialysis; HD, hemodialysis; RDA, recommended dietary allowance.

Mineral and vitamin intake

An LPD also limits phosphate intake as foods rich in proteins are also rich in phosphate. Phosphate intake should be in the range of 8–10 g/kg per day with GFR between 25 and 70 ml/min and the intake can be lowered in the range of 5–10 g/kg per day, with GFR <25 ml/min. Phosphate binders might be needed to control phosphate concentration. The limiting of dairy products to avoid a protein or phosphate excess may compromise calcium intake. Calcium supplementation is therefore necessary to reach an amount of 1400–1600 g/day. Zinc and selenium deficiencies may develop from long-term LPD, but supplements are not usually recommended.

Low protein regimens also increase the risk of water-soluble vitamin deficiencies (mainly riboflavin, thiamine, pyridoxine, folate, and vitamin C). Therefore these vitamins may require supplementation. Pyridoxine intake should be in the range of 5 mg/day since the metabolism of this vitamin is altered in CRF patients. Vitamin C supplementation should be kept below 60 mg/day to avoid the risk of oxalosis. Folate requirements are higher during the first period of erythropoietin therapy. Supplementation may be needed at this time and possibly in patients with high homocysteine levels.

The supplementation of 1,25-dihydroxycholecalciferol (calcitriol) (0.25 μg each day or every second day) will help to prevent hyperparathyroidism. The risk of developing hypercalcemia must be carefully monitored.

13.4 Diabetic nephropathy

Diabetic nephropathy can complicate both type 1 and type 2 diabetes. Clinical features are microalbuminuria in the first stages, then progressing to proteinuria, hypertension, and progressive CRF. Treatment is aimed at a strict glycemic and blood pressure control. The issue of the opportunity of prescribing an LPD is not fully resolved. Many experimental studies demonstrate that LPDs have a protective effect on renal function by decreasing proteinuria and reducing the rate of deterioration of GFR in diabetic nephropathy. In type 1 diabetic patients a low-protein (0.6 g/kg per day) and low-phosphorus (500–1000 mg/day) diet was able to delay the deterioration of GFR from 0.0168

to 0.0043 ml/min per month. Albumin excretion was also reduced by an LPD.

A meta-analysis of the studies on patients with type 1 diabetes mellitus concluded that the data from available studies 'are not a strong justification for the use of protein dietary restriction in routine clinical practice. Nevertheless, on the basis of clinical judgment, dietary protein restriction should be recommended to selected diabetic patients' (Toigo G et al., 2000). A similar effect on GFR and albumin excretion rate has recently been described in patients with type 2 diabetes mellitus.

13.5 Nephrotic syndrome

Nephrotic syndrome is a condition where high amounts of protein (>3 g/day) are lost in the urine. Classic features of the nephrotic syndrome are:

- Proteinuria (>3 g/day)
- Hyperlipidemia
- Hypoalbuminemia
- Edema

Patients with nephrotic syndrome are often malnourished: they characteristically present low plasma albumin levels and a derangement of plasma lipid concentrations (high VLDL, LDL, and IDL plasma levels). However, a severe derangement of muscle metabolism has also been described. In the past, the nutritional treatment of nephrotic syndrome was a high protein intake. The theory was that increasing nitrogen intake through the diet could compensate for the heavy protein loss in the urine. However, in experimental models, higher protein intakes induced an increase in albumin synthesis, while causing increased proteinuria, a negative nitrogen balance, and a worsening of hypoalbuminemia.

The reduction of protein intake in patients with the nephrotic syndrome lowers proteinuria, probably through a reduced production of renin and its gene expression. In some nephrotic patients without renal insufficiency, VLPDs supplemented with essential amino acids have been found to have a positive effect on the clinical course of the disease. Recently it has been shown that nephrotic patients treated with diets providing 0.8 g/kg per day are able to maintain a positive nitrogen balance, by means of a reduction in protein catabolism and stimulation of protein synthesis.

In conclusion, a relatively LPD (0.8–1.0 g/kg per day) without replacement of proteinuria, and 35 kcal/kg per day or more, according to the physical activity levels, produce the best protective effect on renal function without risk of malnutrition. In subjects with renal failure on a 0.6 g/kg per day protein restriction, it is recommended that dietary protein should be supplemented with 1 g HBV protein for each gram of protein lost in the urine. The diet should be high in complex carbohydrates, but low in fat and sodium.

13.6 Renal replacement therapy

When the GFR drops to below about 10 ml/min, patients are usually described as being at end stage renal disease (ESRD) and usually require renal replacement therapy (RRT). This can be in the form of hemodialysis or continuous ambulatory peritoneal dialysis (CAPD). RRT changes a patient's requirements for protein, energy, minerals, and vitamins.

Malnutrition has been reported in 10–70% of hemodialysis and 18–51% of CAPD patients.

Causes of malnutrition

The start of dialysis requires changes in both protein and fluid intake. These modifications may be difficult for some patients to implement and may lead to an overall reduction of nutrient and energy intake. Some patients also seem to restrict their nutrient intake during interdialytic days for fear of excessive weight gain.

Furthermore the dialysis treatment can worsen PEM for a number of reasons. A single hemodialysis session causes a significant loss of free amino acids (from 4 to 9 g per session) and of peptides (2–3 g per session). Dialysis treatment can cause protein catabolism, but the exact mechanism for this is not known. The use of bio-incompatible cuprophane membranes, in comparison to the use of more bio-compatible synthetic membranes, and the reuse of the dialysis filters seem to be at least partially responsible for these metabolic changes. Damage caused to blood cells by the membranes could lead to the liberation of proteolytic leukocyte enzymes, or of proinflammatory cytokines. High levels of cytokines have been associated with anorexia, protein catabolism, malnutrition, inflammation, atherosclerosis, and ischemic heart disease.

In CAPD patients the protein losses from the peritoneum are larger than in hemodialysis patients, ranging from 5 to 15 g/day, while the amino acid and peptides in dialysis fluid are lower (1.2–3.4 g/24 h). If mild or severe peritonitis develops, protein loss can be doubled. Anorexia can be worsened by the continuous absorption of glucose from the peritoneum. The abdominal distension resulting from the presence of CAPD fluids in the abdomen can further lower food intake. CAPD patients tend also to be physically inactive, due to the time involved in exchanging dialysis fluid. As a consequence of a relatively high energy intake and a negative nitrogen balance a severe kwashiorkor-like malnutrition can develop and frequent nutritional follow-up is mandatory.

The maintenance of an adequate nutritional status in RRT patients is related to the adequacy of the dialysis sessions. Insufficient dialysis has been shown to be associated with low protein intake. Therefore the prescription of dialysis dose and quality needs to be individualized and monitored, for example with the calculation of the ratio between the dialyzer urea clearance (k) multiplied by total treatment time (t) and the total body urea distribution volume (V), i.e. kt/V.

RRT patients show also gastrointestinal disturbances and changes in energy-regulating hormones with increased levels of leptin and cholecystokinin (CCK). Comorbid conditions such as diabetes mellitus, cardiovascular disease, depression, stressful conditions, unfavorable socioeconomical factors, and medications can contribute to an inadequate nutrient intake. The presence of inflammation is another factor able to influence not only the nutritional status but also the efficacy of treatment. Protein–energy malnutrition (PEM) and inflammation are frequently both present in RRT patients, and the association between the two conditions has been called malnutrition–inflammation complex syndrome (MICS). Patients with high levels of C-reactive protein have lower albumin concentrations, greater weight loss, and a reduced response to nutritional interventions and dialysis treatment. Furthermore MICS may be responsible for increased risk of cardiovascular atherosclerotic disease, erythropoietin hyporesponsiveness, and higher hospitalization and mortality rates.

Assessment of nutritional status

Nutritional indices

To assess nutritional status the usual array of clinical, anthropometric, biochemical, and functional indices may be used. The NKF recommends SGA application in the assessment of the nutritional status of RRT patients. SGA showed a direct relation with various components of nutritional status. The reproducibility of the test is adequate and also the ability to discriminate between well-nourished and malnourished subjects; however, it has a low sensitivity in detecting the levels of PEM severity. Recently a number of studies have proposed modifications of SGA such as the DMS (Dialysis Malnutrition Score) and the MIS (Malnutrition and Inflammation Score) which include also laboratory data or body composition measurements to overcome the limitations derived from subjective medical judgment.

Prealbumin levels in CRF are modified by renal functions and therefore not useful indicators of nutritional status in predialysis patients. When renal function is lost, as in RRT patients, prealbumin can be used as nutritional marker. Values <30 mg/dl are indicative of PEM. It should be noticed that this cut-off value is lower than in subjects with normal renal function (10–40 mg/dl).

Special considerations in the nutritional assessment of RRT patients

Many factors related to RRT may affect the results of nutritional assessment and must be taken into account to obtain reliable results.

As fluid overload can affect body weight and BMI calculation, measurement of weight should be always done at the end of the hemodialysis session or post emptying of the peritoneal cavity in CAPD patients (dry weight). As energy intake may be in excess in CAPD patients from absorption of glucose from the dialysate fluid, a normal or increased body fat can mask the loss of muscle or body cell mass. Therefore in these cases body composition assessment can be useful to define nutritional status.

In dialysis patients, UNA is calculated during the interdialytic interval (Box 13.2).

In RRT patients all biochemical indices should be measured before the hemodialysis session or after the equilibration phase in CAPD. In dialyzed patients, since there is no renal excretion, serum creatinine, measured before dialysis, is an index of intake of creatine-rich foods and of endogenous production in muscle. Therefore a low predialysis creatinine can reflect muscle wasting but also a low dietary protein intake. Low serum cholesterol may also be an index of both malnutrition and/or low dietary intake.

Prognostic relevance of nutritional indices

Several nutritional indices have prognostic value in RRT patients (Box 13.6).

Both BMI and body composition indices are strong predictors of mortality. The protective effect of a higher BMI is observed in patients with normal or high skeletal muscle mass. In dialysis patients albumin serum levels correlate very poorly with indices of nutritional status, including lean body mass or SGA and show a negative correlation with C-reactive protein, diabetes, and cardiovascular diseases. Serum albumin should therefore not be used as a nutritional marker in RTT, although it is a sensitive prognostic index. A progressively increasing risk for mortality in dialysis has been found for albumin plasma levels ranging from normal levels (4.0–4.5 g/dl) to very low (<2.5 g/dl). The worst prognosis is associated with albumin levels lower than 3 g/dl, although values between 3.0 and 3.5 g/dl are also associated with a bad outcome. Carnitine concentrations have also been shown to correlate with clinical outcome parameters.

During dialysis treatment, the patients with UNA higher than 80% of reference normal values have a 4.1 times lower probability of death within 12 months than patients with body nitrogen lower than 80%.

Box 13.6 Nutritional factors related to outcome in renal replacement therapy patients

- Reduced nutrient intake
- Low levels of negative acute phase proteins (serum albumin, transferrin, prealbumin)
- Increased levels of inflammation indices (serum C-reactive protein, amyloid, cytokines)
- Predialysis serum creatinine (as index of muscle mass)
- Low plasma urea or urea nitrogen appearance (as indices of protein intake)
- Low serum cholesterol
- Reduced total lymphocyte count
- Body composition changes (reduction of BMI, skinfold thickness, arm muscle circumference, lean body mass, fat mass)
- Worsening in nutritional scores as SGA, Prognostic Nutritional Index (PNI), etc.

Hand grip strength determination and lean body mass measured by dual-energy X-ray absorptiometry (DXA) have been shown to have prognostic value in male but not in female patients.

Beginning of RRT and nutritional status

Renal replacement therapy can worsen PEM developed during the predialytic phase. Therefore the presence of PEM is a poor prognostic factor for patients beginning RRT. Both quality of life and survival are lower in patients who have:

- low protein and energy intake,
- low body weight,
- low muscle mass,
- reduced levels of serum proteins, or
- impaired immune function.

Thus it is important to maintain the nutritional status of patients with advanced renal insufficiency prior to RRT in order to prevent severe PEM from developing.

Usually RRT is started with a GFR of 5–10 ml/min. The worst prognosis shown by patients who begin RRT with PEM suggests to start dialysis at GFR >20 ml/min if there is evidence of a worsening of the nutritional status, in the absence of other concomitant causes of malnutrition and in spite of a correct nutritional intervention. In 2000, the National Kidney Foundation gave these guidelines about levels of PEM to be considered at risk:

(1) More than a 6% involuntary reduction in edema-free usual body weight or to less than 90% of standard body weight (according to NHANES II) in <six months.
(2) A reduction in serum albumin greater or equal to 0.3 g/dl and to less than 4 g/dl, in the absence of acute infection or inflammation.
(3) A worsening of SGA scoring by one category.

Medical nutrition therapy for RRT patients

The beginning of dialysis requires important dietary changes, especially about protein intake. The main guidelines are reported in Table 13.3.

Dietary prescription for hemodialysis patients
Protein intake
A frequent association has been found between PEM and low protein intake. However, exact protein requirements for hemodialysis patients are still not established (Table 13.3). Studies on nitrogen balance have not always taken into account the unmeasured nitrogen losses, the quality of the nitrogen administered, or the energy intake. The available data seem to indicate that 1–1.2 g/kg per day (at least 50% HBV) are adequate to maintain a neutral nitrogen balance in most patients. ESPEN Guidelines recommend a protein intake of 1.2–1.4 g/kg ideal body weight per day (50% HBV). K/DOQI Guidelines suggest an intake of 1.2 g/kg per day (at least 50% HBV) with higher intakes up to 1.3 g/kg per day, in acutely ill patients. If the protein intake is lower than 1.2 g/kg per day the risk of developing PEM increases and the nutritional status should be closely monitored. If PEM develops,

Table 13.3 Guidelines for dietary treatment of patients with chronic renal failure on dialysis treatment

	ESPEN (Toigo G. *et al.*, 2000)	K/DOQI Guidelines (2000)	Kopple *et al.* (2004)
Hemodialysis			
Energy, kcal/kg body weight per day	35 or more in undernourished patients	35 30–35 (if age >60 years)	35 30–35 (if age >60 years)
Protein, g/kg body weight/day	1.2–1.4 (50% HBV)	1.2 (≥50% HBV)	1.2 (≥50% HBV) 1.3 in patients with acute illness
Peritoneal dialysis			
Energy, kcal/kg per day including energy from dialysate	30–35 adapted if patients over- or underweight	35	35
Protein, g/kg per day	1.2–1.5 (or more if peritonitis occurs)	1.2–1.3 (≥50% HBV)	1.2–1.3 (≥50% HBV)

HBV, high biological value.

dietary counseling should be increased and/or nutritional support initiated.

Energy intake

The energy intake for patients with a normal BMI should be 30–35 kcal/kg per day in relation to the level of daily activities. According to the K/DOQI, from the age of 60 years it should kept in the lower range. The presence of hypertriglyceridemia may require a reduction in the energy intake from carbohydrate and a higher fat intake (up to 35–40% of total energy) with limitations of simple sugars. As for patients with CRF the indications from the Third Report of the National Cholesterol Education Program (NCPE) Expert Panel may need to be applied to control the cardiovascular risk (http://www.nhlbi.nih.gov/guidelines/cholesterol/index.htm).

Fluid, electrolyte, and vitamin intake

Fluid volume should be restricted to 500–800 ml/day (including the water in foods) plus an amount equal to the residual diuresis. Sodium intake should be limited to 60–100 mEq/day. While there is still some residual renal function potassium intake needs to be only moderately restricted. Attention should be paid to factors that might lead to a high serum potassium level (hyperkalemia) such as excessive intake, use of certain drugs (e.g. non-steroidal anti-inflammatory drugs (NSAIDs) and angiotensin-converting enzyme (ACE) inhibitors), metabolic acidosis, or catabolic stress. Generally dietary potassium should be kept around 60–70 mEq/day or <1 mEq/kg per day with high predialysis plasma levels (>6 mEq/l).

High potassium foods include many fruits and vegetables, including potatoes, and of course salt substitute containing potassium chloride. Potassium content in vegetables can be reduced by boiling them in plenty of water which should be discarded after cooking. Phosphate intake needs to be kept low (8–17 mg/kg ideal body weight). Further restriction of phosphorus intake is not feasible because of the higher protein requirements of these patients (foods rich in proteins are also rich in phosphate). Even with this level of phosphate restriction, phosphate binders are usually necessary. With the use of calcium-containing phosphate binders, dietary calcium intake should be maintained below 1 g/day and a dialysate with a lower calcium content may be necessary. With the use of phosphate binders without calcium, calcium intake needs to be around 1200–1600 mg/day. Calcium and phosphate levels require careful and frequent monitoring.

Hemodialysis causes loss of water-soluble vitamins. Vitamins C and B_6 and folic acid should be supplemented to reach a total intake of 60–90 mg, 10 mg, and 1 mg or more/daily respectively.

Carnitine

In addition, in dialysis patients, plasma carnitine is often low. Carnitine is necessary for fatty acid transport to the sites of beta-oxidation within the mitochondria. Therefore a role for carnitine deficiency in the pathogenesis of dyslipidemia has been hypothesized. The results of carnitine supplementation on lipid pattern of patients with CRF are not univocal. However, some recent studies have found a positive effect of carnitine supplementation on oxidative metabolism during exercise, and improvement of muscle weakness and quality of life. Recommended dosages are 10–20 mg/kg given i.v. at the end of each dialysis, three times a week or 0.5 g/kg per day per os. The bioavailability by the oral route however may be inadequate.

Dietary prescription for CAPD patients

The dietary regimens for CAPD patients are somewhat different from those prescribed to hemodialysis patients.

Protein intake

Protein intake should be 1.2–1.5 g/kg per day, at least 50% of high biological value (HBV), according to the nutritional status and to the amount of proteins lost in the dialysate. An additional 0.1–0.2 g/kg per day may need to be prescribed if peritoneal inflammation occurs. According the NKF K-DOQI indications, daily protein intake should be at least 1.2 g/kg body weight to ensure that the supply is adequate in most subjects.

Energy intake

The glucose absorption from the dialysate fluid must be taken into account. The total energy requirement, as in hemodialysis patients, is 35 kcal/kg per day, including the energy absorbed from the dialysate. Glucose absorption can be in the order of 100–200 g/day. This is one of the causal factors of the severe hypertriglyceridemia that is often present in these patients. In these cases fat supply can be increased to 35–40% of total energy intake while simple sugars should be restricted. A less hypertonic dialysate may need to be used in obese patients.

Fluid, electrolyte, and vitamin intake

Indications are similar to those for hemodialysis patients. Pyridoxine and vitamin C supplements are recommended.

Nutritional support in RRT patients

See also Chapter 8. Nutritional support should be considered for those who are underweight or have increased metabolic needs (infections, operations, etc.). Oral supplements, enteral nutrition, or parenteral nutrient administration can be used.

Dietary supplements might be an easy way of increasing the nutrient intake. However, even though their usefulness has been assessed with retrospective studies, no randomized studies have been conducted to confirm their clinical efficacy.

Special nutritional supplements, specifically designed for patients with CRF, either on conservative treatment or on dialysis, are commercially available and can be an optimal source of energy or protein. However, the cost of such supplements is not always covered by the health system, and patients often complain about the low palatability of the products.

Parenteral administration of concentrated nutrients may be necessary in dialysis patients who are unable to receive a complete oral or enteral nutrition. Guidelines for the provision of TPN to chronically uremic dialyzed patients have been recently published by the American Society for Enteral and Parenteral Nutrition (ASPEN). Energy and nitrogen intake are calculated based on the degree of hypercatabolism and nutritional status. Fluid volume needs to be limited and adjusted on the fluid loss during dialysis. Fat intake should be around 20–30% of total energy. Plasma concentrations of electrolytes, (especially potassium, phosphorus, and calcium) should be monitored carefully and adjusted accordingly. Water-soluble vitamins may be lost during the dialysis sessions and should be measured if possible and supplemented. Several lipid-soluble vitamins require specific consideration (risk of accumulation of vitamin A, need of long-term supplementation of vitamin D, weekly administration of vitamin K).

In hemodialysis patients, beside TPN, nutrients can be supplied by intradialytic parenteral nutrition (IDPN). Indications for this treatment include, beside inadequate nutrient intake and a body weight <90% of normal, a progressive weight loss and serum albumin levels <3.4 g/dl. Since IDPN is administered during the hemodialysis session, the nutrients can only be provided for 3–4 h, three times a week. Fifty grams of amino acid and 1000 kcal (50–60% glucose) or more can be infused during a single session and are generally well tolerated, provided that fluid overload, hyperglycemia, and hyperlipidemia are prevented by appropriate ultrafiltration and metabolic monitoring. This amount of nitrogen and energy is clearly not providing full nutritional requirements and must only be used as a supplement to oral and/or enteral nutrition. Improvements in nutritional status, immunocompetence, and survival have been described in controlled and non-controlled studies, and in retrospective reviews. However long-term, well-conducted studies do not currently exist.

In CAPD patients feeding can be supported by intraperitoneal nutrition. The intraperitoneal infusion of amino acids was tested in the early 1980s, but results were disappointing. New solutions are now available (1.1%, amino acid formula, 40 mmol/l lactate), and good results have been reported with an improved nitrogen balance and protein plasma levels. The treatment with intraperitoneal amino acid solutions seems to be a very promising nutritional treatment. In the future new studies are needed to better identify the patients who may benefit most from these interventions.

13.7 Transplantation

Renal transplantation largely or partially restores renal function, and the dietary restrictions imposed on patients during the dialysis period are no longer needed. Nevertheless, uremic patients both immediately before and after surgery need to be followed carefully from the nutritional point of view. Indications about the nutritional management of these patients are reported in Table 13.4.

Pretransplant nutritional management

In the pretransplant period it is very important to screen patients in order to identify risk factors that may reduce survival or the chances of a successful transplant. In particular, diabetics, obese, and elderly patients should be adequately assessed and monitored. Severe malnutrition should be corrected if necessary

Table 13.4 Guidelines for dietary treatment of renal transplanted patients

	ESPEN (Toigo *et al.*, 2000)	ASPEN (2002)
Pretransplant		
Energy and protein intake	To correct malnutrition	
Early post-transplant		
Energy, kcal/kg per day	30–35	35[a]
Protein, g/kg per day	1.3–1.5	1.5–2[b]
Late post-transplant		
Energy, kcal/kg per day	To maintain ideal body weight	
Protein, g/kg per day	1.0	

[a]Requirements may transiently increase as a result of sepsis or acute rejection.
[b]Protein requirement may decrease to 1 g/kg per day, as the dose of corticosteroids is reduced to maintenance level.

by nutritional support. Particular attention should be paid to the treatment of hypertension and dyslipidemia. In diabetic patients the glycemic control must be optimal, and patients must be motivated to stop smoking. Control of energy intake may be encouraged in obese patients.

Bone metabolism, which may be rapidly impaired by post-transplant steroid therapy, should be assessed by bone mineral density (DXA) and by measuring the levels of calcemia, phosphorus, and PTH levels. A schedule of regular physical exercise should be prescribed to improve glucose and lipid metabolism, blood pressure, and bone density.

Early post-transplant nutritional management

This is the most delicate phase for the prognosis both of the patient and of the transplanted kidney. Although surgery usually produces a mild degree of trauma, a state of severe PEM may develop as a result of the presence of a previously impaired nutritional state and/or of steroid therapy. For this reason nutritional status of the transplanted patient needs to be carefully monitored. Generally it is not necessary to start artificial nutrition, as bowel function resumes rapidly and patients can feed themselves spontaneously orally. Development of Cushing syndrome can be slowed by a hyperproteic diet. Despite the fact that renal function is rapidly restored, correction of pre-existing malnutrition is very slow. Three months after the transplant the muscle still shows the typical alterations of uremia, and, after one year, the electrolyte and protein metabolism changes typical of chronic uremia are still present. Only after some years does muscle metabolism seem to become normalized.

Energy intake at this stage should be in the range of 30–35 kcal/kg per day and should be adjusted for the malnourished or obese patient. Protein intake should be moderately high due to the hypercatabolism seen post surgery and therefore 1.3–1.5 g protein/kg ideal body weight per day or more in highly catabolic patients are generally required.

The frequent development of diabetes mellitus after renal transplant is mainly due to the use of steroid therapy, and appropriate dietary measures may be necessary (see Chapter 12). Often diabetes or impaired glucose tolerance resolve within one year from the renal transplant.

Due to the frequent low phosphorus plasma levels, normal to high phosphate dietary intake is allowed in the early post-transplant phase. Attention should also be paid to the low levels of magnesium induced by some medications such as the cyclosporins.

Late post-transplant nutritional management

During this period renal function stabilizes and protein metabolism becomes normalized. However, the patient can remain hypercatabolic especially if the treatment with corticosteroids continues. At this stage a protein intake within normal limits is usually recommended (1 g/kg per day). Energy intake should be tailored to the patient's age and level of physical activity in order to maintain an ideal body weight.

The most frequent metabolic problem in this phase is hyperlipidemia, characterized above all by increased LDL cholesterol. This depends on multiple causes, such as renal insufficiency proteinuria, overweight, type of diet, lack of physical activity, and use of immunosuppressive therapy. The dietary recommendations of the National Cholesterol Education Program and an increase in physical activity may be an adequate approach.

Beside modification of dietary fat and weight reduction, the intake of *n*-3-rich fish oil is effective in reducing high lipid concentration in transplanted patients as much as simvastatine.

13.8 Future perspectives

There is need to further improve screening and assessment tools of nutritional status for early identification of PEM and to predict outcome. The goals of MNT will focus on retarding the progression of kidney disease, improve PEM, reduce the morbidity and mortality of cardiovascular disease and of kidney failure. New therapeutic approaches must be tested but offer new possibilities in the care process of kidney patients. Features that require further investigations are the role of lipids (quantity and quality) on kidney failure progression and the possible effects of dietary fatty acid manipulations on inflammation and immune responses. The relation between hyperhomocysteinemia and intake of folate and vitamins B_{12} and B_6 on the control of cardiovascular disease also needs further clinically controlled studies. The studies on the effects on the nutritional status of anabolic or antinflammatory agents have already shown promising results.

Anabolic agents

To treat patients with ongoing catabolism in spite of apparently adequate MNT, a number of anabolic agents have been tested. Recombinant human growth hormone (rhGH) is a well-established therapy for chronically uremic children with growth retardation, and the side effects of its administration are limited. rhGH has also been proposed for improving protein metabolism in malnourished patients: faster amino acid transport, stimulation of protein synthesis, and inhibition of amino acid oxidation have been described. However, the possible positive effects of rhGH in adult uremic patients treated with hemodialysis or peritoneal dialysis have not yet been definitively demonstrated and are under investigation.

In hemodialysis patients the administration of rhGH was associated with a better nitrogen balance. Similarly in CAPD patients rhGH administration caused a sustained anabolic response, as suggested by decreased blood urea nitrogen and urea nitrogen appearance, as well as by increased plasma concentration of arginine, histidine, lysine, threonine, tryptophan, and valine. In hemodialysis administration of rhGH determined an increase in muscle protein synthesis without affecting muscle catabolism. However, in non-uremic acutely ill patients treated with rhGH an increased mortality rate has been described. This was possibly caused by a growth hormone-mediated decrease in glutamine availability for protein synthesis in tissues with rapidly dividing cell turnover. For these reasons the supplementation of GH in acutely ill uremic patients is at the moment not recommended.

Results found in hemodialysis patients on bone collagen metabolism and mineral content after long-term treatment with rhGH are not univocal. Resistance to GH and to IGF-1 administration is present in uremic patients with uncorrected acidosis. Disturbed expression of hepatic GH receptor and IGF-1 genes, as well as increased synthesis of IGF-binding proteins, might be related to the GH and IGF-1 resistance in chronic uremia. In CAPD patients the protein metabolism was improved by the administration of large doses of rhIGF-1.

A positive effect of nandrolone decanoate on fat-free mass and functional status of male adult patients receiving hemodialysis has been recently described. Low-dose administration of megestrole acetate in chronically uremic patients induced an increase of dry weight and of plasma albumin concentration, probably related to increased nutrient intake: however, a close monitoring of potentially severe side effects has been recommended.

Anti-inflammatory and antioxidant agents

In patients with inflammation associated with high C-reactive protein levels and low albumin serum concentration, nutritional interventions are less efficient. In these cases treatment of inflammation may lead to improvement of nutritional status and prevent complications. Antibiotics are of course needed in the presence of infections. Other means to control inflammation are increased intake of antioxidants such as vitamin E. Vitamin E-coated hemodialysis membranes have been shown to ameliorate endothelial function and to influence mononuclear cell apoptosis and neutrophil activation and LDL oxidation. Hemolipodialysis is a special technique of vitamin E and C administration in the dialysate. Vitamin E is added in liposomes which are particles big enough not to cross the dialysis membranes. Treatment with statins, beside lowering CRP levels, had positive effects on the nutritional status of hemodialysis patients.

References and further reading

ASPEN Board of Directors and the Clinical Guidelines Task Force. Guidelines for the use of parenteral and enteral nutrition in adult and pediatric patients. *JPEN J Parenter Enteral Nutr* 2002; 26(1 Suppl): 74–76SA.

Beto JA, Bansal VK. Medical nutrition therapy in chronic kidney failure: Integrating clinical practice guidelines. *J Am Diet Assoc* 2004; 104: 404–409.

Bosutti A, Barazzoni R, Savoldi S *et al*. Interleukin-10 genotype and gene expression affect the severity of inflammatory state in haemodialysis patients. *Clin Nutr* 2003; 22(Suppl 1): S39.

Cianciaruso B, Brunori G, Kopple JD *et al*. Cross-sectional comparison of malnutrition in continuous ambulatory peritoneal dialysis and hemodialysis patients. *Am J Kidney Dis* 1995; 26: 475–486.

Fedorak RN, Madsen KL. Probiotics and prebiotics in gastrointestinal disorders. *Curr Opin Gastroenterol.* 2004; 20: 146–155.

Guarnieri G, Toigo G, Situlin R, Carraro M, Tamaro G. The assessment of nutritional status in chronically uremic patients. *Contrib Nephrol* 1989a; 72: 73–103.

Guarnieri GF, Toigo G, Situlin R *et al*. Nutritional state in patients on long-term low-protein diet or with nephrotic syndrome. *Kidney Int* 1989b; 36: S195–S200.

Guarnieri G, Toigo G, Fiotti N *et al*. Mechanisms of malnutrition in uremia. *Kidney Int* 1997; 52(S62): 41–44.

Guarnieri G, Situlin R, Biolo G. Carnitine metabolism in uremia. *Am J Kidney Dis* 2001; 38(Suppl 1): S63–67.

Guarnieri G, Antonione R, Biolo G. Mechanisms of malnutrition in uremia. *J Ren Nutr* 2003; 13: 153–157.

Heimburger O, Qureshi AR, Blaner WS, Berglund L, Stenvinkel P. Hand-grip muscle strength, lean body mass, and plasma proteins as markers of nutritional status in patients with chronic renal failure close to start of dialysis therapy. *Am J Kidney Dis* 2000; 36: 1213–1225.

Kalantar-Zadeh K, Ikizler TA, Block G, Avram MM, Kopple JD. Malnutrition-inflammation complex syndrome in dialysis patients: causes and consequences. *Am J Kidney Dis* 2003; 42: 864–881.

Kopple JD. Massry SG. *Kopple and Massry's Nutritional Management of Renal Disease*, pp. 379–414. Philadelphia: Lippincott, Williams & Wilkins, 2004.

Kumar P, Clark M, editors. *Clinical Medicine*. Renal Disease, pp519–95. Edinburgh: Saunders, 1998.

Modification of Diet in Renal Disease Study Group. Short term effects of protein intake, blood pressure, and antihypertensive therapy on glomerular filtration rate in the Modification of Diet in Renal Disease Study. *J Am Soc Nephrol* 1996; 7: 2097–2109.

Nathens AB, Curtis JR, Beale RJ *et al*. Management of the critically ill patient with severe acute pancreatitis. *Crit Care Med.* 2004 ;32: 2524–2536.

National Kidney Foundation K/DOQI, Clinical practice guidelines for nutrition in chronic renal failure. *Am J Kidney Dis* 2000; 35(Suppl. 2): S1–S140

National Kidney Foundation K/DOQI, Clinical practice guidelines for chronic kidney disease: evaluation, classification, and stratification. *Am J Kidney Dis* 2002; 39(Suppl 1): S17–S31.

Qureshi AR, Alvestrand A, Danielsson A *et al*. Factors predicting malnutrition in hemodialysis patients: a cross-sectional study. *Kidney Int* 1998; 53: 773–782.

Toigo G, Aparicio M, Attman P *et al*. Consensus Report: Part 1. Expert working group report on nutrition in adult patients with renal insufficiency. *Clin Nutr* 2000; 19: 197–207.

Toigo G, Aparicio M, Attman P *et al*. Consensus Report: Part 2. Expert working group report on nutrition in adult patients with renal insufficiency. *Clin Nutr* 2000; 19: 281–291.

Young GA, Kopple JD, Lindholm B *et al*. Nutritional assessment of continuous ambulatory peritoneal dialysis patients: an international study. *Am J Kidney Dis* 1991; 17: 462–471.

14
Nutritional and Metabolic Support in Hematologic Malignancies and Hematopoietic Stem Cell Transplantation

Maurizio Muscaritoli, Gabriella Grieco, Zaira Aversa, and Filippo Rossi Fanelli

Key messages

- Patients with hematologic malignances are at increased risk of malnutrition so it is important that all patients are nutritionally assessed and receive nutritional counseling at diagnosis, and during the course of treatment.
- To prevent the negative impact on nutritional status of high-dose radio- and chemotherapy, artificial nutrition is frequently indicated in hematologic malignancy.
- Mucositis of the gastrointestinal tract represents the main indication for artificial nutrition in hematologic malignancy.

- Hematopoietic stem cell transplantation (HSCT) may negatively affect oral food intake and nutrient absorption and increase nutrient and energy needs. Nutritional and metabolic intervention should be considered as an integral part of supportive care of HSCT patients.
- Parenteral nutrition (PN) still represents the main tool to provide nutritional support to patients undergoing HSCT. Enteral nutrition should be attempted as soon as gastrointestinal impairment resolves.

14.1 Introduction

The impact of hematologic malignancies on nutritional status is extremely variable, and is essentially a function of disease- and treatment-related impairment in nutrient absorption, nutrient losses, and altered energy and protein metabolism. Until recently, however, little attention has been drawn to the nutritional implications of hematologic malignancies. Unlike solid tumors, which have a dramatic impact on a person's metabolic homeostasis and nutritional status, hematologic malignancies are, at least initially, rarely associated with a significant deterioration of nutritional status. The advent of aggressive antineoplastic regimens involving the use of high-dose combination chemotherapy, followed or not by hematopoietic stem cell transplantation (HSCT) in order to achieve high disease remission rate and longer disease-free survival, has disclosed a new scenario where nutritional and metabolic impairment occur as a consequence not of the underlying disease, but rather of the deleterious side effects of antineoplastic treatments. Therefore, patients initially well nourished (as most hematologic patients are), may acutely become at risk of malnutrition or overtly malnourished, making nutritional intervention necessary (Table 14.1).

The novelty of this clinical problem reflects in the lack of precise guidelines for the appropriate nutritional approach to patients with hematologic diseases. This chapter will mainly focus on the nutritional sequelae of the therapeutic regimens for hematologic diseases, including HSCT.

14.2 Hematologic malignancies

Hematologic malignancies represent a heterogeneous group of diseases, including leukemia and other myeloproliferative disorders and lymphomas.

Table 14.1 Disease-dependent and treatment-dependent nutritional risks in hematologic malignancies

Diseases	Disease-dependent nutritional risks	Treatment-dependent nutritional risks
Myelodisplastic syndromes		✓
Acute myeloid leukemia		✓
Chronic myeloid leukemia	✓	✓
Acute lymphocytic leukemia		✓
Chronic lymphocitic leukemia		✓
Hodgkin's lymphoma	✓	✓
Non-Hodgkin's lymphoma	✓[a]	✓

[a]Weight loss is more frequent in high-grade lymphomas.

Myeloproliferative disorders

Myeloproliferative disorders are caused by acquired clonal abnormalities of the hematopoietic stem cells. They produce characteristic syndromes with well-defined clinical features including polycythemia vera, essential thrombocytemia, myelofibrosis, myelodysplastic syndromes, and leukemias. Although progress has been made in the management of these conditions, most patients fail to respond or relapse after an initial response to therapy.

Nutritional intervention is most frequently indicated for patients with myelodysplastic syndromes and leukemias.

Myelodysplastic syndrome (MDS)

MDS is characterized clinically by a hyperproliferative bone marrow, reflective of ineffective hematopoiesis, and is accompanied by one or more peripheral blood cytopenias. Bone marrow failure results, leading to death from bleeding and infection in the majority, while transformation to acute leukemia occurs in up to 40% of patients. Besides transfusions and hormonal therapy (androgens, danazol), chemotherapeutic agents including fludarabine and cytosine arabinoside are employed, alone and in combination, in a variety of regimens ranging from attenuated low-dose schedules to the more conventional antileukemic myelotoxic type strategies. The use of high-dose chemotherapy followed by either bone marrow or peripheral blood stem cell (PBSC) infusion has been utilized in a limited fashion.

Acute myeloid leukemia

Acute myeloid leukemia (AML) is the most common variant of acute leukemia occurring in adults, comprising approximately 80–85% of cases of acute leukemia diagnosed in individuals over 20 years of age. Currently, more than 80% of young adults and 60% of all patients can achieve complete remission. The French-American-British (FAB) morphologic classification names the AML according to the normal marrow elements that they most closely resemble (M0–M7 and hybrid leukemias).

Most patients with AML present with anemia, thrombocytopenia, and leukocytosis (median white blood cell count 10 000–20 000/μl). Patients with AML generally present initially with symptoms related to complications of pancytopenia, including weakness, easy fatigability, infections of variable severity, or hemorrhagic findings such as gingival bleeding, ecchymoses, epistaxis, or menorrhagia. Combinations of these symptoms are common. Although increased resting energy expenditure has been described in pediatric and adult patients with AML, nutritional status is usually good upon diagnosis. Protein turnover is also increased.

Changes in plasma free amino acid concentration have been described in AML that only partially resemble those observed in solid tumors. In a study performed in 40 AML patients upon diagnosis, a significant increase in glutamic acid, ornithine, free tryptophan, and glycine plasma concentrations was reported, while serine, methionine, and taurine were significantly reduced with respect to control subjects. When patients were stratified according to their response to chemotherapy and their status at 18 months after chemotherapy, it was shown that taurine and its precursor serine and methionine tended to be even lower in patients who had not responded to or had relapsed after high-dose chemotherapy. Thus, it would appear that taurine deficiency may have some relevance in the clinical outcome of AML, since it has been previously demonstrated that taurine is the most abundant intracellular free amino acid in AML, and that its plasma concentrations drop after chemotherapy, while its intracellular content correlates to the chemosensitivity of a leukemia cell line.

The therapy of AML has traditionally been divided into stages: induction, postremission therapy of varying intensity and duration, and postrelapse therapy.

- Induction therapy is designed to produce rapid clearing of leukemic cells from the peripheral blood with subsequent marrow aplasia, and is achieved with combined therapy including daunorubicin and ara-C, causing severe mucosal damage.
- Postremission therapy is based on high-dose cytarabine and daunorubicin chemotherapy; both allogeneic and autologous HSCT have been advocated for selected patients in first remission.
- Relapsed and refractory AML are usually treated with single drug or combining chemotherapy. A transient reduction of energy expenditure may be induced by chemotherapy. However, fever, immunosuppression, and consequent opportunistic infections may again increase metabolic rate and protein wasting, particularly in the neutropenic period.

Chronic myeloid leukemia

Chronic myeloid leukemia (CML) is a clonal myeloproliferative disorder of a pluripotent stem cell with a specific cytogenetic abnormality, the Philadelphia (Ph) chromosome, involving myeloid, erythroid, megakaryocytic, B lymphoid cells, and sometimes T lymphoid cells, but not the marrow fibroblasts. The first phase of the disease, the chronic phase, terminates in a second, more acute or abrupt course, called the blast phase. Symptoms and signs usually develop insidiously and include fatigue, anemia, progressive splenomegaly, and leukocytosis. In the chronic phase, the white blood cell count approximates 2 000 000/μl. The myeloid cells in the peripheral blood show all stages of differentiation, but the myelocyte predominates. Therapeutic options include recombinant interferon-gamma (rIFN-γ) combined with chemotherapy.

Acute lymphocytic leukemia (ALL)

Acute lymphocytic leukemia (ALL) comprises 80% of the acute leukemias of childhood. The peak incidence is between three and seven years of age. It also occurs in adults, causing approximately 20% of acute adult leukemias. Adults with ALL are treated with combination chemotherapy including daunorubicin, vincristine, prednisone, and asparaginase. This treatment produces complete remission in 80–90% of patients. After complete remission, central nervous system prophylaxis is performed. High-dose chemotherapy plus bone marrow transplantation represent an alternative therapeutic option.

Postremission consolidation is achieved with variably myelosuppressive doses of cytarabine and other chemotherapeutic agents in varied combinations, while no standard approach has been devised for relapsed or refractory ALL.

Allogeneic HSCT (the transfer of marrow from a donor to another person) can cure a considerable fraction of patients with ALL in relapse or in second or subsequent remission. Autologous HSCT (the use of the patient's own marrow) can also be of some benefit in children who have relapsed. Although HSCT can be recommended for patients who have relapsed, the benefits of transplantation for patients in first remission are controversial.

Chronic lymphocytic leukemia (CLL)

Chronic lymphocytic leukemia (CLL) is characterized by a progressive accumulation of monoclonal B lymphocytes. During the initial asymptomatic phase, the patients are able to maintain their usual lifestyle, but during the terminal phase, the performance status is poor, with recurring need for hospitalization. The most frequent causes of death are severe systemic infections (especially pneumonia and septicemia), bleeding, and malnutrition with cachexia.

Most cases of early CLL require no specific therapy. Standard treatment with chlorambucil is well tolerated and usually effective, and does not cause any nutritional impairment.

Lymphoproliferative disorders

The malignant lymphomas are neoplastic transformations of cells that reside predominantly within lymphoid tissues. Although Hodgkin's and non-Hodgkin's lymphomas (NHLs) are among the most sensitive malignant neoplasms to radiation and cytotoxic therapy, their response rates are markedly different (nearly 75% for Hodgkin's lymphomas and 35% for NHLs).

Hodgkin's lymphoma

Hodgkin disease is a group of lymphoproliferative disorders characterized by the pathognomonic finding of

Reed–Sternberg cells, with varying degrees of normal reactive and inflammatory cells and fibrosis within involved lymph nodes.

The disease has a bimodal age distribution with one peak in the 20s and a second over age 50. Presenting symptoms include fever, weight loss, night sweats, generalized pruritus, and the occurrence of a painless mass, generally in the neck. Patients with stage I–II Hodgkin's disease with favorable prognostic factors are candidates for radiotherapy alone or for modified radiotherapy and chemotherapy. Patients with unfavorable prognostic factors should receive chemotherapy (adriamycin, bleomycin, vincristin, and daunorubicin; ABVD) and radiotherapy as initial treatment. ABVD is also the treatment of choice in advanced disease. For patients who fail to achieve remission with primary chemotherapy the best therapeutic option is autologous bone marrow transplantation. Allogeneic bone marrow transplantation has been performed in patients with relapsed Hodgkin's disease, with disappointing results.

Non-Hodgkin's lymphoma

Non-Hodgkin's lymphomas are a heterogeneous group of neoplasms of lymphocytes. The pathogenesis of these disorders has been widely clarified with the aid of molecular biology. Although classification of the lymphoma is a controversial area in continuous evolution, lymphoma classification schemas are mainly based on lymph node architecture, cytologic classification of the neoplastic cells, and on lymphoid cell immunophenotype.

Unlike patients with Hodgkin's disease, who present with weight loss, fever, or night sweats, patients with NHL generally do not present with systemic complaints, but mainly with painless peripheral lymphadenopathy.

The appropriate therapeutic regimen is strictly dependent upon the histology and extent of disease. The patient's age and the presence of comorbid diseases also influence the treatment choice. Patients with early-stage NHL usually undergo either involved field irradiation, extended field irradiation, with a limited number receiving total lymphoid irradiation, while those with advanced-stage NHL are treated by systemic both single-agent and combination chemotherapy, although fractionated total body irradiation (TBI) also provides up to 85% complete remission rate in some cases of stage III/IV disease. High-dose therapy and

autologous HSCT are employed for patients evolving into a more aggressive histology.

Early-stage aggressive NHL is treated with involved field radiation therapy followed by adjuvant chemotherapy, while aggressive first and second generation combination chemotherapy is highly effective in advanced-stage aggressive NHL.

The treatment of high-grade lymphomas (such as lymphoblastic, Burkitt's, and Burkitt's-like lymphomas) involve the use of high-dose combined chemotherapy regimens. Disease relapse is treated by supralethal doses of chemotherapy, often in combination with radiation therapy, syngeneic, allogeneic, or autologous stem cell transplantation in order to circumvent myelosuppression.

14.3 Rationale for nutritional intervention in hematologic malignancies

As stated previously, patients with hematologic malignancies should be considered at high risk of developing malnutrition despite their good initial nutritional status. In fact, nutritional impairment in this heterogeneous group of clinical conditions is essentially a consequence of therapeutic intervention, i.e. radiotherapy, chemotherapy, and HSCT. The rationale for nutritional and metabolic support in hematologic malignancies is illustrated in Figure 14.1.

Mucositis of the gastrointestinal tract

This condition represents one of the main indications for artificial nutrition in patients undergoing chemotherapy for hematologic malignancies. The rapidly proliferating cells of the oropharyngeal and gastrointestinal mucosa are particularly vulnerable to the cytotoxic effects of both chemotherapy and radiotherapy (Figure 14.2). Combined aggressive chemotherapy favors serious gut impairment enhanced by concomitant myelosuppression, particularly if methotrexate is used. Within 7–10 days following remission-induction regimens, patients almost invariably develop oro-esophageal mucositis and gastrointestinal impairment. These two conditions may cause decreased oral intake, nausea, vomiting, diarrhea, decreased nutrient absorption, and loss of nutrients from the gut (especially amino acids) secondary to the altered transmembrane transport of nutrients.

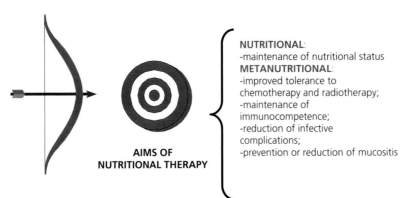

Figure 14.1 Rational for nutritional therapy.

CHEMOTHERAPY

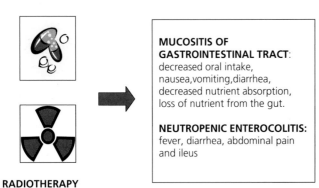

RADIOTHERAPY

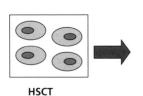

HSCT

Figure 14.2 Treatment-related nutritional problems.

Although both the severity and duration of gastrointestinal impairment may greatly differ among individuals, food intake and absorption are significantly reduced for up to 2–3 weeks following chemotherapy or radiotherapy initiation. Diarrhea is common after TBI or bowel irradiation or after chemotherapy administration with cisplatin, carboplatin, and other chemotherapy agents. Adequate hydration must be maintained and antiemetics that do not have diarrhea as a side effect may be indicated. Mild diarrhea is controlled with opioid drugs such as loperamide and diphenoxylate atropine and by lowering the fiber content of food.

When immunosuppression is present, infectious pathogenesis should also be considered. Neutropenic enterocolitis is a serious complication of chemotherapeutic regimens administered in the treatment of both acute leukemias and lymphomas (Figure 14.2). This acute inflammatory disease may involve the terminal part of the ileum, cecum, and colon. Although the precise etiology of this seldom fatal condition is still unknown, neutropenia, infections, and drug-induced alterations of the bowel mucosal surface have been proposed to have a role. Ileotyphlitis is a life-threatening complication of neutropenic enterocolitis frequently occurring in neutropenic patients receiving high-dose idarubicin-containing chemotherapy. Its clinical picture is characterized by fever, diarrhea, abdominal pain, and ileus.

The diagnosis of ileotyphlitis may be delayed because the presenting clinical features (fever, diarrhea, and/or abdominal pain) are not specific and may suggest other abdominal diseases, such as chemotherapy-induced mucositis, antibiotic-related colitis, cytomegalovirus colitis, *Salmonella* spp. gastroenteritis, or cryptosporidiosis. Computed tomography or ultrasonography of the abdomen yield characteristic findings, such as dilated bowel loops and thickening of the bowel wall >8 mm, reflecting the pathology of the disease, consisting of transmural inflammation, mucosal ulceration, wall edema, necrosis, teleangectasia, and formation of intramural hematomas.

Although most patients with ileotyphlitis undergo surgical observation, abdominal surgery has no therapeutic role in this syndrome, which is routinely treated with bowel rest achieved by total parenteral nutrition, and antibiotic therapy.

Hematopoietic stem cell transplantation

Hematopoietic stem cell transplantation (HSCT) is a therapeutic procedure consisting in the administration of high-dose chemo-radiotherapy followed by intravenous infusion of hematopoietic stem cells, aimed at restoring lymphohematopoiesis in patients with damaged or defective bone marrow, reconstituting marrow function after marrow ablating chemo- or

Box 14.1 Diseases treated by bone marrow transplantation

Hematologic malignancies
- Acute myelogenous leukemia
- Chronic myelogenous leukemia
- Acute lymphocytic leukemia
- Chronic lymphocytic leukemia
- Myeloproliferative disorders
- Multiple myeloma
- Non-Hodgkin's lymphoma
- Hodgkin's disease

Solid tumors
- Breast cancer
- Testicular cancer
- Ovarian cancer
- Glioma
- Neuroblastoma
- Small cell lung cancer
- Non-small cell lung cancer

Other pathologic conditions
- Severe aplastic anemia
- Beta-thalassemia
- Severe combined immunodeficiency
- Autoimmune disorders
- Amyloidosis
- Hereditary metabolic disorders

radiotherapy, and at treating a number of genetic and non-malignant disorders.

HSCT is a well-established therapy, administered to thousands of patients every year in the world (Box 14.1). The source of hematopoietic stem cells may be bone marrow (by BMT), peripheral blood, or umbilical cord blood. For this reason, the term bone marrow transplantation is currently being replaced by the term HSCT.

Types of HSCT
At present, two types of HSCT can be performed: allogeneic HSCT (allo-HSCT) and autologous HSCT (a-HSCT). Recently, cord blood stem cells transplantation (cord blood transplantation; CBT) from both related and unrelated donors has been employed for the treatment of patients with hematologic disorders.

Allogeneic bone marrow transplantation (allo-BMT)
Allo-BMT involves the transfer of marrow from a donor to another person (the recipient). Best results are seen after BMT from HLA-genotypically matching

sibling donors, but only 30% of patients have such a donor. BMT from HLA-phenotypically identical unrelated donor or from cord blood are alternative for patients who lack a donor in the family.

After the donor has been identified, the patient has to undergo high-dose radiotherapy and/or chemotherapy in order to:

- induce immunosuppression necessary to avoid destruction of the allograft by residual, immunologically active cells of the host;
- destroy any residual cancer cells and provide space for the new marrow to grow.

Preparative (or conditioning) regimens to allo-HSCT usually consist of radiotherapy combined with alkylating agents, etoposide and cytarabine. The major advantages of an allogeneic graft include the absence of malignant cells, the potential for an immunologic anticancer effect of the graft (the graft-versus-tumor effect), and the ability to treat both malignant and non-malignant diseases. The major disadvantages of allo-HSCT include the difficulty in finding an appropriate HLA-matched donor, and the occurrence of graft-versus-host disease (GVHD).

GVHD represents a serious complication of allo-HSCT, occurring when immunocompetent cells in the graft target antigens on the cells in the recipient. It is manifested primarily by symptoms and signs involving skin, gastrointestinal system, and liver. GVHD can be divided into two distinct clinical entities: acute GVHD (a-GVHD), occurring within 1–3 months after HSCT, and chronic GVHD, occurring more than 100 days after transplantation. GVHD prophylaxis is usually accomplished by combination of immunosuppressive drugs as corticosteroids, cyclosporine, and methotrexate. Since the incidence of GVHD increases with age, allo-HSCT is largely limited to patients under 60 years old.

Autologous bone marrow transplantation

Autologous BMT (a-BMT) involves the use of the patient's own marrow to re-establish hematopoietic cell function after the administration of high-dose chemotherapy. The major advantages of autologous transplantation include the ready availability of a stem cell product and the absence of GVHD, which translate into lower morbidity, mortality, and cost. The major disadvantages of a-BMT include the potential for tumor cell contamination within the graft, with a higher risk of relapse, and the lack of a graft-versus-tumor disease.

Peripheral blood progenitor cell transplant

Peripheral blood progenitor cell transplant (PBPCT) consists of autologous or allogeneic infusion of hematopoietic stem cells collected from peripheral blood. The cells are collected after the administration of hematopoietic growth factors, associated or not with chemotherapy. Potential advantages of PBPCT over a-BMT include stem cell collection without the need for general anesthesia or repeated painful bone marrow aspirations, more rapid engraftment, particularly for platelets, and less tumor contamination. For these reasons PBPCT can be safely performed also in older patients. PBPCT has been recently proposed as a possible treatment for severe intractable autoimmune diseases such as multiple sclerosis, systemic lupus erythematosus, rheumatoid arthritis, and others.

Cord blood transplantation

Cord blood transplantation (CBT) consists of infusion of hematopoietic stem cells harvested from cordal and placental blood immediately after delivery. Umbilical cord blood cells are phenotypically different, functionally more immature and with higher proliferative potential with respect to bone marrow progenitor cells.

At present, CBT from HLA-matched, mismatched, or even unrelated donor, is performed mainly in children, but also in adults, to treat leukemia, and other hematologic diseases. The incidence and severity of GVHD appears to be less after CBT than after BMT. Patients candidate to CBT also receive conditioning regimens consisting of radio-chemotherapy; prophylaxis of GVHD is achieved with cyclosporine and corticosteroids.

Nutritional and metabolic support in HSCT

Irrespective of the type of HSCT employed, conditioning regimens have tremendous and deleterious consequences on the anatomic and functional integrity of the gastrointestinal tract (Figure 14.2). However, relevant differences exist in the impact on nutritional status exerted by autologous or allogeneic transplantation. In fact, although patients receive high-dose chemotherapy prior to BMT, peripheral stem cell utilization and the use of growth factors have significantly reduced the time to engraftment, the duration of profound neutropenia (<7 days) and, consequently, the duration of neutropenic mucositis.

Indeed, in these patients sufficient oral food intake is rather frequent, which may significantly reduce the need for parenteral nutrition, unless severe complications occur.

Conversely, allo-HSCT patients receive conditioning regimens combining high-dose chemotherapy with total body irradiation (TBI), in order to induce profound immunodepression. TBI is an extremely toxic procedure, inducing a severe and prolonged mucositis. Moreover, the occurrence of a-GVHD, as early as 10–12 days after engraftment, may represent an insult of major proportions, primarily involving the gut, with abdominal pain and severe diarrhea, for up to 20 days in patients who do not respond to immunosuppressive therapy. Chronic GVHD occurs in about 50% of long-term survivors, 3–6 months after allo-HSCT. In about 20% of patients with chronic GVHD there is no history of previous a-GVHD. The use of high-dose steroid drugs for the management of GVHD as well as of antiviral drugs used to prevent infectious complications, further contribute to the onset of malnutrition.

The main complications of HSCT and their nutritional implications are detailed below.

Acute (a-) and chronic graft-versus-host disease (GVHD)

The occurrence of a-GVHD could be regarded as a positive event, since it usually implies a graft-versus-leukemia effect. Indeed, patients developing a-GVHD have a lower incidence of leukemia and lymphoma. However, this is a major complication, which may occur from 7–10 days up to three months after allo-HSCT in 30–60% of patients. When severe a-GVHD involves the skin, large fluid and protein losses may occur. When the liver is involved, severe cholestasis occurs, as a result of small bile duct destruction. Serum bilirubin concentrations are frequently elevated, with concomitant impairment of other liver function tests. Intestinal GVHD is characterized by diarrhea with or without nausea, vomiting, and abdominal pain. Occasionally ileus occurs, resulting from the destruction of intestinal crypts. As a consequence, mild to severe gastrointestinal impairment may develop, ranging from profuse secretory mucous diarrhea with consequent severe nitrogen loss, to mucosal ulcers with possible perforations and need for emergency surgical treatment.

Hepatic GVHD-induced steatorrhea secondary to bile salt synthesis and enterohepatic circulation derangements may further worsen diarrhea. Interestingly, mucosal absorptive capacity may remain abnormal even after apparent healing of the intestinal mucosa.

Chronic GVHD also has deleterious consequences on nutritional status or normal growth if it occurs in pediatric patients. Oral (mucositis, sicca syndrome), esophageal (strictures, dysphagia), hepatic (cholestasis, hyperbilirubinemia), and intestinal involvement (mucositis, malabsorption) may impair both nutrient oral intake and intestinal nutrient absorption.

Altered metabolism

Administration of HSCT may have a dramatic impact on the recipient, affecting protein, energy, micronutrient, and vitamin metabolism. An overall decrease in body cell mass with no changes in body fat or lean body mass has been described in allo-BMT recipients, these patients showing an increase in extracellular fluid, and a significant decrease in intracellular fluid. Negative nitrogen balance is a common feature in BMT patients, as a consequence of both intestinal losses with diarrhea and the catabolic effects on skeletal muscle initially exerted by the underlying disease, then by conditioning regimens, and subsequently by the possible HSCT complications such as sepsis and GVHD. Although data on energy expenditure following HSCT or BMT are not conclusive, it is generally assumed that BMT patients have increased energy needs.

Steroid and/or cyclosporine administration or the occurrence of septic complications may negatively affect carbohydrate metabolism and induce impaired glucose tolerance. BMT per se might negatively affect pancreatic beta-cell function and induce glucose intolerance or overt diabetes.

Abnormalities in lipid metabolism are uncommon in the initial phases following BMT, while elevated serum cholesterol and triacylglycerol concentrations frequently occur in patients maintained on long-term cyclosporine therapy for chronic GVHD.

Vitamin status may be altered in BMT patients due to poor intake and malabsorption of both water- and lipid-soluble vitamins secondary to intestinal mucositis or hepatic GVHD. The use of cyclophosphamide and radiation has been reported to increase the need for antioxidant vitamins such as tocopherol and beta-carotene.

Malabsorption and increased needs for bone marrow reconstitution may induce trace element deficiency. In particular, zinc deficiency has been shown to correlate with mortality after BMT. Trace element deficiency may be prevented in some patients receiving plasma and/or blood derivative transfusions.

Veno-occlusive disease (VOD) of the liver

This is a serious and often fatal event which may complicate both a-HSCT and allo-HSCT, occurring in about 20% of cases. VOD is, however, not exclusive of HSCT patients, since it may also complicate high-dose cyclophosphamide and busulfan, without TBI. VOD is histologically characterized by narrowing and occlusion of hepatic venules and injury to hepatocytes due to the toxic effects of chemotherapy. The clinical manifestations of VOD appear within 2–4 weeks after high-dose conditioning regimens, more frequently during the phase of profound pancytopenia, before bone marrow recovery, and include right upper quadrant abdominal pain, hepatomegaly, jaundice, elevation of serum transaminase activities, often followed by oliguria, sodium and water retention and ascites, liver failure, and hepatic encephalopathy. The pathogenesis of this severe clinical picture is yet to be fully elucidated, although a possible role might be played by the obstruction of the hepatic venules by endothelial cell injury and thrombosis, the shift of albumin- and electrolyte-rich fluid to the extravascular space and the consequent reduction in renal blood flow, with activation of the renin–angiotensin axis and retention of sodium and fluid.

Assessment of nutritional status in patients receiving HSCT

Nutritional assessment and evaluation of nutritional risk is mandatory in all patients undergoing HSCT. Evaluation of nutritional status does not represent a problem prior to HSCT, particularly in hematologic patients, but the evaluation of the efficacy of nutritional support on nutritional status is more difficult. In fact, immunologic indices are not of great value because of the underlying disease or the effects of chemotherapy. Biochemical indices do not accurately reflect changes in nutritional status of BMT recipients. In fact BMT patients frequently develop acute complications (sepsis, GVHD, etc.) that may influence *per se* the concentrations of plasma proteins. Anthropometric measurements may be influenced by fluid and electrolyte disturbances.

Nitrogen balance is considered the most accurate way to perform nutritional assessment in HSCT patients, since it is the direct expression of the imbalance existing between protein breakdown and synthesis. However, in the clinical setting of BMT patients, urine collection may be difficult, while vomiting and diarrhea may make calculations of nitrogen losses less accurate.

14.4 Nutritional and metabolic support following HSCT

HSCT is largely used in the treatment of both solid tumors and hematologic malignancies, including leukemia and lymphomas. The impact on nutritional status varies depending on the indication for HSCT. Hematologic patients are usually well nourished at the time of BMT, while patients with solid tumors exhibit malnutrition more frequently. Impaired nutritional status before transplantation represents a negative prognostic factor for outcome after BMT. Irrespective of nutritional status prior to BMT, it is well recognized that patients undergoing high-dose chemotherapy are at risk of developing malnutrition. Therefore, nutritional support is frequently given routinely following BMT, in order to prevent malnutrition secondary to either drug-induced side effects or increased nutritional requirements.

Energy and nutrient demands are increased because of the induced catabolic state due to the cytoreductive therapy, the presence of sepsis or, in allo-HSCT, GVHD. Optimal blood cell reconstitution is also thought to increase nutritional requirements.

In recent years, indications for parenteral nutrition have markedly decreased in favor of enteral nutrition. However, high-dose chemotherapy, followed or not by HSCT, represent a major field for parenteral nutrition utilization, mainly because of the gastrointestinal sequelae of the preparative cytoreductive chemotherapy, total body irradiation, infections, or GVHD. High-dose chemotherapy-induced gastrointestinal impairment precludes optimal nutrient intake and absorption. Nausea, vomiting, and oro-oesophageal mucositis make placement of nasogastric tubes difficult. Furthermore, the majority of patients undergoing

HSCT have a central venous catheter placed, through which parenteral nutrition can be given (via a dedicated lumen). Finally, parenteral nutrition allows more accurate modulation and provision of fluids, electrolytes, and macronutrients, which has pivotal importance, especially when complications of HSCT occur, such as a-GVHD or VOD.

HSCT patients should be assessed and monitored and nutritional support prescribed on an individual basis. This prescription may change during the course of the post-HSCT period. For all these reasons controlled trials on the effects of enteral nutrition in HSCT patients are to date still scanty.

Energy expenditure may differ between a-HSCT and allo-HSCT patients, but consensus exists that energy requirements in HSCT recipients may reach 130–150% of the predicted basal energy expenditure. Therefore, 30–35 kcal/kg body weight per day are usually administered. Lipids (long-chain triglycerides (LCT) or long- and medium-chain triglyceride (LCT/MCT) admixtures) should provide 30–40% of non-protein energy. Lipids may be particularly useful in achieving the energy target if hyperglycemia develops as a consequence of steroid treatment or infection or when fluid restriction is warranted.

Increased protein needs may be satisfied by provision of 1.4–1.5 g/kg body weight per day of a standard amino acid solution. What remains less well defined is when artificial nutrition should be started in these patients. Parenteral nutrition is often considered to be an expensive procedure and is therefore started only 'when it becomes necessary,' i.e. after severe mucositis develops, significantly affecting oral nutrient intake. This may occur variably after transplantation, depending on the underlying disease, type of HSCT, and conditioning regimen. Most of the studies performed to date aimed at evaluating the effects of parenteral nutrition on outcome of HSCT patients; many patients were allowed oral food intake. In the well-known study from Weisdorf, including both allo- and a-BMT patients, for example, parenteral nutrition was initiated prior to chemotherapy and irradiation and continued up to day 28 after BMT, with patients being allowed oral food intake. This makes the effect of parenteral nutrition hard to evaluate.

In the Department of Hematology at our institution, parenteral nutrition is routinely initiated on day +1 after allo-BMT and continued for 15–21 days according to intensity and duration of mucositis. Oral intake is not allowed during the parenteral nutrition period, in order to minimize the risk of both gut contamination from food, and diarrhea. Parenteral nutrition is not routinely administered to a-BMT patients, unless complications occur, such as prolonged mucositis. This is consistent with the evidence that the pathologic milieu as well as the impact of a-BMT and allo-BMT on nutritional status may be substantially different.

14.5 Perspectives on the future

The first evidence that prophylactic standard parenteral nutrition could significantly improve outcome of BMT patients was provided by Weisdorf, who showed that the three-year survival rate of parenteral nutrition-treated patients was improved with respect to those who did not receive any nutritional support.

Since then, artificial nutrition has rapidly moved from simple supportive care (mainly aimed at the maintenance of nutritional status) to adjunctive therapy, on the basis of the potential 'meta-nutritional' benefits deriving from a specialized nutritional intervention. Several effects not directly deriving by the maintenance or improvement of nutritional status could, at least theoretically, be obtained through an optimal specialized nutritional approach to patients undergoing BMT (Figure 14.3).

Artificial nutrition support is in fact provided following BMT, during the delicate phase of bone marrow engraftment and reconstitution; it is therefore conceivable that metabolically active substrates administered during this period may influence biologic responses such as time to and success of engraftment itself, occurrence and severity of mucositis, GVHD, VOD, thus potentially affecting the outcome of BMT patients.

It is in fact known that some nutritional substrates may interfere with certain physiologic and pathophysiologic mechanisms or otherwise protect the gastrointestinal tract from radio- and chemotherapy-induced mucosal injuries.

In this respect, lipid substrates and glutamine (GLN) would appear the more promising nutrients for optimal nutritional and metabolic support to HSCT patients.

Exogenously administered essential fatty acids have been shown to interfere with the synthesis of biological effectors of immunity and inflammation such as

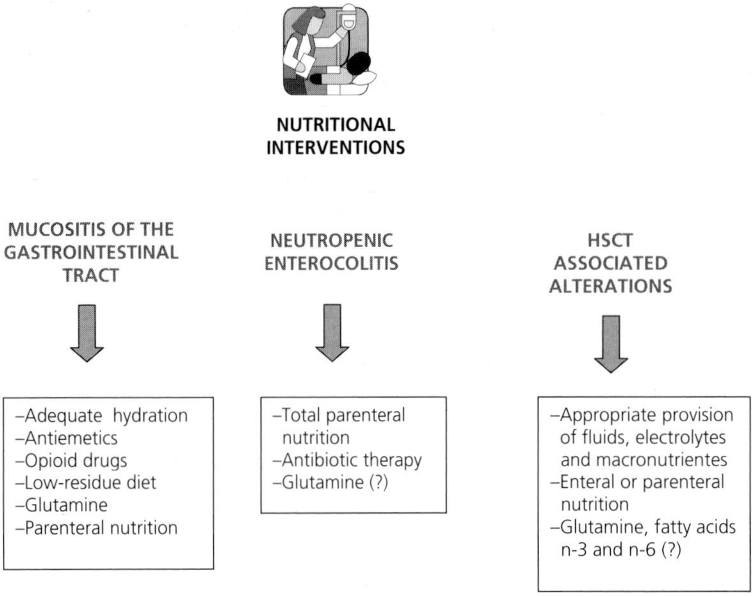

**NUTRITIONAL
INTERVENTIONS**

MUCOSITIS OF THE GASTROINTESTINAL TRACT	NEUTROPENIC ENTEROCOLITIS	HSCT ASSOCIATED ALTERATIONS

–Adequate hydration
–Antiemetics
–Opioid drugs
–Low-residue diet
–Glutamine
–Parenteral nutrition

–Total parenteral nutrition
–Antibiotic therapy
–Glutamine (?)

–Appropriate provision of fluids, electrolytes and macronutrientes
–Enteral or parenteral nutrition
–Glutamine, fatty acids n-3 and n-6 (?)

Figure 14.3 Strategy for nutritional interventions. HSCT, hematopoietic stem cell transplantation.

prostaglandins and leukotrienes, via their incorporation into cell membranes and might therefore play an additional role in affecting the outcome of HSCT patients. The provision of a lipid-based parenteral nutrition was associated with lower incidence of lethal a-GVHD in allo-BMT patients. To explain these findings it could be hypothesized that the increased availability of arachidonic acid and of its metabolite prostaglandin E2 (PGE2), secondary to exogenous long-chain n-6 triacylglycerol administration, would lead to decreased interleukin 1 (IL-1) and tumor necrosis factor (TNF) macrophage production, reduced expression of major histocompatibility complex antigens, increased T-suppressor activity, and decreased peripheral blood lymphocyte IL-2 production.

The role of fish oil-derived n-3 fatty acids in the metabolic support of HSCT is yet to be entirely explored. The ability of these lipid compounds to modulate inflammatory and immune responses could have a role in improving the outcome of BMT recipients, at least on a theoretical ground; n-3 fatty acid administration has been in fact shown to reduce vasoconstriction and platelet aggregation, and to have a profound influence on cell–cell signaling during immunologic events, by inhibiting cytokine secretion as well as lymphocyte activation and differentiation. It could therefore be hypothesized that n-3 fatty acid supplementation following HSCT might prove beneficial in the prophylaxis and management of BMT-related complications such

as GVHD and VOD. Clinical trials aimed at verifying this intriguing hypothesis are lacking.

The rationale for administering GLN-supplemented nutrition to BMT patients was initially based on the concept that GLN represents a primary fuel for the enterocytes and for gut-associated lymphoid tissue and that its administration by the enteral or parenteral route could prevent or mitigate treatment-induced gastrointestinal impairment. A number of clinical trials have been performed to evaluate the effect of GLN administration on gastrointestinal impairment in BMT, which failed to demonstrate a clear preventive or curative effect of this amino acid on intestinal mucositis. Based on the conflicting results, recent American Society for Enteral and Parenteral Nutrition (ASPEN) guidelines formally discourage the use of pharmacologic doses of GLN in HSCT patients. It should be underlined, however, that the majority of the studies evaluating the efficacy of GLN were performed in non-homogeneous patients undergoing either allo-BMT or a-BMT for solid tumors or hematologic malignancies, which renders the interpretation of these negative results rather difficult.

Further studies are warranted including homogeneous patients and evaluating possible differences exerted by the route of administration of GLN.

Glutamine administration following BMT was indeed shown to exert positive effects on nitrogen balance, incidence of infectious complications, survival, duration of hospital stay, and need for parenteral nutrition, although not in all cases. The potential for the use of GLN in the prevention or treatment of VOD deserve particular attention. Preliminary data would indeed suggest that GLN infusion during BMT preserves hepatic function. The likely mechanism of such action is the maintenance of hepatic glutathione concentrations, which would protect hepatocytes from the oxidant stress of high-dose conditioning regimens. Glutamine supplementation may have a beneficial role in hepatic protection from VOD both as prophylactic agent and as a possible treatment. Nutritional and metabolic support to patients undergoing HSCT has recently been reviewed.

Further reading

ASPEN Board of Directors and the Clinical Guidelines Task Force. Guidelines for the use of parenteral and enteral nutrition in adult and pediatric patients. *JPEN J Parenter Enteral Nutr* 2002; 26(1 Suppl): 1–138.

Coghlin Dickson TM, Wong RM, Offrin RS *et al.* Effect of oral glutamine supplementation during bone marrow transplantation. *JPEN J Parenter Enteral Nutr* 2000; 24: 61–66.

Eghbali H, Soubeyran P, Tchen N, de Mascarel I, Soubeyran I, Richaud P. Current treatment of Hodgkin's lymphoma. *Crit Rev Oncol Hematol* 2000; 35: 49–73.

Herrmann VM, Petruska PJ. Nutrition support in bone marrow transplant recipients. *Nutr Clin Pract* 1993; 8: 19–27.

Isaacson PG. The current status of lymphoma classification. *Br J Haematol* 2000; 109: 258–266.

Miller KB. Myelodysplastic syndromes. *Curr Treat Options Oncol* 2000; 1: 63–69.

Multani P, White CA, Grillo-Lopez A. Non Hodgkin's lymphoma: review of conventional treatments. *Curr Pharm Biotechnol* 2001; 2: 279–291.

Muscaritoli M, Conversano L, Petti MC *et al.* Plasma amino acid concentrations in patients with acute myelogenous leukemia. *Nutrition* 1999; 15: 195–199.

Muscaritoli M, Greco G, Capria S, Iori AP, Fanelli FR. Nutritional and metabolic support in patients undergoing bone marrow transplantation. *Am J Clin Nutr* 2002; 75: 183–190.

Passweg J, Gratwohl A, Tyndall A *et al.* Hematopoietic stem cell transplantation for autoimmune disorders. *Curr Opin Hematol* 1999; 6: 400–405.

Schulte C, Reinhardt W, Beelen D, Mann K, Schaefer U. Low T3-syndrome and nutritional status as prognostic factors in patients undergoing bone marrow transplantation. *Bone Marrow Transplant* 1998; 22: 1171–1178.

Tabbara IA, Zimmerman K, Morgan C, Nahleh Z. Allogeneic hematopoietic stem cell transplantation. Complications and results. *Arch Intern Med* 2002; 162: 1558–1566.

15
The Lung

Annemie MWJ Schols and EFM Wouters

Key messages

- Patients with chronic obstructive pulmonary disease (COPD) demonstrate classic signs of undernutrition. A low body mass, weight loss, and decrease in lean body mass have been associated with impaired functional status and increased risk of mortality.
- Compromise of nutritional status imposes major limits on respiratory function in disease, including weakened respiratory muscles, reduced ventilatory drive, and impaired immune function.
- A low body mass index and recent weight loss have been identified as important factors for the outcome of acute exacerbations of COPD including frequency of admission and time spent on mechanical ventilation.
- In the majority people with COPD, adverse consequences of weight loss, and in particular muscle wasting, are at least partly treatable by protein–energy supplementation.
- The association of cytokine-induced inflammatory markers in COPD patients suggests that interventions aimed at controlling cytokine production may be required to reverse the cachexia syndrome and improve functional status.

15.1 Introduction

Malnutrition can be caused by diseases of the respiratory system, but malnutrition can also affect the respiratory system. It causes loss of lung tissue, as well as respiratory muscle tissue, including diaphragmatic tissue. The respiratory muscles become weaker and suffer from fatigue earlier than normal muscles. In patients with borderline respiratory function this can precipitate respiratory failure or delay weaning from a ventilator. The effects of malnutrition on the respiratory system may be more subtle. For example, starvation can reduce the sensitivity of the respiratory center to hypoxic stimuli, and this too may delay weaning of patients off mechanical ventilation.

The spectrum of respiratory diseases is large and the clinical problems vary with the disease. The conditions may be acute, such as asthma and pneumonia, or more chronic, such as chronic obstructive airways disease (COPD) and pulmonary fibrosis. Some patients may require artificial ventilation either because their respiratory muscles fail or because lung function is inadequate. In those with CO_2 retention, an increase in tidal volume and/or respiratory rate with artificial ventilation may wash out the CO_2. In those who are hypoxic, an increase in the inspired oxygen concentration (this may exceed 60%) may also help. There are also special modes of ventilation that help prevent collapse of airways, especially in the presence of viscous secretions, and weaning from artificial ventilators.

Respiratory diseases may also place considerable demands on the respiratory muscles. Although the energy cost of breathing is only about 2% of basal metabolic rate in normal subjects, it may rise to 20% in those with acute respiratory distress syndrome and this can precipitate respiratory muscle fatigue. The lungs may be affected by diseases of other organs and systems. For example heart failure may lead to pulmonary edema, with consequent respiratory failure. In contrast, chronic lung disease may also cause right-sided heart failure (cor pulmonale).

In this chapter emphasis will be placed on COPD, not only because it is a common condition, which frequently causes malnutrition, but also because it helps to illustrate some of the clinical and nutritional principles of care.

Interest in the nutritional management of chronic respiratory disease, in particular COPD, has changed remarkably over the past two decades. COPD is a disease state characterized by the presence of airflow obstruction due to emphysema or intrinsic airway disease classically typified as chronic bronchitis. The airflow limitation is generally progressive, and largely irreversible. Emphysema is defined pathologically as an abnormal permanent enlargement of the air spaces distal to the terminal bronchioles, accompanied by destruction of their walls, without fibrosis. Chronic bronchitis is defined clinically as the presence of a chronic productive cough for three months in each of two successive years in patients in whom the other causes of chronic cough have been excluded.

Weight loss has long been recognized as a symptom of COPD. In the late nineteenth century Fowler and Goodlee first described the association between weight loss and emphysema. Interestingly, attempts to describe different COPD classifications found that body weight might be an important discriminating factor. This led to the classical description of the pink puffer (emphysematous type) and the blue bloater (bronchitic type) (Plate 5). The pink puffing patient is characteristically thin, breathless with marked hyperinflation of the chest. The blue and bloated patient may not be particularly breathless, at least when at rest, but has severe central cyanosis, a bluish-purple discoloration of the skin and mucous membranes, resulting from a deficiency of oxygen in the blood. Although these extreme types can indeed be seen, most patients present a mixed picture.

Traditionally weight loss was considered to be an inevitable and irreversible terminal progression of the disease process. It was thought that nutritional support might even adversely influence the disease by inducing an additional metabolic and ventilatory stress on the pulmonary system. Studies into the disturbed energy balance during weight loss in COPD, however, challenged this approach. Furthermore, the concept of COPD as a systemic disorder (Figure 15.1) gave further insights into the role of nutrition in the disease. Nutritional depletion contributes to disability (dyspnea, exercise capacity) and handicap (health status), independent of the impaired lung function. In the majority of the patients these adverse consequences of weight loss and in particular muscle wasting are (partly) treatable by protein–energy supplementation. However, under certain circumstances nutritional and metabolic abnormalities are not only limited to a disturbed energy balance but may also affect substrate metabolism.

15.2 Prevalence and consequences of weight loss and muscle wasting

To understand the role of nutrition support in respiratory disease, an insight into the consequences and underlying mechanisms of nutritional abnormalities in COPD is needed. In COPD, consequences of weight loss are specifically related to the decrease in body cell

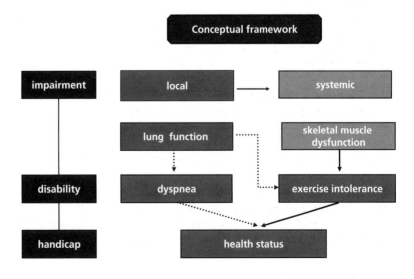

Figure 15.1 Conceptual framework for disease management in COPD.

mass (BCM). The body cell mass is defined as the active metabolizing (organs) and contracting (muscle) tissue. Independently of the underlying disease state or condition, a loss of BCM up to 40% is inevitably associated with death.

Muscle function and exercise performance

The prominent symptoms of COPD are dyspnea (shortness of breath) and exercise intolerance (Figure 15.1). Besides airflow obstruction and loss of alveolar structure, skeletal muscle weakness is an important determinant of these symptoms. Skeletal muscle dysfunction is predominantly determined by skeletal muscle mass in COPD. Muscle mass is the single largest tissue of body cell mass and can be assessed indirectly in clinically stable COPD patients by measurement of fat-free mass (FFM) (see chapter 2 in *Introduction to Human Nutrition* in this series). Besides effects on muscle strength, FFM is also a significant determinant of exercise capacity and exercise response. Patients with a depleted FFM are characterized by lower peak oxygen consumption, peak work rate, and early onset of lactic acid compared with non-depleted patients. The functional consequences of nutritional abnormalities are therefore not only related to muscle wasting *per se*, but also to intrinsic alterations in muscle morphology and energy metabolism towards early anaerobic metabolism. Indeed, the activity of key enzymes involved in oxidative metabolism such as citrate synthase and succinate dehydrogenase as well as energy-rich phosphates (ATP, creatine phosphate) are decreased in some patients with COPD. Furthermore, derangement in muscle electrolyte status such as decreases in potassium, magnesium, and phosphorus and an increase in sodium may occur, occurring more profoundly in the presence of nutritional depletion.

Autopsy studies have clearly shown that nutritional depletion not only leads to peripheral skeletal muscle wasting, but also decreases diaphragm muscle mass. In COPD the effects of nutritional depletion on respiratory muscle function cannot be separated from the mechanical influences on the diaphragm due to hyperinflation. In severely depleted anorexia nervosa patients, free of any other disease, the influence of nutritional depletion on the diaphragm was illustrated by a severely depressed diaphragm contractility that increased significantly by 42% after 30 days of nutrition-

al support. During this period body weight increased by 13% and FFM by 9%.

Mortality and morbidity in COPD

The relationship between weight loss and underweight with mortality in COPD has been studied since the 1960s. In the early years a significant association was reported between weight loss and survival. Five-year mortality was 50% in weight-losing patients compared with 20% in weight-stable COPD patients. Several retrospective studies using different COPD populations from the USA, Canada, Denmark, and the Netherlands reported a relationship between low body mass index (BMI) and mortality independent of disease severity. In all these studies a decreased mortality risk was observed in overweight patients not only compared with underweight patients but also with normal weight subjects (Figure 15.2). This remarkable observation could be related to the fact that depletion of FFM is not only a

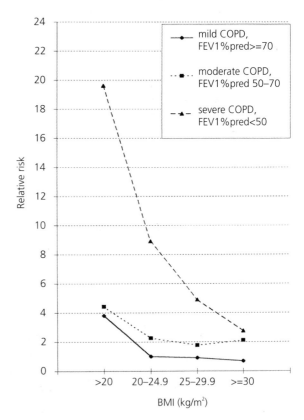

Figure 15.2 COPD-related mortality by BMI in 2132 subjects with mild, moderate, and severe COPD. Reproduced with permission from Landbo *et al.* (1999).

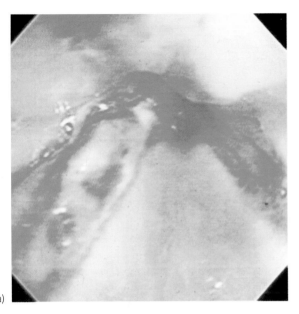

(a)

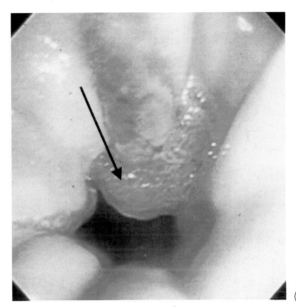

(b)

Plate 1 Endoscopic appearances in food-allergic gastroesophageal reflux in infants. Both cases show endoscopic evidence of esophagitis, with linear reddening of the mucosa and contact bleeding. The case on the right demonstrates an esophageal 'pearl' (arrowed), which is found on histological assessment to contain multiple eosinophils. Both cases failed to resolve with conventional medical therapy, but normalized on exclusion diet.

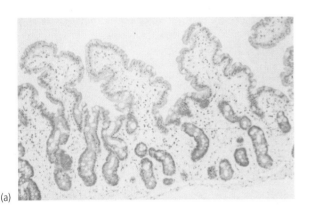

(a)

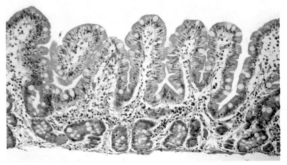

(b)

(c)

Plate 2 Histological changes occur within the small intestine in food-sensitive enteropathy. In (a), which is from a non-allergic child with poor growth who did not eventually have a gastroenterological diagnosis (i.e. as near to a normal control as you can ethically get), there are long villi with no lengthening of the crypts, and no evidence of excess inflammatory infiltrate within the epithelium or lamina propria. Specimen (b) was obtained from a child with cow's milk sensitive enteropathy. There are subtle abnormalities, including some shortening and blunting of the villi and a modest increase in lymphocyte density within the lamina propria. However it is easy to see why specimens are sometimes labeled 'within normal limits,' particularly in centers where there are no pediatric pathologists. Specimen (c), by contrast, is grossly abnormal and shows the characteristic features in celiac disease, with complete loss of villous architecture and lengthening of the crypts (crypt hyperplastic villous atrophy). There is a dense infiltrate of lymphocytes and plasma cells.

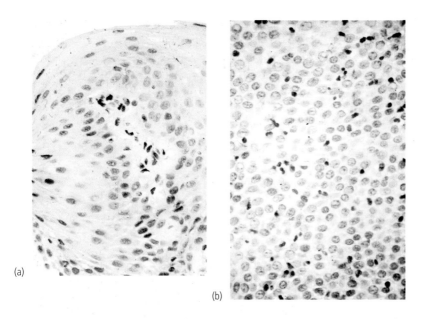

(a)

(b)

Plate 3 Histological findings in the esophagus in food allergic dysmotility. (a) Infiltration of lymphocytes within the papillae, from the lamina propria underlying the epithelium. (b) Large numbers of eosinophils, showing their characteristic red cytoplasm, within the epithelium.

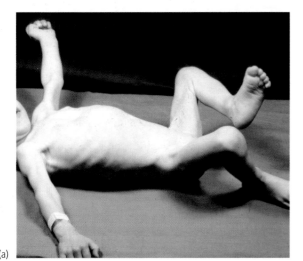

(a)

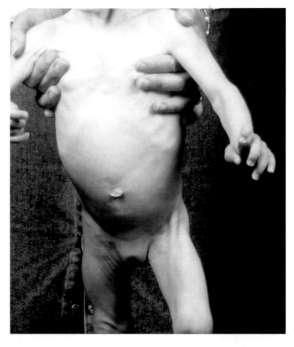

(b)

Plate 4 Potential severe nutritional consequences of dietary allergies. The child on the left, who suffered from cow's milk sensitive enteropathy, shows severe wasting without abdominal distension. The child on the right, who has celiac disease, shows gross wasting with the classical abdominal protruberance. The majority of cases of celiac disease show much less obvious abnormality, hence the phrase 'the celiac iceberg' – most cases are hidden out of sight.

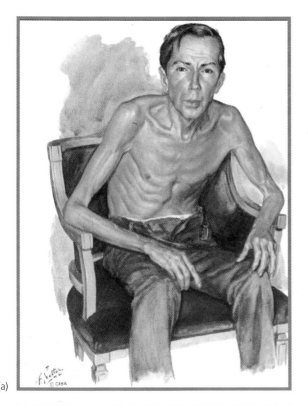

(a)

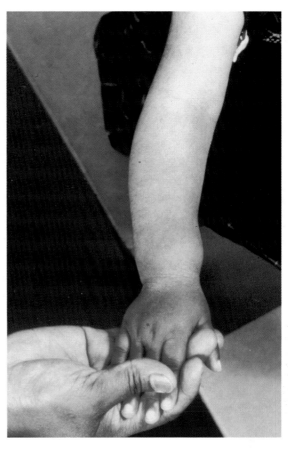

Plate 6 An 18-month-old boy with vitamin D deficiency rickets, showing moderate skin pigmentation and wrist swelling.

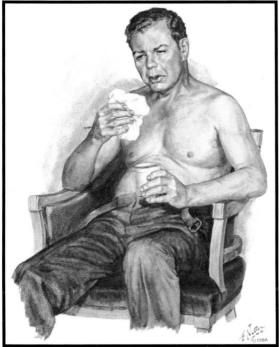

(b)

Plate 5 Classical description of the pink puffer (emphysematous type) and the blue bloater (bronchitic type).

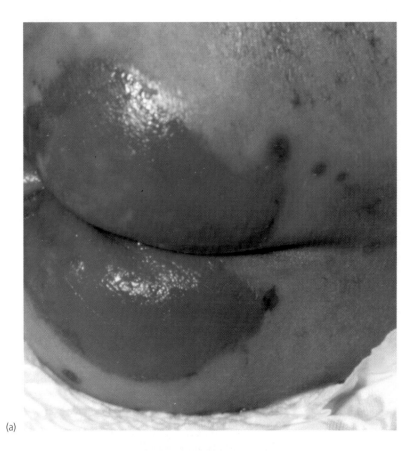

(a)

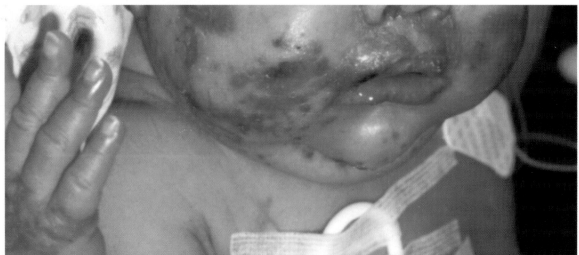

(b)

Plate 7 Zinc deficiency. The characteristic desquamation over the hands, mouth and anus can be seen. The rash healed quickly with zinc supplementation.

consequence of weight loss, but may also occur in normal weight patients with a relatively high fat mass. Specific investigation into the relationship between FFM and mortality showed a significantly increased mortality risk in patients with depleted FFM, independent of the BMI. The independent effect of weight loss on mortality in COPD was strengthened by the results of a nutritional intervention study showing a positive association between weight gain after nutritional supplementation and decreased mortality risk.

Many patients with COPD suffer from acute disease exacerbations requiring hospitalization. A low BMI, as well as recent weight loss, have been identified as important factor for predicting the outcome of acute exacerbations as indicated by the frequency of hospital readmissions, the need for mechanical ventilation, and the inability to wean from the ventilator.

Prevalence of malnutrition in COPD

In clinically stable patients with moderate to severe COPD, depletion of FFM has been reported in 20% of COPD outpatients and in 35% of those eligible for pulmonary rehabilitation. Limited data are available regarding the prevalence of nutritional depletion in mild COPD. Weight loss and a low BMI are more frequently observed in emphysematous patients compared with those with chronic bronchitis. Any observed difference in body weight between the two COPD subtypes is usually due to a difference in fat mass. Depletion of FFM with all its adverse consequences, also occurs in chronic bronchitis.

Health-related quality of life

The functional consequences of underweight and particularly of depletion of FFM are not only reflected at the disability level in exercise tests, but also in a decreased health related quality of life measured by the disease-specific St George's Respiratory Questionnaire (www.atsqol.org/george.asp).

15.3 Causes of weight loss and muscle wasting

Weight loss, and particular loss of fat mass, occurs if energy expenditure exceeds dietary intake. Muscle wasting is a consequence of an imbalance between pro-

tein synthesis and protein breakdown. An imbalance between energy and protein balance may occur simultaneously, but can also be dissociated due to altered regulation of substrate metabolism.

Energy metabolism

Total daily energy expenditure is usually divided into three components:

(1) resting energy expenditure (REE) comprising sleeping metabolic rate and the energy cost of arousal,
(2) diet-induced thermogenesis, and
(3) physical activity-induced thermogenesis.

Based on the assumption that REE is the major component of total energy expenditure in sedentary persons, several studies have measured REE in COPD. After adjustment for the metabolically active FFM, REE was found elevated in 25% of the COPD patients. The increased resting metabolic rate seen in COPD patients is probably due to the greater respiratory muscle work necessary to maintain the higher ventilation rate than seen in healthy controls of comparable age and gender. However, at rest this increased energy cost will only slightly contribute to hypermetabolism. Beta-2-agonists (such as nebulized salbutamol) are used as inhaled bronchodilators in the treatment of many patients with COPD and these may stimulate metabolic rate. However, no significant acute metabolic effects of this treatment were shown in elderly COPD patients in comparison with an age-matched healthy controls.

Another factor contributing to hypermetabolism in COPD is systemic inflammation. Elevated levels of various inflammatory markers like tumor necrosis factor alpha (TNFα) and soluble TNF receptors were found in patients with COPD, particularly in those experiencing weight loss. Several studies have shown an association between markers of systemic inflammation and REE. Despite the increased REE seen in COPD and other chronic inflammatory diseases, total energy expenditure (TEE) often remains unaltered due to the compensatory factor of reduced activity-induced energy expenditure.

In contrast to other chronic diseases, a study of patients with COPD reported an increase in total daily energy expenditure (TDEE), which might be ascribed to inefficient ventilation, inefficiency in leg exercise, and possible impaired oxidative metabolism. However, another study in underweight patients with COPD did not find an overall increase in TDEE, although the results were variable.

Altered substrate metabolism

Until now investigations have mostly focused on energy metabolism in COPD. FFM depletion in weight-stable patients despite a normal or even high fat mass, indicates that there is an altered regulation of substrate metabolism in COPD. Preliminary observations confirm this hypothesis. In normal weight COPD patients whole body protein turnover (protein synthesis and protein breakdown) is increased. In addition, some normal weight emphysematous patients with depleted FFM appear to have a reduced lipolytic response.

Reduced dietary intake

Dietary intake in weight-losing patients is lower than in weight-stable patients both in absolute terms as well as in relation to measured REE. The reasons for the relatively low dietary intake seen in COPD are not completely understood. Patients with COPD may eat suboptimally due to the changes in breathing pattern and low oxygen saturations seen with chewing and swallowing. Indeed in hypoxemic patients a rapid decrease in SaO_2 (percentage saturation of hemoglobin with oxygen in arterial blood) is seen, which slowly recovers after completion of the meal. The decrease in SaO_2 is related to increased dyspnea sensation. The severity of the drop may differ depending on the composition of the meal. Gastric emptying time of a meal may also af-fect dietary intake since gastric filling in COPD patients reduces the functional residual capacity and leads to an increase in dyspnea. Simple dietary practices may help to overcome these problems (Table 15.1).

Systemic factors may also affect dietary intake. Recent studies suggest that appetite regulation may be adversely affected by systemic inflammation. The adipocyte-derived hormone leptin represents the afferent hormonal signal to the brain in a feedback mechanism regulating fat mass. Circulating leptin levels are increased in some patients. This increased plasma leptin level is positively related to an increase in some of the markers of systemic inflammation and inversely related to dietary intake adjusted for REE. These clinical data are in line with experimental animal studies showing that administration of endotoxins or cytokines produced a prompt increase in serum leptin levels and a decrease in appetite and dietary intake.

15.4 Outcome of nutritional intervention

The first clinical trials investigating the effectiveness of nutritional intervention consisted of nutritional supplementation by means of oral liquid supplements or enteral nutrition. All short-term studies of 2–3 weeks duration showed a significant increase in body weight and respiratory muscle function. The effect of refeeding and weight gain on the immune response has been less investigated, but has been associated with a significant increase in total lymphocyte count and with an increase in reactivity to skin test antigens after 21 days of refeeding.

Table 15.1 Simple dietary practices that may help the patient with COPD

Respiratory symptom	Dietary modification
Dypsnea (shortness of breath)	Small, frequent meals and snacks
	Soft meals to reduce work of chewing and swallowing
	Sit up for meals and out of bed if possible
Oxygen therapy	Wear nasal prongs instead of oxygen mask when eating
Dry mouth	Moist meals
	Artificial saliva
Constipation	Increase fluid and fiber intake
Dysphagia	Speech and language therapy review
Taste alterations	Provide meals and drinks with strong flavours
CPAP/BiPAP	Nasogastric feeding
Regurgitation of meals	Post-pyloric enteral feeding
Immobility	Social review regarding home help and help with shopping and meal preparation

CPAP, continuous positive airway pressure; BiPAP, bilevel positive airway pressure.

Significant improvements in respiratory and peripheral skeletal muscle function, exercise capacity, and health-related quality of life have been shown after three months of a daily oral supplement of about 1000 kcal. However, several other studies have not been able to demonstrate this effect, possibly due to the fact that energy requirements were not accurately measured, or that patients were taking the supplements instead of, rather than in addition to their meals.

The progressive nature of weight loss in COPD requires appropriate feeding strategies to allow sustained weight gain. Nutritional supplementation alone has been shown to be of little effect in improving physiological function. This is in part due to a weight gain of fat mass. This limited therapeutic impact of isolated aggressive nutrition support could be related to the absence of a comprehensive rehabilitative strategy. From a functional point of view it is obvious to combine nutritional support with some form of exercise therapy in order to provide an anabolic stimulus. A daily nutritional supplement as an integrated part of an eight-week pulmonary rehabilitation program resulted in significant weight gain (0.4 kg/week).

The combined treatment of nutritional support and exercise not only increased body weight but also resulted in a significant improvement of FFM and respiratory muscle strength. Weight gain and an increase in respiratory muscle strength have been associated with significantly increased survival rates. A comprehensive evaluation of the implementation of nutritional support in a pulmonary rehabilitation program also showed statistically and clinically significant effects in peripheral skeletal muscle strength, exercise capacity, and health status.

Composition of nutritional supplements

Nutrition and ventilation are intrinsically related as oxygen is required for optimal energy exchange. Meal-related dyspnea and limited ventilatory reserves may restrict the quantity and composition of nutritional support in patients with respiratory disease. It was long believed that patients with respiratory disease should consume a fat-rich diet to decrease carbon dioxide load, since the respiratory quotient of fat oxidation is 0.7 relative to 0.83 for protein and 1.0 for carbohydrate oxidation. Scientific evidence supporting this theory is scarce, however, and not convincing.

More recent reports show that patients experience less dyspnea after a carbohydrate-rich liquid supplement than after an equicaloric fat-rich supplement. This result is not surprising as gastric emptying time is significantly longer after an equicaloric fat-rich than following a carbohydrate-rich supplement. Protein requirements have not yet specifically been investigated in COPD. Based on data in other chronic wasting conditions, daily protein intake should be at least 1.5 g/kg body weight to allow optimal protein synthesis.

Skeletal muscle serves as an important reserve system in maintaining supplies of amino acids for metabolism and protein synthesis. Alterations in plasma and muscle amino acids profile have been observed in COPD. Specifically, disturbances in leucine metabolism have been reported and at the muscular level consistently decreased levels of glutamate are found. Intracellular glutamate is known to be an important precursor for the antioxidant glutathione as well as glutamine synthesis in muscle. Indeed muscle glutamate is strongly associated with glutathione in COPD, though not with glutamine. Avoiding depletion of intracellular glutamate possibly by specific nutritional intervention may therefore be important in the prevention of oxidative stress in the skeletal muscle of COPD patients.

Nutritional modulation of muscle metabolism by amino acids or other substrates and cofactors in energy metabolism may not only be relevant in wasted patients, but also as anabolic stimulus to enhance efficacy of exercise training. This approach is already common practice with elite athletes. Besides, evidence is accumulating that, independent of nutritional state, the metabolic response to exercise is altered in COPD patients. In a recent study 20 min of submaximal constant work rate exercise caused a reduction in the levels of most amino acids in muscle, whereas an increase was found in several plasma amino acids compared with normal. This suggests elevated release of amino acids from muscle during exercise in COPD.

The effects on protein metabolism and exercise performance of specific amino acid supplementation prior to or immediately after exercise to balance this response are unknown.

Timing of nutritional support

The effects of nutritional supplementation have mostly been studied in clinically stable patients. In some patients weight loss follows a stepwise pattern, associated with acute infectious exacerbations. There is often negative energy balance at the time of acute exacerbations due to the sudden reduction in energy intake. These patients may also have increased protein breakdown. Factors contributing to weight loss and muscle wasting during acute exacerbation include an increase in symptoms, flare-up of the systemic inflammatory response, alterations in leptin metabolism, and the use of high doses of glucocorticoids.

Indeed a significant inverse association was shown between daily glucocorticoid dose and nitrogen balance during hospitalization for acute exacerbations. A positive effect of nutritional support was shown on well-being and some lung function measurements, but more research is needed to evaluate the effectiveness of nutritional support during an acute exacerbation relative to the role of nutrition support in the clinically stable patient.

Practical implementation of nutritional supplementation

The relationships between nutritional depletion and outcome in patient care are summarized in the flowchart for nutritional screening and therapy shown in Figure 15.3. Simple screening can be performed based on repeated measurements of body weight. Patients are characterized by body mass index and the presence or absence of involuntary weight loss. In view of the high mortality risk, nutritional supplementation is indicated for all patients with a BMI <21 kg/m² with moderate to severe COPD. Involuntary weight loss in patients with a BMI <25 kg/m² should also be treated to prevent further deterioration; involuntary weight loss in patients with a BMI >25 kg/m² should be monitored to assess whether it is progressive.

If possible, measurement of FFM may provide a more detailed screening of patients, since this allows

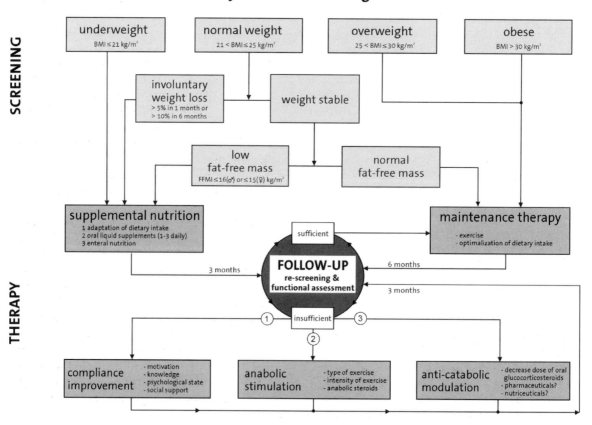

Figure 15.3 Flowchart for nutritional screening and therapy.

identification of normal weight patients with a depleted FFM who, even despite a normal body weight, should be considered for diet therapy.

Depending on the underlying cause of energy imbalance (decreased dietary intake or increased nutritional requirements) initial nutritional therapy can include adaptations of the dietary behavior and food patterns, followed by the use of oral nutritional supplements. Nutritional supplements should be given well divided during the day to avoid loss of appetite and adverse metabolic and ventilatory effects resulting from a high caloric load. Note that for some patients a supplement of 500 kcal may already cause early satiety and acute adverse effects on exercise capacity. Where possible, patients should be encouraged to attend a pulmonary rehabilitation program. For the severely disabled patients unable to perform exercise training, even simple strength maneuvers combined with training of daily activities and energy conservation techniques may be effective. Exercise not only improves the effectiveness of nutritional therapy, but also stimulates appetite.

After 8–12 weeks, response to therapy can be determined. If weight gain and functional improvement have occurred, the caregiver and the patient can decide whether further improvement by a similar strategy is possible. It may then also be worthwhile to add or alter the exercise training program (i.e. intensity or type). If functional improvements and weight gain cannot be demonstrated, issues relating to compliance, lack of motivation, lack of knowledge, decreased cognitive functioning, lack of social support, anxiety, and depression may need to be addressed. A multidisciplinary team is useful for the respiratory patient in this regard.

15.5 Acute lung injury

Acute lung injury ranges from simple localized lung infections to diffuse alveolar damage seen in adult respiratory distress syndrome. The general goal of nutrition therapy in acute lung injury is to meet the increased requirements in the hypercatabolic state to prevent protein breakdown.

Symptoms of anorexia, fatigue, malaise, cough, and dyspnea all compromise oral intake. If mechanical ventilation is necessary, artificial nutrition support should be started in the majority of patients to minimise muscle breakdown. A negative nitrogen balance reduces respiratory muscle strength and ventilatory drive and compromises immune function, which in turn has long-term effects on outcome and recovery. For more on nutrition support see Chapter 8.

15.6 Perspectives on the future

Further characterization and understanding of the altered substrate metabolism in COPD and the underlying molecular mechanisms may change the perspective for nutritional intervention in the future. By targeted nutritional modulation of specific problems in subgroups of COPD patients, at either physiological or pharmacological dose, nutritional management of these patients may be maximized.

The interaction between nutritional depletion and systemic inflammation has drawn attention to the potential beneficial effects of anticatabolic agents in modulating the systemic inflammatory response. Several agents such as *n*-3 fatty acids and non-steroid anti-inflammatory agents, have been investigated in other wasting conditions such as HIV, cancer, and sepsis with encouraging results on proinflammatory mediators and weight response. These agents may become an interesting therapeutic alternative for some patients with COPD. It has been shown that COPD patients responding inadequately after nutritional supplementation and exercise therapy with or without the use of anabolic steroids, are characterized by a elevated systemic inflammatory response as reflected by enhanced levels of soluble TNF receptors, circulating leptin, and acute phase proteins.

As well as effects of inflammation on energy balance and protein metabolism, recent experimental *in vitro* studies point towards a direct effect of inflammatory mediators on aspects of the muscle cell cycle such as differentiation and apoptosis. In the future, further unraveling of the molecular mechanisms of these effects to explore novel nutritional and pharmacological intervention strategies to reverse the wasting process may be possible. Within two decades, the role of nutrition in chronic respiratory disease has thus moved from ignorance and merely supportive care to targeted intervention of the functional consequences and health status.

References and further reading

Brug J, Schols A, Mesters I. Dietary change, nutrition education and chronic obstructive pulmonary disease. *Patient Educ Couns* 2004; 52: 249–257.

Creutzberg EC, Wouters EFM, Mostert R, Weling-Scheepers CAPM, Schols AMWJ. Efficacy of nutritional supplementation therapy in depleted patients with Chronic Obstructive Pulmonary Disease. *Nutrition* 2003; 19: 120–127.

Landbo C, Prescott E, Lange P, Vestbo J, Almdal TP. Prognostic value of nutritional status in chronic obstructive pulmonary disease. *Am J Respir Crit Care Med* 1999; 160: 1856–1861.

Rogers RM, Donahoe M, Constatino J. Physiologic effects of oral supplemental feeding in malnourished patients with chronic obstructive pulmonary diseases, a randomized control study. *Am Rev Respir Dis* 1992; 146: 1511–1517.

Schols AM, Slangen J, Volovics L, Wouters EF. Weight loss is a reversible factor in the prognosis of chronic obstructive pulmonary disease. *Am J Respir Crit Care Med* 1998; 157: 1791–1797.

Schols AM. Nutritional and metabolic modulation in chronic obstructive pulmonary disease management. *Eur Respir J Suppl* 2003; 46: 81s–86s.

16
Nutrition and Immune and Inflammatory Systems

Bruce R Bistrian and Robert F Grimble

Key messages

- The immune system may become activated by microbial invasion, as well as a wide range of stimuli and conditions. The immune response exerts a high metabolic and nutritional cost upon the body.
- Nutrition has a two-way influence on the immune system. The activities of the immune system exert a deleterious influence on nutritional status and alterations in nutrient intake modulate the intensity of the various activities of the immune system.
- Proinflammatory cytokines have far-reaching metabolic effects throughout the body, including changes in protein, fat, and trace element metabolism, alteration of body temperature and appetite, and changes in liver protein synthesis.

- An individual's nutritional status and intake of specific nutrients can modify cytokine biology in ways which have major implications for health and well-being.
- Antioxidants may suppress inflammatory components of the response to infection and trauma and enhance components related to cell-mediated immunity.
- The unsaturated fatty acid and cholesterol content of the diet also plays a role in the inflammatory response. While n-6 polyunsaturated fatty acids (PUFAs) and cholesterol exert a proinflammatory influence, n-3 PUFAs and monounsaturated fatty acids exert the opposite effect.

16.1 Introduction

Humans live in the presence of many types of microorganisms, which exert pathological effects if they succeed in penetrating the surface defenses of the body. Once entry is gained, rapid multiplication occurs which, if unchecked, can end in death. However, we possess an immune system that has a great capacity for immobilizing invading microbes, creating a hostile environment for them and bringing about their destruction. Humans and warm-blooded animals have survived because their immune systems have the ability to focus a range of lethal activities upon the invader. This biological property is important since many microbes can multiply at least 50 times faster than the cells of the system. The immune system must therefore become rapidly effective once invasion has occurred. The immune system can also become activated, in a similar way to the response to microbial invasion, by a wide range of stimuli and conditions; these include burns, penetrating and blunt injury, the presence of tumor cells, environmental pollutants, radiation, exposure to allergens, and the presence of chronic inflammatory diseases. This latter group of stimulatory conditions includes such diseases as rheumatoid arthritis, Crohn's disease, asthma, and psoriasis. The strength of the response to this disparate range of stimuli may vary of course, but it will contain many of the hallmarks of the response to invading pathogens. In the normal response to perturbation the immune system goes from a state of activation to deactivation as the body becomes repaired from the effects of the invasion. However, in chronic inflammatory disease the initial activation continues unabated.

As will be seen later, the immune response exerts a high metabolic and nutritional cost upon the body.

Inappropriate prolongation of the response will exert a deleterious effect upon the nutritional status of the patient.

16.2 The response of the immune system to activation

The immune system is located throughout the body. It consists of clearly recognized structures, such as the spleen, thymus, and lymph nodes, and diffuse populations of cells. Examples of the latter component of the system are lymphocytes which circulate around the body via the bloodstream and lymphatic circulation. In addition macrophages (cells capable of engulfing foreign particles, bacteria, viruses, and fungi) populate the linings of lungs and together with lymphocytes occupy areas deep in the walls of the small and large intestine. There is also a network of immune cells (dendritic cells) within the skin which form an important part of overall immune defense. Thus virtually every part of the body comes under the vigilance of the immune system.

In general terms the reaction of the immune system to activation can be divided into two components: an innate response which is unaffected by whether the subject has encountered a particular pathogen before but is rapid, non-specific, and is the main mediator of the inflammatory response, and a specific immune response which 'remembers' a previous encounter with a pathogen and produces a much enhanced response on each subsequent exposure (Figure 16.1).

The specific immune response is further subdivided into a cell-mediated and humoral response. The first of these involves T lymphocytes which have originated from the bone marrow and have undergone further development in the thymus. The second involves B lymphocytes which have originated from the bone marrow and when stimulated with molecules that are foreign to the body (antigens), develop into cells capable of producing antibodies (immunoglobulins (Ig)). These are highly specific to the antigen and aid in its destruction.

While potentially thousands of discretely different immunoglobulins can be produced (one for each antigenic substance/organisms that might be encountered by the body), they fall into five main classes, depending upon their gross structure. The classes are labeled G, M, A, D, and E. For example, IgA has the ability to cross cell epithelial cell layers and is thus found in tears, saliva, gut secretions, and milk. IgE on the other hand has

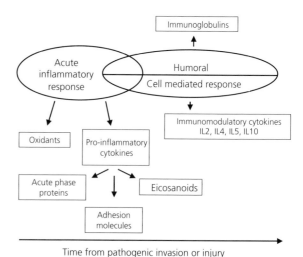

Figure 16.1 The response to infection and injury.

the ability to attach to mast cells and when activated leads to the release of histamine and other chemicals associated with allergy.

B cells also come under the influence of a type of T cell called helper T cells. These forms of lymphocytes and macrophages secrete a range of proteins called cytokines which act as the 'hormones of the immune system.' Within this group are the interleukins (IL), tumor necrosis factors (TNF), and interferons (IFN). The cytokines act in an apocrine, paracrine, and endocrine manner and modify many activities of the immune system (Table 16.1).

Table 16.1 Some examples of cytokines and their effects

Cytokine	Major effects
Interleukin 1[a]	Fever, muscle protein loss, raised blood glucose, changes in blood trace element concentration
Tumor necrosis factor-alpha[a]	Fever, appetite loss, muscle protein loss, raised blood lipids, changes in blood trace element concentration. Stimulates oxidant production
Interleukin 6[a]	Stimulates acute phase protein production by liver
Interleukin 2	Stimulates T lymphocyte proliferation
Interleukin 8	Causes attraction of immune cells – chemotaxis
Interleukin 10	Inhibits proinflammatory cytokine production

[a]There are varying degrees of overlap between the actions of these proinflammatory cytokines

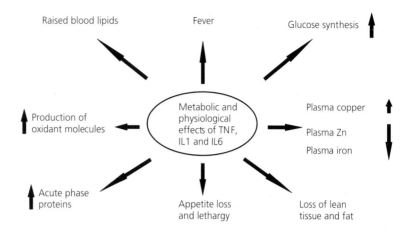

Figure 16.2 General physiological and metabolic effects of proinflammatory cytokines.

In addition to their direct influence on immune cells the cytokines IL-1, IL-6, and TNF have widespread metabolic effects upon the body and stimulate the process of inflammation. These cytokines are thus subclassified as proinflammatory cytokines. Key features of the effects of this group of molecules are shown in Figure 16.2.

Nutrition has a two-way influence on the immune system. The activities of the immune system exert a deleterious influence on nutritional status and alterations in nutrient intake modulate the intensity of the various activities of the immune system. Experimental studies and clinical observation have shown that many aspects of the immune response can be modified by alteration in the intake of protein, specific amino acids, lipids, and micronutrients.

16.3 The effects of proinflammatory cytokines

Many of the signs and symptoms experienced after infection has occurred, such as fever, loss of appetite, weight loss, negative nitrogen and mineral balance, and lethargy are caused directly and indirectly by proinflammatory cytokines (Figure 16.2). The indirect effects of cytokines are mediated by actions upon the adrenal glands and endocrine pancreas, resulting in increased secretions of the catabolic hormones epinephrine (adrenaline), norepinephrine (noradrenaline), glucococorticoids, and glucagon. Insulin insensitivity occurs in addition to a 'catabolic state.'

The diverse range of metabolic changes caused by the proinflammatory cytokines can be seen as a coordinated response (Figure 16.3) designed to:

- create a hostile environment for the invading organism,
- provide nutrients, from within the body, to support the actions of the immune system, and
- enhance the defence systems of the body to protect healthy tissue from the potent actions of the inflammatory response.

Changes in protein and fat metabolism

The biochemistry of an infected individual is thus fundamentally changed in a way that will ensure that the immune system receives nutrients from within the body to perform its tasks. Muscle protein is catabolized to provide amino acids for synthesizing new cells and proteins for the immune response. Furthermore, amino acids are converted to glucose (a preferred fuel for the immune system). The extent of this process is highlighted by the major increase in urinary urea excretion, ranging from 9 g/day in mild infection to 20–30 g/day following major burn or severe traumatic injury. Fat is catabolized and the fatty acids released help to satisfy the increased energy needs of the infected person (the resting metabolic rate increases by 13% for every 1°C rise in body temperature).

Alteration of body temperature and appetite

The rise in temperature is part of the body's attempt to create a hostile environment for the invader. In past centuries physicians have often advocated steam baths for treatment of infection. It is also interesting to note that when infected, cold-blooded animals, which are unable to raise body temperature by endogenous

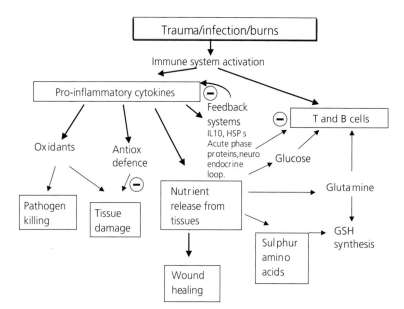

Figure 16.3 The physiological and metabolic consequences of proinflammatory cytokine production.

means, often move to hotter areas of their immediate environment in an attempt to create hostile conditions for the invading organisms.

In mammals, the changes in temperature are mediated by the interaction of proinflammatory cytokines with specialized neurons in the hypothalamus. There is some debate over whether the cytokines gain access directly to the hypothamalus by crossing the blood–brain barrier, or whether circulating cytokines are excluded by the barrier but induce cytokine production within the hypothalamus. The interaction of cytokines with the hypothalamus also brings about a loss of appetite. This may be transient in nature, or prolonged and profound, as is the case in chronic infections such as tuberculosis or during cancer. It is interesting to note that the body fat regulatory hormone leptin is induced by TNF, but as of yet no direct role for leptin in the significant weight loss during infection and cancer, has been found.

Changes in trace element metabolism

Major changes occur in plasma cation concentration, such as those of iron, copper, and zinc. These changes in iron and zinc are often misinterpreted as indicating mineral deficiency but are very likely to be due to major redistribution of these elements within the body in an attempt to 'starve' blood-borne microbes

of nutrients or to foster certain beneficial aspects of the systemic inflammatory response in specific organs. However, micronutrient deficiency can be precipitated by the response to infection as urinary loss of many micronutrients is accelerated following infection and injury. The resultant deficiencies in zinc, iron, and copper have deleterious effects on general immune function and wound healing. The cytokines also stimulate the synthesis of potent oxidant molecules (hydrogen peroxide, nitric oxide, hydroxyl radical, hypochlorous acid, and superoxide anion) which damage the cellular integrity of the invading organism.

Changes in liver protein synthesis

Specialized proteins called acute phase proteins, which focus the actions of the immune system on the invader and help to protect healthy tissue from 'collateral damage' in the 'battle' with pathogens, are synthesized in increased amounts by the liver. Important acute phase proteins and their respective functions are highlighted in Table 16.2. The liver focuses its activities on acute phase protein synthesis by shutting down the synthesis of its main protein product, serum albumin, and also a number of other secretory proteins such as prealbumin, retinol-binding protein, and transferrin. This latter group of proteins are termed 'negative acute phase reactants.'

Table 16.2 Biological functions of major acute phase proteins

Acute phase protein	Function
Alpha-1-proteinase inhibitor Alpha-1-antichymotrypsin Alpha-2-macroglobulin	Inhibition of proteinase released during the inflammatory response
C-reactive protein Serum amyloid A	Removal of antigens from the host
C-reactive protein C3 complement	Activation of the immune response
Proteinase inhibitors Alpha-1-glycoprotein	Suppression of the immune response
Ceruloplasmin Alpha-1-acid glycoprotein	Antioxidant properties
Ceruloplasmin Haptoglobin Transferrin Alpha-1-acid glycoprotein	Binding and transport of metals and biologically active compounds

Serum albumin concentration is often regarded as an index of protein nutritional status. Thus the fall in albumin concentration that occurs during infection and inflammatory disease is often misunderstood as a sign of protein deficiency and complicates the assessment of protein status in patients. In virtually every instance, clinically, a low serum albumin reflects the presence, or recent occurrence, of a systemic inflammatory response. The response produces malnutrition by inducing anorexia, decreasing voluntary activity, and reducing the metabolic efficiency of endogenous and exogenous protein utilization. However, low serum albumin concentrations is not specifically a measure of nutritional status, since only an unattainably low protein intake, in conjunction with an adequate energy intake, will even modestly affect serum albumin concentrations. For instance patients with very severe anorexia nervosa, with losses of body weight in excess of 30%, will have normal concentrations of serum albumin.

Many of these complex metabolic changes result in the balance being swung from being in favor of the invading organism to being in favor of the infected individual.

16.4 Control systems for cytokines

Proinflammatory cytokines also induce the production of a cascade of production of other cytokines from lymphocytes. The cascade has modulating actions on lymphocyte function (IL-2 stimulates lymphocyte proliferation, IL-8 attracts immune cells to the site of invasion, IL-4 alters the class of antibodies produced). It is of interest to note that cytokines are also capable of autoregulation, IL-10 with IL-4, produced in response to proinflammatory cytokines, suppress production of proinflammatory cytokines.

Conceptually there is evidence that there can be a poor outcome from an excessive systemic inflammatory response. This syndrome is referred to as the systemic inflammatory response syndrome (SIRS) and is manifest by increased TNF concentrations in sepsis or following burn injury. However, there is a compensatory anti-inflammatory response syndrome (CARS), reflected in increased production of IL-4 and IL-10, which if excessive can also have a deleterious outcome. It has been hypothesized, from a growing body of research data, that the relative balance between SIRS and CARS has an impact on survival. This is probably why attempts to block proinflammatory cytokine production with monoclonal antibodies have met with little success in reducing mortality.

Nutritional modulation that affects both sides of the SIRS/CARS equation offers a greater promise of success. A class of proteins called heat shock proteins (HSP), which were originally identified in heat-stressed cells, are also produced by cells exposed to proinflammatory cytokines. HSPs have a general anti-inflammatory influence and suppress cytokine production. These autoregulatory mechanisms are very important biological phenomena, because, while cytokines are essential for effective operation of the immune system, they exert a high metabolic cost on the body and can exert damaging and lethal effects (Figure 16.3). Conceptually the systemic inflammatory response should be viewed as a general benefit in most instances, but to have the potential for harm through excessive or prolonged activation of SIRS or CARS. These adverse impacts can result as a consequence of excessive inflammation, immunodepression, and/or the development of protein–energy malnutrition.

16.5 Damaging and life-threatening effects of cytokines

Although cytokines are essential for the normal operating of the immune system when produced at the right time and in the right amounts, they play a major damaging role in many inflammatory diseases such as rheumatoid arthritis, inflammatory bowel disease, asthma, psoriasis, multiple sclerosis, and in cancer. They are also thought to be important in the development of atheromatous plaques in cardiovascular disease. In conditions such as cerebral malaria, meningitis, and sepsis, they are produced in excessive amounts and are an important factor in increased mortality. In these diseases the cytokines are being produced in the wrong biological context.

The end stages of many chronic conditions have, as a root cause, an on-going systemic inflammatory response which has been documented by either elevated plasma cytokines, their soluble receptors, IL-1 receptor antagonist, IL-6, spontaneous or stimulated release of cytokines from peripheral blood mononuclear cells, or elevated acute phase protein concentrations, particularly C-reactive protein (CRP). These conditions include end stage liver disease (TNF), end stage renal disease (IL-6, CRP, soluble cytokine receptors), congestive heart failure (TNF), weight-losing chronic obstructive pulmonary disease (IL-6), as well as elevated CRP concentrations in poorly controlled diabetes and obesity. Furthermore concentrations of this acute phase protein have been associated with higher risk of coronary or cerebrovascular disease.

Adverse effects of an individual's genotype

It has recently become apparent that single base changes (single nucleotide polymorphisms (SNP)), usually in the promoter region of genes responsible for producing the molecules involved in the inflammatory process, exert a modulatory effect on the intensity of inflammation. *In vitro* production of TNFα by peripheral blood mononuclear cells (PBMCs) from healthy and diseased subjects stimulated with inflammatory agents shows remarkable individual constancy in men and postmenopausal women. This constancy suggests that genetic factors exert a strong influence. A number of studies have shown that SNPs in the promoter regions for the TNFα and lymphotoxin-α (LT-α) genes are associated with differential TNFα production. The *TNF2(A)* and *TNFB2(A)* alleles (at −308 and +252 for the TNFα and LTα genes, respectively), are linked to high TNF production, particularly in homozygous individuals.

A large body of research has indicated that SNPs occur in the upstream regulatory (promoter) regions

of many cytokine genes (e.g. IL-6 −174, IL-1β −511). Many of these genetic variations influence the level of expression of genes and the outcome from the inflammatory response. Both pro- and anti-inflammatory cytokines are influenced by the differences in genotype.

In a study on inflammatory lung disease, caused by exposure to coal dust, the *TNF2* (LTα +252A) allele was almost twice as common in miners with the disease than in those who were healthy. Development of farmer's lung, from exposure to hay dust, was 80% greater in individuals with the *TNF2* allele than in those without the allele. The *TNF2* allele was also twice as common in smokers who developed chronic obstructive pulmonary disease (COPD) than in those who remained disease free.

In addition to disease progression, genetic factors have important effects on mortality and morbidity in infectious and inflammatory disease. In a study on malaria, children who were homozygous for *TNF2* had a sevenfold increase in the risk of death or serious pathology than children who were homozygous for the *TNF1* allele. In sepsis, patients possessing the *TNF2* allele had a 3.7-fold risk of death than those without the allele and patients who were homozygous for the LTα +252A allele had twice the mortality rate and higher peak plasma TNFα concentrations than heterozygotic individuals. The *TNF2* allele has also been found in increased frequencies in systemic lupus erythromatosus, dermatitis hepetiformis, and insulin-dependent and non-insulin-dependent diabetes mellitus.

Genetic factors also influence the propensity of individuals to produce oxidant molecules and thereby influence nuclear transcription factor kappa B (NFκB) activation. Natural resistance-associated macrophage protein 1 (NRAMP1) has effects on macrophage functions, including TNFα production and activation of inducible nitric oxide synthase (iNOS), which occurs by cooperation between the NRAMP1, TNFα, and LTα genes. There are four variations in the NRAMP1 gene, resulting in different basal levels of activity and differential sensitivity to stimulation by inflammatory agents. Alleles 1, 2, and 4 are poor promoters, while allele 3 causes high gene expression. Hyperactivity of macrophages, associated with allele 3, is linked to autoimmune disease susceptibility and high resistance to infection, while allele 2 increases susceptibility to infection and protects against autoimmune disease.

SNPs also occur in genes for anti-inflammatory cytokines. There are at least three polymorphic sites

(−1082, −819, −592) in the IL-10 promoter which influence production. In intensive care patients the occurrence of *1082*G* high producing allele for IL-10 was present in those who developed multiorgan failure with a frequency one-fifth of that of the normal population.

Thus it now appears that each individual possesses combinations of SNPs in their genes associated with inflammation corresponding to 'inflammatory drives' of differing intensities when microbes or tissue injury are encountered. At an individual level this may express itself as differing degrees of morbidity and mortality.

In general, men are more sensitive to the genomic influences on the strength of the inflammatory process than women. In a study on LTα genotype and mortality from sepsis it was found that men possessing a *TNFB22* (LTα +252AA) genotype had mortality of 72% compared with men who were *TNFB11* (LTα +252GG), who had a 42% mortality rate. In female patients the mortalities for the two genotypes were 53% and 33% respectively. In a study on patients undergoing surgery for gastrointestinal cancer it was found that postoperative CRP and IL-6 concentrations were higher in men than women. Multivariate analysis showed that men possessing the *TNF2* (TNFα −308A) allele had greater responses than men without it. The genomic influence was not seen in women. Furthermore, possession of the IL-1 −511T allele was associated with a greater length of stay in hospital in old men admitted for geriatric care. Women were unaffected by these genetic influences.

Many studies have shown a clear link between obesity, oxidant stress, and inflammation. The link may lie in the ability of adipose tissue to produce proinflammatory cytokines, particularly TNFα. There is a positive relationship between adiposity and TNF production. Leptin has been shown to influence proinflammatory cytokine production. Thus plasma triglycerides, body fat mass, and inflammation may be loosely associated because of these endocrine relationships.

In an investigation of cytokine production in healthy men, one of the authors found that, in the study population as a whole, there were no statistically significant relationships between BMI, plasma fasting triglycerides, and the ability of PBMCs to produce TNFα. However individuals with the LTα +252AA genotype (associated with raised TNF production) showed significant relationships between TNF production and BMI and fasting triglycerides. Thus despite the study population

being comprised of healthy subjects, within that population were individuals with a genotype that resulted in an 'aged' phenotype as far as plasma lipids, BMI, and inflammation were concerned.

Adverse effects of proinflammatory cytokines on body composition

Experience worldwide shows that infections are a potent inhibitor of growth. The actions of IL-1, IL-6, and TNF exert a high metabolic cost to the body. Substrate released from muscle, skin, and bone under their influence will undoubtedly nourish the immune system and help wound healing; however, in a growing child a conflict of interests occurs and nutrients will be diverted away from growth. The metabolic cost of cytokine action has potentially deleterious effects also in adults. In malaria, tuberculosis, sepsis, cancer, human immunodeficiency virus (HIV) infection, and rheumatoid arthritis, the cytokines bring about a loss of lean tissue, which can seriously debilitate the individual. It is a well-known phenomenon that infection is accompanied by a raised body temperature and an increased output of nitrogenous excretion products in the urine. The loss of nitrogen from the body of an adult during a bacterial infection may be equivalent to 60 g of tissue protein and in a period of persistent malarial infection over 500 g of protein.

There are four clinical conditions that cause maximal protein catabolism: (a) major third-degree burns of more than 30% of body surface area, (b) multiple trauma, (c) closed head injury with a low Glasgow Coma Score, and (d) severe sepsis. They result in losses of nitrogen of up to 30 g/day, which is equivalent to 200 g tissue protein. The latter translates into losses of 900 g lean tissue/day, at the usual conversion figure of 30 : 1 for lean tissue to grams of nitrogen.

Important endocrine changes occur during the systemic inflammatory response that impact upon growth and tissue composition. There is a reduction in anabolic stimuli for growth including a reduction in testosterone and insulin resistance. Despite increases in growth hormone, which enhances fat mobilization and gluconeogenesis, the hormone fails to promote insulin-like growth factor 1 (IGF-1) production by the liver, which is responsible for the growth-promoting actions of growth hormone. Furthermore insulin resistance in carbohydrate metabolism fosters an increase in hepatic glucose production and a reduced up-take by skeletal muscle.

These changes, which at first sight appear detrimental, may be beneficial during the systemic inflammatory response, primarily because they result in an increase in blood glucose. Glucose is an ideal metabolic fuel because, having no charge and small size, it is easily diffusible and because it can be either oxidized to easily excreted products (carbon dioxide and water), or can uniquely be metabolized to produce ATP without a requirement for oxygen by anaerobic glycolysis. This latter process is particularly important in ischemic tissues and in macrophages and fibroblasts, which are facultative anaerobes.

Other beneficial results of the systemic inflammatory response are the release of glutamine from muscle, which is important for cells of the immune system and other rapidly dividing cells. In addition, the creation of ammonium ions from deamination of glutamine assists in acid–base balance.

Potential damage from the interaction of oxidants with cytokine production

There are further characteristics of cytokine biology that can damage an infected individual indirectly. The oxidant molecules produced by the immune system to kill invading organisms may also activate the important cellular control molecule NFκB. This factor is a control switch for biological processes, not all of which are of advantage to the individual. Activated NFκB migrates to the nucleus where it switches on genes for cytokine, glutathione, and acute phase protein production. Unfortunately, however, it also increases HIV replication. This sequence of events accounts for the ability of minor infections to speed the progression of individuals who are infected with HIV towards the acquired immune deficiency syndrome (AIDS) (Figure 16.4).

During the last decade it has become increasingly clear that an individual's nutritional status and intake of specific nutrients can modify cytokine biology in ways that have major implications for health and well-being.

16.6 Influence of malnutrition on key aspects of the cytokine response

Malnutrition has a major effect upon the normal operation of the immune and inflammatory components of the immune system. In a sense, malnutrition was the first known 'acquired immune deficiency' disease; the effects of malnutrition have much in common with the later recognized AIDS due to HIV infection. Malnutrition influences virtually all of the components of the immune response. The most obvious ones are a reduction in cell number and function of the lymphocytes associated with cell-mediated immunity, shrinkage or impaired development of the organs of the immune system (thymus, spleen, and gut-associated lymphoid

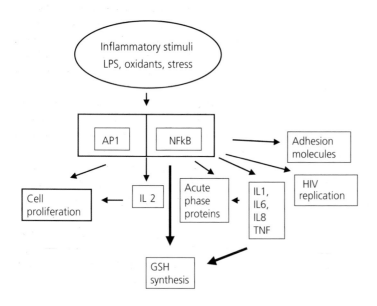

Figure 16.4 Effect of inflammatory stimuli on cell biology via activation of transcription factors. AP1, activator protein 1; NFκB, nuclear factor kappa B; IL, interleukin; GSH, reduced form of glutathione.

tissue), and suppression of some aspects of the inflammatory response.

Influence of protein–energy malnutrition

Children hospitalized with protein–energy malnutrition often show no fever when they are experiencing bacterial, viral, and parasitic invasion. As nutritional rehabilitation proceeds the children become febrile and may develop an overwhelming inflammatory response marked by oxidant damage and 'shock-like' symptoms. It is unknown whether the afebrile state is due to impaired cytokine production, or to changes in the responsiveness of the central nervous system. Studies in rats, rabbits, and guinea-pigs have shown that protein-deficient diets reduce the ability of macrophages to produce cytokines. In monkeys, other macrophage functions such as the ability to engulf and kill microorganisms have also been shown to be depressed.

Pure protein deficiency in humans does not exist as a discrete entity, but occurs in combination with deficiencies of other nutrients. However it was shown in 1982, by studies in Boston, that circulating white blood cells from malnourished elderly patients had an impaired ability to produce inflammatory cytokines and that normal function could be restored by dietary protein and energy supplements. Paradoxically, chronic food deprivation in previously healthy subjects has been reported to enhance TNF production by monocytes stimulated by phytohemagglutinin (PHA). A similar phenomenon has been found in basal TNF production in patients with anorexia nervosa.

Influence of vitamin A deficiency

Vitamin A intake has a potent effect on immune function in malnourished populations. Supplementation studies have shown reductions of approximately 30% in childhood mortality in many countries where vitamin A deficiency is endemic. The mechanisms for the increased effectiveness of the immune system is not fully understood; however, it seems likely that the effects of the nutrient on improving epithelial barriers and IgA production may play a role. In addition, vitamin A supplements have been shown to enhance IL-1 production in malnourished children. Supplemental zinc has also been shown to have a restorative effect on immune function in malnourished experimental animals and individuals. Further details of the effect of

micronutrients on immune function are described in chapters 8 and 9 of the *Introduction to Human Nutrition* textbook in this series.

16.7 Antioxidant defenses and their impact on immune and inflammatory systems in patients

The increase in oxidant production which occurs in the presence of cytokines carries the risk that healthy tissues within the body may become damaged as well as invading organisms. When glutathione synthesis was blocked in rats by injection of diethyl maleate, a sublethal dose of TNF became lethal. The onset of sepsis in patients (going on to develop multiple organ failure) leads to a transient decrease in the total antioxidative capacity of blood. The capacity returns to normal values over the following 5 days. However this was found not to be the case for patients who died, for whom values remained well below the normal range. Oxidants enhance the production of a number of cytokines by the activation of nuclear transcription factors, such as NFκB and activator protein 1 (AP1). A change in cell redox status results in activation of these factors and migration into the nucleus where they initiate transcription of a wide range of genes associated with inflammation and cell proliferation (Figure 16.4).

A number of components of antioxidant defense are enhanced by proinflammatory cytokines. Glutathione synthesis and the activities of superoxide dismutase (SOD), catalase, glutathione peroxidase, and reductase are increased. Gamma-glutamyl cysteine synthetase, the rate-limiting enzyme in the biosynthetic pathway for glutathione, has an NFκB-activated domain in the promoter region for its gene.

Normally, the ability of cytokines to raise the level of antioxidant defenses offers a measure of protection to host tissues. Nonetheless there is evidence of oxidative damage in a wide range of clinical conditions in which cytokines are produced. Lipid peroxides and increased thiobarbituric acid-reactive substances (TBARS) are present in the blood of patients with septic shock, asymptomatic HIV infection, chronic hepatitis C, breast cancer, cystic fibrosis, diabetes mellitus, and alcoholic liver disease. Peroxides also increase following cancer chemotherapy, open heart surgery, bone marrow transplantation, and hemodialysis.

A pivotal role for glutathione in antioxidant defense

While all antioxidants are important in maintaining robust antioxidant defenses, glutathione is a pivotal member of this group of compounds due to its multifunctional role in maintaining other antioxidants (alpha-tocopherol, ascorbate) in a reduced state, by acting as a reservoir of sulfur amino acids for acute phase protein synthesis, and by functioning as an immunomodulator.

In addition to its important role as a component of antioxidant defense, glutathione can influence aspects of immune function that are related to T lymphocytes. T cell functions can be potentiated by glutathione administration *in vivo*. However the relationship between cellular concentrations and cell numbers is complex. In healthy subjects the numbers of helper (CD4+) and suppressor (CD8+) T lymphocytes increased in parallel with intracellular glutathione concentrations of up to 30 nmol/mg protein. A 7% increase in CD4+ and a 50% increase in CD8+ occurred over the concentration range. However numbers of both subsets declined at concentrations between 30 and 50 nmol/mg protein. When the subjects of the study engaged in a program of intensive physical exercise daily for four weeks, a fall in glutathione concentrations occurred in liver, muscle, and blood. Individuals with glutathione concentrations in the optimal range before exercise, who experienced a fall in concentration after exercise, showed a 30% fall in CD4+ T cell numbers. The decline in T cell number was prevented by administration of *N*-acetyl cysteine, which did not arrest the decline in glutathione concentration. The studies therefore suggest that immune cell function may be sensitive to a range of intracellular sulfhydryl compounds including glutathione and cysteine.

In HIV-positive individuals and patients with AIDS, a reduction in cellular and plasma glutathione has been noted. It is unclear at present whether the depletion in lymphocyte population is related to this phenomenon.

Antioxidant defenses are depleted by infection and trauma

As indicated earlier, the enhancement of antioxidant defenses that occurs during the inflammatory process may not be able to completely protect the subject from tissue damage. Furthermore, a decrease in some components of antioxidant defense may occur in some diseases. Observations in experimental animals and patients indicate that antioxidant defenses become depleted during infection and after injury. In mice infected with the influenza virus there were 27%, 42%, and 45% decreases in the blood levels of vitamin C, vitamin E, and glutathione, respectively. In asymptomatic HIV infection substantial decreases in glutathione in blood and lung epithelial lining fluid have been noted.

In patients undergoing elective abdominal operations the glutathione content of blood and skeletal muscle fell by over 10% and 42% respectively, within 24 h of the operation. While values in blood slowly returned to preoperative values, concentrations in muscle were still depressed 48 h postoperatively. Furthermore reduced tissue glutathione concentration have been noted in hepatitis C, ulcerative colitis, and cirrhosis. In patients with malignant melanoma, metastatic hypernephroma, and metastatic colon cancer, plasma ascorbic acid concentrations fell from normal to almost undetectable levels within 5 days of commencement of treatment with IL-2. In patients with inflammatory bowel disease, substantial reductions in ascorbic acid concentrations occurred in inflamed gut mucosa.

Risks of oxidant damage posed by parenteral feeding with solutions containing PUFAs

Many lipid sources in total parenteral nutrition (TPN) formulations are rich in polyunsaturated fatty acids (PUFAs). Requirements for the antioxidant vitamin E are related to PUFA intake as these fatty acids are susceptible to peroxidation. The risk of increased peroxidation is apparent in patients receiving home TPN. When healthy volunteers and home TPN patients were given a linoleic acid-rich infusion there was a marked rise in breath pentane, indicating increased lipid peroxidation. The intake of vitamin E was 45 mg/day.

Evidence of depleted antioxidant defenses and increased lipid peroxidation in patients receiving home parenteral nutrition has also been shown in a study in which *n*-6-rich TPN was given. Serum malondialdehyde (an index of lipid peroxidation) was positively correlated with *n*-6 PUFA given and negatively correlated with plasma alpha-tocopherol. Clinical measures to improve iron status may unwittingly increase oxidant stress. Normally free iron concentrations are kept at very low levels in tissues by sequestration with binding proteins during inflammation, since the ion catalyzes free radical production. Thus provision of iron to patients experiencing a SIRS is often likely to be harmful.

It can be seen that the antioxidant defenses of the body do not offer complete protection for host tissues against the oxidative molecules produced by the immune system. There is therefore the potential to improve antioxidant defenses. The capacity of the host for enhancement of antioxidant defenses will depend upon the previous and concomitant intakes of nutrients. Synthesis of acute phase proteins and glutathione is influenced by protein intake, sulfur amino acid sufficiency, and glutamine supplementation. The intake of micronutrients such as copper, zinc, and selenium influences the activity of antioxidant enzymes. Other components of the antioxidant defenses are derived directly from the diet and include ascorbic acid, tocopherols, beta-carotene, and a number of less well-characterized phytochemicals (see chapter 14 in *Nutrition and Metabolism*).

Immunomodulation by manipulating antioxidant defences

Without doubt antioxidant defenses provide a potentially effective target for immunomodulation. An impressive number of studies in animal models of infection and trauma in healthy subjects and hospitalized individuals indicate that a wide range of nutrients are able to modulate the functioning of the immune system. These include protein, specific amino acids, PUFAs, copper, zinc, and iron, vitamins B_6, C, E, and riboflavin. All of these nutrients directly or indirectly are linked to antioxidant defense or the ability of the patient to produce an oxidative environment within their tissues. As illustrated in Figure 16.5 the mechanisms whereby the nutrient brings about immunomodulation via changing the antioxidant status varies from nutrients which clearly operate via this mechanism (vitamin C and E) to nutrients which alter the oxidant/antioxidant environment of the cell to a smaller extent as part of their immunomodulatory influence via changes in this cellular characteristic (PUFAs, vitamin B_6, iron, and zinc).

Antioxidant defenses are interlinked and interactive

Many of the components of antioxidant defense interact to maintain the antioxidant capacity of the tissues.

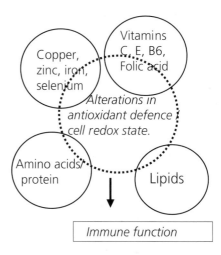

Figure 16.5 Nutrients which modulate immune function by partially influencing antioxidant defenses and cellular redox state.

For example, when oxidants interact with cell membranes, the oxidized form of vitamin E is restored to the antioxidant form through reduction by ascorbic acid. Dehydroascorbic acid formed in this process is reconverted to ascorbic acid by interaction with the reduced form of glutathione. Subsequently, oxidized glutathione formed in the reaction is reconverted to the glutathione by glutathione reductase. In healthy subjects, a daily dose of 500 mg ascorbic acid for six weeks resulted in a 47% increase in glutathione content of red blood cells. Vitamins E and C and glutathione are thus intimately linked in antioxidant defense. Vitamin B_6 and riboflavin, which have no antioxidant properties *per se*, also contribute to antioxidant defenses indirectly. Vitamin B_6 is a cofactor in the metabolic pathway for the biosynthesis of cysteine. Cellular cysteine concentration is rate limiting for glutathione synthesis. Riboflavin is a cofactor for glutathione reductase, which maintains the major part of cellular glutathione in the reduced form (Figure 16.6).

Many potentially immunomodulatory nutrients and pronutrients may operate by enhancing glutathione status. In Figure 16.7 it can be seen that glutathione synthesis might be altered by changes in the supply of the three precursor amino acids by an increase in cysteine supply from *N*-acetyl cysteine treatment, or from an increase in metabolic flux through the transmethylation and transulfuration pathway, assisted by vitamin B_6 and folic acid and from provision of L-2-oxothiazolidine-4-carboxylate (pro-cysteine).

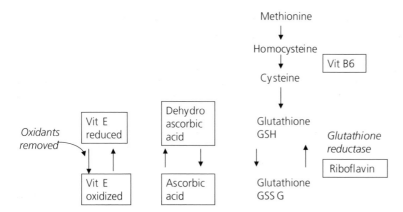

Figure 16.6 Major components of antioxidant defense and their metabolic interrelationships.

The anti-inflammatory and immuno-enhancing influence of antioxidants

There is a growing body of evidence that antioxidants suppress inflammatory components of the response to infection and trauma and enhance components related to cell-mediated immunity. The reverse situation applies when antioxidant defenses become depleted.

Influence of vitamin E intake

Vitamin E exerts modulatory effects on both inflammatory and immune components of immune function. In general, vitamin E deficiency and low tissue vitamin E content enhance components of the inflammatory response and suppress components of the immune response. Dietary vitamin E supplementation brings about the opposite effect. When elderly subjects were supplemented with 800 IU of alpha-tocopherol for 30 days there was a 50% increase in the delayed-type hypersensitivity response, a 65% increase in IL-2 production, and a decrease in oxidative stress as indicated by a major decrease in plasma lipid peroxides and increased TBARS.

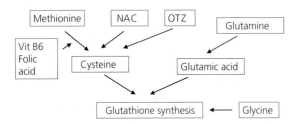

Figure 16.7 Nutrients and pronutrients which contribute to glutathione synthesis. NAC, *N*-acetyl cysteine; OTZ, L-2-oxothiazolidine-4-carboxylate (procysteine).

Studies in animals have demonstrated that vitamin E deficiency impairs cellular and humoral immunity and is associated with an increased incidence of disease. Supplementation of the diet with vitamin E at levels that are several-fold greater than requirements increases resistance to a number of pathogens. Resistance of chickens and turkeys to *Escherichia coli* and of mice to pneumococci was enhanced by vitamin E supplementation. A similar phenomenon may also occur in humans, since epidemiological evidence shows lower incidence of infectious disease in subjects with high plasma alpha-tocopherol concentrations. Rats consuming diets that were deficient in vitamin E and given injections of endotoxin showed a greater degree of anorexia and greater concentrations of plasma α_1-acid glycoprotein and IL-6 than animals consuming adequate amounts of the vitamin. In smokers, a low intake of vitamin E was associated with an increased intensity of the inflammatory response to cigarette smoke. Plasma concentrations of α_1-acid glycoprotein was 50% higher in subjects in the lowest tertile of intake compared with the values for subjects in the highest tertile.

In healthy subjects and smokers, a four-week period of supplementation with 600 IU of alpha-tocopherol resulted in a significant reduction in TNFα production from PBMCs stimulated with endotoxin. Intense exercise of healthy young and elderly subjects results in the appearance of a mild inflammatory response characterized by raised blood IL-1, IL-6, and acute phase protein concentrations. A twice daily supplement of 400 IU of alpha-tocopherol inhibited the response.

Influence of vitamin C intake

The effect of vitamin C status on immune function has been studied extensively. High concentrations of the vitamin are found in phagocytic cells. While the role of the vitamin as a key component of antioxidant defense is well established, most studies have shown only minor effects upon a range of immune functions. Unlike deficiencies in vitamins B_6, E, and riboflavin, deficiency of vitamin C does not cause atrophy of lymphoid tissue. Studies in guinea-pigs have shown that the humoral response is unaffected by vitamin C deficiency but cell-mediated responses are reduced. The function of phagocytic cells is influenced by vitamin C status. While the ability of neutrophils from guinea-pigs affected by scurvy to produce H_2O_2 and kill staphylococci is similar to those from well-fed animals, peritoneal macrophages from animals with scurvy are smaller and have a decreased ability to migrate. However no defect in phagocytic ability of the cells has been noted.

The effect of vitamin C status and large doses of ascorbic acid on the response of healthy volunteers to the common cold virus has been studied in great detail. Only minor effects on immune function have been observed, although a reduction in the severity of symptoms has been noted. In a study of ultra marathon runners, dietary supplementation with 600 mg/day reduced the incidence of upper respiratory tract infections after a race by 50%. It is interesting to note that strenuous exercise has been shown to deplete tissue glutathione content. The interrelationship between glutathione and ascorbic acid may therefore play a role in the effect of exercise on immune function.

When immunological parameters and antioxidant status were measured in adult males fed 250 mg/day of vitamin C for 4 days followed by 5 mg/day for 32 days, plasma ascorbic acid and glutathione decreased and impairment of antioxidant status became evident from a doubling in semen 8-hydroxydeoxyguanosine concentration. A fall in vitamin content in PBMCs was noted and the delayed-type hypersensitivity reactions to seven recall antigens was reduced.

An unconfirmed study has reported that vitamin C supplementation results in clinical improvement in AIDS patients. An in vitro study also showed that a thymocyte cell line infected with HIV, when incubated with calcium ascorbate, glutathione, and N-acetyl cysteine, showed inhibition of HIV replication. The clinical usefulness of this observation is unclear since intravenous administration of ascorbic acid would be necessary to achieve the intracellular concentrations that were shown to be effective in inhibiting viral replication in vitro.

Ascorbic acid may exert its most potent effects upon the inflammatory component of the immune response. In rats that have been made congenitally unable to synthesize ascorbic acid elevated concentrations of acute phase proteins occur in the absence of any applied inflammatory stimulus. The inflammatory influence of cigarette smoke is partly modulated by vitamin C intake. Individuals consuming less than 80 mg/day of vitamin C had plasma ceruloplasmin and CRP levels that were 10% and 59% greater than in individuals with a higher intake of the vitamin.

Influence of vitamin B_6

Although it has no antioxidant properties, vitamin B_6 plays an important part in antioxidant defenses because of its action in the metabolic pathway for the formation of cysteine, which is the rate-limiting precursor in glutathione synthesis. Vitamin B_6 status has widespread effects upon immune function. Animal studies have clearly demonstrated that a deficiency of the vitamin results in large effects on lymphoid tissues. Thymic atrophy occurs and lymphocyte depletion in lymph nodes and spleen has been found in monkeys, dogs, rats, and chickens. Antigen processing was normal; however, the ability to make antibodies to sheep red blood cells was depressed. In human studies the ability to make antibodies to tetanus and typhoid antigens is not seriously affected unless the diet is also deficient in pantothenic acid.

Various aspects of cell-mediated immunity are also influenced by vitamin B_6 deficiency. Skin grafts in rats and mice survive longer during deficiency, and guinea-pigs exhibit decreased delayed-hypersensitivity reactions to bacille Calmette–Guérin (BCG).

Deficiency of vitamin B_6 is rare in humans but can be precipitated with the anti-tuberculosis drug isoniazid. However, experimental deficiency in elderly subjects has been shown to reduce total blood lymphocyte numbers and decrease the proliferative response of lymphocytes to phytohemagglutinin (PHA) and ConA. Likewise, IL-2 production is reduced by vitamin deficiency. Restoration of vitamin B_6 intake to normal by dietary supplements restores immune function. However, intakes that are higher than current recommended values are required to normalize all immune functions, suggesting that optimal immune function can only be achieved in this way. It is unclear, at present, whether a similar situation occurs in younger subjects.

One mechanism for the effect of vitamin B_6 on immune function may be due to the importance of the vitamin in cysteine synthesis, as outlined earlier. Deficiency of the vitamin may limit the availability of cysteine for glutathione synthesis. In rats, vitamin B_6 deficiency resulted in decreases of 12% and 21% in glutathione concentrations in plasma and spleen respectively. In healthy young women large doses of vitamin B_6 (27 mg/day for two weeks) resulted in a 50% increase in plasma cysteine content, presumably by increased flux through the transulfuration pathway of methionine metabolism. As cysteine is a rate-limiting substrate for glutathione synthesis, these findings may have implications for the response to pathogens because of the importance of glutathione in lymphocyte proliferation and antioxidant defense (see Section 16.7). However, while vitamin B_6 has cellular effects on the immune system, evidence is lacking of any effect upon the inflammatory response.

Mechanisms for the anti-inflammatory immuno-enhancing effects of antioxidants

There are a number of candidate mechanisms for the immuno-enhancing, anti-inflammatory actions of antioxidants. Oxidant damage to cells will, indirectly, create a proinflammatory effect by the production of lipid peroxides. This situation may lead to upregulation of NFκB activity, since the transcription factor is activated in endothelial cells cultured with the main dietary n-6 PUFA linoleic acid, and the effect is inhibited by vitamin E and N-acetyl cysteine. A change in the redox state of the cell towards more oxidative conditions will directly lead to activation of NFκB. By 'quenching' oxidants, antioxidants will counteract the trend towards NFκB activation.

Differential effects of oxidants and antioxidants on transcription factor activation

Evidence is emerging that not all transcription factors respond to the effects of antioxidants in the same way. In an *in vitro* study on HeLa cells and cells from human embryonic kidney, both TNF and hydrogen peroxide resulted in activation of NFκB and AP1. Addition of the antioxidant sorbitol to the medium resulted in suppression of NFκB activation (as expected) but activation of AP1 (Figure 16.8). Thus the antioxidant en-

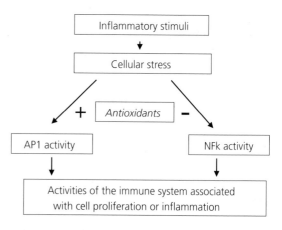

Figure 16.8 An hypothesis to explain the anti-inflammatory and immuno-enhancing effects of antioxidants. AP1, activator protein 1; NFκB, nuclear factor kappa B.

vironment of the cell might exert opposite effects upon transcription factors closely associated with inflammation (e.g. NFκB) and cellular proliferation (AP1).

Further evidence for this biphasic effect is seen when glutathione was incubated *in vitro* with immune cells from young adults. A rise in cellular glutathione content was accompanied by an increase in IL-2 production and the mitogenic response to ConA, and a decrease in production of the inflammatory mediators prostaglandin E2 (PGE2) and leukotriene B4 (LTB4). As indicated earlier, supplementation of elderly subjects with large doses of alpha-tocopherol not only improves IL-2 production and cell-mediated immunity but decreases TBARS in plasma, which could have arisen from a proinflammatory state. Indeed it has been noted by that in healthy elderly subjects there is an increase in proinflammatory cytokine production, which may be linked with the loss of lean tissue that occurs during the aging process.

Modification of the glutathione content of liver, lung, spleen, and thymus in young rats by feeding diets containing a range of casein contents changed immune cell numbers in lung. It was found that the number of lung neutrophils decreased with dietary protein intake and tissue glutathione content in unstressed animals. However, in animals given lipopolysaccharide (LPS), cell numbers related inversely with tissue glutathione content. Addition of methionine to the protein-deficient diets normalized glutathione content and restored lung neutrophil numbers to those seen in unstressed animals fed a diet of adequate protein content.

Thus it can be hypothesized that antioxidants exert an immuno-enhancing effect by activating transcription factors that are strongly associated with cell proliferation (e.g. AP1) and an anti-inflammatory effect by preventing activation of NFκB by oxidants produced during the inflammatory response (Figure 16.8).

16.8 Immunomodulatory effects of lipids

Lipids have been shown to be potent modulators of inflammation – not a surprising fact given that a large number of the modulatory compounds cited earlier are derived from the hydrolysis of membrane phospholipids by the action of phospholipase A2 (prostaglandins, thromboxanes, and leukotrienes), phospholipase C (diacylglycerol (DAG)), phospholipase D (phosphatidic acid), and sphingomyelinases (ceramide). Many of these lipid mediators modulate the activity kinases in the intracellular signaling pathways (e.g. MAP kinases) or transcription factors (e.g. NFκB)

Mode of action of fatty acid composition on cytokine biology

The fats consumed in diets contain widely differing amounts and proportions of unsaturated fatty acids. Many vegetable oils (e.g. corn, safflower, and sunflower oils) are rich in the n-6 PUFA linoleic acid (LA). Saturated animal fats, such as those of beef, lamb, and butter, contain low concentrations of linoleic acid, as does coconut oil. All other fats of plant origin are rich in linoleic acid. Maize, palm, and olive oils and butter contain substantial quantities of the monounsaturated fatty acid oleic acid. Oils from fatty fish are rich in the long-chain n-3 PUFAs eicosapentaenoic acid (EPA) and docosahexaenoic acid (DHA). The n-3 PUFA linolenic acid (LNA) can act as a precursor for EPA and DHA. LNA is derived from leafy vegetables, although none except linseed oil is particularly rich in this nutrient.

The most likely site in the cell where lipids might modulate inflammation is the cell membrane. Dietary unsaturated fatty acids can alter the composition of the fatty acyl chains of membrane phospholipids. Fatty acids may be incorporated into any of the various classes of phospholipids within the membrane: phosphatidyl choline (PC), phosphatidyl ethanolamine (PE), phosphatidyl serine (PS), phosphatidyl inositol (PI), and sphingomyelin (SPH). Thus the nature of the substrate for PG, LT, DAG, phosphatidic acid, and ceramide production may be changed.

The changes in fatty acid composition may also exert a biophysical influence on membrane structure by altering the fluidity characteristics of the membrane. Theoretically changes in fluidity may influence the activity of membrane-associated enzymes important in controlling cytokine production. For example fluidity changes may alter G protein activity, thereby altering the activity of enzyme systems which are influenced by G proteins (e.g. adenylate cyclase, phospholipase A2 (PLA2), and phospholipase C activity). Alterations in membrane phospholipids will also directly influence the synthesis of lipid-derived mediators such as the eicosanoids, DAG, phosphatidic acid, ceramide, and platelet-activating factor.

The fatty acid composition of all of these mediators will reflect membrane phospholipid composition. The pattern of eicosanoid production will be influenced by the fatty acid incorporated into the sn-2 position, as activation of PLA2 will release fatty acid from this location for eicosanoid synthesis. The position is usually occupied by unsaturated fatty acids. Arachidonic acid (AA) is the parent compound of prostanoids and leukotrienes of the 2 and 4 series respectively, whereas EPA is the precursor of the less potent prostanoids and leukotrienes of the 3 and 5 series respectively. Eicosatetraenoic acid (ETA), which is produced under conditions of essential fatty acid deficiency, does not serve as an eicosanoid precursor and thereby dramatically reduces 2-series prostaglandins, protacyclins, and thromboxanes and 4-series leukotrienes. Dietary fat composition may thus modulate the proportions of all three eicosanoid precursors (Figure 16.9).

Influence of fats on responses to inflammatory agents and diseases

In theory, fats may influence inflammation by altering the production of cytokines and other inflammatory mediators, or by changing the sensitivity of target tissues to inflammatory mediators, or by acting at both levels. Lipids also have substantial and profound effects on cellular and humoral aspects of immunity. These aspects are dealt with in detail in chapter 5 of *Nutrition and Metabolism* in this series of textbooks.

In general terms n-3 PUFAs downregulate or inhibit T cell proliferation and function. Mononunsaturated fatty acids may have a similar but less potent effect.

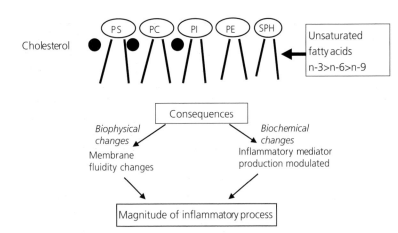

Figure 16.9 The consequences of differential incorporation of unsaturated fatty acids into the membranes of cytokine-producing and cytokine-responsive cells. PS, phosphatidyl serine; PC, phosphatidyl choline; PE, phosphatidyl ethanolamine; PI, phosphatidyl inositol; and SPH, sphingomyelin.

Studies have investigated the influence of lipids upon the responses of animals to bacteria, bacterial extracts, burns, and other forms of injury, and injections of recombinant proinflammatory cytokines. In addition, studies have examined the effects of lipids on *in vivo* and *in vitro* proinflammatory cytokine production, from cells of the immune system. The ability of lipids to modify the gross inflammatory process in both animal models and disease states in humans has also been examined.

Influence of fats on responses to proinflammatory cytokines and inflammatory agents

Numerous studies have shown that fats rich in *n*-3 PUFAs exert a generalized anti-inflammatory influence. Guinea-pigs fed fish oil for six weeks experienced a smaller fever in response to IL-1 than animals fed safflower oil. Likewise rats fed fish oil exhibited a lesser degree of anorexia in response to IL-1 and TNF than animals fed corn oil.

Olive oil and butter, which, like coconut oil, have a low content of linoleic acid, almost without exception suppress both the effects of inflammatory agents that are clearly mediated by eicosanoids, such as anorexia and fever, and those that are not, such as elevation of plasma acute phase protein concentrations and increases in protein synthetic rates in liver, lung, and kidney. Olive oil and butter contain substantial amounts of the monounsaturated fatty acid oleic acid, which may bestow anti-inflammatory properties on these fats.

Addition of olive oil to the diet of rats almost totally suppressed metabolic responses to an endotoxin injec-

tion. Conversely, diets rich in linoleic acid had a proinflammatory influence in animal models of inflammation. The inflammatory response to burn injury in guinea pigs was enhanced by safflower oil when it constituted 30–50% of dietary energy. In rats the degree of anorexia, fall in body temperature, elevation of ceruloplasmin, and increase in liver protein and zinc content in response to endotoxin injections was increased in a stepwise manner when maize oil was included in their diets in amounts of 50, 100, and 200 g/kg.

Although oleic acid is capable of inhibiting incorporation of linoleic acid and arachidonic acid into membrane phospholipids, it is improbable that it is exerting its influence on visceral protein responses by modulating eicosanoid metabolism. *In vitro* studies have shown that oleic acid is also able to activate protein kinase C, which has been implicated in the downregulation of receptors for TNF.

Cholesterol may exert a proinflammatory effect by enhancing cytokine production. Studies on rabbits show that IL-1 and TNF synthesis in the aorta wall in response to an LPS injection was enhanced by inclusion of cholesterol (3 g/kg) in diets containing maize oil. Cholesterol may also exert a more generalized proinflammatory effect. *In vitro* studies on monocytes showed that incubation with cholesterol increased expression of HLA-D subregion products. Cholesterol was also shown to increase the proliferative response of human peripheral blood lymphocytes to PHA.

In summary, it would seem that the intensity of many of the metabolic changes that are part of the inflammatory process is influenced by the unsaturated fatty acid and cholesterol content of the diet. While *n*-6 PUFAs and cholesterol exert a proinflammatory influence, n-3 PUFAs and monounsaturated fatty acids exert the opposite effect.

Influence of fats on cytokine production

Relatively few studies have examined the modulatory effects of lipids on the ability of cells to produce cytokines. In human volunteers supplementation of the diet for six weeks with 18 g/day of a fish oil concentrate rich in EPA and DHA reduced the ability of monocytes to produce IL-1α and β and TNFα and β by at least a third. The effect was still evident 10 weeks after cessation of dietary supplementation. A similar suppressive effect of dietary supplementation with fish oil on IL-1 production by stimulated monocytes was noted in rheumatoid patients and on IL-1, IL-6, and TNF production in young and old women. In the study on rheumatoid patients, olive oil supplements were given to the control group. A fall in ability to produce IL-1 was noted in this group also. The effect did not reach statistical significance; however, the effect is interesting in view of the anti-inflammatory nature of olive oil in animal studies and the suggestion that rheumatoid arthritis is less common in Mediterranean regions of Europe than elsewhere.

Studies on rats, in which the ability of a range of fats with differing unsaturated fatty acid contents to alter cytokine production from peritoneal macrophages was examined, indicated that production of IL-1 related positively to the n-6 PUFA intake and IL-6 production correlated with the total intake of unsaturated fatty acids. The study in rats was partly paralleled by the results of an investigation on the influence of a cholesterol-lowering diet on immune function of middle-aged subjects. A change in n-6 PUFA intake from 6.6 to 8.8% of dietary energy resulted in a 62 and 47% increase in IL-1 and TNF production respectively, from stimulated monocytes. Addition of 0.54% of energy as n-3 PUFAs counteracted this effect and resulted in decreases of 40 and 7% in the production of the two cytokines, respectively.

Influence of fats on inflammatory responses in disease in animal models and humans

Inflammatory symptoms in rheumatoid arthritis, psoriasis, asthma, Crohn's disease, and ulcerative colitis are ameliorated by fish oil. The substantial weight loss which occurs in pancreatic cancer is prevented by a daily supplement of fish oil. A 5-day period of ad-

ministration of TPN containing a mixture of soybean oil, medium-chain triglycerides (MCT), olive oil, and fish oil (SMOF) to surgical patients was found to lower LTB4/LTB5 ratios and shorten hospital stay by 7 days. Fish oil supplementation has been shown to produce a beneficial outcome following renal transplantation in terms of reduced rejection episodes and improved transplant function. It also improves outcome in the rare and generally fatal condition IgA nephropathy.

There are many animal models of acute and chronic inflammation in which fats have been shown to modulate these processes. Fish oil protected pigs, rats, and guinea-pigs from the lethal effects of endotoxin. The oil exerted protective effects in experimental colitis in rats. The oil also reduced the metabolic response to burn injury in guinea-pigs, the number of polymorphonuclear cells in air pouches of rats challenged with bovine serum albumin, and the degree of anorexia and weight loss in mice given the MAC16 colon adenocarcinoma. Diets rich in MCTs produced similar ameliorative effects in the same cancer cachexia model.

Mechanisms whereby fats modulate immune function: observations from experimental studies

The most likely manner in which lipids might modulate proinflammatory cytokine biology is by changing the fatty acid composition of the fatty acyl chains of the phospholipids in cell membranes. The fatty acids compete for incorporation into the phospholipid structure. The affinity for incorporation is in the order linolenic acid > linoleic acid > oleic acid. Furthermore, dietary arachidonic acid and EPA may be incorporated into phospholipids. EPA is incorporated with the highest affinity of all unsaturated fatty acids. Studies in rats indicate that EPA exerts an anti-inflammatory effect by displacing arachidonic acid from the membrane. Other n-3 PUFAs such as DHA and alpha-linolenic acid are much less effective at exerting an anti-inflammatory influence.

The n-6 PUFA gamma-linolenic acid also exerts an anti-inflammatory effect by suppressing IL-1β and TNFα from human PBMCs. This effect has shown clinical efficacy in studies on patients with adult respiratory distress syndrome given the fatty acid in an enteral feed.

Conversion of the n-3, n-6, and n-9 fatty acids to precursors of eicosanoids occurs after they have become attached to the *sn*-2 position of membrane phospholipids. As a consequence of the changes in the fatty acid component of membrane phospholipids, two interrelated phenomena may occur, namely alteration in membrane fluidity and in the products which arise from the hydrolysis of membrane phospholipids.

Changes in fluidity may alter the binding of cytokines and cytokine-inducing agonists to receptors. They may also alter components of the signal transduction process, which leads to alterations in cytokine production or effects.

Changes in membrane fluidity

In theory, a decrease in membrane fluidity would be expected to increase the intensity of the immune/inflammatory response, since in a more rigid membrane cytokines might be able to make contact and bind with greater affinity to their receptors due to a slower velocity of receptors within the membrane. Inclusion of cholesterol in the diets of rabbits, which might be expected to reduce membrane fluidity, enhanced IL-1 and TNF expression in aorta. However both ethanol, which increases fluidity, and sterols, which decrease fluidity, have been shown to inhibit IL-2 production.

When both lateral and rotational fluidity were measured in membranes from peritoneal macrophages and hepatocytes from rats fed a wide range of fats, it was found that in general fluidity assessed by either method is influenced in a similar manner in membranes from both types of cell. There was, however, no consistent relationship between membrane fluidity and the intensity of inflammation. Fish and coconut oils resulted in high lateral fluidity and suppressed proinflammatory cytokine production and responsiveness of tissues to inflammatory agents. However, butter and maize oil resulted in low lateral fluidities but had opposing effects on these parameters of inflammation. Thus the precise nature and significance of alterations in membrane fluidity induced by fat on cytokine-producing and cytokine-sensitive cells requires further investigation.

Implications of experimental observations on lipids and inflammation for inflammatory disease in human populations

With the major decline in infectious disease in populations in industrialized countries attention has been focused on other diseases in which inflammation plays

a part, such as atherosclerosis, rheumatoid arthritis, asthma, inflammatory bowel diseases, and the end stages of heart, lung, kidney, and liver disease.

In many industrialized countries, such as the UK, the USA, and Australia, large increases in the intake of *n*-6 PUFAs have occurred in the last 30 years. In the UK the dietary polyunsaturated to saturated fatty acid ratio doubled between 1972 and 1988. The intake of *n*-6 PUFAs has risen from 4% of dietary energy in the early 1970s to 6% at present. It has been suggested that the upsurge of asthma that has been observed in the UK, Australia, and New Zealand is related to these increases in PUFA intake. For example, the incidence of asthma is lower in Scotland and the more industrialized north of England, than in the south. Intakes of *n*-6 PUFAs are highest in the south of England. Likewise, the incidence of asthma was lower in the eastern part of Germany (where intakes of *n*-6 PUFA were lower and atmospheric pollution is higher) than in the western parts of the country (where larger quantities of *n*-6 PUFA were consumed).

In southern Finland the incidence of asthma in rural children is over three times higher than in children from the more industrialized east of the country. The levels of *n*-6 PUFAs in plasma cholesterol esters are significantly greater in the former region, thus confirming a higher intake of *n*-6 PUFAs. In Japan, where a steady increase in fat intake from 16% to 24% of dietary energy, and a change in the relative amount of *n*-6 to *n*-3 PUFAS in the diet has occurred as a result of 'westernization of the diet' between 1966 and 1985, major rises in the incidence of Crohn's disease have been observed. An epidemiological study reported that an increase in *n*-6 : *n*-3 PUFA ratio from 3.3 to 3.8 was associated with a doubling in the number of newly diagnosed cases of the disease. The unexplained increase in the incidence of eczema and allergic rhinitis, and regional differences of inflammatory disease within countries, may relate to *n*-6 PUFA intake.

While the impact of changes in dietary fat intake on the incidence of inflammatory disease in populations has played little part in the recommendations of governmental committees, recommendations from a recent COMA report (1994), although targeted at coronary heart disease, may have a beneficial influence on the burden of inflammatory disease in the population. The document recommends that 'no further increase in the average intakes of *n*-6 PUFAs occur' and that 'the proportion of the population consuming in excess of about 10% of energy (as *n*-6 PUFAs) should not increase.' For *n*-3 PUFAs it is recommended that 'the population average consumption of long chain *n*-3 PUFAs (should increase) from 0.1 g/d to about 0.2 g/d.'

The incidence of atherosclerotic heart disease is reduced by about 30% in individuals consuming two fish meals per week, reflecting these modest intakes. However, to achieve the dramatic effects in altering disease outcomes in studies previously quoted generally takes at least 1 g of *n*-3 PUFA intake daily. This amount would be present in approximately 3 g of oil from cold water fish.

Possible role of conjugated linoleic acid as an anti-inflammatory and immuno-enhancing agent

Conjugated linoleic acid (CLA) appears particularly in milk fat as the result of hydrogenization of linoleic acid by bacteria in the rumen, resulting in the formation of a number of isomers. CLA enters the bloodstream and is extracted by the mammary gland and incorporated into milk fat. The amount of CLA varies according to the diet of the milk-producing animal. A number of animal feeding studies have shown that CLA has widespread effects upon the actions of the immune system. CLA increases phagocytosis of rat and chicken lymphocytes, increases IL-2 production by lymphocytes from mice, and suppresses TNF and IL-6 production from rat macrophages. The effect on IL-2 may indicate that CLA could be used as an immuno-enhancing agent in patients. The effect on TNF and IL-6 may indicate that it could be used in patients to suppress inflammation. Research still remains to be done in this area.

16.9 Route and content of nutritional provision and immune function and patient outcome

The massive wasting of lean tissue and immunosuppression which can follow trauma and sepsis continues to be a matter of concern in those caring for hospitalized patients. Individuals with these characteristics have increased risk of serious infection and mortality. It is generally thought that a normally nourished individual can manifest an optimal systemic inflammatory response of moderate severity for 7–10 days and accompanying semi-starvation. Beyond this period, and earlier in those with pre-existing malnutrition, exog-

enous nutritional support to meet energy, protein, and other essential nutrient needs are necessary to avoid the consequences of developing malnutrition.

The pioneering work of Dudrick, Rhoads, and co-workers in the USA in the 1970s showed that these outcomes could be influenced by intravenous administration of nutrients by the process of parenteral nutrition. There are many choices to be made in the administration of nutrients by the parenteral route:

- continuous or bolus feeding,
- complete profiles of nutrients administered in 'all-in-one bags' or as separately infused components,
- various lipid emulsions based on natural oils or on reconstructed triglycerides,
- pure amino acid solutions of various composition including essential amino acids only, branched chain amino acid-enriched, branched chain amino acid-enriched with low aromatic amino acids, or glutamine-enriched, complete nutrient mixes, or
- mixtures enriched with nutrients with potential 'nutriceutical' properties.

These developments have arisen from observations in experimental studies which indicate that immune function can be enhanced, or at least preserved, the rate of tissue wasting arrested, or at least slowed, and the number of postoperative complications reduced by specific nutrient provision.

Comparative risks and benefits of enteral and parenteral feeding

There is much debate over whether enteral or parenteral feeding is the more effective in feeding patients. A number of studies have suggested that enteral nutrition produces a better patient outcome in terms of lower rates of infection and shorter hospital stay. An often cited reason for this difference in outcome that has been proposed is the difference in nutritional status of the gut epithelia. In animal models atrophy of the mucosa occurs in animals fed by TPN. However, evidence for a similar phenomenon in humans is weak. In animals, increased bacterial translocation across the gut wall and survival in gut-associated lymph nodes has been noted. Again evidence for a similar phenomenon in patients is lacking.

A more careful review of comparisons of parenteral versus enteral nutrition in randomized clinical trials in trauma patients reveals a serious flaw in study execution. In each study, substantially and significantly more energy was provided in the parenteral arm of the study and substantial hyperglycemia was noted. Given the effect of a blood glucose >220 mg/dl to markedly increase the risk of nosocomial infection, it is reasonable to conclude that this was the likely reason for the differences seen. When similar amounts of energy was provided enterally and parenterally in multiple trauma or severe head injury as well as in routine postoperative care following major abdominal surgery in the malnourished patient, there was no difference in outcome. However, given the relative cost differences and perhaps greater risk of complications of parenteral nutrition in less skilled hands, enteral nutrition, if possible, is preferred.

There is no doubt that TPN is a life-saving therapy in patients who cannot be fed by the enteral route; however, its effects on patients may be less than ideal in certain circumstances.

Adverse effects of total parenteral nutrition

In the early days of TPN it was recognized that reticulo-endothelial cells might become engorged with fat during TPN and that this condition impaired immune function. Most of the evidence was based on animal models with a small amount of data from studies on patients. This phenomenon requires careful consideration since there are data from studies in patients both to support and refute it. In a prospective, crossover study on 23 surgical patients in which two iso-nitrogenous TPN regimens were used (one containing soybean oil, the other lipid free), in vitro IL-2 production and lymphocyte cytotoxicity were increased by inclusion of lipid in the regimen. There was no effect of lipid inclusion on patient outcome. However, a recent report of a prospective randomized study on the effects of inclusion of lipid in TPN on outcome in 60 trauma patients indicates that inclusion of lipid in TPN resulted in increased length of hospitalization (39 days versus 27 days). Length of stay in intensive care also increased (29 days versus 18 days), more days were spent on ventilation, and suppression of T-cell function occurred. Twice as many infections were experienced in the group receiving TPN containing lipid as in the group receiving lipid-free TPN.

The mechanisms for the immunosuppression in the above study is unclear. The immunosuppressive effects of PGE2 were not responsible as PGE2 production by

both stimulated and unstimulated peripheral blood lymphocytes were similar in the two dietary groups.

Overcoming the problems associated with total parenteral feeding

A study in non-surgical patients with HIV infection compared the effect of long-chain triglycerides (LCTs) and a mixture of LCTs/MCTs on immune function. While the LCT infusion decreased the response of lymphocytes to PHA, the LCT/MCT mixture had no effect and resulted in a small but statistically non-significant rise in CD4+/CD8+ ratio. A study on bone marrow transplant patients examined the effect of TPN containing high (25–30%) or low (6–8%) concentrations of lipid on bacteremia and fungemia. The incidence was almost identical in each dietary group, 54 and 55% respectively. A review of many of these studies has suggested that it is the rate of LCT administration that is the likely cause of adverse outcomes. As long as the infusion rates are below 0.11 g/kg per h adverse effects were not seen. This is equivalent to 1 liter of 10% fat (100 g) over 12 h.

In many comparative studies in patients as suggested above, significantly more calories were provided to the parenteral groups and this may have resulted in overfeeding, thereby increasing complication rates. Certainly overzealous provision of nutrients by the parenteral route to critically ill patients is associated with substantial metabolic problems:

- Infusion of glucose at rates greater than 5 mg/kg per min is associated with hyperglycemia, hyperinsulinemia, and increased CO_2 production.
- Administration of more than 2 g of lipid/kg body weight per day results in fatty deposition in liver, hepatomegaly, elevated serum transaminase concentrations, impaired phagocytosis, and neutrophil chemotaxis, and in some studies exaggerated proinflammatory and vasoconstrictive eicosanoid production.
- Administration of more than 2 g protein/kg body weight per day results in increased ureagenesis and impaired renal function if there is pre-existing renal disease.

At least one of the complications, hyperglycemia, increases the risk of nosocomial infections.

Furthermore it is likely that both parenteral and enteral feeding will only show beneficial effects if patients are malnourished when feeding starts. This is not an altogether surprising finding because the metabolic processes which follow trauma and infection, as were outlined earlier (Section 16.3), result in the release of substrate from endogenous sources to supply the immune system. In a well-fed individual these resources would be plentiful. This would not be the case in a malnourished subject. However overfeeding is not helpful in this setting and can be harmful. Thus parenteral nutrition can be looked upon as an effective form of nutrition, when used appropriately, but one which carries with it a higher risk of error than feeding by the enteral route.

Finally in these studies, cited above, two important variables must be considered – the presence of malnutrition and severity of the systemic inflammatory response. Where malnutrition existed nutritional support was more likely to be efficacious, and the sicker the patient the more likely nutritional benefit could be achieved. Parenteral and enteral nutrition are about equally effective if one or both of these conditions are met.

16.10 Perspectives on the future

Evidence to date strongly supports the effectiveness of parenteral or enteral nutrition to improve outcome in the malnourished and/or the seriously stressed patient. Given that nutritional repletion is not possible in the stressed patient and that overfeeding can be harmful, strong evidence is developing that modest energy intakes at 75–100% of energy expenditure and protein intakes at 1.2–1.5 g/kg will optimally support the systemic inflammatory response while limiting the risk of adverse consequences related to overfeeding. It was recently shown that 1 liter of 7% amino acids and 20% dextrose providing 70 g protein and about 1000 kcal is as effective clinically in critically ill patients for the first 10 days of hospitalization as energy provided to meet estimated energy needs with somewhat less risk of feeding-related complications.

A second major development is the commercial availability of immune-enhancing diets containing various mixtures of *n*-3 PUFAs, arginine, glutamine, and ribonucleic acids. These enteral formulas have demonstrated efficacy in postoperative feeding of malnourished cancer patients and in the more seriously stressed trauma patients. In a metanalysis of more than 1000 patients, the use of these diets was shown to reduce the length of stay in hospital by 2.9 days, reduce the time spent on requiring support on a ventilator by 2.6 days, and to result in a reduction in infection rates. These results are clearly encouraging. Given the limited efficacy demonstrated, so far, of a variety of pharmacologic agents in adult respiratory distress syndrome or sepsis in the critically ill, these positive benefits of simple nutritional therapy confirm the importance of nutritional support in the critically ill.

For the future, two strategies that may bear fruit in improving the efficacy of immunonutrients are first, to develop active nutrients that influence patient outcome and secondly, to understand the precise relationship between the genetic characteristics of patients and their responsiveness (or not) to immunonutrients.

References and further reading

Bistrian BR. Novel lipid sources in parenteral and enteral nutrition. *Proc Nutr Soc* 1997; 56: 471–477.

Bistrian BR. Acute phase proteins and the systemic inflammatory response. *Crit Care Med* 1999; 27: 452–453.

Bistrian BR, Schwartz J, Istfan NW. Cytokines, muscle proteolysis, and the catabolic response to infection and inflammation. *Proc Soc Exp Biol Med* 1992; 200: 220–223.

COMA (Committee on Medical Aspects of Food Policy). Nutritional aspects of cardiovascular disease. Report of the Cardiovascular Review Group. *Rep Health Soc Subj (Lond)* 1994; 46: 1–186.

Gadek J, DeMichele S, Karlstad M *et al.* Effect of enteral feeding with eicosapentaenoic acid, gamma-linolenic acid and antioxidants in patients with acute respiratory distress syndrome. *Crit Care Med* 1999; 27: 1409–1420.

Grimble RF. Interaction between nutrients, pro-inflammatory cytokines and inflammation. *Clin Sci* 1996; 91: 121–130.

Grimble RF. Effect of antioxidative vitamins on immune function with clinical applications. *Int J Vitamin Nutr Res* 1997; 67: 312–320.

Grimble RF. Dietary lipids and the inflammatory response. *Proc Nutr Soc* 1998; 57: 1–8.

Paoloni-Giacobino A, Grimble R, Pichard C. Genomic interactions with disease and nutrition. *Clin Nutr* 2003; 22: 507–514.

17
The Heart and Blood Vessels

Stephen Wheatcroft, Brian Noronha, and Mark Kearney

Key messages

- Nutrition and diet play a key role in the development of atherosclerosis, hypertension, and heart failure.
- These diseases are currently the leading cause of death in developed countries and are set to become the most common cause of death worldwide in the next two decades.
- The amount and type of dietary fat consumed in the diet play a fundamental role in the development and management of atherosclerosis.
- An increased plasma concentration of low-density lipoprotein (LDL) cholesterol is a key risk factor for the development of coronary heart disease, and reducing LDL levels, by diet or drugs, is a fundamental goal of disease prevention.

- Lifestyle changes such as dietary modification are useful adjuncts to antihypertensive drug therapy in individuals with hypertension and, if adopted on a large scale, may reduce the incidence of coronary heart disease and stroke in the population.
- Malnutrition (cancer cachexia) can be seen in up to 30% of patients with severe chronic heart failure.
- Although the results of trials using vitamin and mineral supplements have been disappointing, achieving a high intake of beneficial micronutrients through diets rich in fruit and vegetables such as the 'Mediterranean style diet' may contribute to the reduced incidence of coronary heart disease.

17.1 Introduction

Diseases of the heart and blood vessels are the commonest causes of death in developed countries, and over the next 20 years will become the most important cause of death worldwide. The evidence that nutritional factors are central to the etiology of cardiovascular disorders such as atherosclerosis, hypertension, and cardiac failure is compelling. Diet therefore plays a key role in their management.

Atherosclerosis underlies the majority of vascular disorders as illustrated in Figure 17.1. Atherosclerotic diseases, and in particular coronary heart disease, form the focus of this chapter. Knowledge of the pathobiology of atherosclerosis is vital to understanding the ways in which nutrients may be implicated in its development and the chapter begins with a review of the processes involved.

Dietary fats are the most important nutritional determinants of coronary heart disease and the evidence for the principal role of saturated fat is discussed in depth. The evolving roles of monounsaturated and polyunsaturated fatty acids are also explored. Plasma lipoproteins are thought to be integral to the link between dietary fats and vascular disease and a summary is provided of lipoprotein types, lipoprotein metabolism, and the common dyslipidemias. An overview of lipid-lowering drugs is accompanied by a summary of

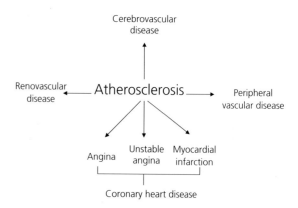

Figure 17.1 The central role of atherosclerosis in cardiovascular disorders.

the landmark clinical trials that support the benefits of these agents.

Recent studies highlight the importance of factors other than dietary saturated fats and plasma lipids in the prevention of coronary heart disease. The roles of antioxidants, proteins, and alcohol are discussed. In particular, the evidence for a protective effect of a Mediterranean-style diet and a diet high in fish oils is discussed.

This chapter also summarizes the role of dietary factors in the etiology of hypertension, stroke, and peripheral vascular disease and discusses the nutritional aspects of chronic heart failure, one of the most frequent sequelae of coronary heart disease. The chapter concludes with an outline of the contribution of micronutrients to cardiovascular disorders.

17.2 Atherosclerosis

Atherosclerosis is the pathological process that underlies the majority of vascular diseases. The atherosclerotic plaque is a collection of lipid, inflammatory cells, smooth muscle cells, and fibrous tissue within the vessel wall. Atherosclerotic plaques may lead to clinical problems by two principal mechanisms. First, bulky plaques encroach upon the vessel lumen, restricting blood flow by reducing the vessel internal diameter and lead to ischemia in organs and tissues supplied by that vessel. Secondly, plaques may rupture and stimulate localized platelet aggregation and clot formation, which cause symptoms either by embolizing and occluding smaller vessels downstream, or by occluding the vessel at the site of the plaque and causing ischemia or infarction of the target organ.

The arterial wall consists of three layers: the intima, media, and adventitia (see Figure 17.2). Atherosclerosis is primarily a disease of the innermost layer, the intima, which comprises smooth muscle cells lined by a single layer of endothelial cells. The endothelium provides a barrier between the constituents of circulating blood and the remainder of the vessel wall. The importance of the endothelium, however, far exceeds its role as a physical barrier. Endothelial cells maintain vascular homeostasis by secreting a number of locally acting substances, which exert effects on neighboring cells in the vessel wall and cells within the vessel lumen. Endothelial production of substances such as nitric oxide, which promote vasodilatation and inhibit platelet aggregation, is of vital importance in maintaining vessel health.

The presence of coronary heart disease risk factors leads to the loss of the protective actions of the endothelium, triggering the development of atherosclerosis. One of the earliest events in this process is the adhesion of circulating leukocytes (monocytes) to dysfunctional/damaged endothelium. This process is facilitated by the expression of binding proteins known

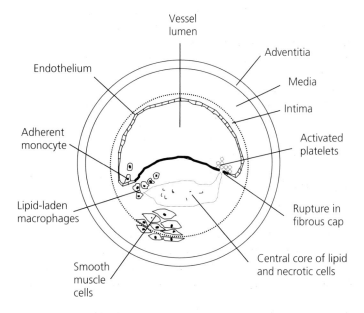

Figure 17.2 The atherosclerotic plaque.

as adhesion molecules on the surface of dysfunctional endothelial cells. Once bound, adherent monocytes migrate into the intima and transform into macrophages and are joined by other leukocytes, such as T lymphocytes, in mediating a complex inflammatory response. The macrophages within the intima avidly take up lipid and change into lipid-laden foam cells, giving rise to a lesion known as the fatty streak. Fatty streaks are the earliest visible manifestation of atherosclerosis and are detectable in the aorta and coronary arteries in humans from a very young age.

Inflammatory cells within fatty streaks secrete cytokines and growth factors that fuel the gradual progression of the fatty streak to a mature atherosclerotic plaque. Platelets adhering to adjacent endothelium provide another source of cytokines and growth factors. Smooth muscle cells migrate from the media to the intima in response to growth factors and form the bulk of the plaque. Macrophages continue to accumulate lipid, principally in the form of cholesterol esters. The cholesterol is taken up into the vessel wall from the circulation, where it is carried by specialized proteins known as lipoproteins.

Low-density lipoprotein (LDL) is the most atherogenic circulating lipoprotein. This is most avidly taken up by macrophages in the plaque after it has been oxidized. LDL oxidation, therefore, is a crucial step in atherosclerosis and increased 'oxidant stress' in the vascular wall is a feature of many pro-atherosclerotic states (such as diabetes mellitus, smoking, and hypertension).

A mature atherosclerotic plaque consists of a connective tissue cap, smooth muscle cells, macrophages, and other inflammatory cells, and a central core of lipid-rich, necrotic debris (see Figure 17.2).

Two main types of plaque are described. 'Stable' plaques have a thick (often calcified) fibrous cap, they have a low propensity to rupture, and form a chronic obstruction to blood flow. 'Unstable' plaques have a thin, friable cap, which is prone to rupture, exposing the potent thrombogenic lipid core to blood within the vascular lumen. When plaques rupture, platelet aggregation and initiation of the clotting cascade leads to thrombus formation. Unstable plaques are typically less bulky and encroach less upon the vessel lumen than stable plaques and may be asymptomatic until plaque rupture occurs. Following rupture, however, thrombus may completely occlude the vessel and lead to infarction in the territory supplied by that vessel.

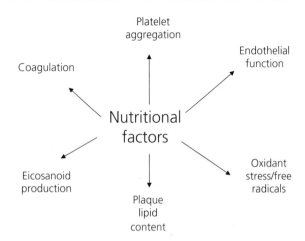

Figure 17.3 The role of nutritional factors in atherosclerosis.

Figure 17.3 illustrates the way in which nutritional factors may interact with the multiple biological processes involved in the development of atherosclerosis.

17.3 Dietary lipids and coronary heart disease

There is compelling evidence that dietary lipids play a fundamental role in the development of atherosclerosis. These data have accrued over many years from a combination of epidemiologic studies revealing an association between dietary fat consumption and the incidence of coronary heart disease, experimental studies showing that feeding lipids to animals causes atherosclerosis, and studies in which changing lipid consumption in humans reduces the risk of disease.

Before these are discussed, it is necessary to review the principal types of dietary fats and how these are classified.

Types of dietary lipids

Lipids are hydrocarbon-based organic molecules that are insoluble in water. Figure 17.4 illustrates the way in which lipids are classified as 'simple' or 'complex' depending on whether they are unmodified or have been esterified by the addition of a molecule containing an alcohol group. Simple lipids are further divided into saturated, monounsaturated, and polyunsaturated forms depending upon the number of double bonds within their structure (see Figure 17.4).

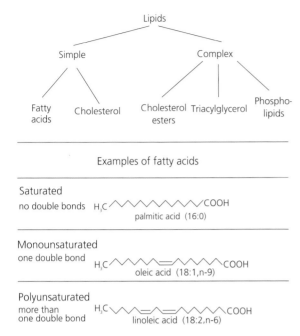

Figure 17.4 Types of lipids.

Table 17.1 shows the main dietary sources of these fats.

Biochemically, fatty acids are described by a numerical code which defines the following:

- the number of carbon atoms within the molecule,
- the number of double bonds, and
- the position of the first double bond as counted from the terminal carbon atom.

Table 17.1 Food sources of types of dietary fats

Type of fat	Food source
Saturated fats	Dairy products
	Beef
	Lamb
	Poultry
	Pork
Monounsaturated fats	Olive oil
	Canola oil
Polyunsaturated fats	Margarines
	Vegetable oils (corn, sunflower, safflower, soy)
	Fatty fish and fish oils
Cholesterol	Egg yolks
	Meats
	Dairy products

For example, oleic acid is described as (18:1,*n*-9) because it contains 18 carbon atoms and 1 double bond, with the double bond situated 9 carbon atoms from the terminal end.

The link between saturated fat consumption and coronary heart disease

Epidemiology

Cross-population studies allow the identification of factors which may predispose to coronary heart disease in groups with substantially different diets and rates of coronary heart disease. The Seven Countries Study, which began in 1958, was a classic cross-population study in which the relationship between dietary composition and coronary heart disease mortality was assessed in more than 12 000 men (aged 40–59 years), living in Japan, Italy, Greece, the Netherlands, the former Yugoslavia, Finland, and the USA. The study demonstrated that mortality from coronary heart disease is strongly related to the mean serum cholesterol level in a population, which in turn is strongly associated with the average intake of saturated fat (Figure 17.5).

Comparing coronary heart disease rates between populations suffers from a number of potential confounding effects, including genetic differences between the populations studied. This was addressed by the Ni Hon San Study, which followed migrants from Japan (Nippon) to Hawaii (Honolulu) and California (San Francisco). Japanese migrants living in Honolulu and San Francisco consumed significantly greater proportions of total fat in the diet, and had higher mean total cholesterol levels, than Japanese natives. This was associated with a significant increase in coronary heart disease mortality rates in the migrants (Figure 17.6).

Further studies performed within populations are consistent with cross-population studies in showing a significant correlation between consumption of total and saturated fat and coronary heart disease mortality. Within-population studies have also been instrumental in determining which individual risk factors predispose to coronary heart disease. For example, long-term follow-up of residents of Framingham, a small town in the USA, has identified several important predictors of increased coronary heart disease risk. These include total cholesterol, LDL cholesterol, HDL cholesterol (inversely related to coronary heart disease), hypertension, smoking, and diabetes. Framingham

(a)

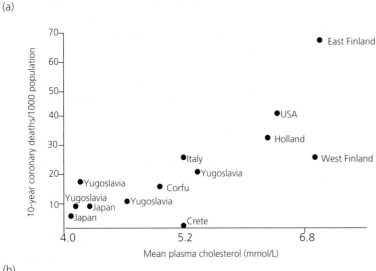

(b)

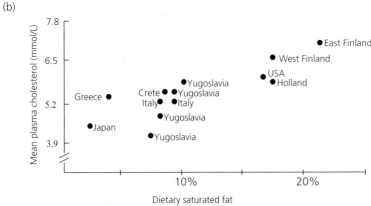

Figure 17.5 The Seven Countries Studies.

data have been used to construct risk factor charts and scoring systems to predict the risk of coronary heart disease in a given individual. Whilst caution must be employed in extrapolating data from a single population to other, potentially different populations, such tools have proved extremely useful in clinical practice.

A number of other within-population studies have strengthened the evidence of an association between plasma cholesterol levels and coronary heart disease. The Multiple Risk Factor Intervention Trial (MRFIT) is of particular relevance as it studied over 360 000 men. The data demonstrate convincingly that there is a continuous and graded relationship between serum total cholesterol and coronary heart disease mortality (Figure 17.7).

The British Regional Heart Study followed 7735 men chosen at random from general practices in 24 towns in England, Scotland, and Wales to assess the impact of variations in personal, economic, and social factors on coronary heart disease. Again, there was strong, graded association between total cholesterol and the risk of a major coronary event, even after adjustment for other risk factors.

Experimental evidence

Further support that dietary fats play a role in the development of atherosclerosis comes from studies in animals, which demonstrate a direct link between consumption of saturated fat, increased plasma cholesterol levels, and atherosclerosis. Feeding animals such as rabbits and non-human primates a diet high in saturated fat leads to predictable elevations of total and LDL cholesterol and the subsequent development of vascular intimal lesions characteristic of human

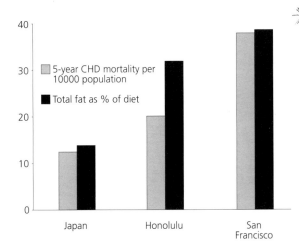

Figure 17.6 The Ni-Hon-San Study.

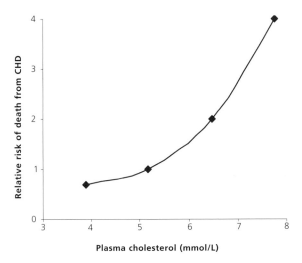

Figure 17.7 The relationship between plasma cholesterol and death from coronary heart disease (the MRFIT Study). Reprinted with permission from Elsevier (*The Lancet* 1986, **ii**, 933–936).

atherosclerosis. Furthermore, reduction of blood cholesterol levels by dietary modification leads to regression of established atherosclerosis in these animals.

Animal studies also show that certain fats, particularly the long-chain saturated fatty acid stearic acid, are able to induce platelet aggregation and thrombus formation. In contrast, diets rich in (*n*-3) polyunsaturated fatty acids reduce the incidence of arterial thrombosis in animals and lower the predisposition to fatal cardiac rhythm disturbances in models of coronary artery occlusion.

The effect of reducing saturated fat consumption on the risk of coronary heart disease

Although epidemiological and experimental studies provide persuasive evidence for a major role of saturated fat in the development of coronary heart disease, proof of its involvement requires that dietary modification, such reducing the consumption of saturated fat, leads to a decrease in the incidence of coronary heart disease.

In fact, a large number of clinical trials performed over the last half century have demonstrated that diets low in saturated fat reduce the incidence of coronary events. As it is difficult in clinical trials to precisely regulate the food intake of free-living subjects in the community, many diet-intervention studies have been centered on residents living in institutions or hospitals. Table 17.2 illustrates a selection of intervention trials of dietary modification.

In the first large-scale trial of an experimental diet, the Finnish Mental Hospital Study, over 10 000 patients in psychiatric hospitals were given a diet low in saturated fat. This led to a significant reduction in plasma cholesterol and coronary heart disease mortality.

The Los Angeles Veterans Administration Study randomly assigned men living in a war veteran's home to an experimental diet low in saturated fat or to control diet. Subjects consuming the experimental diet experienced a 31% decrease in cardiovascular events.

The Oslo trial investigated the effects of dietary and smoking advice in 1232 healthy men aged 40–49 years. These men, who were at high risk of cardiovascular disease due to a high prevalence of hypercholesterolemia and cigarette smoking, were randomly allocated either to an intervention group, who received dietary and antismoking advice; or to a control group, who did not receive any advice. The recommended diet was low in saturated fat and high in fiber. During the course of the study, there was a 47% reduction in the incidence of myocardial infarction and sudden death in the intervention group.

Not all intervention studies of a diet in saturated fat have yielded positive results. For example, the Minnesota Coronary Survey involved feeding 9057 men and women living in psychiatric hospitals and nursing homes in Minnesota a low saturated fat diet. Despite a reduction of 14% in mean serum cholesterol, there were no significant differences in the rates of myocardial infarction and sudden cardiac death. It is possible

Table 17.2 Selected studies assessing the effects of modified fat diets on cardiovascular outcomes

Study	Date of publication	Subjects	Age (years)	Design	Duration (years)	% Change in total cholesterol	Outcome
Finnish Mental Hospital Study	1968 & 1979	5497 M&F	>15	Crossover Low saturated fat	6	−12 to 18	53% reduction in CHD mortality in men (P < 0.002)
Los Angeles Veterans Administration Study	1968	846 M	50–89	Double-blind Randomized Low saturated fat	5–8	−13	31% reduction in MI, CHD mortality, stroke, ruptured aneurysm, ischemic gangrene (P < 0.01)
Oslo Primary Prevention Trial	1981	1232 M	40–49	Randomized Low saturated fat, high fiber Anti-smoking advice	5	−13	47% reduction in MI and sudden death (P = 0.028)
Minnesota Coronary Survey	1989	9057 M&F	All	Double-blind Randomized Low saturated fat, high polyunsaturated fat	<4.5	−14	No significant difference in MI or sudden death

that the negative results reflect a low baseline cholesterol and young age of the study population.

✳ Moreover, saturated fat intake in this study was replaced by *n*-6 polyunsaturated fatty acids. It is now recognized that increasing consumption of *n*-6 fatty acids without increasing *n*-3 fatty acids may unfavorably disrupt the balance of eicosanoid production and offset the benefits of LDL reduction (see later). Such a diet is no longer recommended.

Analysis of pooled data from all dietary intervention studies with over two years of follow-up reveals that modification of dietary fat intake leads to a modest but important reduction in the risk of coronary heart disease (see Further reading).

The effect of saturated fats on plasma cholesterol and atherosclerosis

The principal way in which saturated fats contribute to atherosclerosis is likely to be by increasing plasma concentrations of LDL cholesterol. This is mediated, at least in part, by a decrease in LDL cholesterol catabolism, possibly by saturated fats inducing a reduction in LDL receptor numbers or decreased cell membrane fluidity. LDL is taken up from the circulation into the vessel wall, where it makes up an important part of the atherosclerotic plaque. Macrophages within the plaque become activated after acquiring oxidized LDL and secrete a number of substances, which may further promote atherosclerosis progression.

Saturated fats vary in their ability to raise plasma LDL cholesterol. Myristic and palmitic acids have been reported to possess the greatest cholesterol-raising potential, whereas stearic acid has little effect on plasma cholesterol levels (although interestingly may still be atherogenic).

Dietary cholesterol and coronary heart disease

Cholesterol is a component of a normal diet and is present at high levels in foods such as eggs, dairy products, and red meats. Cholesterol esters form a fundamental part of the atherosclerotic plaque and it has been known for many years that feeding animals with a diet high in cholesterol leads to atherosclerosis. Moreover, epidemiologic studies reveal a strong positive relationship between the intake of dietary cholesterol and the incidence of coronary heart disease in humans. Interpretation of these data, however, is complicated by the fact that cholesterol-rich foods are often also high in saturated fats. The strong association between dietary saturated fats and coronary heart disease has been discussed. In fact, dietary cholesterol appears to be a less potent determinant of plasma cholesterol levels than are the dietary fatty acids, particularly saturated fatty acids. The effect of lowering dietary cholesterol intake independently of changes in saturated fat consumption on coronary heart disease incidence has not been studied.

Nonetheless, most dietary strategies for protection from coronary heart disease recommend a reduction in intake of both saturated fat and dietary cholesterol. It is important, however, to be aware of the distinction between a 'cholesterol-lowering' diet and a 'low-cholesterol' diet.

Dietary polyunsaturated fats and coronary heart disease

Dietary polyunsaturated fats are divided into two main families: *n*-6 and *n*-3, according to the position of the double bond in their molecular structure. Linoleic acid (*n*-6) and alpha-linolenic acid (*n*-3) are found in plants and vegetable oils and are termed essential fatty acids as they are not synthesized by humans. Once ingested, however, these essential fatty acids are biochemically processed (by desaturation and elongation) to form long-chain fatty acids (Figure 17.8). Long-chain polyunsaturated fatty acids are also contained in the diet in, for example, fish oils.

Long-chain polyunsaturated fatty acids are important in the synthesis of eicosanoids – potent biologically active substances which act locally within cells and tissues to regulate processes such as vessel tone, inflammation, and platelet aggregation. *n*-6 and *n*-3 fatty acids compete for enzymes in each other's metabolic pathways, so that high levels of linoleic acid, for example, may inhibit the conversion of linolenic acid to its longer chain forms. The relative abundance of *n*-6 and *n*-3 polyunsaturated fatty acids in the diet, therefore, may determine the relative production of pro- and antiatherosclerotic eicosanoids. The balance between dietary *n*-6 and *n*-3 fatty acids is also important as the two families compete for incorporation into cell membranes. *n*-3 fatty acids exert beneficial effects on membrane fluidity and ion transport, and may lead

n-6 family	n-3 family
18:2,n-6 Linoleic acid	18:3,n-3 Linolenic acid
↓	↓
18:3,n-6	18:4,n-3
↓	↓
20:3,n-6	20:4,n-3
↓	↓
20:4,n-6 Arachidonic acid	20:5,n-3 Eicosapentaenoic acid
↓	↓
18:2,n-6	22:5,n-3
↓	↓
18:2,n-6 Docosapentaenoic acid	22:6,n-3 Docosahexaenoic acid

Figure 17.8 Families of polyunsaturated fatty acids.

to clinically relevant cardioprotective effects (see Fish, n-3 fatty acids, and sudden death, page 286).

Polyunsaturated fatty acids have traditionally been used as substitutes for saturated fatty acids in low saturated fat diets. When the potential health implications of reducing saturated fat intake first became apparent, the food industry replaced many traditional sources of fat (such as lard and butter) with vegetable oils and margarines. These were principally derived from sunflower, safflower, and corn oils, which are high in linoleic acid. The n-6 fatty acid content of the UK diet, therefore, has risen substantially over the last 20 years without a corresponding increase in n-3 fatty acids. Although such a pattern is effective in reducing plasma LDL cholesterol, there are concerns that a high ratio of dietary n-6 to n-3 fatty acids may not reduce cardiovascular risk where the overall intake of n-3 fats is low. The benefits of increasing the intake of n-3 fatty acids have become apparent in the light of recent clinical trials (see Fish, n-3 fatty acids, and sudden death).

Foods rich in n-3 fatty acids include seed oils (e.g. linseed oil, rapeseed oil, soya oil, walnut oil), nuts (e.g. walnuts, peanuts), meat (e.g. beef), green leafy vegetables (e.g. spinach), and oily fish (such as tuna, salmon, mackerel, sardines, and herring).

Dietary monounsaturated fats and coronary heart disease

Monounsaturated fatty acids contain one double bond in their molecular structure and are found in all animal products and vegetables. Rich dietary sources include olives, rapeseed, avocado, nuts, meat, and peanut oil. Early studies suggested that dietary monounsaturated fatty acids had a neutral effect on plasma lipoprotein levels. More recently, however, it has become apparent that monounsaturates, when substituted for dietary saturated fatty acids, lead to reductions in LDL cholesterol and triacylglycerols (TAGs) and small increases in HDL cholesterol.

Oleic acid is present in large amounts in olive oil, an important source of dietary lipid in Mediterranean countries. The long life expectancy and low risk of coronary heart disease in some Mediterranean countries, such as Crete, has led to the promotion of a Mediterranean-style diet as being cardioprotective. The Mediterranean-style diet is dealt with in detail later in this chapter.

Dietary trans-fatty acids and coronary heart disease

Fatty acids exist in two molecular configurations known as cis- or trans-isomers. Vegetable oils largely comprise cis-fatty acids, where the hydrogen groups are on the same side of the carbon chain (Figure 17.9). In contrast, trans-isomers contain hydrogen moieties on opposite sides of the carbon chain. Trans-fatty acids are present naturally at low levels in the diet but the majority are formed artificially by the hydrogenation of vegetable oils. Hydrogenation converts liquid vegetable oils to a semi-solid state and is widely used in the manufacture of hard margarines and other processed foods. Diets high in trans-fatty acids do not have a beneficial effect on the lipoprotein profile and may,

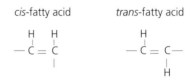

Figure 17.9 cis- and trans-fatty acids.

in fact, lead to elevation of LDL and reduction of HDL cholesterol levels. For this reason, it is recommended that the consumption of hydrogenated vegetable oils is kept to a minimum and margarines low in *trans*-fatty acids are preferred.

17.4 Plasma lipoproteins

An increased plasma concentration of LDL cholesterol is a key risk factor for the development of coronary heart disease, and reducing LDL levels, by diet or drugs, is a fundamental goal of disease prevention. In recent years, the importance of more subtle changes in the plasma lipid profile has emerged. Although a detailed description of plasma lipoproteins is beyond the scope of this chapter, a basic knowledge of their structure and metabolism is integral to understanding the mechanisms of cardiovascular risk reduction.

The two major lipids in plasma, cholesterol and TAG, are insoluble in an aqueous environment and therefore circulate in association with specialized proteins (apoproteins) in complexes known as lipoproteins. Lipoproteins consist of a central lipid core of cholesterol esters and TAGs, surrounded by an outer layer comprising phospholipids, free cholesterol, and apoproteins (Figure 17.10). Apoproteins play an important role in lipoprotein metabolism by interacting with cellular receptors and enzymes.

Plasma lipoproteins are classified in to five groups according to their density, which determines the way the lipoproteins separate when subjected to ultracentrifugation. Table 17.3 shows the way in which lipid distribution and apoprotein composition varies between the lipoprotein classes.

- *LDL cholesterol* makes up approximately 70% of total serum cholesterol. It contains a single apoprotein,

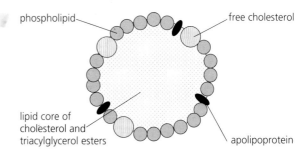

Figure 17.10 Lipoprotein structure.

apo B. LDL is the major atherogenic lipoprotein, and delivers cholesterol to the vessel wall where it is incorporated into atherosclerotic plaque. Oxidation of LDL significantly increases its atherogenicity.
- *HDL cholesterol* normally makes up 20–30% of the total serum cholesterol. HDL levels are inversely correlated with the risk of coronary heart disease. HDL helps to protect against atherosclerosis, mainly by carrying cholesterol away from the vessel wall to the liver in a process known as reverse cholesterol transport.
- *Very low density lipoproteins* (VLDL) are TAG-rich lipoproteins, but contain 10–15% of serum cholesterol. VLDL are produced by the liver and are precursors of LDL. VLDL may be degraded in the circulation to form VLDL remnants, which are rich in cholesterol and may contribute to atherosclerosis.
- *Intermediate density lipoproteins* (IDL) are produced by the catabolism of VLDL. Their role in atherosclerosis is not well defined. In clinical practice, IDL is measured as part of the LDL fraction.
- *Chylomicrons* are TAG-rich lipoproteins, which are formed in the intestine from dietary fat and pass into the bloodstream. When partially degraded, chylomicrons (then known as chylomicron remnants) may carry some atherogenic potential.

Table 17.3 Composition of plasma lipoproteins

| | Composition (%) | | | | | |
	Cholesterol (free)	Cholesterol (esters)	Triacylglycerol	Phospholipid	Protein	Major apolipoproteins
Chylomicrons	1	3	85	9	2	B_{48}, E, C-II
VLDL	7	13	50	20	10	B_{100}, E, C-II
IDL	12	22	26	22	8	B_{100}, E
LDL	8	37	10	20	25	B_{100}
HDL	2	5	4	24	55	A-I, A-II

17.5 Lipoprotein metabolism

The plasma lipoproteins transport fats within the circulation. These have either been absorbed from the intestine, or manufactured endogenously. Lipoprotein metabolism is characterized by complex interactions between lipoproteins of different classes, regulatory enzymes, and cellular receptors. These may be simplified by considering three main areas: the exogenous pathway, the endogenous pathway, and reverse cholesterol transport. These are illustrated in schematic form in Figure 17.11.

Exogenous pathways

After digestion, dietary cholesterol and fatty acids are absorbed within the intestine and re-esterified to form TAGs and cholesterol esters in intestinal mucosal cells. Here they are packaged with apoproteins, phospholipids, and cholesterol to form chylomicrons. Apolipoprotein B-48, essential for chylomicron formation, is added by the action of microsomal transfer protein.

Chylomicrons are secreted into intestinal lymphatics and carried by the thoracic duct into the bloodstream.

Once in the bloodstream, TAGs within chylomicrons are rapidly hydrolyzed to free fatty acids and glycerol by lipoprotein lipase, an enzyme bound to vascular endothelial cells within muscle and adipose tissue. The resulting fatty acids are either delivered to muscle as fuel or re-esterified and stored as TAGs in adipose tissue. During the process of TAG hydrolysis, chylomicrons acquire cholesterol ester from other lipoproteins, such as mature HDL, in exchange for TAGs by the action of cholesterol ester transfer protein. The particles become progressively depleted in TAGs and enriched in cholesterol esters and acquire apoprotein E from HDL to become chylomicron remnants. These remnants are rapidly cleared from the circulation by the liver, after binding to hepatocyte receptors which recognize apoprotein E.

Endogenous pathway

Cholesterol and TAGs are synthesized by the liver and

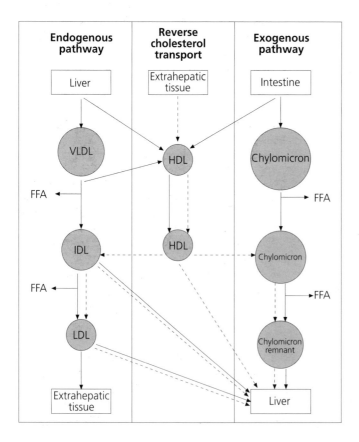

Figure 17.11 Overview of lipoprotein metabolism.

secreted in VLDL particles for transport to peripheral tissues. Cholesterol is manufactured by a complex synthetic pathway using acetyl CoA derived from fatty acid oxidation and carbohydrate metabolism. The rate of cholesterol synthesis is determined by the enzyme hydroxymethyl glutaryl (HMG) CoA reductase. Hepatic TAGs are produced from fatty acids originating from adipose tissue or by lipogenesis from carbohydrates. Newly synthesized TAGs combine with those acquired by chylomicron remnant uptake to be secreted in VLDL. VLDL particles, like chylomicrons, are formed by the packaging together of TAGs, cholesterol esters, cholesterol, phospholipids, and apolipoproteins. Apolipoprotein B-100, the major apolipoprotein of VLDL, is added by microsomal transfer protein.

After release into the bloodstream, TAGs in VLDL are rapidly hydrolyzed by lipoprotein lipase to release free fatty acids. During this process, VLDL particles exchange lipids with HDL to form cholesterol-rich IDL particles. IDL particles are either taken up by LDL receptors on the liver, or further metabolized by hepatic lipase to form LDL.

LDL constitutes the major cholesterol-carrying lipoprotein, serving to deliver cholesterol to peripheral cells and remaining in the circulation for 2–3 days. LDL is taken up from the circulation by the interaction of its B-100 apolipoprotein with cell surface LDL receptors. Around 75% of LDL is cleared by the liver and 25% by peripheral tissues. Receptor-mediated LDL uptake is of crucial importance in regulating plasma cholesterol concentrations. After binding, the receptor/LDL complex is delivered to the cytoplasm, where cholesterol esters are hydrolyzed to form free cholesterol. The LDL receptor recycles to the cell membrane, whereas the increased intracellular cholesterol concentration maintains cholesterol homeostasis by a number of mechanisms. HMG CoA reductase is inhibited, reducing *de novo* cholesterol synthesis; the enzyme acyl CoA:cholesterol acyl transferase is activated, promoting re-esterification of cholesterol to cholesterol esters; and, in addition, LDL receptor expression is downregulated.

Reverse cholesterol transport

Cholesterol surplus to cellular requirements is returned from peripheral tissues to the liver by HDL in a process called reverse cholesterol transport. HDL particles are the smallest of the lipoproteins and are synthesized in the liver and intestine as bilayer disks containing apoprotein A and phospholipids. Newly formed HDL avidly takes up cholesterol from cell membranes and other lipoproteins to become a cholesterol-rich spherical particle. Free cholesterol within HDL particles is rapidly esterified to cholesterol esters by the enzyme lecithin cholesterol acyl transferase, which circulates along with HDL. Mature HDL particles are heterogeneous and interact with lipoproteins of other classes. In doing so, cholesterol esters within HDL particle are transferred to particles such as IDL and chylomicrons, in exchange for TAGs, by cholesterol ester transfer protein.

A minority of cholesterol-rich HDL is taken up directly by the liver. The majority of cholesterol within HDL particles, however, returns to the liver indirectly after transfer to lipoproteins of lower density.

Types of dyslipidemia

Abnormalities of the plasma lipid profile may arise as a primary defect or may occur secondary to an underlying condition or drug therapy. Primary dyslipidemias include rare inherited lipid disorders, often arising as a consequence of single gene mutations, and the common type of dyslipidemia, frequently seen in clinical practice, which has a polygenetic background.

Secondary causes of dyslipidemia are summarized in Box 17.1.

Lipid-modifying drugs and coronary heart disease

Coronary heart disease prevention has been revolutionized in recent years with the widespread availability of safe, effective drugs that modify the lipid profile. Large, well-designed studies have conclusively shown that the addition of lipid-modifying drugs to diets low in saturated fat leads to substantial reductions in coronary heart disease events and mortality.

The main classes of lipid-modifying drugs, and their effects on plasma lipoproteins, are summarized in Table 17.4.

Resins

Resins (such as cholestyramine), bind bile acids in the intestine and prevent their reabsorption. An increased amount of cholesterol is therefore diverted to bile acid synthesis in the liver and hepatic LDL receptors are upregulated, thus lowering plasma LDL. There is limited

- Diabetes
- Insulin resistance syndrome
- Hypothyroidism
- Obesity
- Alcohol excess
- Renal failure
- Liver disease
- Gout
- Eating disorders (anorexia nervosa and bulimia nervosa)
- Pregnancy
- Drugs (e.g. cyclosporin, antiretroviral drugs for HIV, anticonvulsant drugs)

evidence from clinical trials of a reduced incidence of coronary heart disease events with cholestyramine (see Table 17.5).

Resins, which are administered as powders, are not generally used in the prevention of coronary heart disease, due the inconvenience of administration and gastrointestinal side effects.

Nicotinic acid derivatives

Nicotinic acid (niacin) is a vitamin which at high doses causes reductions in LDL and TAGs. It is particularly effective in hypertriglyceridemia, where large falls in TAG levels are accompanied by elevations of HDL. Nicotinic acid reduces the flux of fatty acids from adipose tissue to liver. This action inhibits hepatic output of VLDL and reduces hepatic TAG synthesis. The use of nicotinic acid is limited due to side effects such as flushing, pruritus, nausea, and glucose intolerance. These are less troublesome with the nicotinic acid derivative acipimox, though this compound is far less potent.

Fibrates

The fibrates (or fibric acid derivatives) have complex actions, including an enhanced clearance of TAGs from the circulation by stimulation of lipoprotein lipase.

Their main effect is to reduce TAG levels, although consistent increases in HDL and variable reductions in LDL are also clinically relevant. They are first-line drugs for the treatment of hypertriglyceridemia. Their role in the prevention of coronary heart disease had been eclipsed by the statins, although there has been recent interest in their potential to increase HDL.

Early trials of fibrates (using clofibrate) were complicated by drug-induced gallstone formation and an unexplained increase in non-cardiac deaths (see Table 17.5). In a secondary prevention trial, bezafibrate failed to reduce coronary events, although there was a significant reduction in events in patients with high TAG levels.

Two recent studies using gemfibrozil produced more encouraging results. In the Helsinki Heart Study (HHS), a major primary prevention trial, 4082 men were randomized to a lipid-lowering diet alone or diet plus gemfibrozil. After five years follow-up there was a 35% reduction in the primary end point of combined non-fatal and fatal myocardial infarction in the gemfibrozil group.

The potentially beneficial effect of using fibrates to raise HDL was explored in the Veterans Affairs High-Density Lipoprotein Intervention Trial (VA-HIT). In this secondary prevention trial, subjects with low HDL levels were randomized to receive gemfibrozil or placebo. After five years there was a significant 22% reduction in the combined end point of non-fatal myocardial infarction and death from coronary heart disease in the fibrate-treated group. Statistical analysis suggested that the majority of the beneficial effect was mediated by an increase in HDL.

In current clinical practice, the focus with respect to lipids and the prevention of coronary heart disease is on achieving target levels of total cholesterol or LDL by the use of diet and statin drugs. With increasing recognition of HDL as an important cardiovascular risk factor, however, fibrates and other interventions designed to increase HDL are likely to receive greater prominence in future.

Statins

The statins are potent, specific inhibitors of the enzyme HMG CoA reductase, which catalyzes the rate-determining state in hepatic cholesterol synthesis. By inhibiting cholesterol synthesis, statins increase hepatic LDL receptor activity and increase the uptake of LDL with a consequent reduction in plasma LDL levels.

Table 17.4 Lipid-modifying drugs and their effects on plasma lipids

	LDL Cholesterol	HDL Cholesterol	Triacylglycerol
Resins	↓↓	↑	↑↓
Nicotinic acid	↓	↑	↓↓
Fibrates	↓	↑↑	↓↓
Statins	↓↓	↑	↓

Table 17.5 Selected trials assessing the effect of a combination of diet and lipid-modifying drugs on cardiovascular outcomes

Study	Year of publication	Subjects	Age (years)	Design	Follow-up (years)	Lipids outcome	Clinical outcome
WHO Cooperative Trial of Clofibrate	1978	10 000 M, TC in upper 1/3 of normal distribution	30–59	RCT, Diet + clofibrate (1.6 g/day) versus placebo	5.3	TC −8%	25% reduction in non-fatal MI. Increase in total mortality
Lipid Research Council Coronary Primary Prevention Trial	1984	3806 M, TC >95th centile for population	35–59	RCT, Diet + cholestyramine (24 g/day) versus placebo	7.4	TC −9%, LDL −13%	19% reduction in CHD death or non-fatal infarction
Helsinki Heart Study	1987	4082 M, Non-HDL cholesterol >5.2 mmol/l	40–55	RCT, Diet + gemfibrozil (1.2 g/day) versus placebo	5	TC −10%, LDL −11%, TAG −35%, HDL +11%	35% reduction in non-fatal and fatal MI
West of Scotland Coronary Prevention Study (WOSCOPS)	1995	6595 M, TC >6.5 mmol/l, LDL >4 mmol/l	45–65	RCT, Diet + pravastatin (40 mg/day) versus placebo	4.9	TC −20%, LDL −26%, TAG −20%, HDL +5%	31% reduction in death from CHD and non-fatal MI
Air Force/Texas Coronary Atherosclerosis Prevention Study (AFCAPS/TexCAPS)	1998	5608 M, 997 F, Average TC and LDL. Below average HDL	45–73 M, 53–73 F	RCT, Diet + lovastatin (20–40 mg) versus placebo	5.2	LDL −25%, HDL +6%	37% reduction in major coronary events
Scandinavian Simvastatin Survival Study (4S)	1994	3572 M, 872 F, TC 5.5–8.0 mmol/l	35–70	RCT, Diet + simvastatin (20–40 mg/day) versus placebo	5.4	LDL −35%, TAG −10%, HDL +8%	44% reduction in major coronary events, 30% reduction in all cause mortality
Cholesterol and Recurrent Events Study (CARE)	1996	3577 M, 582 F, TC<6.2 mmol/l, LDL 3–4.5 mmol/l	21–75	RCT, Diet + pravastatin (40 mg/day) versus placebo	5	LDL −28%, TAG −14%, HDL +5%	24% reduction in CHD death or non-fatal MI
Long-Term Intervention with Pravastatin in Ischaemic Disease Study (LIPID)	1998	7498 M, 1516 F, TC 4–7 mmol/l	31–75	RCT, Diet + pravastatin (40 mg/day) versus placebo	6.1	TC −28%, LDL −25%, TAG −11%, HDL +5%	24% reduction in death from CHD, 22% reduction in total mortality
Veterans Affairs High-Density Lipoprotein Intervention Trial (VA-HIT)	1999	2531 M, HDL<1.0 mmol/l, LDL<3.6 mmol/l	<74	RCT, Diet + gemfibrozil (1.2 g/day) versus placebo	5.1	TC −4%, LDL no change, TAG −31%, HDL +6%	22% reduction in CHD death or non-fatal MI
Bezafibrate Infarction Prevention Study (BIP)	2000	2885 M, 267 F, TC 4.7–6.5 mmol/l, HDL <1.2 mmol/l	45–74	RCT, Diet + bezafibrate (400 mg/day) versus placebo	6.2	LDL −5%, TAG −21%, HDL +18%	No difference in fatal or non-fatal MI and sudden death (40% reduction in subgroup with TAG >2.3 mmol/l)
Heart Protection Study	2002	20 536 M&F, TC >3.5 mmol/l	40–80	RCT, Diet + simvastatin (40 mg/day) versus placebo	5	LDL −1.0 mmol/l, HDL +0.03 mmol/l, TAG −0.3 mmol/l	18% reduction in death from coronary heart disease

M, male; F, female; RCT, randomized controlled trial; TC, total cholesterol; LDL, low density lipoprotein cholesterol; HDL, high density lipoprotein cholesterol; TAG, triacylglycerol.
Full references are available in Further Reading section at www.nutritiontexts.com

Statins also lead to a small increase in HDL and modest reduction in TAGs. They are first-line treatment for familial hypercholesterolemia but are mostly used as an adjunct to diet in the prevention of coronary heart disease. Their widespread use in this capacity follows the demonstration of their efficacy and excellent safety record in a series of large, well-designed, randomized controlled clinical trials.

In the primary prevention setting, significant reductions in coronary events were observed in the West of Scotland Coronary Prevention Study (WOSCOPS) (Table 17.5). This showed that a combination of dietary advice and statin therapy in a high-risk population with moderately elevated cholesterol levels reduced the risk of fatal and non-fatal myocardial infarction, cardiovascular mortality, and total mortality.

In another primary prevention trial, the Air Force/ Texas Coronary Artery Prevention Study (AFCAPS/ TexCAPS), the population studied was at much lower baseline risk, with average LDL levels but low HDL. Even in this group, diet and statins significantly reduced the incidence of first major coronary events.

Extrapolation of AFCAPS/TexCAPS findings to the general population suggests that large numbers of people might benefit from statin therapy. The widespread adoption of such a policy, however, has huge cost implications and is unlikely to be financially tenable. Current primary prevention strategies, therefore, take into account other risk factors such as age, sex, smoking status, hypertension, and diabetes, and recommend statin therapy only if the calculated risk exceeds a threshold level.

The important role of statins in the secondary prevention of coronary heart disease is now established unequivocally. Three large randomized trials have revealed significant reductions in coronary events with the combination of diet and statins in patients with established coronary heart disease (Table 17.5).

The Scandinavian Simvastatin Survival Study (4S) showed a 44% reduction in major coronary events and a 30% reduction in total mortality with diet and statin treatment in high-risk patients with prior myocardial infarction or angina and elevated cholesterol levels.

The Cholesterol and Recurrent Events Study (CARE) study went on to assess whether lowering plasma cholesterol reduces the risk of recurrent coronary events in patients with average baseline cholesterol levels.

Treatment with dietary measures and pravastatin in survivors of myocardial infarction with LDL levels of 3–4.5 mmol/l reduced the primary end point of fatal coronary events and non-fatal myocardial infarction by 24%. The subjects in the CARE study were typical of the majority of survivors of myocardial infarction.

The Long-Term Intervention with Pravastatin in Ischaemic Disease (LIPID) Study also enrolled patients with a broad range of cholesterol levels (4.0–7.0 mmol/ l) but, in contrast to CARE, both unstable angina and myocardial infarction were included as entry criteria. Diet and statin treatment in the LIPID study led to a significant 24% reduction in mortality from coronary heart disease and reduced all-cause mortality by 22%.

The recent Heart Protection Study enrolled over 20 000 men and women who were at increased risk due to established cardiovascular disease, peripheral vascular disease, diabetes, or hypertension. Regardless of plasma cholesterol levels, dietary advice and statin treatment reduced the risk of death from coronary heart disease by 18%.

Given the impressive reductions in coronary event rates in these landmark trials, there is a strong argument to recommend a combination of dietary modification and a statin in virtually all patients at increased risk of coronary heart disease, regardless of their plasma cholesterol levels.

Although a reduction in LDL cholesterol is integral to the cardioprotection mediated by statins it is likely that other properties also contribute to their beneficial effects. These include inhibition of smooth muscle proliferation and platelet aggregation, enhancement of endothelial function, and anti-inflammatory effects.

Summary of evidence supporting positive relationship between dietary saturated fats, plasma cholesterol levels, and coronary heart disease

Epidemiological studies reveal a strong association between intake of saturated fat, plasma cholesterol levels and incidence of coronary heart disease.

Experimental studies in animals and in humans show that consumption of saturated fats leads to increased plasma cholesterol levels and promotes the development of atherosclerosis.

Clinical trials show that lowering cholesterol levels by a diet low in saturated fat and/or by drugs leads to a reduction in the incidence of coronary events.

Other lipid risk factors and coronary heart disease

High-density lipoprotin

It has been recognized for many years that HDL cholesterol is inversely associated with the risk of coronary heart disease. The Framingham Heart Study, for example, convincingly showed that HDL is inversely related to coronary heart disease incidence in men and women, an effect that is independent of LDL. The Prospective Cardiovascular Munster (PROCAM) Study, which recorded major coronary events in almost 20 000 individuals aged 16–65 years, found that after eight years of follow-up, the incidence of major coronary events was significantly higher in individuals with an HDL <0.9 mmol/l than in those with HDL >0.9 mmol/l.

The magnitude of protection predicted by HDL levels is substantial. Analysis of pooled data from four large prospective studies shows that for every 0.3 mmol/l increase in HDL, the predicted incidence of coronary events decreases by 20% in men and 30% in women.

HDL protects against atherosclerosis by carrying out reverse cholesterol transport and, perhaps, by delivering endogenous antioxidant enzymes, such as paroxonase, to the vessel wall.

Low HDL levels are associated with type 2 diabetes, obesity, cigarette smoking, and lack of regular exercise. Weight loss may increase HDL levels, as there is a linear inverse relationship between body mass index and HDL. This should be achieved by a combination of reduced energy diet and increased physical exertion, as exercise increases HDL in its own right. Smoking cessation also increases HDL by a modest amount.

The role of drugs such as fibrates and statins has been discussed.

HDL may be increased by:

- Weight loss
- Increase in physical activity
- Smoking cessation
- Fibrates.

Triacylglycerols

Many, though not all, prospective epidemiological studies have reported a positive relationship between serum TAG levels and the incidence of coronary heart disease. Early multivariate analyses, however, failed to identify TAG as an independent risk factor, probably because of the close interrelationship between TAG and other lipid risk factors.

Recent studies, however, have helped to clarify matters and have established TAG levels as an independent risk factor for coronary heart disease. For example, multivariate analysis after eight years follow-up in the large PROCAM study, discussed above, demonstrated that TAGs are an independent risk factor for major coronary events, even after adjustment for LDL, HDL, and other classical cardiovascular risk factors.

Furthermore, recent meta-analyses of this and other studies have confirmed that TAG are an independent risk and that each 1 mmol/l increase in serum TAG levels increases the relative risk of cardiovascular disease by 14% in men and 37% in women.

It is unclear whether the observed association between TAGs and coronary heart disease represents a direct atherogenic effect of TAGs themselves or an indirect effect, mediated by changes in other lipoproteins.

Four potential ways in which TAGs may promote atherosclerosis are highlighted below:

- Reduction in HDL levels
- Formation of atherogenic chylomicron remnants
- Formation of small, dense LDL – a highly atherogenic form of the LDL fraction, which is associated with a significant increase in coronary heart disease risk
- Predisposition to thrombosis by interaction with coagulation factors.

There is increasing recognition that subtle abnormalities of post-prandial TAG metabolism may be equally as important as fasting TAG levels in predicting cardiovascular risk. Prolonged exposure to TAGs after a meal results from overproduction of TAG-rich lipoproteins by the intestine and the liver or from a decrease in their clearance. Even in patients without overt fasting hypertriglyceridemia, an abnormal post-prandial response to a fat challenge predicts an increased incidence of coronary heart disease.

The causes of elevated TAG levels are summarized in Box 17.2.

Elevated TAG levels may be lowered by a combination of lifestyle changes and drug treatment. Weight reduction, physical exercise, and smoking cessation fa-

Box 17.2 Causes of elevated triacylglycerols

- Obesity
- Alcohol excess
- Physical inactivity
- Very high carbohydrate diets
- Diabetes
- Renal failure
- Nephrotic syndrome
- Bulimia
- Pregnancy
- Drugs (thiazide diuretics, estrogens, beta blockers, corticosteroids, protease inhibitors for HIV)
- Genetic

Box 17.3 Dietary antioxidants

Vitamins
- Vitamin E
- Vitamin C
- Beta-carotene

Trace elements
- Zinc
- Copper
- Manganese
- Selenium

Others
- Flavanoids (fruit, berries, tea, wine)
- Isoflavones (soybean)
- Phenolic compounds (olive oil)

vorably modify multiple risk factors including TAGs. Lipid-modifying drugs have been discussed.

17.6 Other dietary factors and coronary heart disease

Antioxidants

Oxidative stress is thought to play an important role in the development of atherosclerosis. Endogenous oxidizing agents and free radicals within the vessel wall have multiple adverse actions, including increasing the atherogenicity of LDL, impairing endothelial function, and promoting inflammation, smooth muscle cell proliferation, plaque rupture, and thrombosis. The diet, however, contains many antioxidant compounds which, once ingested and transported to the vessel wall, may offset these harmful effects. Common antioxidants present in the diet are listed in Box 17.3.

Observational, case–control, and cohort studies show that high antioxidant intake is associated with reduced risk of coronary heart disease. The most convincing evidence is for a protective effect of vitamin E, which, as it is lipid soluble, is readily able to reduce the oxidation of LDL.

Despite the convincing evidence of a protective effect of antioxidants in epidemiological studies, the results of randomized, controlled trials of antioxidant supplements have been disappointing. Several large primary and secondary prevention studies have assessed the potential of antioxidants including vitamin E, vitamin C, and beta-carotene, alone and in combination, to reduce the rates of coronary events. Despite long follow-up periods, antioxidant supplementation failed to effectively reduce the risk of coronary heart disease events or mortality in these studies.

The reasons for the lack of success are unknown but questions have been raised about the methodology of these studies and the type, combinations, and doses of antioxidant supplements used. It has also been suggested that because atherosclerosis develops slowly and the vessel wall is exposed to oxidant stress for many years, antioxidant treatment may need to be started at a very young age to prove effective.

There is insufficient evidence at present to recommend the use of antioxidant supplements in the prevention of coronary heart disease. However, consumption of a diet rich in fruit and vegetables (and hence natural antioxidants) is supported by epidemiological data and should be encouraged.

Fiber

Prospective observational studies show an inverse association between the intake of fiber from fruits, vegetables, and cereals and the risk of coronary heart disease. The mechanism appears to be a modest cholesterol-lowering effect of soluble fibers such as pectin, psyllium, and guar gum, attributed to their ability to bind bile acids within the gut. High-fiber diets may also reduce insulin levels and improve insulin sensitivity and blood clotting parameters.

There is a lack of clinical trials supporting the benefits of fiber in coronary heart disease prevention. Nonetheless, the consumption of fiber is certainly safe and may help to replace high fat, high cholesterol foods in the diet.

Soy protein

Data from early animal studies suggest that diets rich in proteins of vegetable origin, such as soy, are less atherogenic than those rich in proteins of animal origin. Replacement of animal protein with soy protein in humans leads to a modest reduction in LDL cholesterol and TAGs, particularly in subjects with high baseline cholesterol levels. Proposed mechanisms for the cholesterol-lowering properties of soy include enhanced bile acid excretion, increased LDL receptor activity, potential estrogen-like effects of soy-based isoflavones, and modulation of other hormones affecting cholesterol metabolism. The role of soy protein in the prevention of coronary heart disease has not been assessed in a randomized trial.

Alcohol

Epidemiological studies show an inverse association between morbidity and mortality from coronary heart disease and the moderate consumption of alcohol. Potential mechanisms mediating the cardioprotective effects of alcohol include an increase in HDL cholesterol and inhibition of platelet aggregation. In addition, red wine contains antioxidant polyphenols, such as catechin, quercetin, and resveratrol. It has been suggested that red wine may offer greater protection that the consumption of other types of alcohol but the data are conflicting. Moreover, cardioprotective actions of alcohol require the consumption of modest amounts on several days per week. This pattern is typical of the consumption of wine with meals in Mediterranean countries.

Higher levels of alcohol consumption and binge drinking are associated with increased mortality. In terms of coronary heart disease prevention, it is reasonable to recommend moderate drinking to those who already consume alcohol. The evidence does not, however, justify the recommendation of alcohol intake to a non-drinker for its cardioprotective effect.

Plant sterols and stanols

Plant sterols and stanols are incorporated into foods as 'functional foods' which lower plasma cholesterol levels. They are members of the phytosterol family of compounds, which occur naturally in a variety of plants and vegetable oils such as soy, corn, and wheat. Stanols are saturated sterols with no double bonds in their molecular structure, they are present in nature only in trace amounts and are manufactured by the hydrogenation of plant sterols.

The chemical structure of plant sterols and stanols is very similar to that of cholesterol, allowing them to inhibit cholesterol absorption in the intestine and thereby lower plasma cholesterol levels. Plant sterols and stanols themselves are poorly absorbed.

Recently, spreads enriched with plant sterol/stanol esters have become commercially available. When consumed on a regular basis these lead to significant reductions in plasma total cholesterol and LDL levels of around 10%. The absorption of fat-soluble vitamins is not affected by plant sterol/stanol intake, though some studies reveal a reduction in carotenoid levels. This may be offset by increasing the intake of fruit and vegetables.

Plant sterol/stanol-enriched spreads may be useful adjuncts to a diet low in saturated fat in terms of lowering plasma cholesterol levels. When used in conjunction with statins, the cholesterol-lowering effects are additive.

Tea

Tea has been suggested to have cardioprotective properties due to its high content of flavonoids and other antioxidants. Epidemiologic studies suggest a lower risk of coronary heart disease in subjects with a high intake of flavonoids from tea and other sources, though the evidence is conflicting. Consumption of black tea has been shown, in studies, to improve endothelial function and is associated with reduced mortality following myocardial infarction in recent studies. Further data are required before tea consumption can be recommended as a definitive strategy in the prevention of coronary heart disease.

Garlic

Garlic contains a variety of active compounds that may protect against atherosclerosis by a number of mechanisms including, inhibition of cholesterol synthesis, suppression of LDL oxidation, and inhibition of platelet aggregation and thrombus formation. Pooled data from clinical studies reveal that garlic or garlic extracts are able to lower plasma cholesterol and reduce blood pressure by a modest degree. There is, however, insufficient evidence from robust clinical trials to support an important role for garlic at the moment in coronary heart disease prevention.

Fish, n-3 fatty acids, and sudden death

Interest in a potentially cardioprotective role of dietary fish dates back to the 1950s with recognition of the fact that Inuit Eskimos had very low rates of coronary heart disease, despite consuming a diet high in fat. It subsequently became clear that long-chain n-3 fatty acids, present in fish and fish oils, possess important cardioprotective effects and their consumption in large amounts by the Inuits may explain the 'Eskimo Paradox.' More recently, several large epidemiologic studies have demonstrated an inverse relationship between the intake of long-chain n-3 polyunsaturated fatty acids and mortality from coronary heart disease. Cardioprotective actions have been attributed not only to long-chain n-3 fatty acids (eicosapentenoic acid and docosahexanoic acid) present in fish oil but also to the essential n-3 fatty acid linolenic acid, present predominantly in soybean, flax seed, and canola oils.

n-3 fatty acids protect from coronary heart disease by a number of mechanisms that inhibit atherosclerosis, prevent vessel occlusion, and reduce the predisposition to malignant cardiac arrythmias, a common cause of sudden death. Replacing dietary saturated fats with long-chain n-3 polyunsaturated fatty acids reduces TAG levels and tends to increase HDL levels. The protective effects of these changes in the lipid profile have been previously discussed. Moreover, increasing dietary n-3 fatty acid content shifts the balance of eicosanoid production, favoring the synthesis of vasodilatory and anti-aggregatory metabolites in the vessel wall. These effects promote endothelium-dependent vasodilatation, lower blood pressure, and reduce platelet aggregation. In addition, n-3 fatty acids reduce the production of proatherosclerotic growth factors by mononuclear cells.

Interestingly, epidemiologic studies suggest that n-3 fatty acids may offer particular protection from sudden cardiac death. In animal studies, n-3 fatty acids reduce the predisposition to ventricular fibrillation, a fatal cardiac arrhythmia that is a common cause of sudden death in humans. It is thought that incorporation of n-3 fatty acids into the cell membrane of heart muscle cells provides resistance to arrythmias, perhaps by modulating the electrical conductance of membrane ion channels.

Support for a clinically important cardioprotective action of n-3 fatty acids derives from two recent randomized, controlled secondary prevention trials. The Diet and Reinfarction Trial (DART) allocated 2033 male survivors of myocardial infarction to advice on three dietary changes. These were:

(1) a reduction in total fat intake with an increased ratio of polyunsaturated to saturated fats;
(2) an increase in fish intake (as fatty fish or fish oil capsules); or
(3) an increase in cereal fiber intake.

No reduction in coronary events was seen in the groups who reduced their total fat intake or consumed more fiber. In contrast, consumption of fatty fish or fish oil supplementation led to a significant 29% reduction in all-cause mortality, with a 29% reduction in coronary heart disease mortality.

The GISSI (Gruppo Italiano per le Studio della Sopravvivenza nell'Infarto Miocardico) trial randomized 11 324 patients surviving a recent myocardial infarction to a Mediterranean-style diet supplemented with n-3 fatty acids (1 g daily), vitamin E (300 mg daily), both, or none, for 3.5 years. Treatment with n-3 fatty acids reduced the risk of death, non-fatal myocardial infarction, and stroke by 15%, whereas vitamin E had no effect. Secondary analyses revealed that the mortality benefit was largely attributable to a 45% reduction in sudden death.

Taken together, the available evidence suggests that increasing dietary n-3 polyunsaturated fatty acids, by consumption of fatty fish or fish oil supplements, has a protective effect against mortality from coronary heart disease and, in particular, sudden death. Whether the consumption of a Mediterranean-style diet, as in the GISSI study, has additional protective effects is discussed in the following section.

The Mediterranean Diet

Traditionally, the total energy content of diets low in saturated fat has been maintained by replacing saturated fats by complex carbohydrates. In recent years, however, it is becoming clear that the type of fat in the diet, as well as the total amount, is important in determining cardiovascular risk. Mediterranean-type diets, in which saturated fats are replaced with unsaturated fats, are not low in total fat but there is substantial evidence that such diets offer significant protection from coronary heart disease.

Interest in the potential benefits of a Mediterranean-type diet was triggered by the Seven Countries Study, published in the 1960s, in which low rates of coronary heart disease and long life expectancy were noted in Mediterranean countries. This prompted the hypothesis that protection from coronary events in such countries may be due to the type of diet consumed at that time. The traditional Mediterranean diet, typical of Crete, Greece, and southern Italy in the early 1960s, contained an abundance of plant food (fruit, vegetables, breads, cereals, potatoes, beans, nuts, and seeds) and low to moderate amounts of fish, poultry, meat, dairy products, and eggs. Olive oil was the main source of dietary fat and alcohol was consumed in moderate amounts. Such a diet was rich in fiber and antioxidants and had a high proportion of monounsaturated fats, principally oleic acid from olive oil.

It is well established that replacement of saturated fats by monounsaturates, rather than carbohydrates, lowers LDL cholesterol without an adverse effect on HDL or TAG levels. In addition, monounsaturated fatty acids possess a number of other favorable properties. Olive oil consumption enriches LDL particles with oleic acid. Oleic-acid enriched LDL is more resistant to oxidation and is therefore less atherogenic. Dietary monounsaturates also improve endothelial function, reduce the expression of adhesion molecules, decrease the tendency to thrombosis, and, in some studies, lower blood pressure to a small degree.

It is likely, however, that constituents other than monounsaturated fatty acids contribute to the protective effects of a Mediterranean diet. Antioxidants are supplied in abundance, largely by fruit and vegetables, but also as constituents of olive oil and wine. Insulin sensitivity and glycemic control may be improved by the ingestion of complex carbohydrates and fiber. As discussed earlier, moderate alcohol consumption has been shown in epidemiologic studies to potentially protect against coronary heart disease.

Support for the recommendation of a Mediterranean-style diet to prevent coronary heart disease in clinical practice comes from the Lyon Heart Study, a large randomized secondary prevention trial designed to test whether such a diet, compared with a prudent western diet, may reduce the recurrence of coronary events after a first myocardial infarction. After 46 months of follow-up in a total of 605 participants, there was an impressive 65% reduction in coronary heart disease mortality, and a 56% reduction in all-cause mortality in the group consuming a Mediterranean-style diet. The composition of the experimental diet is summarized in Table 17.6. Participants were recommended to eat more bread, root vegetables, green vegetables, fish, and fruit and to reduce their intake of red meat, replacing it with poultry. A special margarine was supplied to replace butter and cream, and exclusive use of olive oil and rapeseed oil was recommended for salad and cooking. The margarine had a similar fatty acid composition to olive oil, but was supplemented with linoleic acid and, to a larger extent, alpha-linolenic acid.

The experimental diet was very similar, therefore, to the traditional Mediterranean diet consumed in Crete in the 1960s, with the exception of a greater amount of n-3 polyunsaturated fatty acids. This is important, as alpha-linolenic acid possesses many beneficial properties that may have contributed to the favorable outcome of this trial. To date, no trials have assessed whether Mediterranean-type diets are effective in the primary prevention of coronary heart disease. Nonetheless, there is reasonable evidence from epidemiological studies and the Lyon Heart Study to support the use of such diets in coronary prevention.

17.7 Diet and hypertension

Idiopathic (essential) hypertension significantly increases the risk of coronary heart disease, stroke, and

Table 17.6 The Lyon Heart Study Diet

		% of total calories
Total calories	1947	
Total fat		30.4
Saturated fat		8.0
Polyunsaturated fat		4.6
18:1, n-9 (oleic acid)		12.9
18:2, n-6 (linoleic acid)		3.6
18:3, n-3 (linolenic acid)		0.84
Alcohol		5.8
Protein		16.2
Fiber (g)	18.6 g	
Cholesterol	203 mg/day	

Reproduced from de Lorgeril *et al.* (1999) with permission of Lippincott Williams and Wilkins.

promotes left ventricular hypertrophy, heart failure, renal failure, aortic dissection, and peripheral vascular disease. In many cases, hypertension is associated with the presence of other risk factors such as obesity, insulin resistance, and lipid abnormalities and constitutes the 'insulin resistance (or metabolic) syndrome.'

There is a continuous, graded, near-linear relationship between blood pressure and the incidence of coronary events and stroke. Clinical guidelines attempt to target treatment to those at significantly increased risk by defining thresholds of blood pressure above which blood pressure lowering is recommended. Many hypertensive subjects require drug treatment to achieve satisfactory reductions in blood pressure and antihypertensive drugs have been shown to substantially lower the risk of stroke and, to a lesser extent, coronary heart disease, in clinical trials.

Smaller but important decreases in blood pressure, however, may also be achieved by lifestyle changes such as weight loss, physical exercise, and dietary modification. The etiology of hypertension is multifactorial, depending on an interaction between genetic and environmental factors. A substantial body of evidence suggests that a variety of nutritional factors are implicated in blood pressure regulation. Lifestyle changes such as dietary modification are useful adjuncts to antihypertensive drug therapy in individuals with hypertension and, if adopted on a large scale, may reduce the incidence of coronary heart disease and stroke in the population.

Nutritional factors involved in blood pressure regulation

A number of nutritional factors are implicated in the pathophysiology of hypertension. Those most studied include the minerals sodium, potassium, calcium, and magnesium, and other factors such as fatty acids, vitamins, and antioxidants.

Sodium intake is weakly associated with blood pressure in population studies. The effect of reducing sodium intake varies between individuals and is most pronounced in the elderly or those of Afro-Caribbean origin, who often have low renin levels. Pooled data from clinical trials show that dietary sodium restriction leads to small but significant reductions in blood pressure. In a recent randomized trial, the Dietary Approaches to Stop Hypertension (DASH) Study, the ad-

dition of sodium restriction to a diet designed to lower blood pressure led to a further hypotensive effect. Achieving a large reduction in sodium intake can be difficult as salt is a 'hidden' ingredient in many manufactured foodstuffs and a very low sodium diet can be unpalatable. Moderate reductions, however, are more readily achieved.

Sodium acts in concert with other minerals in influencing blood pressure regulation and intake of potassium, magnesium, and calcium are all inversely (but weakly) correlated with hypertension in population studies. However, trials of potassium, magnesium, and calcium supplements in hypertension have yielded inconsistent results.

As discussed, polyunsaturated fatty acids of the n-3 and n-6 groups are essential precursors in the synthesis of eicosanoids, a family of vasoactive molecules with vasoconstrictor and vasodilator properties. Increased consumption of fish oils rich in n-3 fatty acids has been shown to decrease blood pressure in some, though not all, studies – probably by promoting the synthesis of vasodilator eicosanoids.

Vascular production of oxidants and free radicals is increased in hypertension and impairs endothelium-dependent vasodilatation. A number of antioxidants including vitamin C and vitamin E have been shown to reduce blood pressure in hypertensive subjects. Vitamin C, in particular, leads to improvements in endothelial function. As discussed previously, however, antioxidants have proved disappointing in reducing coronary heart disease in clinical trials.

The role of other vitamins in blood pressure regulation is less clear. Vitamin D may play a role through is effect on calcium homeostasis. Vitamin B_6 is implicated in the central control of the sympathetic nervous system and its deficiency leads to hypertension in animal studies. Human data, however, are currently lacking.

Reduction of blood pressure by diet

Given the close relationship between obesity and hypertension, weight loss is a fundamental part of blood pressure reduction in obese and overweight individuals and has been shown to lower blood pressure and the requirement for antihypertensive drugs in clinical trials. Reduction in alcohol consumption may decrease blood pressure in those who drink to excess.

The ability of a specific combination of dietary changes to lower blood pressure was assessed in the recent Dietary Approaches to Stop Hypertension (DASH) Study. In this trial, 459 participants (with baseline diastolic blood pressure of 80–95 mmHg and systolic blood pressure of 120–160 mmHg) were provided with a diet high in fruit and vegetables, a specially designed 'DASH diet,' or a control diet for eight weeks. The DASH diet was rich in potassium, magnesium, fiber, calcium, and protein, and was low in saturated fat and cholesterol. In those randomized to the DASH diet, systolic blood pressure fell by 5.5 mmHg and diastolic blood pressure by 3 mmHg after eight weeks. Smaller, though significant, reductions in blood pressure were seen in the group consuming a diet high in fruit and vegetables. In an extension of the DASH study, the DASH-sodium study showed that addition of sodium restriction to the DASH diet led to further falls in blood pressure. The composition of the DASH diet is shown in Box 17.4.

17.8 Diet and stroke

Stroke is the most common life-threatening neurological disorder and is a major cause of death and disability in developed countries. Most strokes are due to cerebral infarction with the remainder caused by primary intracerebral hemorrhage or subarachnoid hemorrhage. Cerebral infarction arises from occlusion of a cerebral artery either by thrombosis of an atherosclerotic cerebral vessel, or by embolism of thrombus from a proximal site. As atherosclerosis underlies a significant proportion of strokes, it is not surprising that nutritional factors may be implicated. The evidence for an association between the intake of dietary fat, plasma lipids, and the incidence of stroke is, however, weaker than that for coronary heart disease. Epidemiologic studies fail to show a consistent relationship between saturated fat intake or plasma cholesterol levels and the incidence of stroke. Pooled data from large trials of diet and statins in the primary and secondary prevention of coronary heart disease, however, show a significant ~30% reduction in the incidence of stroke. It is unclear whether the benefit stems from cholesterol reduction or other properties of statins such as anti-inflammatory or antioxidant effects.

Stroke incidence is negatively correlated with the intake of antioxidant vitamins in epidemiologic studies.

Box 17.4 The DASH Diet

High in:
- Fruit
- Vegetables
- Low fat diary products
- Fish
- Poultry
- Whole grains
- Nuts

And low in:
- Red meats
- Fats
- Sugar-sweetened foods
- Sugar-sweetened beverages

Randomized trials of antioxidant supplements, however, have consistently failed to demonstrate an effect on the risk of stroke.

Mineral intake is important in the control of blood pressure and the relationship between sodium intake and hypertension, itself a major risk factor for stroke, has been discussed. There is some evidence that increased potassium and magnesium intake may reduce stroke risk independently of blood pressure changes. Data linking fish consumption with risk of stroke are conflicting. Alcohol consumption increases the risk of hemorrhagic stroke in a dose-dependent fashion but studies of alcohol intake and ischemic stroke are inconsistent.

In general terms, therefore, observational studies suggest that certain dietary factors play a role in the predisposition to stroke. In contrast to coronary heart disease, however, there is a lack of large interventional studies to support the general recommendation of dietary modification as a means of stroke prevention.

17.9 Diet and peripheral vascular disease

Peripheral vascular disease (atherosclerotic disease) often coexists with coronary heart disease and shares the same risk factors. Very few studies have assessed the contribution of dietary factors to the pathogenesis or treatment of peripheral vascular disease in isolation from other manifestations of atherosclerotic disease. Nonetheless, it is reasonable to assume that dietary modifications that reduce the incidence of coronary heart disease, hypertension, and diabetes will decrease the burden of peripheral vascular disease in the population.

17.10 Diet and chronic heart failure

Chronic heart failure is a clinical syndrome in which cardiac output is insufficient to meet the body's needs, leading to fatigue, breathlessness, and fluid retention. Most cases of heart failure are characterized by impaired myocardial contractile function accompanied by increased activity of the sympathetic nervous and renin–angiotensin–aldosterone systems. Myocardial dysfunction often occurs as a consequence of coronary heart disease, hypertension, or diabetes. Genetic factors and viral infections are important causes of heart failure in a not insignificant proportion of patients.

Diet is important in the pathophysiology and treatment of heart failure for four main reasons.

(1) Dietary factors are implicated in the etiology of many cases of chronic heart failure as they predispose to coronary heart disease, hypertension, and diabetes.
(2) Sodium retention contributes to fluid retention and edema in many individuals. Restriction of dietary sodium intake, therefore, may be required.
(3) A variety of micronutrients are involved in the regulation of myocardial function and supplementation may improve symptoms in some individuals. This will be discussed later in this chapter. Heart failure as a consequence of overt nutrient deficiency is rare in developed countries but does occur (for example thiamine deficiency).
(4) Patients with chronic heart failure may lose weight and muscle bulk in a process called 'cardiac cachexia.' Dietary modification may help to avoid this process.

Nutrition and cardiac cachexia

Cardiac cachexia denotes an undernourished state, which affects up to a third of patients with severe chronic heart failure and is associated with a poor prognosis. Several mechanisms are thought to contribute to the loss of lean body mass in these individuals.

Energy requirements often increase in chronic heart failure due to an increased resting metabolic rate and a shift toward catabolism. Energy intake, however, usually falls due a combination of anorexia and reduced nutrient absorption. Appetite is decreased by a number of mechanisms, including central nervous system effects, side effects of drugs, or dyspepsia and early satiety caused by hepatic and splanchnic venous congestion. Edema of the gut wall may reduce the ability to absorb digested foods, vitamins, and other micronutrients. Skeletal muscle bulk is lost by a decrease in physical activity and by the effects of poor cardiac output on nutrient and oxygen supply to the tissues. Malnutrition may affect the myocardium directly and further impair cardiac performance. Finally, increased circulating levels of catecholamines and proinflammatory cytokines, such as tumor necrosis factor alpha (TNFα), promote a catabolic state.

There are no specific recommendations for nutritional support in chronic heart failure as opposed to other chronic conditions characterized by undernutrition. A high-energy, limited-sodium diet is recommended and meals should be small and frequent. Clinical trials of high-energy diets in chronic heart failure are small in number and reveal increases in weight with variable effects on function.

17.11 Micronutrients and cardiovascular disease

Micronutrients are implicated in the predisposition to atherosclerosis and in maintaining the contractile function of the heart. Support for an important role of vitamins and minerals in the pathogenesis of coronary heart disease, hypertension, peripheral vascular disease, stroke, and chronic heart failure is provided by observational and case–control studies. Further evidence derives from experimental studies in animals and humans, which emphasize the importance of micronutrients in the biochemical and pathological processes underlying cardiovascular disease. It is also increasingly recognized that subclinical deficiency in certain micronutrients is common in the general population. Randomized clinical intervention trials, however, fail to show a reliable ability of many micronutrient supplements to reduce the incidence of disease. Nonetheless, adequate levels of 'beneficial' micronutrients must be regarded as an essential component of a balanced diet. Achieving high levels of 'beneficial' micronutrients through diets rich in fruit and vegetables, as with the Mediterranean-style diet, may contribute to the reduced incidence of coronary heart disease in recent trials.

Vitamins

Vitamin A
Carotenoids such as beta-carotene are antioxidants, which may reduce the oxidation of LDL. However, an association between dietary intake of beta-carotene and the risk of coronary heart disease is not supported by prospective observational studies. Moreover, beta-carotene supplements fail to reduce coronary heart disease events in primary prevention studies.

Vitamin B_1
Vitamin B_1 (thiamine) is essential for carbohydrate metabolism. Severe thiamine deficiency leads to heart failure in the condition known as beriberi. Diuretic therapy may reduce thiamine levels and inhibit thiamine uptake in the heart. It is unclear whether subclinical thiamine deficiency contributes to myocardial dysfunction in chronic heart failure. Limited evidence suggests that thiamine supplements may increase cardiac performance and symptoms in patients with moderate to severe heart failure.

Vitamin B_6, B_{12}, and folate
Vitamin B_6, B_{12}, and folate are required for the metabolism of homocysteine, an amino acid whose levels are strongly correlated with the risk of coronary heart disease, peripheral vascular disease, and stroke. Increased homocysteine levels predispose to atherosclerosis by promoting LDL oxidation, damaging the endothelium, and adversely affecting platelet function and coagulation. Homocysteine levels are regulated by its conversion to cysteine, in a reaction requiring vitamin B_6; or its remethylation to form methionine in a reaction requiring vitamin B_{12} and folate. Dietary levels of vitamin B_6, B_{12}, and folate are inversely associated with the risk of coronary heart disease. Folate supplementation, either alone or in conjunction with B vitamins, leads to significant reduction in homocysteine levels. Whether this translates in to a reduced risk of vascular disease remains unclear.

Vitamin C
Vitamin C intake is inversely correlated with the risk of stroke and coronary heart disease in some, but not all, observational studies. Vitamin C promotes endothelial nitric oxide production and improves endothelium-dependent vasodilatation in animals and humans, probably through antioxidant effects. Supplementation has not been shown to reduce the incidence of coronary heart disease in randomized controlled trials.

Vitamin D
Vitamin D is closely implicated in calcium homeostasis and may have effects on the regulation of blood pressure. Its role in cardiovascular disorders has not been fully assessed.

Vitamin E
Vitamin E is a powerful lipid-soluble antioxidant, which may protect against atherosclerosis by reducing the oxidation of LDL cholesterol and decreasing platelet aggregation. Consumption of vitamin E is inversely associated with the risk of coronary heart disease in epidemiological studies. Large-scale randomized controlled trials of vitamin E supplementation, however, have failed to show a beneficial effect.

Minerals

Sodium
Increased sodium intake leads to extracellular volume expansion and stimulation of the sympathetic nervous system. Its role in blood pressure regulation has been discussed.

Potassium
Potassium acts along with other minerals to regulate cellular ion balance and vascular tone. Dietary potassium consumption is inversely related to the incidence of hypertension and stroke. The role of supplementation as a preventative measure is controversial. Potassium deficiency or excess may predispose to cardiac rhythm disturbances.

Calcium
The degree of hardness of drinking water is inversely related to coronary heart disease incidence in epidemiologic studies. Since water hardness is partly determined by its calcium content, it has been suggested that calcium has protective effects. There is some evidence that higher calcium intake is associated with lower blood pressure and lower plasma TAG in observational studies, and dietary calcium reduces platelet aggregation in animal studies, perhaps by interfering

with the absorption of saturated fats. Low levels of calcium predispose to cardiac rhythm disturbances and may cause a cardiomyopathy, particularly in children. Calcium supplementation has not been studied in prospective trials with respect to coronary heart disease prevention.

Copper

Copper is a constituent of cellular enzymes, including copper–zinc superoxide dismutase and cytochrome c oxidase. Copper deficiency is rare in humans but marginal levels potentially contribute to heart failure and atherosclerosis and elevate plasma cholesterol. Copper restriction in animals leads to myocyte damage and cardiomyopathy.

Magnesium

Epidemiologic studies show an inverse association between magnesium intake and the risk of coronary heart disease and stroke. Magnesium may also be important in blood pressure regulation by modulating vascular tone. Low magnesium levels are common in heart failure, may be promoted by diuretic use, and are associated with a worse prognosis. Magnesium deficiency can itself lead to heart failure in patients with anorexia nervosa. Low magnesium levels may contribute to cardiac rhythm disturbances and intravenous magnesium is useful in the treatment of ventricular arrhythmias.

Manganese

Manganese is a constituent of the antioxidant enzyme manganese superoxide dismutase. Genetic deletion of this enzyme in mice leads to cardiomyopathy. Reduced levels of manganese superoxide dismutase may also be implicated in the cardiomyopathy induced by the anticancer drug adriamycin.

Zinc

Zinc is a critical component of cell membranes and antioxidant enzymes and blocks apoptotic (programmed) cell death. It maintains endothelial cell integrity and protects against inflammation. Low serum zinc levels are found in heart failure and may reflect diuretic use. Its antioxidant properties may be beneficial in atherosclerosis and heart failure.

Selenium

Selenium is a component of the antioxidant enzyme glutathione peroxidase. Selenium deficiency predisposes to peripartum cardiomyopathy and is the cause of Keshan disease, an endemic cardiomyopathy in China. Selenium deficiency may also cause a cardiomyopathy in patients on long-term parenteral nutrition. Its antioxidant properties are thought to protect against atherosclerosis and low selenium levels have been linked to coronary heart disease and peripheral vascular disease. There is, however, insufficient evidence at present to recommend selenium supplementation in the general population.

Lead

Chronic exposure to low levels of lead has been suggested to cause hypertension in animals and humans. The mechanism is thought to involve increased production of reactive oxidant species.

Arsenic

Arsenic is a toxic mineral, which can promote atherosclerosis. Contamination by arsenic of drinking water wells in Bangladesh and Taiwan causes hypertension and 'blackfoot disease,' a form of peripheral vascular disease, in the affected population.

Others

Coenzyme Q_{10}

Coenzyme Q_{10} (ubiquinone) is a vitamin-like fat-soluble quinone found in mitochondria, where it acts as an electron carrier in oxidative phosphorylation. It also has antioxidant and membrane-stabilizing properties. It is thought that coenzyme Q_{10} depletion may contribute to heart failure, in which low myocardial levels are associated with increased mortality. Statins reduce the production of coenzyme Q_{10}, raising a theoretical concern over their use in patients with chronic heart failure. Limited studies of coenzyme Q_{10} supplements in heart failure have produced inconsistent results.

Carnitine

Carnitine is an organic amine that is involved in fatty acid oxidation. It is administered to treat carnitine deficiency, but its ability to increase energy production and remove toxic metabolites suggests a putative role in the treatment of heart failure, coronary artery disease, and peripheral vascular disease. This has not been adequately assessed in trials.

L-Arginine

The amino acid L-arginine is the precursor of nitric oxide, an endothelium-derived free radical with potent vasodilatory and antiatherosclerotic properties. Although intracellular L-arginine levels are not usually limiting, treatment with exogenous L-arginine has been shown to increase nitric oxide production and improve vasodilatation in animals and humans. A potential role in the prevention and treatment of coronary heart disease has not been tested in large, randomized trials.

17.12 Perspectives on the future

Our understanding of the role of dietary factors in diseases of the heart and blood vessels continues to improve, with important practical implications. Key dietary factors in the prevention of coronary heart disease are summarized in Box 17.5. Recognition of the association between dietary saturated fat, plasma cholesterol levels, and coronary heart disease risk has led to the adoption of cholesterol-lowering measures as the cornerstone of preventive strategies. Large randomized controlled trials have vindicated this approach but more work is needed to ensure that all those who might benefit receive appropriate advice and treatment. New functional foods, such as plant sterol/stanol spreads, provide a useful adjunct to other dietary measures in the reduction of plasma cholesterol. Interest is also turning to other modifiable risk factors, such as HDL and TAG, as targets for intervention. Recognition that other types of dietary fat, such as n-3 polyunsaturated fatty acids, exert cardioprotective effects has led to important recent nutritional studies. Trials of a diet high in fatty fish, for example, have been found to lead to impressive reductions in coronary heart disease risk.

The importance of complex interactions between nutrients in the diet is increasingly apparent. Whilst

> **Box 17.5** Key dietary factors in the prevention of coronary heart disease
>
> - Maintenance of an ideal body weight (BMI 20–25 kg/m²)
> - Reduction in the consumption of saturated fats
> - Use of unsaturated fats, including olive oil or rapeseed oil, for cooking
> - Consumption of fruit and vegetables several times per day
> - Consumption of moderate amounts of complex carbohydrates
> - Consumption of dietary fiber, particularly soluble fiber
> - Increased intake of fatty fish
> - Reduction in salt intake
> - Moderation of alcohol intake

antioxidant supplements have proved disappointing, the adoption of a balanced diet rich in antioxidants is well supported by the evidence. The Mediterranean-style diet may approach the ideal standard of the 'cardioprotective' diet.

References and further reading

Conlin PR. Dietary modification and changes in blood pressure. *Curr Opin Nephrol Hypertens* 2001; 10: 359–363.

Fairfield KM, Fletcher RH. Vitamins for chronic disease prevention in adults: scientific review. *JAMA* 2002; 287: 3116–3126.

Hooper L, Summerbell C, Higgins J et al. Reduced or modified dietary fat for preventing cardiovascular disease (Cochrane Review). In: *The Cochrane Library*. Oxford: Update Software, 2002.

Keys A. *Seven Countries: a multivariate analysis of death and coronary heart disease*. London: Harvard University Press, 1980.

Kromhout D, Menotti A, Kesteloot H et al. Prevention of coronary heart disease by diet and lifestyle: evidence from prospective cross-cultural, cohort, and intervention studies. *Circulation* 2002; 105: 893–898.

de Lorgeril M, Salen P, Martin JL et al. Mediterranean diet, traditional risk factors, and the rate of cardiovascular complications after myocardial infarction: final report of the Lyon Diet Heart Study. *Circulation* 1999; 99: 779–785.

Renaud S, Lanzmann-Petithory D. Coronary heart disease: dietary links and pathogenesis. *Public Health Nutr* 2001; 4: 459–474.

Schaefer EJ. Lipoproteins, nutrition, and heart disease. *Am J Clin Nutr* 2002; 75: 191–212.

Witte KK, Clark AL, Cleland JG. Chronic heart failure and micronutrients. *J Am Coll Cardiol* 2001; 37: 1765–1774.

18
Nutritional Aspects of Disease Affecting the Skeleton

Christine Rodda

Key messages

- Bone health is the result of complex interactions between genetic determinants of peak bone mass, lifestyle factors (including nutrition and exercise), hormonal milieu, and vitamin D status.
- Adequate sun exposure is the most important determinant of vitamin D status.
- Vitamin D deficiency due to poor sun exposure in at risk individuals, leading to rickets in infants and children and osteomalacia in adults, is entirely preventable.

- Age-specific issues need to be considered with regard to nutritional requirements to ensure normal bone growth during infancy, childhood, and adolescence, and for the maintenance of bone mass throughout adulthood.
- Osteopenia and osteoporosis are frequent complications of chronic systemic disease and may be exacerbated by dietary mineral ion and protein undernutrition, and vitamin D deficiency.

18.1 Introduction

The skeleton is a complex structure comprising mineral ions, which precipitate on a predominantly collagen framework of bone matrix proteins, to form the rigid, strong structure characteristic of normal bone. This chapter will review the basic concepts of calcium homeostasis and bone metabolism, with particular emphasis on relevant dietary aspects in health and disease, from conception to senescence.

Bone growth during infancy, childhood, and adolescence ceases once bone growth plates fuse; however, ongoing bone turnover, with resorption of old bone and formation of new bone, continues throughout life. Normal mineral ion homeostasis involves multiple organ systems, namely the parathyroid glands, skin, gastrointestinal system, liver, and kidney, and perturbations of any of these organ systems may affect mineral ion homeostasis and bone metabolism. Consequently, nutritional deficiencies and various chronic diseases may have profound effects on skeletal health, and the complex interactions involved between mineral ion nutrition, protein/calorie nutrition, and vita-

min D status will be discussed together with aspects of diagnostic imaging techniques and laboratory testing relevant to assessment of the skeleton.

18.2 Overview of mineral ion homeostasis and bone metabolism

Bone metabolism

Throughout life bone, like skin and the lining of the gut, is continually turned over in processes referred to as 'modeling' in growing children and 'remodeling' in adults. Bone-resorbing cells (osteoclasts) resorb bone and their action is coupled with that of bone-forming cells (osteoblasts) which lay down new bone (Figure 18.1); osteoblast/osteoclast coupling is mediated via a complex paracrine hormonal interplay between these two cell types, and involves hormones such as RANK ligand, fibronectin, and osteoprogerin.

During normal growth in childhood bone formation exceeds net bone resorption, and bone mass steadily increases during childhood through to adolescence, during which approximately 40% of bone mass ac-

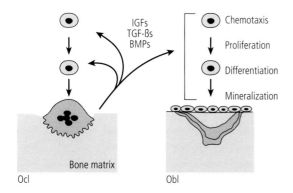

IGFs
TGF-ßs
BMPs

Chemotaxis

Proliferation

Differentiation

Mineralization

Bone matrix

Ocl

Obl

Figure 18.1 Diagram showing the cellular interactions between osteoblasts and osteoclasts. Reproduced from Mundy *et al.* (2003) with permission of the American Society for Bone and Mineral Research.

crual occurs through the peripubertal years. By the beginning of the third decade of life peak bone mass has been attained and bone mass reaches a steady state, and in otherwise healthy young adults bone resorption occurs in balance with bone formation, until menopause in women and late middle age in men, when bone resorption starts to exceed net bone formation, leading to osteoporosis over the ensuing decades.

The major determinants of peak bone mass are listed in Box 18.1.

Osteocytes are the most numerous type of bone cells. They intercommunicate via cellular processes and are considered to be osteoblasts that have become buried within bone. Osteocytes are thought to act as 'strain gauges' within bone, sensitive to weight bearing and shearing forces applied to bone. Weight-bearing exercise is an important determinant of bone strength and, conversely, immobilization due to prolonged bed rest or in more recent years 'weightlessness' in prolonged space travel has been shown to result in bone loss.

The nutritional and hormonal (autocrine, paracrine, and endocrine) influences on bone formation and resorption are complex, and involve parathy-

---

Box 18.1 Determinants of peak bone mass

- Genetic influences
- Hormonal factors, including sex hormones (estrogen and testosterone from puberty through to middle age) and insulin-like growth factor 1 (IGF-1)
- Dietary calcium intake
- Lifestyle factors such as weight-bearing exercise, alcohol intake, tobacco smoking

---

roid hormone (PTH), 1,25-dihydroxy vitamin D_3 $(1,25(OH)_2D_3)$, IGF-1 and 2, transforming growth factor beta (TGFβ), fibroblast growth factor (FGF), sex hormones, and various cytokines and lymphokines. Nutritional factors, malabsorption syndromes, anorexia nervosa, systemic disease such as cystic fibrosis, chronic renal failure, and pregnancy and lactation, particularly in adolescent mothers, also affect bone metabolism.

Mineral ion homeostasis

Mineral ion homeostasis is important for both normal metabolism and structural skeletal rigidity, and the major ions concerned are calcium and phosphorus. Bone osteoid comprises bone matrix proteins, predominantly collagen, which are laid down in a complex helical structure and provide tensile strength to bone. The mineral ions calcium and phosphorus precipitate within this helical structure as hydroxyapatite crystals $(Ca_{10}(PO_4)_6(OH)_2)$, to form a strong, rigid structure characteristic of mature bone.

In growing infants and children, this process predominantly occurs at the metaphyseal growth plates, within the long bones. Once these growth plates have fused and growth has ceased, bone formation and resorption occurs in a coupled fashion throughout the healthy adult skeleton. Unmineralized osteoid, as occurs in rickets in children and osteomalacia in adults, results in soft, pliable bones. Defective mineralization will result as a consequence of either calcium or phosphate depletion, or a combination of both.

Calcium

The adult skeleton contains 1–1.5 kg calcium (20–25 mg/kg fat-free tissue) and represents 99% of total body calcium. Less than 1% of calcium circulates in a soluble form, and it is this fraction that plays a vital role in neuromuscular and cardiovascular function, in coagulation, and as an intracellular second messenger for cell surface hormone action, in addition to its roles in gene transcription, and cellular growth and metabolism. In the presence of dietary calcium insufficiency, circulating blood calcium is maintained at normal concentrations, primarily through the actions of PTH, which maintains circulating calcium at the expense of bone mineralization (Figures 18.2 and 18.3).

Dairy foods are the richest, most bioavailable natural food sources of calcium. The recommended daily

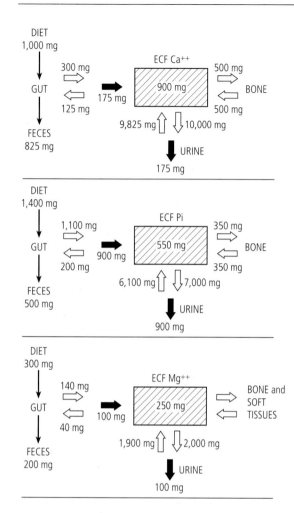

Figure 18.2 Calcium balance.

intakes (RDIs) for calcium are listed in Table 18.1 and dietary sources in Table 18.2. Infant RDI is almost always met as breast milk or formula feeds are the sole dietary intake of infants under three months of age, and should continue to form the bulk of their diet until 9–12 months of age. Calcium intake beyond this age may be inadequate due to cultural food practices, food faddism, or exclusion diets due to cow's milk allergy or lactase deficiency. Fortification of fruit juices, bread, and cereal with calcium may provide alternative dietary sources of calcium for those on such exclusion diets. In the event that the RDI for calcium cannot be met, there are a number of commercially available preparations of calcium supplements.

The effectiveness of calcium absorption from commercial preparations is to some degree dependent on the type of calcium salt, and timing and number of doses. Calcium citrate-malate (CCM) preparations have been found to be absorbed better than calcium carbonate salts, but CCM is not universally available and is unobtainable in some countries. However, overall the benefits of one calcium salt over another is not substantial.

The efficiency of calcium absorption is affected by pH and other components of food such as oxalates and phytates, and calcium supplements are best taken in multiple doses rather than as a single daily dose, to maximize absorption efficiency. However, as the number of daily doses of supplements increase, subject compliance is also likely to decrease.

Reduced gastric acid secretion secondary to atrophic gastritis, which is commonly seen in elderly populations, may also contribute to dietary calcium deficiency in the elderly, and it is important that calcium carbonate supplementation is actually taken with meals to optimize calcium bioavailability under these circumstances.

Calcium retention may be suboptimal due to either decreased calcium absorption such as in vitamin D deficiency or excessive urinary excretion due to a high protein or high salt containing diet. High oxalate (e.g. spinach) and high phytate (e.g. chapatis) diets also reduce calcium absorption. Carbonated drinks with high phosphoric acid content may impair calcium absorption, and may also be preferred to milk drinks. Aluminum in antacids taken in excess may increase urinary calcium excretion. Dietary factors which impair calcium retention are listed in Box 18.2 (page 299).

Phosphorus

The human body contains about 0.8–1 kg of phosphorus (11–14 mg/kg fat-free mass), and, like calcium, less than 1% of this circulates in a soluble form. Unlike calcium, however, only 85% of total body phosphorus is in the skeleton, because it also has a major role in soft tissue growth, with 15% present in muscle and other body tissues. In addition, phosphorus has wide-ranging influences on metabolism, and is an important component of basic molecules such as phospholipids, phosphoproteins, and nucleic acids. Phosphate is also integral to normal muscle function, and has an important role in synthesis and storage of chemical energy as high-energy phosphate bonds such as ATP.

Phosphate is an almost ubiquitous component of food, so dietary deficiency is uncommon unless total

The efficiency of vitamin D synthesis in the skin tends to decrease with ageing, and is a contributory risk factor for vitamin D deficiency in the elderly. The remaining 10% of vitamin D is derived from dietary sources such as cod liver oil, eggs, or oily fish. Skin pigmentation also influences the efficiency of vitamin D_3 production from sunlight exposure, and vitamin D production in the skin is inversely proportional to melanin production, as melanin competes with 7-DHC for UVB protons. Consequently black-skinned individuals need approximately six times the sunlight exposure compared with fair-skinned individuals to maintain equivalent vitamin D status. The amount of UVB exposure from sunlight is also inversely proportional to latitude, so that UVB exposure is greater in equatorial regions compared with that in regions at higher latitudes. Furthermore, UVB exposure is greater during summer than winter at higher latitudes, so that the greatest risk for vitamin D deficiency in such regions is late winter and early spring.

Both dietary vitamins D_2/D_3 and skin-synthesized vitamin D_3 are hydroxylated in the liver to form 25-hydroxy vitamin D_3 (25OH D_3), which is the storage form of vitamin D. This hydroxylation step is largely unregulated. Vitamin D_3 is bound to vitamin D-binding protein and is transported in the bloodstream to the liver where it is hydroxylated. Vitamin D_3 and its metabolites are fat-soluble vitamins, and undergo enterohepatic circulation, by cosecretion of 25OH D_3 and bile salts into the duodenum with subsequent reabsorption of 25OH D_3 within the gut. This reabsorption process may be inhibited by binding of 25OH D_3 to dietary phytates and fiber, or in fat malabsorption syndromes. Further hydroxylation of 25OH D_3 to form $1,25(OH)_2D_3$, occurs in the kidney through the stimulation of 1 alpha hydroxylase by PTH, hypocalcemia (probably indirectly via PTH), and hypophos-

phatemia, with feedback inhibition of PTH secretion by $1,25(OH)_2D_3$ (Figure 18.3).

Gut absorption of both calcium and phosphate is increased by the action of $1,25(OH)_2D_3$ on the gut, both directly and via upregulation of the calcium-binding protein calbindin-D. Although both calcium and phosphate are absorbed throughout the length of the small intestine, the majority of phosphate is absorbed from the jejunum and ileum, and the majority of calcium from the duodenum. To maintain normal mineral ion homeostasis, particularly in growing children, the RDIs of both vitamin D (Table 18.3) and calcium (Table 18.1) must be met. However, the RDI for vitamin D remains controversial given the wide variation in direct sun exposure around the world due to both latitude and lifestyle factors. In Australia there are no national RDIs for vitamin D, as it is assumed that Australians have adequate sunlight exposure for their vitamin D requirements. The RDIs for vitamin D cited in this chapter are based on a number of published recommendations by other authors. Dietary sources of vitamin D are listed in Table 18.4.

Skeletal effects of $1,25(OH)_2D_3$ are complex and beyond the scope of this chapter. However in broad terms, $1,25(OH)_2D_3$ affects both bone formation and resorption in the ongoing modeling/remodeling process of bone. At a cellular level, osteoblasts express $1,25(OH)_2D_3$ receptors and may modulate the synthesis of a number of osteoblast-derived products such as alkaline phosphatase and osteocalcin, in addition to the stimulation of proliferation of osteoblasts themselves. During pregnancy, the placenta is also an extrarenal source of 1 alpha hydroxylase and $1,25(OH)_2D_3$. In disease states such as sarcoidosis, tuberculosis, and neonatal subcutaneous fat necrosis hypercalcemia may

Table 18.3 Age-related recommended daily intake (RDI) for vitamin D

Infants and children	400 IU
Adults	200 IU
Pregnant and lactating women	800 IU

Table 18.4 Dietary sources of vitamin D

Food type	Vitamin D content (IU/100 g)
Cod liver oil	8 000–28 000
Oily fish (e.g. salmon, sardines, tuna)	200–480
Margarine	200–240
Eggs	40–80

develop as a result of extrarenal 1 alpha hydroxylase-induced $1,25(OH)_2D_3$ production.

18.3 Age-appropriate biochemical reference ranges

Specific reference ranges will not be presented; however, it is important to be aware of age-appropriate reference ranges which affect the following biochemical parameters.

Alkaline phosphatase
Alkaline phosphatase (ALP) is mostly bone-derived in infants and children, and consequently is normally up to 3–4 times the upper limit of the normal adult reference range in this age group. The isoenzyme bone-specific ALP (BSAP) may now be readily measured using commercially available assays.

Phosphate
Phosphate tends to directly correlate with growth rate and is highest in premature infants and during the first few months of life, and continues to be higher than adult reference ranges throughout growth.

Insulin-like growth factor 1
Insulin-like growth factor 1 (IGF-1) also tends to directly correlate with growth rate and is highest during the pubertal growth spurt, and continues to be higher than adult reference ranges throughout growth during childhood and adolescence, from the age of two years. IGF-1 is also an important marker of overall nutritional status and will be abnormally low in undernutrition and malnutrition, particularly in children and adolescents.

Others
Osteocalcin, a measure of bone formation, is also age and pubertal stage dependent.

Parathyroid hormone, magnesium, and calcium concentrations do not appear to be age dependent.

18.4 Pharmaceutical agents commonly used in bone disease

Vitamin D preparations used for vitamin D deficiency include ergocalciferol (D_2) and cholecalciferol (D_3) and either preparation is effective in restoring vitamin D stores in vitamin D deficiency.

The active form of vitamin D, $1,25(OH)_2D_3$ (calcitriol) should not be used to treat vitamin D deficiency as it 'bypasses' the regulating step of 1 alpha hydroxylation in the kidney, and may lead to hypercalcemia. Calcitriol is also expensive. However, calictriol is required for treatment of (1) hypoparathyroidism, (2) renal osteodystrophy, (3) X-linked hypophosphatemic rickets, (4) congenital disorders of vitamin D metabolism, and (5) as an adjunct to treatment and prevention of glucocorticoid-induced bone disease. An alternative, less expensive pharmacologic agent used in some countries is 1 alpha hydroxyvitamin D_3, which undergoes rapid hepatic conversion to $1,25(OH)_2D_3$.

Bisphosphonates are a class of therapeutic agents that chemically resemble naturally occurring pyrophosphate, and inhibit bone resorption. Bisphosphonates are commonly used in the treatment and prevention of post-transplant, glucocorticoid-induced, and senile osteoporosis. It is important to ensure dietary calcium intake is adequate to prevent hypocalcemia, particularly immediately following intravenous administration of bisphosphonates.

18.5 Diagnostic imaging assessment of the skeleton

Diagnostic imaging techniques are important in the evaluation of skeletal disease. Although skeletal radiography remains the most useful diagnostic imaging technique in the assessment of rachitic metabolic bone disease, it is insufficiently sensitive for the assessment of bone density. Over the past decade or so, a number of diagnostic imaging techniques have been developed including single- and dual-photon absorptiometry, which have now been superseded by dual-energy X-ray absorptiometry (DXA), quantitative computed tomography (QCT), and ultrasound.

DXA analyses photon absorption at two different energies to calculate the amount of bone mineral as bone mineral content and bone mineral density (BMD). It is able to measure total body BMD, in addition to BMD at regional (clinically relevant) sites such as the lumbar spine, femoral neck and head, and Ward's triangle. DXA also has the advantage of low radiation exposure, equivalent to approximately one-tenth of that for a chest X-ray. BMD measured by DXA is an areal bone density and actually assesses bone 'density' in cross-sectional area, hence is expressed as g/cm^2 and is size dependent. Total body and regional (e.g. vertebral) cross-sectional area increases with increasing height and bone size, so for the same true volumetric bone density (g/cm^3 – see below), a short individual will be expected to have a lower areal bone density than a tall individual.

Adult BMD is expressed as 'T' scores, which are standard deviation scores compared with a sex-matched healthy young adult reference range. According to WHO criteria, a 'T' score of −1.5 to −2.49 standard deviation scores (SDS) is defined as osteopenia, and osteoporosis is defined as a 'T' score of less than or equal to −2.5 SDS.

In growing children, the 'T' score is clearly meaningless, consequently the BMD is compared with age- and sex-matched healthy children, and is expressed as a 'Z' score. However, even this approach has its limitations because areal BMD increases with increasing bone size, so areal BMD increases during growth in childhood and adolescence. The 'Z' score may appear to be within the osteopenic or osteoporotic range, because the child may be smaller than his or her age-matched peers due to constitutional delay in growth and puberty for example, when bone density would be expected to 'catch up' following the onset of puberty.

By assuming a cylindrical shape for the vertebra, for example, a true volumetric bone density may be calculated. It has been shown that true volumetric bone density in normal, healthy growing children and adolescents remains relatively constant during growth.

QCT measures true volumetric bone density and can assess bone quality in more detail than is possible with DXA, as cortical bone volume and trabecular bone volume can be assessed separately. The disadvantages of this method include scant reference data at the present time for children and adolescents, substantially increased radiation exposure compared with DXA, and the limitation to specific skeletal sites, as the lumbar spine only can be measured in a whole body QCT, or other specific sites, (e.g. involving upper or lower limb) need to be assessed using peripheral QCT (pQCT).

Bone ultrasound is another diagnostic imaging technique under development for the assessment of bone density; however, pediatric and adolescent reference data remains limited. Once again, total body bone density cannot be assessed using this technique.

At the present time, however, DXA using specific pediatric software remains the most widely available

and best validated method to assess BMD in children and adolescents, and in fact these features of DXA apply across all age groups, and provided that the underlying assumptions of areal BMD are understood, DXA currently remains the preferred method of clinical assessment of BMD.

18.6 Rickets/osteomalacia (vitamin D deficiency)

There is still no internationally agreed definition of rickets, particularly with regard to a 'cut-off' value for serum 25OH D$_3$ concentrations. In older infants and children, radiological changes (as outlined below) invariably occur with unequivocally low 25OH D$_3$ values, and the presence of rachitic radiological changes confirms a diagnosis of rickets in this age group, irrespective of other biochemical features present.

The definition of osteomalacia, which occurs in adults, is arguably more uncertain, as adults no longer have 'growth plates' so that the characteristic metaphyseal changes seen in children do not occur in adults. In order to prevent vitamin D deficiency, milk products have been routinely fortified in the US since 1957. Although milk had been fortified previously in the mid 1920s to the 1950s with provitamin D$_2$ (ergosterol) and irradiated, this practice was stopped due to the development of hypercalcemia in some individuals as a result of excess vitamin D exposure. Quality control for fortification of milk with vitamin D remains an issue, as hypercalcemia has also occurred in recent years as a result of inadvertently fortifying milk with excessive vitamin D.

Most European countries also now routinely provide vitamin D supplementation to exclusively breast-fed infants, and fortify milk products with vitamin D, although in 'sunny countries' such as Australia, for example, there are no systematic public health measures to provide vitamin D supplementation. Yet in Australia, sun avoidance is increasing due to the risk of skin melanoma from increased exposure to UVB because of development of the 'ozone hole' in the earth's atmosphere. This has prompted the development of 'broad spectrum' sunscreens which block both UVA and UVB from sunlight and with ongoing use these may also reduce skin exposure to UVB sufficiently to cause vitamin D deficiency.

Risk factors

Individuals at risk for vitamin D deficiency include those with

- limited sunlight exposure,
- highly pigmented skin, or
- malabsorption syndromes.

Individuals at risk of vitamin D deficiency due to specific social and cultural settings include:

- those who are institutionalized and 'house bound', especially the elderly and chronically disabled;
- Islamic women who observe the practice of *Hajjab*, in which they are almost entirely covered for reasons of modesty; and
- highly pigmented individuals who are socially isolated, particularly apartment dwellers, who spend minimal time exposed to direct sunlight.

In the absence of vitamin D-fortified foods or vitamin D supplements, individuals living in polluted cities at high latitudes are at increased risk of vitamin D deficiency, and child-bearing women and infants and young children are at greatest risk. For lightly pigmented individuals, just 10–20 min direct sun exposure of face and forearms every day or so over summer should prevent the development of vitamin D deficiency.

Rickets in infants and young children

The association of rickets with sunlight deprivation was not recognized until the early twentieth century, although some physicians had recognized the antirachitic properties of cod liver oil before this. At the beginning of the twentieth century, 85% of children living in northern hemisphere urban industrialized cities had rickets. In industrially developed countries today, rickets most commonly occurs in exclusively breastfed infants born in cities at high latitudes to mothers who are also at risk of vitamin D deficiency due to poor sunlight exposure, unfortified food sources (such as milk), social isolation, increased skin pigmentation, or cultural clothing practices, independently or in combination.

In utero, the fetus receives 25OH D_3 from transplacental transfer from the maternal circulation. Hence neonatal 25OH D_3 levels reflect maternal stores. Premature infants and infants of vitamin D-deficient mothers are at high risk of vitamin D deficiency if vitamin D supplementation is not instituted routinely in the neonatal period.

Clinical features

Hypocalcemic seizures are a common presenting feature of rickets in infants aged less than nine months, but are seen less frequently in older infants and toddlers. Older infants and toddlers tend to present with gross motor delay, leg bowing, or occasionally fragility fractures. However, the diagnosis may be made incidentally on biochemical testing or on chest X-ray performed for other reasons, such as investigation for failure to thrive or fever of unknown origin. The clinical characteristics of rickets include slowing of linear growth, rachitic rosary, wrist and ankle swelling, craniotabes (softening of the skull bones), a widely patent anterior fontanelle, frontal bossing, and reluctance to weight-bear/delayed walking (Plate 6). Rachitic bones are characteristically soft and pliable, as a result of growth of unmineralized bone osteoid. Consequently, wrist and ankle swelling and leg bowing become more marked as infants start weight-bearing through crawling, cruising, and walking.

Rachitic rosary corresponds to the flaring of the costochondral junctions seen radiologically, and may be palpated anteriorly along the 'nipple line,' and is sometimes also visible on the anterior chest wall in infants and children in the setting of failure to thrive.

It is important also to be aware that other dietary deficiencies may coexist in prolonged, essentially exclusively breastfed infants and toddlers through the second and into the third year of life, including iron-deficiency anemia, and if the mother is a vegan, consuming no dairy products, vitamin B_{12} deficiency may also be present. Older infants and children may also have abnormal dentition, due to enamel hypoplasia.

Radiological features

Rachitic X-ray changes include flaring of the costochondral junctions and frayed, cupped long bone metaphyses, with generalized osteopenia. The typical radiological appearances of rickets are shown in Figure 18.4. These radiological changes represent ongoing osteoid being laid down in bone which is then poorly mineralized. Radiologically, gross metaphyseal changes are frequently not seen in infants under three months of age; however, generalized osteopenia remains characteristic, and occasionally 'periosteal reactions' are also seen in the long bone X-rays, giving rise to the radiological differential diagnosis of osteomyelitis or scurvy, which may be excluded on clinical grounds.

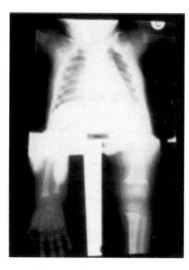

Figure 18.4 Upper limb X-rays of an 18-month-old boy with vitamin D deficiency rickets. Note the expanded metaphyses particularly of the radius and ulnar at the wrist.

Biochemical features

Characteristic biochemical features include:

- raised alkaline phosphatase (bone specific alkaline phosphatase, BSAP), due to increased bone turnover,
- raised PTH, in response to hypocalcemia, and
- low or undetectable 25OH D_3.

Other biochemical changes such as serum 1,25OH D_3, calcium, and phosphate levels are variable, and dependent on the course of the disease. 1,25(OH)$_2$D$_3$ may often be within the upper end of the reference range or frankly elevated. Both serum calcium and serum phosphate may be low or within the normal range, hence measurement of these parameters is unhelpful in diagnosis. Serum phosphate is characteristically decreased in long-standing rickets, due to the phosphaturic action of PTH.

Prevention

Expectant and lactating mothers have an increased vitamin D requirement, 2–4 times the RDI for adults at other times. Identification of pregnant mothers at risk for vitamin D deficiency and providing vitamin D supplementation during pregnancy will protect both the mother and fetus from vitamin D deficiency. Postnatal administration of vitamin D to vitamin D-deficient lactating mothers needs to be approximately six times

the adult RDI to correct their infants' vitamin D deficiency, indicating that it is preferable to give vitamin D replacement to the mother and infant separately. Vitamin D supplementation of 400 IU daily to exclusively breastfed 'at risk' infants or vitamin D-supplemented infant formula feeds totally prevents the development of vitamin D-deficiency rickets in otherwise normal infants.

Osteomalacia in adults

Vitamin D-deficiency osteomalacia in adults is an entirely preventable cause of osteoporotic fracture; however, it is often asymptomatic or individuals may present with vague symptoms of musculoskeletal aches and pains, depression, and lethargy. Occasionally adults may become significantly hypocalcemic and present with carpopedal spasm or fitting. Characteristic biochemical changes and poorly mineralized osteoid on bone biopsy provides confirmation of vitamin D-deficiency osteomalacia in adults.

Vitamin D deficiency in the institutionalized and elderly

Institutionalized individuals with severe chronic physical and/or intellectual disability associated with epilepsy, such as severe cerebral palsy, are at risk from developing vitamin D deficiency rickets or osteomalacia due to both limited direct sunlight exposure and anticonvulsant medication, which reduces vitamin D stores through effects on hepatic metabolism. The institutionalized elderly are also at risk for vitamin D deficiency through reduced direct sun exposure, compounded by aging effects on the skin, which reduces the efficiency of vitamin D production in the skin, and on the gut which results in reduced calcium absorption.

Vitamin D deficiency in fat malabsorption

The 25-hydroxylated form of vitamin D is a fat-soluble vitamin and it is 'recycled' within the enterohepatic circulation (Figure 18.3). Diseases which cause fat malabsorption such as celiac disease and conditions associated with pancreatic exocrine insufficiency such as cystic fibrosis (see Chapter 23), are added risk factors for vitamin D deficiency across all age groups.

Other causes of rickets/osteomalacia

Chronic renal disease

Chronic renal disease generally, and in dialysis and immediately post-transplant patients in particular, is frequently associated with the following disorders:

- Protein–energy malnutrition and loss of lean muscle mass occurs 18–75% of dialysis patients depending on dietary protocols used. Protein restriction in chronic renal failure has been recommended in the past to reduce the degree of uremia and to minimize further renal damage from excessive hyperfiltration. In more recent years, earlier institution of dialysis and renal transplant, especially in children, has improved protein–energy nutritional status in renal patients.
- Calcium deficiency is exacerbated by impaired $1,25(OH)_2D_3$, which results in hyperparathyroidism.

Rickets/osteomalacia occurs in chronic renal disease basically via two mechanisms, either alone or in combination. These two underlying mechanisms causing bone disease in chronic renal disease are characterized by secondary hyperparathyroidism and adynamic renal bone disease.

- Secondary hyperparathyroidism develops due to associated impaired renal $1,25(OH)_2D_3$ production, which results in hypocalcemia, which in turn causes secondary hyperparathyroidism. Hyperparathyroidism in this context is an appropriate response to $1,25(OH)_2D_3$ and dietary calcium deficiency, and may be reversed by ensuring sufficient dietary calcium intake and administration of calcitriol. Prolonged, poorly controlled secondary hyperparathyroidism may then progress to tertiary, or unregulated, hyperparathyroidism, which requires surgical intervention and total parathroidectomy.
- Adynamic renal bone disease resembles senile osteoporosis, as it is characterized by decreased bone turnover associated with low ALP and other bone formation markers, and bone resorption exceeds bone formation. The underlying causes of adynamic renal osteodystrophy are not well understood, but may include: aluminum toxicity in dialysis patients, poor protein/calorie nutrition, and/or inappropriate mineral ion nutrition, hormonal factors such as decreased IGF-1 bioactivity either due to low IGF-1 associated with poor nutritional status or due to increased circulating IGF-binding proteins associated with reduced glomerular filtration rate (GFR) and reduced weight-bearing activity due to lethargy associated with chronic illness.

Severe dietary calcium deficiency in young children

Rachitic features may also be observed after weaning when the children have minimal access to dairy and other calcium-rich foods. Rachitic changes may also develop as a consequence of a combination of vitamin D and calcium deficiency, highlighting the need to take a very careful dietary history of calcium intake when assessing rachitic infants. Vitamin D replacement alone without increasing dietary calcium will result in persistent rachitic changes, radiologically and biochemically, with persisting raised alkaline phosphatase and PTH, in the presence of adequate vitamin D stores ($25OH D_3$ levels).

Genetic disorders

Genetic disorders causing renal phosphate wasting, such as X-linked and autosomal dominant hypophosphatemic rickets, usually present with leg bowing in toddlers and older children, with characteristic rachitic radiological changes, but differ biochemically, as hypocalcemia and secondary hyperparathyroidism do not occur in untreated individuals with this condition. Affected individuals are treated with phosphate supplements and $1,25(OH)_2 D$ (calcitriol).

Genetic abnormalities of vitamin D metabolism are rare, but do need to be considered when children with rickets are clearly vitamin D sufficient. These include the autosomal recessive conditions of 1 alpha hydroxylase deficiency, which may be treated with calcitriol, and vitamin D-resistant rickets, due to genetic mutations within the vitamin D receptor, which may respond to high-dose calcitriol, although severely affected individuals may require parenteral calcium administration as the only means of treatment.

18.7 Mineral ion homeostasis in preterm infants

A proportion of infants born prematurely will develop metabolic bone disease, but it is difficult to provide accurate figures for the true incidence as there are no widely accepted diagnostic criteria. Bone disease in preterm infants is principally due to substrate (calcium and phosphate) deficiency. Additional factors such as the administration of steroids, diuretics, and the effects of immobilization or inactivity also merit consideration for their independent effects on skeletal development.

Bone disease in preterm infants is characterized in the short term by a sequence of events which begins with biochemical evidence of disturbed mineral metabolism, continues with reduced bone mineralization (as assessed by quantitative absorptiometric techniques), and results in abnormal bone remodeling and reduced linear growth velocity. In extreme forms, fractures of ribs and the distal ends of long bones and craniotabes have been reported. In the longer term, height may be reduced, there is a trend towards earlier presentation with fracture (excluding non-accidental injury cases) and bone mineral accretion in later childhood may also be influenced.

Biochemical changes typically observed as part of metabolic bone disease in preterm infants

Whole blood ionized calcium falls within 18–24 h of delivery. This is a physiologic rather than pathologic event reflecting continued calcium accretion into bone in the face of reduced exogenous calcium input, and a postnatal surge in calcitonin production of unknown etiology. An increase in calcitonin will stimulate calcium uptake into bone, resulting in a reduction in calcium in the blood, until milk feeds are established. Hypophosphatemia characteristically develops at between 7 and 14 days of age, with plasma phosphate falling below 1.0 mmol/l, and is accompanied by hypophosphaturia, with tubular reabsorption of phosphorus typically >90%, indicating renal phosphate-conserving mechanisms in the infant.

Plasma ALP activity typically rises over the first three weeks of postnatal life to levels two- to three-fold greater than the maximum of the adult normal range. ALP increases further (from age five to six weeks) in infants who receive diets low in mineral substrate compared with those who receive diets with increased mineral content. In the short term, plasma alkaline phosphatase activity greater than five times the maximum of the adult normal range is associated with progressive slowing of linear growth velocity.

In phosphate-depleted infants both hypercalcemia (plasma calcium >2.7 mmol/l) and hypercalciuria are frequently observed, possibly in response to elevation of $1,25(OH)_2D$. Where routine vitamin D supplementation of milk and cereals is practised, cord blood levels of $25OH\ D_3$ are typically >50 nmol/l, indicating vitamin D sufficiency. Maternal supplementation with vitamin D results in higher cord blood levels of $25OH\ D$, but not $1,25(OH)_2D$. Where maternal vitamin D intake during pregnancy has been poor, or where there is pre-existing maternal vitamin D deficiency, neonatal vitamin D stores may be low, and supplemental vitamin D of more than the normal 400 IU/day may be required.

A number of studies have identified low/borderline plasma $25OH\ D$ and elevated $1,25(OH)_2D$ levels in the plasma of preterm infants fed unsupplemented human milk, suggesting an increased requirement for vitamin D during rapid bone turnover in phosphate-depleted infants. Many studies indicate that vitamin D supplementation does improve calcium absorption and retention, although the magnitude of this improvement is variable, possibly reflecting mineral as well as vitamin D status. There are no data indicating improved long-term outcome for infants receiving higher doses of vitamin D. There is no good evidence suggesting frank vitamin D deficiency in the majority of infants.

Radiological changes seen in preterm infants with metabolic bone disease of prematurity

Radiological abnormalities are occasionally seen at birth in very growth-retarded infants, presumably secondary to inadequate transplacental substrate supply. The majority of infants developing radiological abnormalities (rachitic changes, fractures) either weigh <1000 g at birth, or receive diets grossly deficient in mineral substrate. Such diets include intravenous solutions formulated with inorganic mineral salts and breast milk which is not supplemented with phosphate.

A useful scoring system based on single view radiographs of the wrist or ankle at postnatal ages 5 and 10 weeks was described 20 years ago by Koo, and it has been found that the majority of infants weighing less than 1000 g have evidence of abnormal remodeling using this system. In older reports, epiphyseal cupping, splaying and fraying and craniotabes were observed in up to 50% of the population of infants of less than 33 weeks gestation. Fractures of the ribs and long bones were also widely reported.

Debate continues over the natural history of bone mineral accretion in preterm infants after discharge from hospital. Some suggest a period of rapid 'catch-up' usually by 8–16 weeks post-term age such that appendicular bone mineral content estimated for preterm infants is similar to that of term infants. Increasing the mineral content of the postdischarge diet is associated with improved bone mineral accretion rates. Many infants show a continuing deficit in radial bone mineral content up to age one year. Beyond this time there appears to be a gradual catch-up, and then continued increased mineral accretion (when compared with children born at term) from the age of two years.

Substrate delivery

Ideally an intake of 2 mmol/kg per day of phosphate and 3 mmol/kg per day of calcium should be achieved. Breast milk contains on average 0.5 mmol/100 ml of phosphate and 1 mmol/100 ml of calcium. Volumes of any milk greater than 240 ml/kg per day are rarely given in hospital. Without phosphate supplementation, a phosphate intake close to that needed to sustain normal bone mineral accretion can only be achieved in an infant that has linear growth arrest.

In general, studies show that almost all the phosphate is absorbed whatever kind of milk is given, but that only 30–50% of the calcium is absorbed. The issue is much more critical for phosphate than for calcium, however, since 99% of calcium is in the bones, but only 60–70% of the phosphate. Phosphate is needed for many essential processes in the body, and in the face of phosphate insufficiency, the bones will be broken down to provide more phosphate.

In summary, sick preterm infants, weighing <1000 g, on fluid restriction, diuretics, and steroids are at greatest risk of mineral ion deficiency and osteopenia of prematurity, and require careful attention particularly in their recovery phase to ensure that they receive appropriate mineral ion supplementation, to allow for normal linear growth and bone mineralization.

18.8 Corticosteroid-induced bone disease

Glucocorticoids (GCs) are widely used pharmacologically for diverse diseases such as asthma, malignancy, and a variety of chronic inflammatory conditions. High-dose GCs are also being increasingly used as part of the immunosuppressive therapy required post organ transplant. Unarguably glucocorticoids are very effective therapeutic agents; however, in high dose (equivalent to greater than prednisolone 2 mg/kg per day) they have a variety of actions on calcium homeostasis and bone itself which together contribute to reduced dietary calcium retention and the development of steroid-induced osteoporosis.

Actions mediated by parathyroid hormone

The classical view of the effect of GCs was that they induced renal calcium efflux and inhibited calcium uptake from the intestine, leading to a fall in serum calcium and the development of secondary hyperparathyroidism. Increased peripheral sensitivity to actions of PTH has also been reported. The consequences of continuously elevated PTH levels is to increase bone resorption and reduce bone formation. This pattern of effects has been widely reported immediately after initiating GC therapy, but the increase in bone resorption does not usually continue. There is a relative increase in bone resorption versus formation that suggests reduced osteoblastic activity or reduced osteoblastogenesis.

PTH has specific effects on the growth plate, acting through the PTH/PTHrP receptor to inhibit chondrocyte differentiation. This may contribute to the slowing in growth observed clinically and in *in vivo* model systems. There are also thought to be direct effects of steroids on cartilage cells. Fewer cells exit the resting zone to progress through differentiation in model animal systems of direct steroid infusion into the growth plate area.

Additional effects of glucocorticoid excess on systems that modulate bone remodeling

Sex hormones and estrogen in particular have a major role in maintaining normal bone health. Growth hormone (GH) and IGF-1 are also considered to have an important role in bone growth. Glucocorticoid excess causes reduction of secretion of these hormones via several pathways:

- *Pituitary* – glucocorticoids inhibit secretion of growth hormone, luteinizing hormone/follicle-stimulating hormone, and adrenocorticotropic hormone. Although serum GH and IGF-1 levels are normal, IGF-1 bioactivity is reduced, possibly due to increased IGF-binding protein 1.

- *Gonadal function* – glucocorticoids inhibit synthesis of estrogen by the ovary, testosterone by the testes.
- *Adrenal* – decrease in secretion (due to suppression of ACTH) of adrenal androgens, dehydroepiandrosterone (DHEA), and androstenedione.
- *Cellular transport* – glucocorticoids decrease transport of calcium and phosphate, particularly from the gut.

Direct effects on bone cells

There is debate about the effects of steroids directly on bone cells. Whilst *in vivo* GCs are inhibitory, *in vitro* GCs can either stimulate or inhibit bone formation depending on the model system, the conditions pertaining, and the amount of steroid in the system. It is important to distinguish between the developmental and regulatory effects of GCs on bone formation. GCs may enhance the differentiation of osteoblastic cells thus providing more cells to contribute to new bone formation (but also see below) but in the complete organ will also inhibit the functions of the differentiated cells and may also provoke apoptosis.

In the normal bone-remodeling cycle, bone resorption (which lasts about two weeks in any individual site) is followed by bone formation (which lasts about 2.5 months). In children the amount of bone replaced in each 'packet' is 3% more than that removed, thus maintaining an increase in bone mass as part of skeletal linear growth.

In GC-induced bone disease in animals and humans, bone resorption is initially increased (for about a week after starting therapy), but then continues at the normal rate. However, the amount of new bone which is formed to 'fill in' the defects created by resorption is reduced, reflecting both an apparent reduction in osteoblastogenesis and increased apoptosis of osteoblasts.

Increased osteoblast and osteocyte apoptosis have been widely reported in sections of bone from GC-treated humans and animals. In the light of the recent data on the speed of onset/offset of fracture risk associated with steroid therapy, it has been suggested that preservation of the integrity of the osteocyte network is a critical factor in preventing fractures in GC-treated patients.

Prevention and treatment of steroid-induced osteoporosis

Because dietary calcium absorption and retention is approximately 20% less efficient with high-dose GC therapy, dietary calcium intake should increase accordingly. However, previous studies have failed to show a clear benefit of the use of calcium and vitamin D in the prevention of fractures in GC-treated adult patients. There is some evidence for beneficial effects with calcitriol and calcium in combination. Bisphosphonates are a class of drugs which inhibit bone resorption, and have been found to be useful in the treatment of GC-induced osteoporosis in adults. In organ transplant patients in particular, bisphosphonates have been given before transplant in an attempt to prevent the major increase in bone resorption post transplant. There are no data available for children that indicate either the preferred mode of treatment of established osteoporosis caused by GCs, or prophylaxis in this vulnerable group.

18.9 Post-transplant bone disease

Organ transplants are carried out with increasing frequency and success, due to the development of potent immunosuppressive agents, which include GCs, cyclosporine A, azothioprin, tacrolimus, and newer agents such as rapamycin and mycophenolate mofetil. Post-transplant bone loss is multifactorial, and, as for chronic systemic disease briefly discussed below, prolonged immobilization, poor protein/calorie nutrition, hypogonadism, and underlying disease all contribute. Of the immunosuppressive agents listed above, GCs and cyclosporine A have a major impact on post-transplant bone loss. The mechanisms of GCs are described above. Cyclosporine A causes rapid and severe bone loss by increasing osteoclastic bone resorption markedly in excess of bone formation. A degree of bone loss due to pre-existing disease commonly occurs pre transplant, and in the initial stages post-transplant bone loss occurs rapidly and severely, and then may continue in the long term at slower rates, depending on disease state and doses of long-term immunosuppressive agents required. Thus, prevention and treatment of post-transplant osteoporotic fractures is becoming a major challenge.

Severity of post-transplant bone loss varies according to the organ transplanted. For example, after renal transplant, the rate of bone loss at the spine varies from 6% to 18% per year, with the highest rates occurring within the first six months after transplantation (compared with the average rate of bone loss during aging of 1% per year), with fracture rates of 10–20% during the first year post transplant. However, fractures, particular in small bones, occur in nearly 50% of diabetic patients within the first 1–2 years after renal transplant with or without a pancreatic transplant, implying specific issues in this particular patient group, which may be related to a combination of pre-existing complications, glycemic control, and nutritional issues.

Fracture incidences of ~37% have been reported in lung transplant recipients and ~65% in patients who have received liver transplants for primary biliary cirrhosis. Bone marrow transplantation with adequate sex hormone replacement does not tend to be associated with such severe bone loss and osteoporosis.

Although it remains important to optimize calcium intake and absorption, and adequate protein/calorie nutrition in this setting, the overall the main contributors to post-transplant bone loss would seem to be the use of specific immunosuppressive agents which cause rapid and severe bone loss, and the major improvements in post-transplant bone loss is likely to be through the development of immunosuppressive protocols which use bone-sparing immunosuppressive agents.

18.10 Osteoporosis associated with chronic disease

Reduced sunlight exposure/vitamin D deficiency, immobility, use of GCs and immunosuppressive agents such as cyclosporine A, protein/calorie and mineral ion undernutrition/malnutrition, hypogonadotropic hypogonadism associated with chronic systemic illness all contribute to the development of osteoporosis. Specific issues relate to chronic diseases such as:

- cystic fibrosis, where fat malabsorption with vitamin D deficiency, protein–energy malnutrition, use of GCs, and post lung transplantation are particularly relevant (see Chapter 23);
- connective tissue diseases such as systemic lupus erythematosis and rheumatoid arthritis, and cancer treatments, where the use of immunosuppressive

agents including GCs may be specific issues in rheumatological and malignant conditions; and
- thalassemia, in which untreated hypogonadism and extramedullary erythropoiesis and/or use of chelating agents may contribute to bone loss.

However, in chronic disease generally, the risk of development of osteoporosis in both children and adults may be reduced by ensuring vitamin D adequacy, and optimizing mineral ion and protein/calorie nutrition, together with consideration of the use of bisphosphonates.

18.11 Anorexia nervosa

Anorexia nervosa affects approximately 1% of adolescent girls in industrially developed countries, and is associated with considerable morbidity and mortality in up to 15% of affected individuals (see also Chapter 6). Recovery only occurs in up to 50–70% of affected individuals. Major skeletal effects include failure to accrue bone mass during the immediate postpubertal years and bone loss leading to osteoporosis, and are most marked in persistent, early onset (premenarcheal) anorexia nervosa. Osteoporosis in anorexia nervosa is likely to be due to a combination of overall malnutrition, with both direct effects of protein–energy malnutrition and through the consequences of associated hormonal changes such as low serum IGF-1 levels and hypogonadotropic hypogonadism. Furthermore, these effects are not counterbalanced by increased weight-bearing activity characteristically associated with this condition.

Clinical features

As a result of decreased food intake and increased energy expenditure, with or without self-induced vomiting and purgative abuse, ongoing weight loss of more than 15% below the minimum expected for age and height occurs. Due to food faddism, dietary intake may be inadequate both in quality and quantity. With specific reference to bone health, avoidance of high-fat dairy products may result in significantly reduced calcium intake, and decreased overall protein/calorie intake may result in hypophosphatemia and insufficient protein for optimal bone growth. Other biochemical abnormalities which have a detrimental effect on bone formation include hypercortisolemia, low serum IGF-1 levels, and hypogonadotrophic hypogonadism.

Treatment of anorexia nervosa-associated bone disease

Weight loss due underlying malignancy or other chronic illness must be excluded at the outset, and having established the diagnosis of anorexia nervosa, treatment should result in improved dietary intake, using behavioral techniques and psychotropic drugs either alone or in combination, with institution of nasogastric feeding and strict bed rest if the individual's clinical status becomes life threatening. Restoration of bone health depends on achievement of near normalization of weight for height and once this is achieved menses may also be expected to resume. Recovery from anorexia nervosa is defined as attainment of normal body weight within 15% of that expected for age and height, and resumption of regular menses for three consecutive cycles.

Clinical studies have shown that bone mass improves with recovery from anorexia nervosa. However, calcium replacement alone or in combination with estrogen hormone replacement therapy, in the absence of weight gain indicating overall improvement in protein/calorie nutrition, is ineffective in maintaining or restoring normal bone mass, implying that a combination of restoration of normal gonadal function, together with adequate calcium and protein/calorie nutrition is required to support normal bone growth and turnover.

18.12 Senile osteoporosis

Osteoporosis, characterized by thin and brittle bones, represents a significant public health issue in the elderly, and is defined by WHO as bone density standard deviation score less than −2.5 standard deviations at two or more clinically relevant sites. Osteoporotic bone architecture is characterized by an irreversible destruction of trabecular bone structure. Osteoporotic fractures are characterized by 'fragility' fractures, which occur after trivial trauma or spontaneously, and typically occur at the following sites:

- wrist fractures (characteristically following a fall on an outstretched hand);
- femoral neck fractures (occur either spontaneously or following a fall, and are associated with severe morbidity and commonly lead to death in the elderly); and
- vertebral fractures (usually occur spontaneously).

Multiple vertebral fractures result in kyphosis 'the Dowager's hump.' Vertebral fractures are associated with chronic pain and stiffness, and may be associated with nerve compression syndromes.

With an increasingly aging population in industrially developed countries, 25–35% of women and increasing numbers of elderly men will experience osteoporotic fractures, which result in significant morbidity and mortality, in addition to adding millions of dollars to health care costs. Male osteoporosis is becoming more common as male cardiovascular mortality has decreased, and a greater proportion of men are living beyond their eighth decade.

Pathophysiology

Osteoporosis occurring beyond the sixth decade is likely to be due to a combination of factors including the menopause in women, and numerous lifestyle factors, the most important of which are insufficient weight-bearing exercise and long-standing dietary calcium deficiency occurring over decades. Factors in the elderly leading to reduced calcium bioavailability are shown in Box 18.3.

As a consequence of reduced calcium absorption, PTH levels tend to rise in the elderly, exacerbating osteoporosis.

> **Box 18.3** Factors in the elderly leading to reduced calcium bioavailability
>
> - Reduced sunlight exposure in institutionalized or 'house bound' elderly
> - Aging skin reduces skin production of vitamin D
> - Decreased gastrointestinal absorption due to impaired $1,25(OH)_2D_3$ action on the gastrointestinal tract
> - Increasing incidence of atrophic gastritis with age, resulting in reduced gastrointestinal absorption of calcium
> - Thiazide and loop diuretics increase urinary calcium excretion

Preventative strategies

Established osteoporosis is characterized by irreversible bone loss. Consequently in recent years there has been a major emphasis on osteoporosis prevention through modifying lifestyle factors such as optimizing dietary calcium intake, ensuring vitamin D adequacy, taking regular weight-bearing exercise, and avoidance of excessive alcohol consumption and smoking, together with estrogen hormone replacement therapy in younger postmenopausal women and testosterone replacement in hypogonadal men. Walking is the most appropriate weight-bearing exercise in the elderly, and although swimming may be soothing for arthritic joints and beneficial for cardiovascular health, it is non-weight-bearing and consequently is not helpful in maintaining or improving bone strength.

Screening 'at risk' adults in recent years with the widespread availability of DXA assessment of bone density has enabled identification of individuals with osteopenia and/or ongoing bone loss, so that intervention strategies, particularly with administration of bisphosphonates, may instituted, before the development of established osteoporosis and presentation with osteoporotic fractures, at which stage all current interventions for osteoporosis are much less effective.

Other environmental factors including fluoride deficiency also contribute to enamel hypoplasia in teeth and osteoporosis, prompting water fluoridation in deficient areas. However, fluoride therapy at pharmacological doses did not decrease the rates of osteoporotic fracture in the elderly.

18.13 Perspectives on the future

The interaction between nutrition and metabolic bone disease from infancy to old age has been discussed in broad, general terms, with particular emphasis on the interactions between drugs, lifestyle factors, hormonal factors, and chronic systemic disease. The synergy between mineral ion homeostasis and bone metabolism is finely balanced. There are a number of organ systems directly involved with mineral ion homeostasis, namely the parathyroid glands, skin, liver, gastrointestinal system, and kidneys, and this may be perturbed by dietary mineral ion deficiency, either directly or via vitamin D deficiency, by a number of other factors affecting the above organ systems and by the hormonal milieu of various systemic diseases.

Osteoporosis, the endpoint of a number of chronic systemic diseases, is usually the result of the interplay between a number of factors, and therapeutic interventions likewise need to be multifactorial, not only ensuring adequacy of dietary mineral ion intake and vitamin D status, but also by instituting modification to lifestyle factors such as optimizing weight-bearing exercise, avoiding excessive alcohol and caffeine, and smoking, and appropriate sex hormone replacement, with consideration of the use of bisphosphonate or calcitriol therapy as appropriate. The clinical implications of appropriate prevention and treatment of rickets/osteomalacia and osteoporosis cannot be overemphasized, due to the significant associated long-term morbidity, and with particular emphasis on osteoporosis, increased mortality, particularly in the elderly.

With the increasing aging population, there is a pressing need for nutritional preventative strategies to optimise dietary calcium and protein intake throughout life, in both healthy individuals and in the chronically ill, as one of the many interventions required for the prevention and treatment of osteoporosis, an ever increasing burden on health providers. Despite the widening use of antiresorptive agents such as bisphosphonates in the prevention and treatment of osteoporotic fractures, the challenge remains to develop safe and effective stimulators of bone formation. In recent years, there have been promising results to show the benefit of the use of PTH in the treatment of established osteoporosis in the elderly. However, the wider application of PTH in osteoporosis is currently precluded as there are data from animal experiments to show that the use of PTH may increase the incidence of osteosarcoma.

References and further reading

Bishop N. Rickets today – children still need milk and sunshine. *N Engl J Med* 1999; 341: 602–604.

Chan GM, Mileur L, Hansen JW. Calcium and phosphorus requirements in bone mineralization of preterm infants. *J Pediatr* 1988; 113: 225–229.

Dawson-Hughes Bess. Calcium supplementation and bone loss: a review of controlled clinical trials. *Am J Clin Nutr* 1991; 54: 274S–280S.

De Luca HF. The vitamin D story: a collaborative effort of basic science and clinical medicine. *FASEB J* 1988; 2: 224–236.

Elder G. Pathophysiology and recent advances in the management of renal osteodystrophy (Review). *J Bone Miner Res* 2002; 17: 2094–2105.

Epstein S, Inzerillo AM, Caminis J, Zaidi M. Disorders associated with rapid and severe bone loss (Review). *J Bone Miner Res* 2003; 18: 2083–2094.

Favus M. *The Primer on the Metabolic Bone Diseases and Disorders of Mineral Metabolism*, 5th edn. An official publication of the American Society of Bone and Mineral. Philadelphia: Lippincott-Raven, 2003.

Grindulis H, Scott PH, Belton NR, Wharton BA. Combined deficiency of iron and vitamin D in Asian toddlers. *Arch Dis Child* 1986; 61: 843–848.

Martin TJ, Ng KW, Nicholson GC. Cell biology of bone (Review). *Baillière's Clin Endocrinol Metab* 1988; 2: 1–29.

Mundy G, Chen D, Oyajoni B. Bone remodeling. In: *The Primer on the Metabolic Bone Diseases and Disorders of Mineral Metabolism*, 5th edn (M Favus, ed.), pp. 46–58. An official publication of the American Society of Bone and Mineral. Philadelphia: Lippincott-Raven, 2003.

NIH Consensus Statement. Optimum calcium intake Vol 12, no. 4, June 1994

Peacock M. Calcium absorption efficiency and calcium requirements in children and adolescents. *Am J Clin Nutr* 1991; 54: 261S–265S.

Pittard WB, III, Geddes KM, Sutherland SE, Miller MC, Hollis BW. Longitudinal changes in the bone mineral content of term and premature infants. *Am J Dis Child* 1990; 144: 36–40.

Raisz LG. Local and systemic factors in the pathogenesis of osteoporosis. *N Engl J Med* 1988; 318: 818–828.

Reichel H, Koeffler HP, Norman AW. The role of the vitamin D endocrine system in health and disease. *N Engl J Med* 1989; 320: 980–991.

Rizzoli R, Bonjour JP. Dietary protein and bone health (Editorial). *J Bone Miner Res* 2004; 19: 527–531.

Salle BL, Glorieux FH, Delvin EE. Perinatal vitamin D metabolism. [Review]. *Biol Neonate* 1988; 54: 181–187.

Salle BL, Glorieux FH, Lapillone A. Vitamin D status in breastfed term babies. *Acta Paediatr* 1998; 87: 726–727.

Sambrook PN, Kotowicz M, Nash P *et al.* Prevention and treatment of glucocorticoid-induced osteoporosis: a comparison of calcitriol, vitamin D plus calcium, and aledronate plus calcium. *J Bone Miner Res* 2003; 18: 919–924.

Seeman E, Szmuckler G, Formica C, Tsalamandris C, Mestrovic R. Osteoporosis in anorexia nervosa: the influence of peak bone density, bone loss, oral contraceptive use, and exercise. *J Bone Miner Res* 1992; 7: 1467–1474.

Teegarden D, Lyle RM, McCabe LD *et al.* Dietary calcium, protein, and phosphorus are related to bone mineral density and content in young women. *Am J Clin Nutr* 1998; 68: 749–754.

Thomas MK, Lloyd-Jones DM, Thadhani RI *et al.* Hypovitaminosis D in medical inpatients. *N Engl J Med* 1998; 338: 777–783.

19
Nutrition in Surgery and Trauma

Olle Ljungqvist, Ken Fearon, and Rod A Little

Key messages

- The response to stress involves a cascade of events that interact and influence each other.
- Together these responses can have profound catabolic effects on body metabolism, especially following major surgery or trauma.
- A series of measures need to be taken in the surgical/traumatized patient in order to ensure an adequate provision and tolerance of nutritional support.

- Blood glucose levels should be controlled (if necessary with insulin) to maintain normoglycemia.
- No single action will be sufficient to counteract the stress of injury, but a combination of therapeutic maneuvers need to be undertaken in order to turn the patient from catabolism towards an anabolic phase and hence enhance recovery.

19.1 Introduction

Surgery and trauma constitute a major part of modern medicine. In the western world, every year about 5% of the population have an operation, and some 40% of patients in hospitals undergo an operation as part of their treatment. Accidental major trauma is substantially less frequent, but traumatized patients often require intensive care for prolonged periods of times.

While elective surgery represents a type of treatment in which deliberate actions are undertaken to remove or reconstruct organs and hence can be well planned, trauma represents quite a different situation. In trauma, uncontrolled injuries have occurred, the patient is in a variable state of resuscitation, and the trauma team has to adapt to the situation as best possible. Trauma involves a variety of different injuries and affects different parts of the body in various combinations. The objective of treatment is to preserve as many organs and bodily functions as possible with the minimum further trauma. Although the injuries can be very different, the response to injury in surgery and accidental trauma are quite similar. The difference between the two lies in the ability to prepare the patient for the injury and to control homeostasis and the stress response by different means in the elective surgical patient, while

this is not possible in the traumatized patient. The fact that elective surgery care programs can be proactive, and the surgery performed under well-controlled and planned perioperative conditions opens the possibility of enhancing recovery after elective surgery.

The situation is different in trauma, where many of the proactive initiatives cannot be taken for obvious reasons. Nevertheless, the global strategy for metabolic control, and nutritional support in both situations are similar. In addition, the ultimate goals are the same, to have the patient recover and return to normal life as best and as fast as possible.

19.2 The stress response to trauma and its effects on metabolism

It is now about 70 years ago that Sir David Cuthbertson introduced the terms 'ebb' and 'flow' to describe the metabolic response to long bone fracture (Figure 19.1). His was the first attempt to introduce some chronological order into the response to trauma and to include 'shock' as an integral part of the response rather than as a complication. It is important to recognize that the main features of the metabolic response are initiated at the time of the injury and that this is

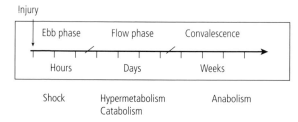

Figure 19.1 Phases of the physiological response to injury. After Cuthbertson (1982).

probably the time at which modulation can be most effective. The mediators of such change include the classical neuroendocrine hormones along with pro-inflammatory mediators.

The complexity of interaction between the different components involved in traumatically induced stress is illustrated in Figure 19.2. The injury caused by the operation initiates an inflammatory response causing the release of cytokines and acute phase proteins, along with the activation of stress hormones. The release of these mediators causes a change of metabolism into a catabolic state. However, even in situations when the inflammatory and endocrine responses are minimized, stress metabolism may occur. This indicates that other mechanisms are likely to be involved in causing the change in metabolism following surgery. The figure also shows that fasting before elective surgery

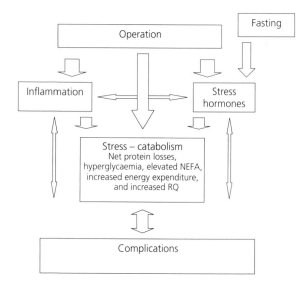

Figure 19.2 Schematic overview of the sequence of events that occurs in response to surgical trauma. NEFA, non-esterified fatty acids; RQ, respiratory quotient.

adds to the stress by enhancing the endocrine stress response. In patients where stress-induced catabolism is pronounced or prolonged, the risk for complications increases. The development of complications will further aggravate the inflammatory and endocrine stress responses and may develop into a vicious circle.

It is perhaps no longer useful to think of the 'ebb' phase as a period of depressed metabolism but rather as the early stage after trauma during which tissue energy production is not limited by oxygen delivery. It is a neuroendocrine response that depends on the magnitude of blood loss and somatic afferent nervous stimuli arising from damaged tissues. These stimuli inhibit homeostatic reflexes subserving both the thermoregulatory and cardiovascular systems. After very serious injuries with failure of oxygen delivery, the 'ebb' phase of altered control mechanisms may be short-lived as the patient enters into the potentially irreversible spiral of cell and tissue death known as 'necrobiosis.' The 'flow' phase is characterized by an increase in body temperature, metabolic rate, and urinary nitrogen excretion associated with net protein breakdown and a reduction in muscle mass and disturbances in energy substrate disposal.

Hypermetabolism

While it has been accepted since Cuthbertson's pioneering studies that hypermetabolism occurs in the 'flow' phase and that the increase was directly related to the severity of injury, there has been a considerable change in our understanding of the magnitude of that increase. In the early 1970s it was believed that the untreated, critically ill, septic, or trauma patient was expending in the region of 5000 kcal/day, creating major problems for those trying to introduce nutrition to the care of such patients. The introduction of clinically useful indirect calorimeters demonstrated that measured energy expenditures were most commonly less than half such predicted values. There was an understandable reluctance to accept these measured values until it was appreciated that a number of the features of critical illness and its treatment would reduce metabolic rate and therefore counterbalance those factors that tended to increase energy expenditure. For example such patients are often in bed for long periods, paralyzed, and ventilated, nursed in a warm environment, receive inadequate feeding, and lose active muscle mass. It is, however, important to ensure that the metabolic rate

dence of benefit from parenteral nutrition under the following conditions:

- As a continuation of preoperative nutritional support in previously malnourished patients.
- In patients with postoperative complications impairing gastrointestinal function and preventing normal oral feeding for more than 5–10 days postoperatively.
- In previously severely malnourished patients undergoing emergency surgery.
- In previously well nourished patients who have suffered major trauma or critical illness and who are unable to tolerate enteral feeding.

The weight of evidence suggests that enteral feeding by the nasogastric, nasoenteral, and jejunal routes or a combination of some enteral and supplementary parenteral feeding are the preferred methods, although, in the presence of prolonged gastrointestinal failure, parenteral feeding may be life saving. There are also some trials indicating that early and adequate oral supplementation in the first week after surgery may improve outcome, particularly in the malnourished patient. A flowchart for the management of postoperative nutrition in surgical patients is shown in Figure 19.3.

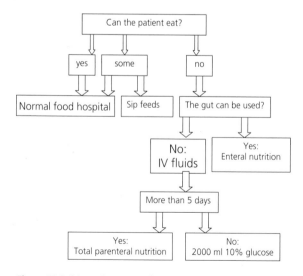

Figure 19.3 Schematic overview of suggested routes to ensure energy and protein intake following surgery.

The importance of glucose control during the nutritional support of the critically ill

There is growing and strong evidence that glucose levels should be maintained at normal levels while feeding the severely stressed surgical patient. Hyperglycemic diabetic patients undergoing surgery have long been known to run a substantially higher risk of complications (mainly infectious) than non-diabetic patients, or those where glucose control has been optimized. Recently, it has been shown that this also holds true for patients without diabetes. It has been demonstrated in a recent study from Belgium that postoperative patients (mainly thoracic surgery) in need of ventilatory support in an ICU setting benefit from intensive insulin treatment to normalize glucose levels (aiming at 4.5–6 mmol/l). Normalizing glucose levels using insulin resulted in marked reductions in septic episodes, renal failure, time on the ventilator, polyneuropathy, and mortality. The results show that insulin action seems to be key to successful immediate postoperative feeding, but also in avoiding complications that will cause further catabolism.

The use of insulin to maintain glucose control is likely to be a better approach than semi-starvation through carbohydrate restriction. Whether the beneficial effects of insulin are confined to the maintenance of normoglycemia or include the previously demonstrated reduction in net protein catabolism and cell membrane function remains to be determined.

Growth hormone has been tested in a series of clinical trials as a method of inducing anabolism in critically ill patients. It is of interest that the increased mortality experienced with the use of growth hormone in critical care patients has been ascribed to growth hormone-induced insulin resistance.

Adverse effects of conventional perioperative care in elective surgery patients

Traditional perioperative surgical practice has focused on prolonged fasting before surgery to reduce the risks of aspiration and after surgery in the face of 'natural' postoperative ileus. In addition, little effort has been made to reduce the classical neuroendocrine stress response which has been accepted as an inevitable consequence of surgical intervention. Finally, patients have been given excess intravenous fluids based on the principle developed in trauma resuscitation that 'wet is best.' Recent evidence has, however, suggested that ad lib administration of intravenous saline results in edema of the gut with delayed gastric emptying, delayed return to normal nutrition, and prolonged hospital stay. The adverse influences of prolonged fasting, unmodulated stress, and saline overload are thought to contribute to the net catabolism, postoperative fatigue, and prolonged recovery time from conventional surgery.

Modern techniques to minimize stress and support nutrition in elective surgery

When endocrine hormones were discovered and became measurable during the last century, early reports showed that even medium-size open surgery (such as uncomplicated open cholecystectomy) evoked marked release of all the classical stress hormones (catecholamines, cortisol, glucagon, and growth hormone). This, in turn, was associated with insulin resistance leading to hyperglycemia, elevated free fatty acid levels, and protein loss caused by increased protein breakdown and reduced protein synthesis. Since then, modern anesthesia, minimal invasive surgery, and other perioperative developments allows the same operation to be performed with almost no or minimal stress response. The difference between the classical responses

to surgery some 10 years ago and what can be achieved using modern techniques is shown in Figure 19.4.

It is important to understand that postoperative metabolic changes still play an important role for the development of secondary complications and for recovery in general. It is therefore not surprising that nutritional regimens play an important role in the postoperative phase. Recovery from surgery requires a reversal of the trauma-induced catabolism and a move towards anabolism. There are several ways by which the catabolic responses can be minimized and anabolism supported. Nutrition, the supply of macro- and micronutrients, represents an essential part of perioperative treatment.

Nutrition in enhanced recovery after surgery programs

'Enhanced recovery after surgery' protocols or 'fast track' surgery programs involve an integrated series of steps aimed to minimize the stress of the surgical operation and to inform and involve the patient in their recovery after the operation. The various events and treatments in the perioperative period have been scrutinized for supportive evidence in the literature and old routines with no scientific backing have been exchanged for routines shown to have positive effects on recovery. These programs have been shown to minimize reduced physiological function and to en-

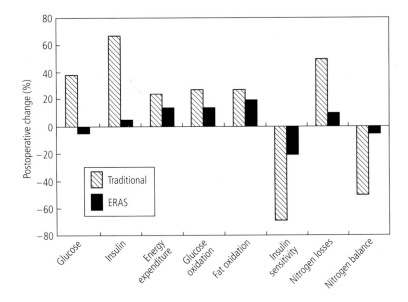

Figure 19.4 The relative changes in different parts of the metabolic response to surgery using traditional perioperative methods compared to perioperative care according to enhanced recovery after surgery (ERAS) programs. The ERAS concept is described in more detail in the text. The figure is used by permission of Mattias Soop, MD, PhD, Thesis Karolinska Institutet, Stockholm, 2003.

hance the return to normal function. A key aspect is the support of normal gastrointestinal function and an early return to normal fluid and food intake. Many of the programs have targeted patients undergoing gastrointestinal (primarily colon) surgery, and have shown clearly that the time of recovery after this type of surgery is prolonged by the use of old traditions and outdated routines.

Preoperative fasting

It has been assumed that the traditional overnight fast preoperatively is useful and not harmful. However, over the last decade many national anesthesia societies have changed preoperative fasting guidelines and now recommend free intake of clear fluids up until 2–3 h before anesthesia for elective procedures. This change has been proven safe and was introduced to reduce the discomfort of thirst. This routine also helps to avoid preoperative dehydration.

It has been shown recently that the metabolic changes that occur during an overnight fast influence the response to stress. In studies where patient's metabolic status has been changed from the overnight fasted state to the carbohydrate fed state by intake of an iso-osmolar carbohydrate-rich drink, marked effects on postoperative insulin resistance were observed. This treatment not only reduces thirst but also hunger and preoperative anxiety. For patients who are excluded from using modern fasting guidelines, intravenous glucose with or without insulin has been shown to have the same benefits. Provided the glucose load is sufficient (5 mg/kg per min often by use of 20% or 30% glucose solutions), the metabolic change from that of overnight fasting to a fed state can be achieved along with glycogen loading. This regimen has been shown to reduce cardiac complications after cardiac surgery.

Continuous epidural analgesia

A central part of the multimodal approach to recovery after surgery is the preoperative placement and activation of a continuous epidural based primarily on the infusion of local anesthetic with or without opiates. For abdominal surgery, the epidural should be placed in the lower thoracic region. This places a block covering the abdominal wall and also the adrenals, hence attenuating the release of catecholamines. By activating

the epidural before the operation, it can be determined that the block covers the region of the proposed incision and that it will function well as the basis for postoperative pain relief.

An effective and functional epidural has several effects. By blocking the adrenals and minimizing catecholamine release, postoperative insulin resistance can be reduced. Effective pain relief also has positive effects on insulin sensitivity. Last, but not least, systemic opioids can be avoided. Opioids have a negative effect on both gastric emptying and gastrointestinal motility in general.

Avoiding fluid overload to support postoperative gastrointestinal function

Overloading the patient with fluids and sodium chloride perioperatively causes edema and delays the return of normal gastrointestinal function. Restricting postoperative maintenance fluids to 2000 ml and NaCl to 77 mmol/day has been shown to enhance substantially gastric motility and speed up recovery. Stopping intravenous fluids on the first postoperative day is one of the key factors in the multimodal approach to enhanced recovery after surgery.

Minimal invasive surgical techniques

With the widespread use of laparoscopic techniques in surgery, it has become evident that minimal invasive techniques play an important role for the recovery of the patient after surgery. Laparoscopic surgery allows the same procedure to be performed with substantially less pain, discomfort, and metabolic derangement. Specifically, the proinflammatory cytokine response is attenuated whereas the neuroendocrine stress response is dampened to a lesser degree. For many procedures laparoscopic surgery has become the method of choice. This is particularly true for upper rather than lower gastrointestinal procedures.

Interestingly, a recent report has shown that patients undergoing laparoscopic cholecystectomy had substantially lower rates of postoperative nausea when given a preoperative dose of corticosteroids well before the onset of the operation. This finding suggests that even with a relatively minor operation, beneficial effects can be demonstrated by blocking the inflammatory response prior to the procedure. Hence, even with minimally traumatic and invasive techniques, multi-modal postoperative care should be considered.

Drains, tubes, and catheters

There is evidence that postoperative 'drip and suck' regimens are used excessively and unnecessarily in traditional patterns of postoperative care. Nasogastric drainage tubes, unless absolutely necessary as in gastric outlet obstruction, have been shown in a large meta-analysis of published studies to be associated with increased complication rates, particularly respiratory infections.

The metabolic effects of a combined treatment program

It has been shown recently that when preoperative carbohydrate-rich drinks and epidural anesthesia are combined with feeding an almost complete enteral diet from the day of surgery onwards, a neutral nitrogen balance can be maintained after major colorectal surgery. In addition, near normal glucose levels (average 5.8 mmol/l) were maintained during ongoing feeding. Postoperative insulin resistance was kept low and comparable with that reported after more minor surgery, such as laparoscopic cholecystectomy or inguinal hernia repair. These data show that if the metabolic response is kept at a minimum, feeding is possible and results in minimal losses of body proteins – a complete transformation of the classical ebb and flow catabolic spiral originally described by Cuthbertson.

19.4 Feeding the severely traumatized patient

The severely traumatized patient represents quite a different situation compared with the elective surgical patient. First and foremost, several organs may have been damaged directly. Key organs in this respect are the thoracic organs, the brain, the liver, and the kidney. Such injuries will potentially have marked impact on the treatment needed to maintain vital organ function and hence subsequent nutritional management. An obvious example is the patient with a head injury demanding ventilatory support, perhaps body tempera-

ture cooling and sedation. These measures will have clear influences on the route of nutrient administration, as well the amounts given.

Another important aspect differing in these patients is that they will have a full-scale stress response, having been injured in the awake state with no preparation possible. Hence, these patients will develop a greater degree of metabolic disturbance and often present with hyperglycemia as a result of marked insulin resistance in response to hemorrhage and other sequelae from the injury. Fluid resuscitation to maintain cardiovascular function will further influence metabolism and nutritional therapy later in the patient's course. Furthermore, many of these patients need surgery in a critical state and various measures needed to maintain vital functions during such procedures will impact on nutritional intake and how well the body tolerates nutrients supplied.

The overall strategy for severely injured trauma patients is to secure vital organ function upon arrival and thereafter during surgery. Once these measures have been stabilized, nutritional support can begin. Pre-emptive planning for postoperative nutrition via the enteral route can be achieved by placement of an enteral feeding tube in the stomach or more often in the jejunum. This will facilitate enteral feeding in the postoperative/post-traumatic phase. Enteral feeding begun in small amounts even within hours after emergency trauma surgery has been shown to be feasible and advantageous. This often needs to be complemented by parenteral feeding. Glucose levels should be kept within the normal range with insulin. However, for patients with multiple injuries a severe degree of insulin resistance may be expected, and for these patients it is necessary to also monitor acid–base balance. Reports from major burn injury have revealed that in severe insulin resistance, glucose may not be fully oxidized due to inhibition of intracellular metabolism and hence there is a risk of excess lactate formation from excessive glucose uptake. In this situation, glucose delivery must be reduced.

Once the patients stabilize and the initial phase is over, the general principles of moving from parenteral to enteral and finally to oral and normal feeding can be employed. During this course, it is may be useful to monitor energy demands by using indirect calorimetry which is available in some intensive care units.

Prescription of feed (see also Chapter 8)

The major aim of perioperative care is the early introduction of normal food. Regular hospital food should be the first choice for nutrition in most postoperative patients. However, it is essential to monitor and record the adequacy of such an intake.

For patients unable to consume sufficient food to meet their needs, the following guidelines can be applied. The supply of nutrients by the enteral route is limited by gastrointestinal tolerance in the postoperative period. For those patients consuming some but not sufficient regular food, sip feeds can be recommended. For patients able to take only minor portions of normal food or none at all, enteral tube feeding using a standard polymeric feed should be used in most cases, starting at 20–30 ml/h and increasing as tolerance improves based on gastric aspirate residuals. Several positive trials of postoperative enteral feeding have used quite low intakes of 18–20 kcal/kg body weight in the first few days, with beneficial results, particularly in terms of infection. Some studies in major trauma and in cancer surgery suggest that immune-enhancing feeds may have some advantage over standard feeds in these conditions.

In a series of recent studies it has been suggested that addition of specific immune-enhancing nutrients such as arginine, n-3 fatty acids, and dietary nucleotides may be of benefit for the patient undergoing major surgery. When these formulas have been given perioperatively, reductions in infectious complications and also reduced length of stay were initially reported. From the design of the studies it is not clear whether the effects were related to the addition of nutrients as such, or the addition of any one of the specific components. Further studies have not shown the same promising results and have even shown an opposite effect. Hence it remains unclear to what extent these formulas may be useful or which component carries the potential effects. Moreover, in the critical care setting there is recent trial evidence suggesting increased mortality associated with the use of particular immunonutrition formulations.

With parenteral nutrition, particular attention should be paid to avoiding too little or too much salt and water and to avoid hyperglycemia. For many patients, insulin may be needed to maintain normoglycemia. Otherwise standard prescriptions can be used to give 25–30 kcal/kg per day with 30–40% of total calories from fat. Intakes of 0.15–0.2 g N/kg per day are usually adequate with an energy-to-nitrogen ratio of approximately 150 : 1. The usual recommended amounts of mineral and micronutrients should also be supplied. The addition of glutamine or glutamine dipeptides to standard TPN has been associated with improved long-term outcome from critical care. Further studies are awaited.

19.5 Perspectives on the future

With adequate precautions against postoperative ileus, most patients undergoing surgery can return to normal oral feeding almost immediately. Several old traditional routines need to be changed. Proper anesthetic techniques for pain control will help to facilitate a return to the use of the oral route for feeding and avoid postoperative ileus. Preoperative feeding improves the outcome from surgery in patients with severe malnutrition and preoperative carbohydrates reduce postoperative insulin resistance and protein catabolism in elective surgery. Postoperative enteral nutrition reduces postoperative complications. There is some evidence of benefit from postoperative enteral and/or parenteral nutrition in previously malnourished patients, in those with postoperative complications and after major trauma or burns. Most importantly, feeding should be part of an integrated protocol of management throughout the patient's clinical course.

References and further reading

Allison SP, Kinney JM. Perioperative nutrition. *Curr Opin Clin Nutr Metab Care* 2000; 3: 1–3.

Beattie AH, Prach AT, Baxter JP, Pennington CR. A randomised controlled trial evaluating the use of enteral nutritional supplements postoperatively in malnourished surgical patients. *Gut* 2000; 46: 813–818.

Cuthbertson DP. The metabolic response to injury and other related explorations in the field of protein metabolism: an autobiographical account. *Scot Med J* 1982; 27: 158–171.

Griffiths RD. Specialized nutrition support in critically ill patients. *Curr Opin Crit Care* 2003; 9: 249–259.

Heyland DK, Montalvo M, MacDonald S, Keefe L, Su XY, Drover JW. Total parenteral nutrition in the surgical patient: a meta-analysis. *Can J Surg* 2001; 44: 102–111.

Kehlet H. Multimodal approach to control postoperative pathophysiology and rehabilitation. *Br J Anaesth* 1997; 78: 606–617.

Kirk HJ, Heys SD. Immunonutrition. *Br J Surg* 2003; 90: 1459–1460.

Knight, David JW. Immunonutrition: increased mortality is associated with immunonutrition in sepsis. *BMJ* 2003; 327: 682-b, 683.

Ljungqvist O, Nygren J, Thorell A. Modulation of postoperative insulin resistance by pre-operative carbohydrate loading. *Proc Nutr Soc* 2002; 61: 1–7.

Lobo DN, Bostock KA, Neal KR, Perkins AC, Rowlands BJ, Allison SP. Effect of salt and water balance on recovery of gastrointestinal function after elective colonic resection: a randomised controlled trial. *Lancet* 2002; 359: 1812–1818.

Soop M. Effects of perioperative nutrition on insulin action in postoperative metabolism. PhD thesis, Karolinska Institutet, Stockholm, 2003.

van den Berghe G, Wouters P, Weekers F *et al.* Intensive insulin therapy in the critically ill patients. *N Engl J Med* 2001; 345: 1359–1367.

20
Infectious Diseases

Nicholas I Paton, Miguel A Gassull, and Eduard Cabré

Key messages

- Advanced human immunodeficiency virus (HIV) infection and tuberculosis are chronic infections that are commonly associated with wasting.
- Reduced nutrient intake is the main cause of wasting although metabolic disturbances may promote lean tissue loss.
- Increasing nutrient intake is the key to treatment although pharmacological management approaches may also sometimes be helpful.

- Anti-HIV drug treatment is frequently complicated by body fat changes and metabolic disturbances.
- Acute infections such as malaria and acute infectious diarrhea have important effects on nutritional status, especially in children, and are an important cause of death in developing countries.
- Malnutrition increases the risk of malaria.
- Rehydration therapy, achieved using the World Health Organization (WHO) rehydration mixture or similar solution, is the key to management of acute infectious diarrhea.

20.1 Introduction

Chronic infections often have profound effects on nutritional status. Two chronic infections are of particular importance in terms of global morbidity and mortality in the early twenty-first century: tuberculosis and human immunodeficiency virus (HIV) infection. The interaction between malnutrition and tuberculosis has long been recognized, although there has been little scientific research in this area. This is in contrast with HIV infection, a relatively new infection, where intense research efforts in the last 15 years have resulted in a body of knowledge about the effects of infection on nutrition and metabolism and the treatment of wasting, that far exceed the existing knowledge accumulated for any other infectious disease. This chapter will therefore focus on HIV infection, and to a lesser extent on tuberculosis, to outline the existing knowledge about the nutritional issues accompanying chronic infections. Many of the principles probably apply to other infectious diseases.

The effects of acute infection on host nutrition and metabolism are similar to those of many other stress conditions, and are largely independent of the causa-tive pathogen. The interaction between nutrition and acute infection is especially important in developing countries where pre-existing malnutrition may increase the frequency and severity of acute infections, and certain acute infections may precipitate malnutrition. Acute gastroenteritis and malaria will be described in this chapter as they are extremely common infections in the developing world, and are both good examples of the infection–nutrition interaction.

Infectious diseases are extremely heterogeneous in their clinical presentation, although a number of nutritional features (such as anorexia, catabolism, increased basal metabolic rate (BMR), decreased physical activity, and increased requirements for some micronutrients) are common to most of them. In addition to these general manifestations, there are other more specific features of some infectious diseases that may have nutritional consequences. Examples include the requirement for special forms of nutritional support in patients with severe infections who require intensive care and mechanical ventilation; the esophageal dilatation and dysmotility of Chagas' disease; and the fluid and electrolyte disturbances of patients with severe gastrointestinal infections such as cholera.

20.2 Human immunodeficiency virus infection

Transmission and epidemiology

HIV is transmitted by sexual intercourse (homosexual or heterosexual), by transfusion of infected blood or blood products, by needles contaminated with blood (usually intravenous drug abusers sharing needles, rarely in the context of accidental injury to health care workers), or vertically (i.e. from mother to baby *in utero*, intrapartum, or by breast milk). Whereas the principal mode of transmission in developed countries is by sexual contact between men, the majority of infections worldwide are acquired by heterosexual transmission and by vertical transmission.

The acquired immune deficiency syndrome (AIDS) pandemic looks set to be among the most devastating events in human history. There were estimated to be 40 million people living with HIV infection at the end of year 2001, more than a million of whom are children. Approximately 5 million new infections are occurring per year. There are an estimated 3 million deaths from AIDS each year, thus placing HIV infection in the same league as the traditional scourges of tuberculosis and malaria as the principal infectious causes of mortality in global terms. The disease has decreased life expectancy by 20 years in some of the worst-affected countries.

Clinical features

The course of HIV infection can be divided into four stages. The seroconversion illness (stage I) occurs in 50–90% of patients, at a average of 2–4 weeks following acquisition of infection. There follows an asymptomatic phase (stage II) without overt clinical manifestations, although active replication of virus and destruction of CD4 cells is continuing. This asymptomatic phase may last indefinitely in a small proportion (less than 5%) of patients, but will progress to symptomatic infection in the majority. The earliest indication of progression to immune failure and symptomatic disease are usually mucocutaneous conditions such as oral candidiasis (thrush) and oral hairy leucoplakia. Persistent generalized lymphadenopathy is the first definitive condition to signify the end of the asymptomatic phase and its occurrence defines stage III disease.

With further depletion of immune function, patients become at risk of opportunistic infections and malignancies. When one of a defined set of indicator conditions develops (such as *Pneumocystis carinii* pneumonia, cytomegalovirus virus colitis, or Kaposi's sarcoma) the patient is deemed to have developed AIDS or stage IV disease. Until the recent advent of highly effective combination antiretroviral therapies, AIDS was invariably fatal within a few years.

Treatment of HIV disease

The therapeutic approach may be divided into prevention of disease progression and treatment of complications that arise. Considerable progress in the development and utilization of antiretroviral drugs has been made in the last few years. Nucleoside analogues, which block the action of the HIV reverse transcriptase enzyme, and drugs that inhibit the HIV protease enzyme have been developed and have a powerful effect in the treatment of HIV. Combination of a protease inhibitor (or alternative drug) with two nucleoside analogues is now regarded as the standard of care in developed nations. This highly active antiretroviral therapy (HAART) has been shown to be effective in halting and even reversing the progression of HIV disease. Widespread adoption of HAART in developed nations has markedly decreased the population rates of progression from asymptomatic HIV disease to AIDS, and the rate of death from AIDS-related illnesses. A retrospective cohort study of nearly 8000 patients in France demonstrated a drop in hospitalization days by 35%, new AIDS cases by 35%, and deaths by 46% within the year following the introduction of HAART into routine usage.

In cases where severe immune compromise has already occurred, prophylactic antibiotics can be used to prevent opportunistic infections such as *Pneumocystis carinii* pneumonia and *Mycobacterium avium* infection. Most of these agents can be discontinued after a period of time on effective antiretroviral therapy. In patients who present for the first time with an episode of acute opportunistic infection, antimicrobial treatment is initially directed towards overcoming the infection.

In developing countries, where antiretroviral therapy is usually unaffordable, the approach to therapy of HIV disease is limited to the treatment of specific complications (especially tuberculosis) and prophylaxis of other infections where affordable agents are available.

Wasting in HIV infection

Definition of HIV wasting syndrome

Involuntary weight loss is a common feature of advanced HIV infection, and 'HIV wasting syndrome' was recognized as one of the conditions that can define a patient as having advanced disease or AIDS. The definition of HIV wasting syndrome is shown in Box 20.1.

Epidemiology of HIV wasting syndrome

Surveillance studies in the US conducted in the early 1990s estimated that between 20 and 25% of patients who had AIDS developed wasting syndrome at some time during the course of their disease. In the late 1990s, the widespread use of HAART had a dramatic effect on the incidence of opportunistic infections and has probably halved the incidence of wasting syndrome in developed countries. Factors contributing to the pathogenesis of HIV-associated wasting are listed in Box 20.2.

The figures for large patient populations are encouraging, and demonstrate convincingly that HAART can prevent wasting. However, it is uncertain whether the

losses of body weight and body cell mass recover fully following the introduction of HAART in patients who have established wasting at the time of initiation of therapy. Few clinical trials of HAART collected even simple body weight measurements, let alone body composition data. Clinical experience suggests that some patients with severe wasting do regain weight but carefully conducted prospective studies are needed to quantify this.

One further important point is that the majority of people infected with HIV live in the developing world and do not have access to combination antiretroviral therapy. HIV-related wasting is therefore likely to remain a significant problem in the populations of developing countries. In some African countries, wasting is such a universal feature of HIV disease that the name 'slim disease' has become synonymous with AIDS.

Definition of HIV-associated wasting

The prevalence of wasting syndrome, as defined above, gives only an approximate indication of the true problem of malnutrition in HIV disease. The definition itself is unsatisfactory as it technically excludes wasting associated with recognized opportunistic infections (which are the commonest cause). Malnutrition is considerably more complex than the clinical concept of wasting syndrome. In one study of HIV patients in Germany, 27% of patients had weight loss of >10% but did not meet the other criteria (fever or diarrhea) for a diagnosis of wasting syndrome. The true incidence of malnutrition in any population of HIV-infected patients will depend on the social, cultural, and medical characteristics of the patients in a practice but it is probably true to say that majority of patients will at some stage experience problems with nutrition.

Thus, due to the inadequacy of the term 'HIV wasting syndrome' which, *sensu strictu*, probably excludes the majority of cases of malnutrition, the term 'HIV-associated wasting' will be used throughout this chapter to refer to the occurrence of weight or lean tissue loss, irrespective of the presence of other clinical symptoms or disease complications. There is no widely accepted definition of HIV-associated wasting, but possible indicators are listed in Box 20.3.

Clinical importance of HIV-associated wasting

There is good evidence that wasting affects survival in HIV-infected patients. One early retrospective study demonstrated that there is progressive depletion of

- 10% unintentional weight loss over a period of 12 months or less
- 10% unintentional body cell mass loss over a period of 12 months or less
- Weight loss with body mass index <18.5 kg/m^2 (for men) and impaired physical function
- Weight loss with body cell mass <35% of body weight (for men) and impaired physical function

body weight and body cell mass up to the time of death in AIDS patients, to a body weight of 66% of ideal and body cell mass (BCM) of 54% of ideal values. These are very close to values prior to death seen in malnourished people in the siege of Leningrad in 1941–1942, and it is therefore likely that in some patients with HIV the timing of death relates to the magnitude of weight and BCM depletion rather than the specific disease process that causes the wasting. Furthermore, some patients die from malnutrition alone without other active complications of HIV infection being apparent.

Other prospective studies have confirmed the relationship between weight loss and survival, and have suggested that even 5% weight loss can have an independent adverse impact on the disease progression. Depletion of BCM appears to have a more direct effect than body weight. A prospective study of BCM measured by bioelectrical impedance in a German cohort has shown that patients with BCM >30% of body weight had significantly longer survival than those with BCM <30% of body weight at baseline (Figure 20.1).

Apart from the effects on survival, loss of lean tissue has been shown to significantly affect physical function in patients with HIV infection. Involuntary weight loss can also cause profound psychological stress to the patient and is often mentioned as one of the most disturbing features of the illness. Patients who have chosen not to disclose their illness to family and friends find it increasingly difficult to maintain the deception, and this therefore may result in social isolation.

The interaction between malnutrition and immune function is well recognized, and wasting may increase morbidity by prolonging recovery from opportunistic infections thereby lengthening hospital stay, and further impairing resistance to non-fatal infections such as oral candidiasis. The consequences of HIV-associated wasting are summarized in Box 20.4.

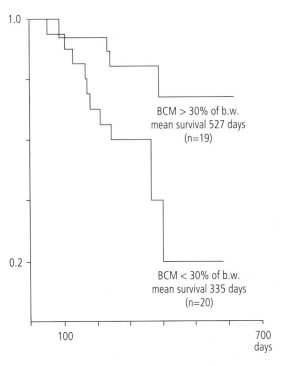

Figure 20.1 Graph of relationship between body cell mass and survival. Reproduced with permission from Suttmann *et al.* (1995).

- Decreased survival
- Decreased physical function
- Decreased quality of life
- Decreased immune function

Patterns of weight change in HIV infection

Weight loss tends to occur in association with disease complications, especially intercurrent infection. A prospective study of weight change in a group of AIDS patients followed for periods of 9–49 months with regular body weight measurement revealed two distinct patterns of weight loss. Episodes of acute rapid weight loss (median 9.1 kg in 1.7 months) were commonly associated with non-gastrointestinal opportunistic infections such as *Pneumocystis carinii* pneumonia (PCP), bacterial chest infections, and septicemia. Episodes of chronic unremitting progressive weight loss (median 13.2 kg in 9.5 months) occurred, usually in conjunction with diarrheal disease such cryptosporid-

(a)

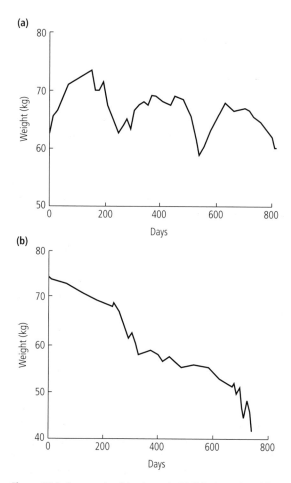

(b)

Figure 20.2 Patterns of weight change in HIV infection. Adapted from Macallan *et al.* (1993). Reproduced with permission from the *American Journal of Clinical Nutrition.* © Am J Clin Nutr, American Society of Clinical Nutrition.

ium infection. Periods of weight stability or weight gain (usually associated with recovery from opportunistic infections) were also observed see Figure 20.2.

Patterns of body composition change in HIV infection

An influential early cross-sectional study in which BCM was measured using total body potassium, demonstrated that BCM was lower in patients with AIDS in comparison with controls. There was a relative increase in extracellular water volume, and body fat mass was also decreased, although this appeared to be to a lesser extent than the BCM loss. This pattern of BCM loss with preservation of fat is indicative of a metabolic basis for the wasting process.

Box 20.5 Body composition in HIV-associated wasting

- Body weight ↓
- Fat mass ↓
- Fat-free mass ↓
- Body cell mass ↓↓
- Extracellular water ↑

Longitudinal studies using dual-energy X-ray absorptiometry (DXA) revealed subsequently that when HIV patients develop wasting they do indeed lose fat, approximately in the proportions that would be expected if calorie restriction were the sole etiology. There also appears to be a sex difference, with HIV-infected women tending to lose a greater proportion of fat than men when they develop wasting. These differences may reflect differences in the baseline fat mass which influence the pattern of weight loss, or perhaps endocrine differences influencing the wasting process. Some of the variability between patients in body composition change may also relate to the specific opportunistic infections from which the patient suffers. One study comparing different opportunistic infections found that patients with protozoal diarrhea had decreased body fat, whereas those with systemic *Mycobacterium avium intracellulare* infection had decreased skeletal muscle mass. Effects on body composition in HIV-associated wasting are listed in Box 20.5.

Energy metabolism in HIV infection

A number of studies have measured one or more components of energy balance in patients with HIV infection. These have shown somewhat conflicting results, but make sense if they are interpreted in conjunction with the clinical characteristics of the patient cohort studied.

In asymptomatic HIV infection, energy intake appears to be normal or slightly increased (by about 15%), possibly as a voluntary or involuntary attempt to compensate for occult malabsorption. This is consistent with the observation of weight stability in early disease. In later stages of HIV disease, energy intake is much more variable, depending on the presence or absence of disease complications at the time the measurement is made. Patients undergoing rapid weight loss (usually in association with an intercurrent infection) have markedly decreased energy intake and those undergoing weight gain (usually following recovery from opportunistic infections) have normal or increased energy intake. Factors causing a reduced food intake are listed in Box 20.6.

Numerous investigators have shown that resting energy expenditure (REE) is elevated in patients with HIV infection. In those free from acute opportunistic infections, mean REE is elevated by an average of 8–12% irrespective of whether the patients have asymptomatic disease, or whether they have experienced prior weight loss and opportunistic infections. Individual patients show greater variability, with some showing reduced REE suggestive of a starvation response. Others measured at the time of secondary infections have been shown to have a mean REE of around 30% above that of controls in some studies. The differing findings may reflect the heterogeneity of advanced HIV disease. One study found that patients with protozoal diarrheal disease had reduced REE, whereas patients with acute PCP and *Mycobacterium avium* infection had raised REE. The differences in REE between infections may also reflect alterations in the amount of body cell mass as well as altered cellular metabolism.

Due to difficulty of measurement, few studies of total energy expenditure (TEE) have been conducted in patients with HIV infection. The definitive study using the doubly labeled water method demonstrated an overall reduction in TEE compared with reference control values for normal men. There was a significant positive relationship between TEE and rate of weight change (i.e. patients with rapid weight loss had the lowest TEE). In the same study, physical activity level (the ratio of TEE/REE) was significantly reduced in patients with rapid weight loss compared with patients with slow weight loss and stable weight (values of 1.3,

1.6, and 1.9 respectively). Thus, increase in TEE cannot be responsible for HIV-associated wasting.

Protein metabolism in HIV infection

Again there is some variability in the findings of studies of whole body protein metabolism in HIV infection. For example a study using the ^{15}N glycine technique demonstrated that asymptomatic patients with AIDS had reduced protein turnover indicative of a starvation-type response. A study using the ^{13}C leucine technique to measure whole body protein metabolism in both the fasted and fed state (using parenteral nutrition) demonstrated that patients with symptomatic AIDS had significantly increased protein turnover compared with controls, with both synthesis and degradation being increased. There was a normal anabolic response to feeding in the HIV-infected patients. The variability of result may reflect the heterogeneity of clinical condition of the patients that were studied.

Fat and carbohydrate metabolism in HIV infection

Various disturbances of fat metabolism have been described in HIV infection. Fasting triglyceride levels increase with progression of disease, lipoprotein lipase activity is decreased, and the clearance of triglycerides is reduced. De novo lipogenesis, the synthesis of fatty acids from other substrates in the liver, is increased. It is unlikely that these changes in triglyceride metabolism have a significant causal role in the wasting process. They are probably an epiphenomenon reflecting increased activity of cytokines in patients with HIV infection.

In contrast to the insulin resistance that usually accompanies infection, it appears that patients with HIV infection (not on HIV treatment) have increased insulin sensitivity and increased rates of insulin clearance. However, insulin resistance is seen frequently in patients receiving antiretroviral drugs.

Endocrine abnormalities and HIV-associated wasting

Hypogonadism has been well documented in HIV infection, occurring in up to 30–50% of men with AIDS, although this appears to be becoming less common in the era of effective HIV drug therapy. Various etiologies have been suggested, including primary testicular disease, the effects of drugs, and hypothalamic dysfunction. It has been shown that androgen levels in hypogonadal men with HIV infection are closely correlated with body cell mass and exercise functional capacity, suggesting that androgen deficiency plays a role in the pathogenesis of HIV wasting.

There is some evidence for disturbance of the growth hormone axis in HIV infection, although the data are conflicting. One study found that HIV-infected adults had insulin-like growth factor 1 (IGF-1) levels at the lower limits of normal and had a blunted response to exogenously administered growth hormone. Another found that growth hormone pulse frequency, amplitude, and area under the curve did not differ between HIV-infected patients and controls.

Cytokines and HIV-associated wasting

It is thought that cytokines may mediate some of the metabolic changes induced by infection, including wasting. Tumor necrosis factor-alpha (TNFα), a cytokine produced by macrophages and monocytes which is a mediator of the immune response, may be responsible for some of the systemic effects of chronic infection. Several studies have found raised levels of serum TNFα or TNF receptors in HIV patients, although others have not. Interleukin-1 (IL-1), interleukin-6 (IL-6), and interferon-alpha have also been proposed as mediators of wasting. Although these cytokines appear to be linked to disturbances in fat metabolism *in vitro* and *in vivo*, the association between serum levels of these factors and the wasting process *in vivo* remains unproven.

Treatment of HIV-associated wasting

General approach to treatment

The aim of treatment is to increase lean body mass (body cell mass, in particular) and thereby improve quality of life, improve physical functioning, and increase survival. The initial step should be to identify and remove any underlying cause for the wasting. Treatment and recovery from opportunistic infection is often accompanied by repletion of body weight. Initiation of treatment for HIV infection with antiretroviral drugs may also result in some weight gain, although this may be offset by lipodystrophy changes.

Given that the predominant cause of wasting is a decrease in energy intake, the first step in the management process must be to increase calorie intake. However, the disturbances in intermediary metabolism which may be present in HIV disease, particularly at the time of opportunistic infections, may have some impact on the efficacy of nutritional interventions. An intervention which just results in the accumulation of fat and water may be deleterious. Assessment of the composition of any weight gain is a critical part of the evaluation of any therapeutic intervention in HIV wasting. A summary of the treatment of wasting is shown in Figure 20.3.

Nutritional therapy
Nutritional counseling

This is likely to be an important first step, although controlled trial evidence for its efficacy is lacking. Alternative diets for 'healthy living' are popular in the HIV community, but may be lacking in important nutrients. Identification of such diets and provision of appropriate advice may result in worthwhile weight gain.

Oral supplements

Many nutritional supplements are available although none have been subjected to controlled trials in comparison with counseling alone. It appears that these supplements do achieve a worthwhile increase in energy intake (i.e. are not simply substituting for energy intake from normal diet), and this increase in energy intake results in body weight gain. One study showed that oral supplementation with 600 kcal daily for six months led to increased weight and lean body mass in clinically stable patients participating in a randomized trial of arginine and omega-3 fatty acids (the 'immunonutrients' themselves had no effect).

Enteral tube feeding

The simplest approach is to use a fine-bore nasogastric tube, but although it is sometimes well tolerated for short periods of time, this can be uncomfortable and unsightly for the patient. Percutaneous endoscopic gastrostomy (PEG) has been demonstrated to be a safe and effective method of providing nutrition in selected situations where conventional nutritional intake is difficult (e.g. patients with swallowing difficulties and patients in intensive care). Several uncontrolled studies have shown that PEG feeding appears to be a useful and relatively safe method of providing long-term

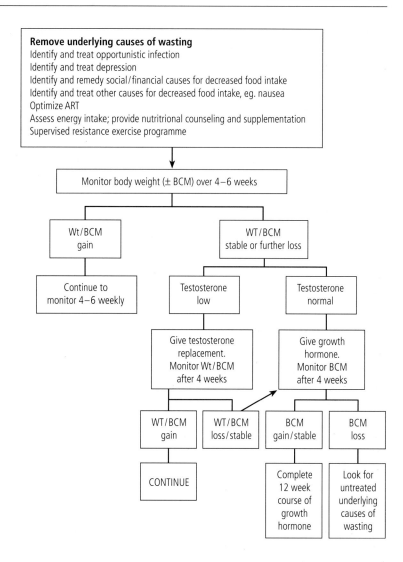

Figure 20.3 Summary of treatment of wasting.

nutritional support in selected AIDS patients. Most of the descriptive studies have documented substantial gains in weight and BCM, without an excessive rate of complications from the procedure.

Parenteral nutrition

This modality of feeding is usually reserved for situations in which the small intestine is inaccessible or non-functional. It is probably not effective for patients with severe ongoing systemic infections (e.g. CMV or *Mycobacterium avium* infection). A prospective controlled multicenter trial of total parenteral nutrition (TPN) versus dietary counseling has been conducted in France. Thirty-one severely malnourished AIDS pa-

tients were randomly assigned to receive either TPN or dietary counseling over a period of two months. Body weight, fat-free mass, and BCM all increased in the TPN group (by 13%, 9%, and 15% respectively) whereas these parameters all decreased in the dietary counseling group (by 6%, 5%, and 12% respectively). The TPN group had better long-term survival. This trial demonstrated that TPN can offer significant benefits in selected patients with AIDS, and the demonstration that a nutritional intervention increases survival is a landmark. The drawbacks of this therapy are that it is costly, logistically difficult to administer for long periods, and may have a net adverse effect on quality of life (this has not been addressed in studies).

improve appearance. There is no treatment available for fat loss in the arms or legs at present.

Central fat gain is perhaps more amenable to therapy. Diet and aerobic exercise should be the first step, and resistance training may also have some beneficial effects. Early reports indicate that growth hormone can decrease dorsocervical fat and intra-abdominal fat in HIV-infected patients with fat accumulation, although the optimal dose of the drug for this indication is unknown. However, growth hormone may worsen insulin resistance.

Lactic acidosis

This is a side effect of nucleoside analogue reverse transcriptase inhibitors which is becoming increasingly recognized. It is defined by elevated venous lactate levels (>2.0 mmol/l) and low arterial pH (<7.3). The main clinical features are nausea, abdominal pain, and shortness of breath. Milder cases may present more subtly with fatigue and weight loss. Underlying liver disease may be a risk factor for the development of drug-induced lactic acidosis. The condition may sometimes be fatal.

Management is uncertain, although some interventions have been used with success in the treatment of other mitochondrial diseases. These include riboflavin and thiamine, antioxidants such as vitamin C, and L-carnitine, although controlled trials of these agents in the treatment of lactic acidosis in the setting of HIV infection are lacking.

Insulin resistance and diabetes

It is apparent that many patients receiving treatment for HIV infection have insulin resistance, although frank diabetes is relatively rare. It is not known whether the insulin resistance will ultimately progress to diabetes, although this is certainly possible. Fasting glucose levels are most often normal and an oral glucose tolerance test, or better the measurement of fasting insulin levels, is needed to make a diagnosis of insulin resistance. The importance of insulin resistance is that it can increase the risk of atherosclerosis (even without raised glucose levels) and is associated with hypertriglyceridemia that is also atherogenic. It is unclear whether the insulin resistance is related to body fat abnormalities, or whether it is mainly related to the use of protease inhibitors that are causing both phenomena.

When considering treatment of insulin resistance, other risk factors for atherogenesis should be looked for (e.g. smoking, high blood pressure, etc.) and modified wherever possible. As with the treatment of type 2 diabetes mellitus, diet and exercise form an essential first component of therapy. The diet should be composed of 50–60% carbohydrate, 30% fat (maximum 10% for saturated fat), and 10–20% protein. Insulin-sensitizing agents such as metformin may be useful.

Hyperlipidemia

Severe increases in total cholesterol, LDL cholesterol, and triglycerides can occur in patients receiving HIV drugs. These appear to be mainly, although not exclusively, related to therapy with protease inhibitors. The consequences of elevated cholesterol and triglycerides are likely to be as great if not greater for HIV-infected people as they are in the HIV-negative patient.

Treatment should mainly be targeted at LDL cholesterol and can follow standard guidelines that are applicable to the HIV-negative population, although attention to triglycerides and reduced HDL is also warranted. Diet and exercise are the most important initial interventions, along with stopping smoking and treatment/reversal of any other risk factors. The diet should involve progressive restriction of dietary fat and total cholesterol until acceptable limits are achieved. Drug therapy may be indicated, and low doses of the statins pravastatin or atorvastatin may be useful. Fibrates (e.g. gemfibrozil) may also be useful, especially where increased cholesterol is combined with increased triglycerides, or in the situation of isolated hypertriglyceridemia. Bile sequestering resins should not be used due to their effects on increasing serum triglycerides and their potential effects to decrease HIV drug absorption.

Micronutrients and HIV

In addition to the marked reductions in intake of macronutrients described above, many HIV-infected patients do not consume the recommended dietary allowance (RDA) of several micronutrients such as B-complex vitamins, vitamin E, and zinc. This situation may be exacerbated by malabsorption, which is common in patients with HIV, especially in the advanced stages of disease. Fat malabsorption may adversely affect the absorption of fat-soluble vitamins. Furthermore, inadequate intake may be further exacerbated by the possibility that the requirements for micronutrients in HIV-infected patients may exceed the RDA in some cases. The prevalence of micronutrient deficiency varies considerably with the patient group, stage of HIV disease, and the setting, but frequencies of up to 65% for vitamin A deficiency (in pregnant women), and 20–30% for deficiency of vitamins E, C, B_6, B_{12}, zinc, and iron have been reported.

A number of studies have linked micronutrient deficiency to accelerated progression of HIV disease. For example, vitamin A deficiency is associated with increased mortality, increased risk of vertical (mother-to-child) transmission of HIV, growth failure in HIV-infected children, and increased HIV in breast milk and the genital tract.

A few clinical trials of micronutrient supplementation have been conducted, but they are generally of small size and the effects may be specific to the population studied. One large-scale study has been conducted and had convincing findings. One thousand pregnant women in Tanzania were randomized to receive a daily multivitamin supplement or a supplement of vitamin A and beta-carotene, or both or neither (all received daily iron and folate). Those who received the multivitamin supplement had a 40% decrease in fetal deaths and low birth weight, and had a significant increase in CD4 counts. The vitamin A and beta-carotene supplement did not appear to have any additional effect. Micronutrient interventions are particularly appealing for developing countries where the prevalence of micronutrient deficiencies is likely to be relatively high and the cost effectiveness and feasiblity of specific interventions is favorable. More data are needed before micronutrient supplementation can be recommended to other groups, although micronutrients are widely consumed by HIV patients in developed countries, at varying and sometimes excessive doses.

Breastfeeding and HIV

See also the chapter on infant feeding in the *Public Health Nutrition* textbook in this series.

HIV can be transmitted from infected mother to uninfected child through breastfeeding, and this route represents one of the major contributors to the HIV epidemic in children. The timing of transmission through breast-milk (early versus late) is hard to define for practical reasons. Several factors may influence the risk of transmission, including the viral load in the breast milk, the presence of mastitis, nipple disease, and variation in feeding practices (such as alternating between bottle and breastfeeding, which seems to increase the risk above that of breastfeeding exclusively).

It is therefore recommended that HIV-infected mothers do not breastfeed their children. Avoidance of breastfeeding has been shown to reduce the transmission of HIV by around 50%. However, complete avoidance of breastfeeding and substitution of formula may not be possible in some developing countries due to financial or practical constraints. Also there is a concern that reliance on formula feeding may increase mortality from other causes that might offset the advantage of reduced mortality from HIV. However, a randomized clinical trial of formula versus breastfeeding for infants of HIV-infected mothers in Kenya showed that the incidence of diarrhea, pneumonia, and overall mortality were similar in the two groups. Furthermore, the rate of survival free of HIV infection at two years was much higher in the formula-fed group, and this would be expected to yield longer term survival benefits in favor of formula feeding. Thus, it appears that formula feeding can be a safe alternative to breastfeeding for HIV-infected mothers in a developing country setting, provided that there is appropriate education and access to clean water.

20.3 Tuberculosis

Epidemiology and importance

It is estimated that approximately one-third of the world's population is infected with *Mycobacterium tuberculosis*, the bacterium that causes clinical tuberculosis. Usually the infection is contained by the immune system so that only a small proportion of the infected people (approximately 15 million) have clinical disease at any one time. However, the disease results in the death of between 1 and 3 million people per year, which places it amongst the most important infectious diseases in global terms. Most of these deaths occur in the developing world, and in many countries the disease has a large social and economic impact. The incidence of tuberculosis started to increase again in the late 1980s and early 1990s, partly due to the advent of HIV infection (which increases TB risk) and partly due to complacency in tuberculosis control programs.

Causative agent and transmission

The tuberculosis bacterium is transmitted mainly by the inhalation of aerosols from individuals suffering from pulmonary disease. The risk factors for infection are proximity to and duration of contact with an infected individual, and so family members and other household contacts of infected individuals are at highest risk. Although vaccination with bacille Calmette–Guérin (BCG) is widely used, the degree of protection offered is variable and certainly not 100%.

Clinical presentation, treatment, and course

Initial infection with tuberculosis is usually asymptomatic. However, a small proportion of infected people develop clinical symptoms such as cough, chest pain, and shortness of breath. Systemic symptoms such as fever, night sweats, and weight loss may also occur. Primary infection may progress to severe lung disease or disseminate throughout the body.

Most cases of tuberculosis are caused by reactivation of infection acquired many years earlier. The trigger for reactivation may be immunosuppression due to disease (e.g. malignancy, diabetes, or HIV infection) or drugs (e.g. in transplant patients). The usual site of disease is the lung. The commonest symptoms of reactivation of pulmonary tuberculosis are cough, fever, night sweats, weight loss, and fatigue. The disease can be diagnosed by chest X-ray and by staining sputum samples to show the mycobacteria. Tuberculosis can reactivate at many sites other than the lungs (e.g. lymph nodes, bones, abdominal viscera, brain, and heart). In addition to the symptoms specific to the region affected, systemic symptoms such as fever and weight loss may sometimes be prominent.

Bloodborne dissemination of *Mycobacterium tuberculosis* can lead to miliary tuberculosis, especially in those people with more severe immunosuppression. Miliary tuberculosis may manifest with symptoms associated with the organs involved (usually several) or as a pyrexia of unknown origin. In chronic cases, cachexia may be prominent and specific clinical signs may be few.

The treatment for tuberculosis is essentially the same, irrespective of the site of disease. Combination

therapy is essential for cure, and direct observation of therapy may also improve the outcome. The usual treatment involves taking a combination of three or four drugs (including rifampicin and isoniazid) for two months followed by continuation of the rifampcin and isoniazid for a further 4–7 months depending on the site of infection and the individual patient's state of immunosuppression. Hepatitis is the main complication of standard combination therapy. Isoniazid interferes with niacin metabolism and this may result in a peripheral neuropathy. This may be prevented by pyridoxine. In malnourished patients, isoniazid may precipitate pellagra.

Nutritional and metabolic effects of TB

Wasting has been recognized for centuries as one of the cardinal signs of tuberculosis: the disease was known to Greek physicians as 'phthisis,' meaning 'to waste away' and in the eighteenth and nineteenth centuries tuberculosis was popularly called 'consumption.' Even in the modern era where prompt diagnosis is possible, patients have often become severely cachectic by the time treatment is initiated. This is especially true in developing countries. A study from Malawi showed that unselected patients presenting for treatment of tuberculosis had body weight reduced approximately 20% below normal values.

In the last 20 years the wasting associated with tuberculosis has been compounded by the fact that many patients with tuberculosis are co-infected with HIV. It is not surprising, given that both are associated with wasting, that the coincidence of the two diseases in the same patient often leads to very severe malnutrition. Indeed, in a post-mortem study of HIV-infected patients dying with 'slim disease,' undiagnosed tuberculosis was found to be present in a large percentage.

Importance of the interaction between malnutrition and tuberculosis

Malnutrition is known to be detrimental to the host immune response to mycobacterial infection, and therefore increases susceptibility to tuberculosis infection. Tuberculosis is a frequent complication of malnutrition, and is a major cause of mortality among malnourished children of developing countries. The reactivation of tuberculosis in the elderly may also be partly the result of malnutrition in this population.

Although it is hard to establish because of many confounding factors, malnutrition is likely to contribute to the increased risk of reactivation of tuberculosis seen in HIV-infected people, alcoholics, and the homeless. Deficiency of vitamin D is known to increase susceptibility to tuberculosis, and there is some evidence that vitamin A and C deficiencies also increase susceptibility to tuberculosis.

As well as increasing the susceptibility to tuberculosis, malnutrition alters the clinical manifestations: malnourished patients have an atypical presentation of tuberculosis. Malnutrition also impairs the recovery from tuberculosis. A study that examined the predictors of mortality in a group of patients who had tuberculosis diagnosed during hospitalization, showed that malnutrition was an independent predictor of death.

Furthermore, surgery (resection of affected lung) is being increasingly employed for the treatment of difficult cases of multidrug-resistant tuberculosis in specialist referral centers. Severe malnutrition is associated with a poor outcome and increased complications following surgery. Patients with multidrug-resistant tuberculosis are also often amongst the most severely malnourished patients as they have endured a prolonged inflammatory process and long courses of toxic drugs.

Etiology of malnutrition in tuberculosis

The etiology of the malnutrition in tuberculosis has not been fully ascertained. A few studies have shown that BMR/REE is slightly increased in tuberculosis, although total daily energy expenditure is unlikely to be greatly raised because physical activity energy expenditure is usually reduced in such patients. Anecdotal experience suggests that the key cause of wasting in tuberculosis is decreased energy intake, as a result of anorexia associated with the infection. However, no studies have formally investigated this aspect of the disease.

The cause of the anorexia associated with tuberculosis has not been established, although several potential mediators can be suggested. One of the most likely is TNF as this cytokine is known to cause cachexia in animal models. Increased production of TNF is known to accompany tuberculosis. Drugs used to treat tuberculosis are frequently associated with gastrointestinal side effects that may further impair food intake.

Body composition in tuberculosis

The nature of body composition changes in tuberculosis have not been well studied. One study has shown a relative increase in extracellular water in patients with tuberculosis. A cross-sectional study of the effects of tuberculosis in patients with underlying HIV infection demonstrated a marked reduction in intracellular water and a relative increase in extracellular water in patients co-infected with tuberculosis compared with those without tuberculosis. The depletion of BCM was severe in patients with tuberculosis. Other markers of nutritional status, such as serum albumin, are also frequently reduced in this disease.

Nutritional therapy for wasting in tuberculosis

There is commonly an improvement in appetite and later a gain in body weight following the initiation of antituberculous therapy. Although clinicians often use weight gain to assess the response to antituberculous chemotherapy, the relationship between weight gain and clinical outcome is uncertain and in one study, microbiological response was not associated with weight gain. Few prospective studies have examined the composition of the weight gain and it may be distorted from normal (e.g. more fat or water gain) by the underlying disease process. One study which used simple anthropometric measurements to investigate the response to therapy found that body weight, arm circumference, and triceps skinfold all improved after two months of chemotherapy in 122 patients with sputum-positive tuberculosis in Malawi, suggesting that at least some fat accrual occurs, but more detailed prospective studies are needed.

In view of the frequency of severe malnutrition, and its importance in adversely affecting the immune response to tuberculosis, optimizing the nutritional status of these patients is likely to confer some benefit on the host and speed of recovery. Although spontaneous nutritional recovery may occur, it is possible that treating both the infection and malnutrition simultaneously will be more successful. However, there are few good data to support the use of nutritional interventions in patients with tuberculosis. Those studies that have been conducted precede modern concepts of study design (i.e. randomized controlled trial), modern techniques of measuring body composition, and the modern era of antituberculous chemotherapy. In general, the studies found evidence of normal response to feeding in tuberculosis and provided evidence of benefit of nutritional therapy in tuberculosis. Whether this influences treatment outcome is uncertain. In one study comparing treatment in a sanatorium (where the nutritional intake was better) with treatment at home found no difference in outcome although there may have been other confounding factors.

The protein requirements are not known. Early work suggested that increasing the protein intake to very high levels might be beneficial. However, increasing nitrogen intake may place additional demands on respiratory function of tuberculosis patients and hence this approach should be avoided in patients with extensive lung damage and respiratory compromise.

Thus in general, the evidence would support attempts to achieve an increased energy intake, with normal or slightly increased protein composition. This can be done most easily by means of dietary alteration, and use of energy and protein supplements. It is important to treat any drug-induced nausea and vomiting with anti-emetics, and use of antipyretics for fever is also likely to help appetite. In severely malnourished patients who are unable to consume sufficient calories and protein by these approaches, use of nasogastric feeding or PEG feeding may be warranted.

Micronutrient supplementation

Vitamin D has been used to treat patients with cutaneous tuberculosis prior to the advent of modern antituberculous drugs. Cod liver oil and sunlight were popular therapies for tuberculosis in the nineteenth century. Consideration should be given to vitamin D supplementation, especially in those who are vegetarians.

Pharmacological treatments for wasting in tuberculosis

A few studies have been conducted of pharmacological treatments to accelerate weight gain. One small study found benefit of using anabolic steroids for patients with tuberculosis, although this needs to be further investigated before it can be recommended. Several studies have found increased weight gain with the use of thalidomide. However, there are no currently accepted

drugs for enhancing weight gain in tuberculosis and treatment is purely nutritional.

20.4 Malaria

Epidemiology and importance

Malaria is the most important protozoal infection in humans, with more than one-third of the world's population exposed to the risk of infection. There are an estimated 300–500 million clinical cases per year, and between 1 and 3 million deaths. The greatest burden of disease is in Africa, and African children account for most of the deaths worldwide.

Malaria control programs that were instituted in the 1950s and 1960s initially had dramatic effects on the incidence of malaria in many areas, but lack of funding and waning enthusiasm led to the collapse of most of these initiatives. Although some areas remain malaria free, in many parts of the world the incidence of malaria has rebounded to high levels again. To add to this bleak picture, drug resistance continues to spread at an alarming rate. The Director General of the World Health Organization has identified malaria as one of the top priorities for action and has instituted a 'roll back malaria' program to address the issues of control of malaria and of the spread of drug resistance.

Clinical presentation and treatment

The main symptom is fever that may become periodic, occurring only every few days, once infection is well-established. Other non-specific symptoms include headache, vomiting, and diarrhea. Although malaria is a mild and self-limiting infection in most cases, patients infected with the *Plasmodium falciparum* parasite can develop a range of complications that may result in death. Common complications include cerebral malaria (manifesting as decreased consciousness, convulsions, or other neurological signs), pulmonary edema, hypoglycemia, anemia, and renal failure. Secondary infections are frequent (e.g. pneumonia, or gram-negative septicemia).

The non-falciparum malarias are treated with chloroquine over a period of 2–3 days followed by primaquine over a period of two weeks to eradicate the liver forms of the parasite. Chloroquine is usually well tolerated. Falciparum malaria is usually treated with quinine for seven days. Quinine can be given orally, although it is not well tolerated. The taste is bitter and quinine often induces a symptom complex called cinchonism (nausea, dysphoria, tinnitus, and high tone deafness). These symptoms are rapidly reversible on stopping therapy. A combination of artesunate and mefloquine is used in areas of South-East Asia where drug resistance is a problem. These drugs are well tolerated and effective.

The role of protein–energy malnutrition in malaria

Early studies suggested that protein–energy malnutrition or protein deficiency protected the host against malaria morbidity and mortality. More recent studies, with more rigorous methods, have indicated the opposite to be the case. Cohort studies have shown that malnutrition is associated with increased rates of infection and increased frequency of clinical attacks of malaria. Studies conducted in hospitalized malaria patients in several African countries have shown that malnourished patients are 1.3–3.5 times more likely to die or have permanent neurological sequelae than normally nourished patients. However, although malnutrition does appear to exacerbate malaria, the impact is smaller than that seen with malnutrition on diarrhea or pneumonia. In addition there may be age-dependent relationships between malnutrition and malaria that may explain some of the inconsistencies in the data. The situation of starvation and famine may present a special case. It has been shown that refeeding humans in situations of famine can reactivate low-grade malaria infections.

Micronutrients and malaria

Multiple nutrients may play a role in protecting against or exacerbating malaria. However, the relationships are complex and the immunological basis unclear. The effects may be due to effects on the host and/or parasite.

A number of cross-sectional studies have shown an inverse relationship between vitamin A levels and the concentration of malaria parasites in the blood. A definitive study on the effects of vitamin A supplementation on clinical malaria was conducted in Papua New Guinea. It showed that giving vitamin A supplemen-

tation reduced the frequency of *P. falciparum* malaria episodes by 30% among preschool children.

Several cross-sectional studies and intervention studies also indicate a relationship between zinc deficiency and malaria. A placebo-controlled trial showed that zinc supplementation reduced the frequency of health center attendance due to falciparum malaria by 38% and reduced the frequency of malaria accompanied by high levels of parasitemia by 69%.

Several studies of iron supplementation in malaria-endemic areas have shown that iron supplementation increases the risk of developing or reactivating malarial illness, while others show no effect. Meta-analysis of all placebo-controlled trials in humans found that iron supplementation resulted in a non-significant increase of 9% in the risk of a malaria attacks and increases in certain malariometric indices (e.g. spleen enlargement). However, the improvements in anemia following iron supplementation were substantial, suggesting that iron supplementation programs in accordance with international dosing guidelines are appropriate for iron-deficient populations residing in malaria-endemic areas.

The effects of folate are unclear. Riboflavin deficiency appears to protect against malaria, although high-dose riboflavin therapy may be advantageous in patients who have clinical malaria. Thiamine deficiency may predispose to more severe malaria. Vitamin E deficiency tends to protect against clinical malaria. The effects of other antioxidants are unknown.

20.5 Gastrointestinal infections

Definition and etiopathogenesis

A large number of pathogens, including bacteria, viruses, and protozoa, can infect the small bowel and colon, mostly causing diarrheal illness such as acute gastroenteritis, food poisoning, and traveller's diarrhea – which are not necessarily clearly distinguishable from each other – and more specific conditions such as typhoid fever, cholera, and dysentery (Box 20.8).

Bacterial diarrhea can be classified into toxigenic and invasive types. The prototype organisms for toxigenic diarrheas are *Vibrio cholerae* and enterotoxigenic *E. coli*. These pathogens do not invade intestinal epithelium, but adhere to the enterocytes, where they

Box 20.8 Organisms causing gastrointestinal infections

Bacteria
- *Vibrio cholerae*
- *Vibrio parahaemolyticus*
- *Aeromonas* spp.
- Enterotoxigenic *E. coli* (ETEC)
- Enteroinvasive *E. coli* (EIEC)
- Enteropathogenic *E. coli* (EPEC)
- Enterohemorrhagic *E. coli* (EHEC)
- Enteroaggregative *E. coli* (EAggEC)
- Diffusely adhering E. coli (DAEC)
- *Shigella* spp.
- *Salmonella* spp.
- *Campylobacter* spp.
- *Yersinia* spp.
- *Staphylococcus aureus*
- *Clostridium perfringens*
- *Bacillus cereus*
- *Lysteria monocytogenes*
- *Clostridium difficile*

Viruses
- Rotavirus (mainly group A)
- Calicivirus (Norwalk virus, Norwalk-like virus)
- Enteric adenovirus
- Astrovirus

Protozoa
- *Giardia lamblia*
- *Entamoeba histolytica*
- *Cryptosporidium*
- *Isospora*
- *Cyclospora*
- *Microsporidium*
- *Balantidium coli*
- *Blastocystis hominis*

produce enterotoxins of the cytotonic type which lead to watery diarrhea and dehydration. Invasive diarrhea is caused by pathogens, such as *Salmonella*, *Shigella*, enteroinvasive *E. coli*, *Campylobacter*, and *Yersinia*. Although some of these organisms can also produce enterotoxins, they cause an intense inflammatory reaction in the intestinal, and mostly colonic, mucosa leading to prostaglandin-mediated diarrhea, often with blood and leukocytes in the feces (dysenteric stools). In some food poisoning (e.g. *Clostridium perfringens*, *Staphylococcus aureus*, *Bacillus cereus*) acute diarrhea is caused by preformed bacterial toxins found in the contaminated food.

Viruses responsible for gastrointestinal infections can be grouped into four categories: rotavirus, calicivirus (including Norwalk virus), enteric adenovirus, and astrovirus. All of them usually produce watery diarrhea, often accompanied by vomiting. Protozoan infections include giardiasis, amebiasis, and infections caused by *Cryptosporidium*, *Isospora*, and *Cyclospora*. Clinical consequences of these infections range from asymptomatic cases or mild diarrhea to severe malabsorption or devastating diarrheal illness.

Epidemiology: The magnitude of the problem

Acute infectious diarrhea is the first or second cause of death in most developing countries, being responsible for 3–4 million deaths annually worldwide, particularly in children. In fact, 20–30% of deaths in infants and children are due to enteric infections. Even in industrialized countries, gastrointestinal infections are a major health problem. In the USA, most children under five years of age experience an average of two episodes of diarrhea per year.

Food poisoning, defined as an illness caused by the ingestion of contaminated food, usually occurs in the form of outbreaks worldwide. Bacteria (or their toxins) cause about 80% of food poisoning outbreaks for which an etiology can be identified. However, it has to be kept in mind that only 40% of such outbreaks fulfil the microbiologic standards for confirmed etiology.

Annually, more than 250 million people travel from one country to another, of which at least 15 million persons go from industrialized to developing countries. Acute diarrhea often occurs among these individuals (traveller's diarrhea) with an attack rate ranging from 25% to 50%. About 30% of patients with traveller's diarrhea are sick enough to be confined in bed, and another 40% of them must alter their planned activities. The etiology of traveller's diarrhea depends on the country, but on average, most cases are due to enterotoxigenic or enteroadherent strains of *E. coli* (ETEC, EAEC), *Campylobacter* spp., and *Shigella* spp. Other bacteria, viruses, and protozoa can also be identified as causative agents. However, in about 40% of cases an individual pathogen cannot be found.

Diarrhea is the most frequent and often most symptomatic gastrointestinal manifestation of AIDS, occurring in 50–90% of these patients. In some cases, diarrhea is due to the so-called 'Idiopathic AIDS enteropathy' that is thought to be due to a combination

Box 20.9 Pathogens most often causing diarrhea in AIDS

Protozoa
- *Cryptosporidium**
- *Microsporidium**
- *Isospora**
- *Cyclospora*
- *Giardia lamblia*

Viruses
- *Cytomegalovirus**
- Herpes simplex
- Rotavirus
- Calicivirus (Norwalk virus)
- Enteric adenovirus
- HIV itself (?)

Bacteria
- *Salmonella* spp.*
- *Shigella* spp.*
- *Campylobacter* spp.*
- *Mycobacterium avium* complex
- *Mycobacterium tuberculosis*

Fungi
- *Histoplasma capsulatum*
- *Coccidioides*
- *Candida albicans*
- *Cryptococcus neoformans*

*Most frequent.

of villus hypoplasia, altered cytokine production, ileal dysfunction, exudative enteropathy, intestinal dysmotility, and bacterial overgrowth. Most often, however, diarrhea is directly related to different intestinal pathogens, particularly protozoa and viruses (Box 20.9). In general, infectious diarrhea is more prevalent and more severe in AIDS patients that in healthy immunocompetent individuals. The effects of gastrointestinal infections associated with AIDS often aggravate the wasting syndrome present in these patients.

Specific (antimicrobial) therapy of gastrointestinal infections

Giving a comprehensive, in-depth description of the specific antimicrobial treatment of all gastrointestinal infections is beyond the scope of this chapter. It is summarized in Table 20.1, and the reader should search for detailed information on this field elsewhere. However, as general guideline, antimicrobial therapy is mandatory in shigellosis, typhoid fever, and some cases of

non-typhoid salmonellosis, cholera, and enteroinvasive *E. coli*. Non-toxigenic strains of *E. coli* should be treated only in infants. Antimicrobial treatment is also advised in giardiasis and amebiasis. A short empirical course of ciprofloxacin in recommended for traveller's diarrhea. Other bacterial diarrheas should be treated with antibiotics only in the presence of bacteremia, as well as in immunodeficient (e.g. AIDS) or seriously ill patients. No drug treatment is recommended for enterotoxigenic *E. coli* or viral diarrhea. There is no satisfactory antimicrobial therapy for some prevalent protozoal infections in AIDS (e.g. *Cryptosporidium*, *Isospora*, *Cyclospora*, and *Microsporidium*).

Nutritional and metabolic management of gastrointestinal infections

Despite the use of antimicrobial therapy when indicated, the management of patients with acute infectious diarrhea mostly relies on dietary and, particularly, supportive rehydration therapy. Appropriate rehydration and replacement of electrolyte losses may be lifesaving particularly in children and in developing countries, where superimposed malnutrition or famine are also frequent.

In chronic diarrhea, daily stool output is usually not greater than 1500 g/day, whereas in acute diarrhea between 1 and 20 kg/day may be passed, the highest amounts occurring in cholera. Normal stools contain relatively low concentrations of sodium (less than 10 mmol/kg) but are high in potassium (90 mmol/kg). As daily stool output increases, fecal sodium concentration rises and potassium falls. At 500 g stool/day they are equimolar (55 mmol/kg), and values approach those of plasma at stool outputs higher than 5 kg/day (130 mmol/kg for sodium, and 4 mmol/kg for potassium).

Oral rehydration solutions

The traditional way to provide fluids and electrolytes has been the intravenous route, but in the recent years oral rehydration solutions (ORS) (Table 20.2) have proven to be equally effective and logistically more practical in developing countries. ORS are based in the reliable physiological principle that glucose (or other organic compounds, such as amino acids) enhance sodium absorption in the small bowel, even in the presence of secretory losses caused by bacterial toxins, and

Table 20.1 Antimicrobial therapy in infectious diarrhea

	Drug of choice	Alternative drugs
Recommended in symptomatic patients		
Shigella spp.	Ampicillin (p.o. or i.v.)	Fluoroquinolones
	TMP-SMX (p.o.)[a]	Nalidixic acid
Clostridium difficile	Metronidazole (p.o.)	
	Vancomycin (p.o.)	
Traveller's diarrhea	Ciprofloxacin (p.o.)	Other fluoroquinolones
		TMP-SMX
EPEC, EAggEC, and DAEC in infants; EIEC	TMP-SMX (p.o.)	
Typhoid fever	Ciprofloxacin (p.o.)	Ceftriaxone
		Amoxycillin
		Chloramphenicol
		TMP-SMX
Cholera	Tetracycline (p.o.)	Doxycycline
		Cipro / Norfloxacin
		Amoxycillin
		TMP-SMX
Salmonella	Ampicillin (p.o.)	Ciprofloxacin
	TMP-SMX (p.o.)*	
Amebiasis	Metronidazole (p.o.), followed by	Tetracycline (p.o.) plus Dehydroemetine (i.m.)
	Iodoquinol (p.o.), or paromomycin (p.o.)	
Giardiasis	Metronidazole (p.o.)	Quinacrine
		Furazolidinone
		Paromomycin
Not recommended, except for immunodeficient, septic, or seriously ill patients		
Campylobacter spp.	Erythromycin (p.o.)	Ciprofloxacin (p.o.)
Yersinia spp.	Fluoroquinolones (p.o.)	Aminoglycosides
	TMP-SMX (p.o.)	Tetracycline
	Chloramphenicol (p.o.)	
Aeromonas spp.	TMP-SMX (p.o.)	Tetracycline
	Cephalosporins (p.o.)	Chloramphenicol
	Fluoroquinolones (p.o.)	
Vibrio (non-cholera)	Tetracycline (p.o.)	
EPEC, EAggEC, and DAEC in adults; EHEC	TMP-SMX (p.o.)	
Not recommended		
ETEC		
Viral diarrhea		

[a]TMP-SMX: trimethoprim-sulfamethoxazole.
*In ampicillin-resistant strains.

Table 20.2 Composition of some oral rehydration solutions

	Electrolytes		Carbohydrates	
	Sodium (mmol/l)	Potassium (mmol/l)	Glucose (g/l)	Rice syrup (g/l)
WHO/UNICEF	75	20	13.5	–
Pedialyte®	45	20	25	–
Rehydralyte®	75	20	25	–
Dioralyte®	60	20	16	–
Glucolyte®	35	20	36	–
Ricelyte®	50	25	–	30
Ceralyte®	70	20	–	40

that in addition colonic pathways for water and electrolyte absorption remain largely intact in acute diarrhea.

Initially used for treating acute infectious diarrhea in children in developing countries, ORS have shown to be useful to manage several types of diarrheal diseases, both in children and adults, and not only of infectious origin (e.g. early stages of short-bowel syndrome, and idiopathic AIDS enteropathy).

For years, the most widely used ORS was the WHO/ UNICEF mixture which was provided in packets containing glucose (20 g) and three salts – sodium chloride (3.5 g), potassium chloride (1.5 g), and either trisodium citrate (2.9 g) or sodium bicarbonate (2.5 g) – to be diluted in 1 liter of water. It has been shown to be lifesaving in mild and moderate diarrhea, but is suboptimal for cholera because, in spite of improving hydration and reducing mortality, it does not shorten the duration of diarrhea.

An early modification of the standard solution was the addition of glycine or other amino acids, but this resulted in little improvement. A subsequent modification was to use some type of starch, usually rice, instead of glucose. A meta-analysis including almost 1400 adult and pediatric patients showed that rice-based ORS reduced stool output in the first 24 h by 36% in adults, and 32% in children with cholera, as compared to the WHO/UNICEF mixture. However, in non-cholera diarrhea, the reduction was only 18%. Other studies have shown no major benefit. Attempts with maltodextrins and cereals have also been disappointing.

Water absorption is more efficient if the gut content is relatively hyposmolar (200–250 mOsm/l) rather than isosmolar (330 mOsm/l). It has been suggested that low osmolarity ORS, in which glucose and sodium concentrations are lowered, improve stool output, duration of diarrhea, as well as the total amount of ORS and intravenous fluids required, both in cholera and non-cholera diarrhea, without inducing hyponatremia. If confirmed, reduced-osmolarity ORS may replace WHO-based solutions in the future.

Diet

Dietary management of acute infectious diarrhea has been influenced more by fads and fancies than by scientific knowledge. The traditional approach is absolute dietary abstinence. However, it is better to eat judiciously during an attack of diarrhea than to drastically restrict oral intake. Soft, easy digestible foods are most acceptable to the patient with acute diarrhea. In the early stages of the disease, a diet based in foods such as rice, carrot, and boiled meat or fish is advisable. Beverages containing caffeine or methylxanthine (coffee, tea, cola) and alcohol should be avoided as they increase bowel motility.

In children, it is important to restart oral feeding as soon as the child is able to accept oral intake. Recent studies indicate that most infants with acute diarrhea could be successfully managed with continued feeding of undiluted non-human milk, and routine dilution of milk or the use of lactose-free products is not necessary.

20.6 Perspectives on the future

The international community has recognized the disastrous consequences that the HIV epidemic is having on the very fabric of society in many of the worst-affected countries. In some countries the depletion of the able-bodied workforce is so severe that it is leading to national decreases in food production and contributing to famine. This exacerbates the nutritional consequences of the disease for those affected, and malnutrition and wasting complicating HIV may become an even more important issue in the coming years. A number of international initiatives have been launched to attempt to bring wider access to HIV treatment for developing countries. The '3 by 5' plan by the WHO intends to provide antiretroviral therapy to 3 million infected people by 2005. The Global Fund to Fight HIV, Tuberculosis, and Malaria plans to channel billions of dollars from international donations to fund treatment programs for these three major diseases.

With wider access to HIV drugs, the metabolic side effects of these drugs may become a problem at the population level, especially in societies where smoking is also prevalent. HIV is fuelling both the rise in tuberculosis and malaria incidence in many countries, and the detrimental interactions between these three infections are likely to increase over time. Increasing rates of drug resistance in tuberculosis are resulting in a greater proportion of patients who have chronic debilitating disease requiring longer treatment, and these patients require more attention to nutritional aspects of their care. Further research work is needed to define appropriate treatment strategies for the management of nutritional and metabolic consequences of these

mately 70% of cancer patients and may be evident at clinical presentation in 10–30% of subjects. It is characterized by anorexia, weight loss, anemia, depletion, and alterations in body compartments, disturbances in water and electrolyte metabolism, and the progressive impairment of vital functions. Specific investigations on the composition of the body compartments of cancer patients have shown an increase in the ratio of total body water to total body potassium compared with normal subjects. Furthermore, a recent study that determined isotopically total body water and total body potassium in cachectic patients, concluded that total body water may be accurately predicted, whereas measured values of total body potassium were significantly lower than predicted. Total body water, therefore, significantly overestimated the metabolically active tissue in weight-losing cancer patients.

Unlike patients with simple anorexia nervosa, in whom weight loss accounts for a more or less proportional decrease in the size of all organs, patients with malignant cachexia have preferential sparing of the liver, kidney, and spleen, as well as significant involvement of other parenchyma. Some experts are now proposing that the emaciation of cancer patients should be more properly defined as 'wasting,' a term meaning a decrease in both body cell mass and weight that is usually associated with poor dietary intake, as opposed to cachexia, which is a decrease in body cell mass even in the presence of stable or increasing weight.

The prevalence and severity of wasting is not always directly related to calorie intake, histological variety, or type of tumor spread; nor are they related to tumor size, since wasting may be present even when the tumor represents less than 0.01% of the total body weight. Several investigations have demonstrated that cachexia represents a major problem at least in terms of prevalence. Patients with malignant tumors have the highest prevalence of malnutrition of any segment of the hospitalized population. In some cancer patients, weight loss may be the most frequent presenting symptom, affecting up to 66% of patients during the course of their disease.

A weight loss greater than 10% of the pre-illness body weight may occur in up to 45% of hospitalized adult cancer patients. The prevalence of malnutrition in different cancer populations is shown in Table 21.1. A relationship exists between weight loss and tumor type. Patients with favorable subtypes of non-Hodgkin's lymphoma, breast cancer, acute non-lymphocytic

Table 21.1 Prevalence of malnutrition in different primary cancers

Tumor type or site	Prevalence of malnutrition (%)
Lung (squamous cell)	50
Breast	36
Sarcoma	39
Colon	54
Prostate	56
Lung (small cell)	60
Lung	61
Pancreas	83
Gastric	83
General cancer population	60
Testicular cancer	25
Colorectal cancer	60
Diffuse lymphoma	55
Sarcoma	66
Head and neck cancer	72
Lung (small cell)	about 50
Neuroblastoma	56
Bronchial carcinoma	66
Breast	9
Rectum	40
Esophagus	79
General cancer population	63

Adapted from Bozzetti (2001).

leukemia, and sarcomas have the lowest prevalence of weight loss (31–41%), while patients with unfavorable non-Hodgkin's lymphoma, colon cancer, prostate cancer, and lung cancer have a 48–61% prevalence of weight loss. Finally, patients with pancreatic or gastric cancer have the highest prevalence of weight loss (83–87%).

In children with cancer, weight loss is determined by the ratio of weight and height compared with an age-adjusted standard (50th percentile for a normal population for each sex). A deterioration in nutritional status is seen in about 23–30% of children. Unlike adults, the worsened nutritional status in children does not seem to correlate with tumor type, with performance status, or with stage of disease.

21.3 Pathophysiology of cancer cachexia

Our understanding of the etiopathogenesis of cancer wasting is limited and based more on the knowledge of abnormalities in nutritional behavior and metabolic patterns than on the identification of specific mediators. Three theories have been suggested:

- Metabolic competition
- Undernutrition
- Alterations of metabolic pathways.

Metabolic competition theory

The metabolic competition theory suggests that neoplastic cells compete with host tissues for amino acids, functioning thereby as a sort of 'nitrogen trap.' This may be true in experimental tumors, where neoplastic tissue accounts for a very high percentage of the carcass weight, but it is unlikely to be an important mechanism in human tumors, where the common experience is the opposite: there are cases of both cachectic patients with tumors of only a few grams, and patients with a rather good general status who have huge abdominal masses. Therefore such a theory cannot explain the nutritional deterioration of the cancer patients except in a very small fraction of them.

Undernutrition

The second theory supports the role of undernutrition as the main cause underlying the development of cancer wasting. The reason for the reduced intake of nutrients in patients with lesions of the upper digestive tract is clear. However, regardless of the tumor's location, anorexia is the most common cause of reduced intake and usually consists of a loss of appetite and/or a feeling of early satiety. Anorexia often precedes the development of malnutrition and anorexia may be a presenting symptom of malignancy in 25% of patients. Abnormalities of food intake and feeding patterns occur in over 50% of newly diagnosed cancer patients. The mechanisms involved in the onset of anorexia are poorly understood. Older studies supported the role of intermediate metabolites (lactate, ketones, low molecular weight peptides, oligonucleotides) coupled with a state of relative hypoinsulinemia.

Parabiotic experiments, in which a non-metastasizing tumor is implanted in an animal whose circulation is connected surgically to that of another non-tumor-bearing animal, demonstrate that anorexia, metabolic changes, weight loss, and cachexia occur in the non-tumor-bearing animals as well, despite the lack of evidence of metastatic tumor at necroscopy. Since the two surgically connected animals only share 1.5% of their total circulation, this suggests the presence of a tumor factor such as a cytokine.

Increased serotoninergic activity within the CNS has been proposed as a possible cause of anorexia. Such activity is secondary to the enhanced availability of tryptophan to the brain since a close relationship between elevated plasma free tryptophan and anorexia was observed in cancer patients with a reduced food intake. The uptake into the brain of tryptophan is competitive with that of branched chain amino acids (BCAAs), and administration of BCAAs by increasing the plasma levels of these competitors at the level of the blood–brain barrier may lead to a decrease in the occurrence of anorexia.

Cytokines may have a pivotal role in long-term inhibition of feeding by mimicking the hypothalamic effect of excessive negative feedback signaling from leptin. This may be achieved by persistent stimulation of anorexigenic neuropeptides such as adrenocorticotropic hormone (ACTH)-releasing factors as well as by inhibition of the neuropeptide Y orexigenic network that consists of opioid peptides and galanin, in addition to the newly identified melanin-concentrating hormone orexin and agouti-related peptide.

As regards leptin – the hormone produced by fat that suppresses appetite and increases energy expenditure to maintain weight stability – initial studies have found its levels to be appropriately low in weight-losing cancer patients.

Reduced intake has also been related to the presence of dysgeusia – a distortion or absence of the sense of taste. The decreased ability to perceive sweet flavors has been linked to anorexia, whereas the decrease in the threshold for bitter flavors has been linked to an aversion to meats rich in bitter substrates (amino acids, purines, polypeptides). Altered smell perception is also related to aversion to food.

In underfed patients there are secondary changes in the gastrointestinal tract, such as a decrease in secretions and atrophy of the mucosa and musculature which may be responsible for the feeling of fullness and delayed emptying, the defective digestion, and the poor absorption of nutrients. Delayed gastric emptying and gastroparesis are also common in patients with advanced cancer.

Alterations of metabolic pathways

The third theory underlying the pathogenesis of cancer cachexia relates to metabolic abnormalities. These span overall energy balance, the individual macro- and micro-nutrients, and the acute phase response.

Energy balance

It is generally accepted that resting energy expenditure (REE) in patients with cancer is more variable than in normal subjects and it is frequently increased by 50–300 kcal per day. The metabolic basis of this increase is poorly understood. One possibility concerns the mass and metabolic rate of malignant tissue. The mass of human tumor rarely exceeds 4% of body weight, so that if it is assumed that the associated metabolic rate (per kilogram of tissue) of this tissue is similar to that of the rest of the body, a large increase in REE would not be expected. However, information about energy expenditure of human malignant tissue *in vivo* is lacking. It is possible that a metabolically active tissue may contribute disproportionally to REE. By analogy, four organs (brain, kidney, heart, and liver), which account for about 5% of body weight, are responsible for about half of the REE in a healthy adult. Another possibility concerns the energy costs of metabolic processes induced by the tumor such as increased gluconeogenesis, increased glucose–lactate recycling, and protein synthesis, all of which require ATP. This increased requirement will be associated with increased heat production.

A further explanation for the alteration in energy expenditure is based on the observation that cancer patients tend to oxidize a higher quantity of non-esterified fatty acids (NEFAs) in comparison to control subjects even in the presence of other energy substrates. This indirectly implies a channeling of carbohydrate intermediates towards lipogenesis before oxidation, which represents a costly metabolism in terms of the consumption of ATP. It has also been reported that protein turnover can account for up to 50% of the REE, with the liver usually accounting for 20–25% of the overall oxygen consumption. Investigations in humans have shown that while the synthesis of muscle protein is diminished in cancer patients, the hepatic synthesis of secretory proteins, acute phase reactants, fibrinogen, glycoproteins, and immunoglobulins can be increased.

The activity of the sympathetic nervous system may also contribute to basal hypermetabolism. It is difficult to explain the large variability in REE by a single metabolic process and it is likely that a combination of metabolic processes are involved, and that the combination of each varies with the type of cancer and stage of disease.

Despite the research emphasis on REE, total energy expenditure (TEE) may not be increased, as shown by tracer studies in free-living patients with cancer and other techniques in other malignancies. The decrease in physical activity, which is very common in malignant (and non-malignant) diseases, offsets or more than offsets any increase in REE. This implies that the loss of energy stores which may eventually lead to cancer cachexia is more likely to be due to a decrease in energy intake than an increase in energy expenditure.

Data on the prevalence and severity of hypermetabolism are shown in Tables 21.2 and 21.3.

Carbohydrate metabolism

Carbohydrate metabolism can be considered as whole body and skeletal muscle glucose metabolism, hepatic glucose metabolism, and tumor glucose metabolism. In this context, the main alterations in carbohydrate metabolism include decreased oral glucose tolerance, which occurs in 37–60% of tumor-bearing patients. By using the intravenous glucose tolerance test, it has been demonstrated that head and neck cancer patients have reduced first phase insulin response similar to that seen in type 2 diabetes and a reduced glucose disposal. This result seems to be directly correlated, at the multiple-regression analysis, not only with acute insulin response but also with triiodothyronine concentration. The reduced glucose disposal indicates that there is insulin resistance, with reduction in the normal ability of the insulin-sensitive tissues (e.g. muscle, gut) to take up glucose.

The investigations with the use of the euglycemic hyperinsulinemic clamp technique have generally shown that there is a significant reduction in glucose utilization when the insulin concentration is in the physiologic range, and that this effect is not overcome with administration of supraphysiologic insulin concentrations. Fasting serum insulin is normal or low. On the whole, these studies imply that glucose may not be utilized in the whole body of the cancer patients as well as lipids or amino acids. Since glucose oxidation appears to be only mildly reduced, the major defect in the glucose utilization probably resides in non-oxidative glucose disposal or in the synthesis of glycogen.

Hepatic glucose metabolism can also be altered during cancer cachexia. Approximately 75% of studies report an increase in the rate of hepatic glucose production in cancer patients. Gluconeogenesis from

Table 21.2 Studies on resting energy expenditure in cancer patients

Year	No. of patients	Type of tumor	% hypermetabolic patients (REE ≥110% PEE)
1869–1924	34	Leukemia	97
1914	33	Gastric carcinoma	45
1924	71	Leukemia	86
1950	41	Leukemia/lymphoma	100
	23	Carcinoma	91
1951	5	Leukemia/lymphoma	5
1956	12	Solid tumors	67
1965	4	Solid tumors	75
1978	10	Miscellaneous	80
1980	65	Miscellaneous	58
1980	42	Gastroenteric tumors	↑ in males
1982	16	Miscellaneous	0
1982	200	Miscellaneous	63
1982	43	Gastroenteric tumors	↑
1983	173	Gastroenteric tumors	54
1983	73	Colorectal carcinoma	30
1983	5	Carcinoma of the lung	100[a]
1984	31	Lung cancer	100
1984	31	Carcinoma of the lung	100
1986a	24	Colorectal carcinoma	0
1986b	98	Miscellaneous	0
1988	7	Sarcoma	100[a]
1988	83	Colon and lung carcinoma	0[a]
1988	58	Colon and lung carcinoma	0[a]
1992	–	Hepatocarcinoma	–

[a]Referred to a control group
REE, resting energy expenditure; PEE, predicted energy expenditure.
Adapted from Bozzetti (2001).

Table 21.3 Resting energy expenditure and type of tumor

Site/type	No. of patients	% patients with increase in REE	Median increase of REE (%)
Lung	5	100	–
	31	100	31
	22	0	–
	38	0	–
Leukemia	133	74	35
Lymphoma	18	–	22
Sarcoma	9	–	14–18
Localized	4	–	33–41
Metastatic	7	100	35
Gastric carcinoma	28	40	10
	7	–	20
Colorectal carcinoma	73	22	20
	24	0	–
	16	–	28
	38	0	–
	45	0	–
Gastroenteric carcinoma	42	–	↑ in males
Local	24	–	4
Metastatic	19	–	8

Adapted from Bozzetti (2001).

several precursors (lactate, alanine, glycerol) has been reported to be increased, as have total glucose production, turnover, and recycling. Cancer patients also have an increased glucose flux, which could consume up to 40% of the carbohydrates ingested and may contribute to the weight loss. The outpouring of lactic acid by some tumors leads to an increase in the conversion of lactate to glucose by the liver. This process – the Cori cycle – is energy-consuming, because the conversion of 2 moles of lactate to glucose requires 6 moles of ATP, whereas only 2 moles of ATP are recovered in the reconversion of glucose to lactate, and it has been estimated to account for 300 kcal of energy loss per day.

Although the Cori cycle normally accounts for 20% of glucose turnover, this rises to 50% in cachectic cancer patients and accounts for disposal of 60% of the lactate. Both glucose production rates were found to be higher in malnourished cancer patients than in non-cancer patients with comparable weight loss. The increase in glucose recycling equivalent to 40% of the daily glucose intake of the cancer patient has been uitin ligase $E_{3\alpha}$ and degraded by the 26S proteasome. Several proinflammatory cytokines, including tumor necrosis factor (TNF), interleukins 1 and 6 (IL-1 and IL-6), and glucocorticoids, stimulate production of ubiquitin mRNA. In muscle loss, pale fibers are affected more than red fibers and predominantly myofibrillar proteins are involved, as shown by measurements of 3-methylhistidine.

As regards hepatic protein metabolism, studies with radiolabeled leucine have shown that while in normal subjects 53% of hepatic protein synthesis derives from muscle, it accounts for only 8% in malnourished cancer patients. Synthesis of structural liver proteins is normal, and that of the acute phase is increased. There is a correlation between hypoalbuminemia and tumor bulk. Studies with labeled precursors have reported a reduction in albumin synthesis, which is partially corrected by increased protein intake, and an increase in the catabolized fraction. However, recent investigations have shown that synthesis of negative acute phase reactants such as albumin is maintained despite reduced circulating concentrations, whereas synthesis of positive acute phase reactants (e.g. fibrinogen) is significantly increased. There is also an increase in transcapillary escape with a decrease in the intravascular and extravascular ratio.

In rare cases, hypoalbuminemia is also due to its sequestration in pathological compartments or loss to the outside (nephrotic syndromes, protein-losing enteropathy, aminoaciduria in acute leukemias). Such findings could explain the frequent occurrence of hypoalbuminemia even when degradation is normal and synthesis is increased, as reported in recent investigations. Chronic administration of TNF in tumor-bearing animals results in a reduction of whole body protein synthesis and net loss of skeletal protein but in an increase in liver protein synthesis.

The tumor itself can interfere with protein metabolism. The metabolic competition theory suggests that the tumor acts as a 'one-way nitrogen trap,' and that this may have an influence on body economy when the mass accounts for 20% of the body weight of the host. However, it has been found that experimental tumors containing less than 6% of total body nitrogen have a protein metabolism equal to 35% of all protein synthesis. In humans it has been demonstrated that when the tumor is localized and resectable (i.e. colorectal cancer), there is no substantial impact on the overall protein kinetics, while the measurement of the differ-

ence in arteriovenous concentrations of amino acids in tumor-bearing limbs versus normal extremities has shown that less than half of the output of amino acids is released in the circulation by the tumor-bearing limb.

Some studies have demonstrated that the amino acid appearance rate is related to tumor bulk. Measurement in tumor tissue of protein metabolism have established that the tissue has a very high fractional protein synthesis rate of 50–90% per day. This is very similar to the liver and contrasts with a rate of 1–3% for skeletal muscle. In a recent study it was found that those cancer patients who had an elevated plasma amino acid appearance rate survived and those with a normal rate died. Although this issue is controversial, it would appear that an adequate acute phase response to tumor may reflect a more effective fight against cancer.

Acute phase response

The development of cancer cachexia may elicit an acute phase response to malignancy, which is a basic defensive and phylogenetically primitive response of the body against injury. This includes reductions in serum iron and zinc levels, alterations in amino acid distribution and metabolism, and increase in acute phase globulin synthesis and gluconeogenesis, negative nitrogen balance, and sometimes fever. This process is due to cytokines secreted by macrophages at the tissue site of tumor which inhibit albumin synthesis and stimulate the synthesis of acute phase proteins.

These include:

- *C-Reactive protein*, which promotes phagocytosis, modulates the cellular immune response, and inhibits the migration of white blood cells into the tissues.
- *Alpha-1-antichymotrypsin*, which minimizes tissue damage due to phagocytosis and reduces intravascular coagulation.
- *Alpha-1-macroglobulin*, which forms complexes with proteases and removes them from circulation, maintains antibody production, and promotes granulopoiesis and synthesis of other acute phase proteins.

An acute phase protein response is seen in a significant proportion of patients bearing tumors that are frequently associated with weight loss (e.g. pancreas, lung, esophagus) and it is more frequent in the advanced stages of disease. The presence of such a response in patients with pancreatic or renal cancer is associated with a shortened survival, perhaps due to the exaggerated muscle breakdown required to supply amino acids for the acute phase response protein synthesis.

Vitamin and mineral deficiencies

Deficiencies in vitamins may be present in some undernorished cancer patients. The most significant include reductions in plasma levels of folate, vitamin A, and vitamin C. Between 19% and 52% of hospitalized patients have been noted to have reduced serum folate levels and 18–35% of patients who die of cancer and subsequent infections have severe liver deficiency of vitamin A at autopsy.

Mineral deficiencies can occur in some cancer patients as part of the cytokine-mediated inflammatory response (in addition to being a consequence of common causes such as poor oral intake, increased dietary requirements, and excessive urinary and stool losses). Zinc concentrations in the blood can drop as an early response to cytokines, which may be elevated in cancer patients. In cancer patients who are hospitalized, a low serum zinc ($<70 \, \mu g/dl$) is not uncommon and usually normalizes after a three-week administration of 50 mg zinc/day. Serum copper is normal or elevated in cancer patients, with a pattern similar to that of serum zinc. Serum iron levels usually fall as result of cytokine-mediated response.

Hormonal milieu

Many patients develop insulin resistance syndrome as a result of cancer, and they exhibit a small but significant elevation in serum insulin concentration. As a consequence, as in the case of diabetes, they have reduced glucose utilization, loss of first phase insulin response, and sometimes increased fasting hepatic glucose production. As already mentioned, the weight-losing cancer patients frequently have an increase in fatty acid oxidation and plasma fatty acid appearance rate. The rate of TAG hydrolysis is much higher than that of fat oxidation so that albumin-bound fatty acids are partially utilized for energy but many are utilized for re-esterification or substrate cycling back to TAGs.

Multiple studies have failed to demonstrate elevation in the counter-regulation of hormones, with the exception of mild elevation in urinary free cortisol secretion. Catecholamines and glucagon are usually normal but growth hormone (GH) was found to be increased at 24-h analysis and by random sampling in malnourished cancer patients. Levels of GH are further increased by the infusion of arginine and insulin. Hypogonadism has been reported in male cancer patients and free triiodothyronine and triiodothyronine concentrations can both be low.

As a normal response to save energy in the injured subject, the body's ability to convert the stored form of a thyroid hormone (thyroxin or T_4) into the active form of thyroid hormones (triiodothyronine or T_3) becomes impaired and T_4 is converted to an inactive form known as reverse-T_3 hormone (rT_3). This process can occur in aggressive cancers when the patient's response is similar to that of an injury response. There is no evidence of increased thyroid hormone levels during refeeding.

Mediators of cancer cachexia

Cytokines

Extensive investigation has failed to identify altered classic hormonal pathways as a cause of cancer cachexia. The most common alterations in hormone profiles include increased cortisol secretion and urinary excretion of epinephrine and norepinephrine, increased glucagon levels and a decreased insulin/glucagon ratio, and changes in thyroid hormones. These alterations can often be attributed to the associated anorexia and cannot be considered the cause of the changes in energy expenditure and body composition.

Recent studies have investigated the role of cytokines, which are produced by immunocytes as an endogenous immune response to the tumor. Cytokines are polypeptide signals produced by the host's cells in response to a growing tumor. They regulate many of the nutritional and metabolic disturbances that occur in the host with cancer, leading to:

- decreased appetite,
- stimulation of the basal metabolic rate,
- stimulation of glucose uptake,
- stimulation of the mobilization of fat and protein stores,
- reduction in adipocyte lipoprotein lipase activity,
- enhanced muscle amino acid release, and
- stimulation of hepatic amino acid transport activity.

Elevated concentrations of tissue and circulating cytokines have been found in cancer patients and

Table 21.4 Cytokine-mediated effects on protein, carbohydrate, and lipid metabolism

Cytokine	Protein	Carbohydrate	Lipid
TNF	Increased muscle proteolysis Increased protein oxidation Increased hepatic protein synthesis	Increased glycogenolysis Decreased glycogen synthesis Increased gluconeogenesis Increased glucose clearance Increased lactate production	Decreased lipogenesis
IL-1	Increased hepatic protein synthesis	Increased gluconeogenesis Increased glucose clearance	Increased lipolysis Decreased LPL synthesis Increased fatty acid synthesis
IL-6	Increased hepatic protein synthesis		Increased lipolysis Increased fatty acid synthesis
IFN-gamma			Decreased lipogenesis Increased lipolysis Decreased LPL activity

LPL, lipoprotein lipase.

enhanced hepatic cytokine gene expression has been found in tumor-bearing animals.

These cytokines include TNF, interleukins 1, 2, 4, and 6, and interferons alpha, beta, and gamma. The clinical effects of the administration of some cytokines to experimental animals are reported in Table 21.4 and are covered in the following section.

Both animal and human studies show that administration of TNFα causes an initial drop in body weight followed by a decreasing response with repeated administration. Acute administration of TNFα causes effects similar to those seen in cancer cachexia, including an increase in metabolic rate (by 30%), plasma TAGs, glycerol turnover (by more than 80%), and NEFA turnover (by more than 60%) as well as in temperature, heart rate, epinephrine and ACTH levels. Similar effects were seen on protein metabolism, where whole body protein turnover and total amino acid efflux and acute phase protein response were increased. It is noteworthy that in human studies where TNF was given to cancer patients intermittently, it did not cause weight loss, perhaps because it was not possible to consistently elevate TNF levels. In these studies, these responses were blunted by ibuprofen despite the absence of changes in the plasma levels of TNFα. However, in chronic administration the alterations were resolved despite continuous administration of TNFα.

Moreover, in no phase I clinical investigation of TNFα was cachexia a major side effect; instead, fluid retention through damage to the vascular endothelium and increased capillary permeability were reported. Only hypertriacylglycerolemia persisted despite the development of tachyphylaxis, but this seems to be unrelated to cachexia since, for instance, hypertriacylglycerolemic AIDS patients maintain their weight for prolonged periods of time.

Experimental studies suggest that the increase in serum TAGs due to TNFα administration is mainly due to hepatic synthesis and secretion of very low-density lipoproteins (VLDLs) rather than from adipose tissue. Depletion of skeletal muscle would be due to the induction of oxidative stress and nitric oxide synthase and consequent decreased myosin creatinine phosphokinase expression and binding activity. It is possible that naturally occurring TNFα inhibitors in the circulation may hide TNFα production by the monocytes of the host. In fact, these inhibitors were found to be circulating freely in healthy volunteers and increased in individuals with ovarian cancer. The inability to detect TNFα in cachectic patients has led to the suggestion that it acts as a paracrine/autocrine mediator rather than as the circulating messenger in cachexia.

Production of TNF by isolated peripheral blood mononuclear cells has been shown to be elevated in weight-losing pancreatic cancer patients with an acute phase protein response, suggesting that local rather than systemic production may be more relevant.

Some investigators did not find elevated TNFα levels in cancer patients, nevertheless, there was a two-fold increase in the relative levels of mRNA for hormone-sensitive lipase in adipose tissue of cancer patients compared with controls. These findings suggest that TNFα may not contribute to the development of cachexia in cancer but indicate a stimulation of lipolysis in adipose tissue. Anti-TNFα antibodies have had minimal effects in tumor-bearing animals even if in a human squamous cell carcinoma of the maxilla, grown as a xenograft in nude mice, anti-TNFα antibodies partially reversed, but did not completely normalize, body weight.

Pentoxifylline has been reported to decrease TNF mRNA levels in cancer patients. However, it failed to show any benefit in a recent trial on cachectic patients with lung or gastrointestinal tumors.

Interleukin-1 has been shown to have many effects similar to those of TNFα, including suppression of lipoprotein lipase and enhancement of intracellular lipolysis. Elevated IL-1 plasma levels are seldom found in cancer patients, but antibodies against an IL-1 receptor mitigate cachectic symptoms in tumor-bearing mice to a similar degree to anti-TNFα antibodies.

Unlike TNFα and IL-1, increased levels of IL-6 are measured in the serum of cancer patients. IL-6 is the main cytokine involved in the induction of acute phase proteins and fibrinogen synthesis, and elevated levels have been reported in 39% of patients with lung or colon cancer and an ongoing acute phase protein response. However, since all of the patients had lost weight, it is difficult to determine whether IL-6 was elevated in cachectic patients alone. Antibodies to IL-6 administered to patients with AIDS-related lymphoma produced weight gain in those losing weight and

stabilized the levels of the acute phase reactant C-reactive protein. The increase in circulating IL-6 is closely related to tumor burden and is thought to originate from tumor cells as well as from various tissues of the cancer-bearing host (e.g. liver, kidney, small intestine, etc.) and to be induced by the IL-1 production of tumor-infiltrating macrophages. Again, local production of IL-6 by peripheral blood mononuclear cells is important and its production seems to be elevated in patients with pancreatic cancer and an acute phase protein response.

Interferon gamma (IFNγ) is known to have effects on fat metabolism similar to those of TNFα, namely the inhibition of lipoprotein lipase and decreased protein synthesis, and polyclonal antibodies anti-IFNγ partly mitigate cancer-induced anorexia and weight loss. Increased serum IFNγ levels have been found in 53% of patients with multiple myeloma. However, no association was observed between level of IFNγ and clinical parameters of the disease. These findings suggest that IFNγ alone may not be responsible for the induction of wasting. Over the long term a vicious cycle is activated that results in anorexia and widespread abnormalities in carbohydrate, protein, and lipid metabolism (Figure 21.1).

The acute response to TNFα in healthy volunteers appears to be a rise in C-reactive protein, a decrease in serum zinc level, and a doubling of the forearm amino acid efflux primarily attributable to increases in the glucogenic amino acids alanine and glutamine. This accelerated nitrogen release may be due to starvation

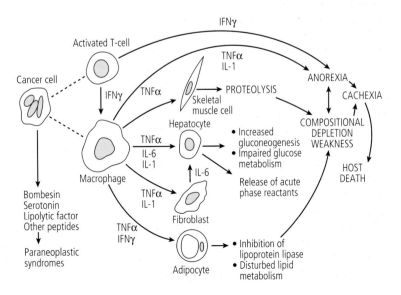

Figure 21.1 Suggested mechanism for cancer cachexia.

effects. These results have been replicated in animals and with IL-1. It is unclear, however, which distal mediators in the cytokine cascade are the key players. The mechanisms underlying host cachexia have been suggested to be due to cytokines, elaborated by activated immunocytes in response to the tumor, and having secondary effects which exhibit an acute phase reaction, rerouting nutrients from the periphery to the liver.

Studies evaluating the effects of cytokine administration on the circulating glucose concentration indicate that the plasma glucose level rises or falls depending on the dose of cytokine administered, the timing of the measurement, and the specific cytokine given. There are experimental data that indicate that TNFα administration can induce a marked increase in whole body glucose utilization even though glucose uptake does not increase equally in all organs or tissues. It is likely that the loss of fat stores in patients with cancer is due in part to the ability of TNFα and IL-1 to mobilize fat stores. In the experimental setting TNFα is able to reduce the adipocyte lipoprotein lipase activity and heparin-releasable lipoprotein lipase activity and to increase the serum TAG levels, which also depend on a stimulation of the hepatic lipid secretion. IL-6 is also able to reduce adipose tissue lipoprotein lipase activity and heparin-releasable lipoprotein lipase activity.

Catabolic factors

In addition to cytokines, some studies have reported circulating human factors that act directly on skeletal muscle and adipose tissues in a hormone-like manner. The most important are the lipid-mobilizing factors (LMFs), and to a lesser extent the protein-mobilizing factors (PMFs). LMFs include the toxohormone-L isolated from the ascitic fluid of patients with hepatoma and that isolated from culture media of the human A375 melanoma cell line. LMFs act directly on adipose tissue with release of free fatty acid and glycerol in a manner similar to that of lipolytic hormones. The mechanism involved could be the continuous stimulation of LMFs on the cyclic adenosine monophosphate (cAMP) that results in the activation of protein kinase which phosphorylates an inactive form of TAG lipase, otherwise known as hormone-sensitive lipase.

In conclusion, there is strong evidence that LMFs produced by tumors are related to the process of cachexia: LMF is absent, or present in reduced amounts, from tumors that do not induce cachexia, and it is absent as well from normal serum even under conditions of starvation. The level of LMFs in the sera of cancer pa-

tients has been found to be proportional to the extent of weight loss, and it is reduced in patients responding to chemotherapy. Following some preliminary *in vitro* investigations showing inhibition of the tumor LMFs by the PUFA eicosapentaenoic acid (EPA), cachectic patients suffering from pancreatic cancer were treated with fish oil capsules containing 18% EPA and 12% docosahexaenoic acid (DHA). This supplementation reversed the weight loss of 2.9 kg/month and led to a weight gain of 0.3 kg/month, which was associated with a temporary reduction of acute phase proteins and stabilization of the REE.

There is some evidence that PMFs play a role in human cancer cachexia. Some investigators found the presence of u- and m-calpains, a group of cytosolic, calcium-dependent proteases able to induce proteolysis when incubated with rat diaphragm, in the serum of cachectic patients, and recently succeeded in isolating the 24 kDa proteoglycan from the urine of cachectic patients, regardless of the tumor type. This factor was able to accelerate the breakdown of skeletal muscle *in vitro* and *in vivo* and to produce weight loss *in vivo* by a process that did not involve anorexia.

Iatrogenic malnutrition

Hypophagia

Anorexia and hypophagia may involve a psychological component that is related to the communication of the diagnosis or of therapeutic decisions such as the need for hospitalization or disabling therapies. In pediatric patients in particular, conditioning mechanisms can lead to anorexia or food aversion. Nutritional changes resulting from iatrogenic lesions of the alimentary tract are also important. Table 21.5 lists the nutritional changes related to the radical resection of organs of the digestive tract. Malnutrition is only rarely related to reduced caloric and protein intake as a result of certain procedures (interference in chewing and swallowing due to glossectomy, dysphagia, total gastrectomy). Instead, it is usually due to malabsorption.

Nutritional complications associated with radiotherapy are frequent (Table 21.6). It has been demonstrated that approximately 90% of patients submitted to intensive treatment in the head and neck region, the abdomen, or the pelvis lose weight unless nutritional support is provided. More than 10% of patients lose over 10% of their usual weight when radiotherapy is continued for a period of 6–8 weeks. The pathophysiology of malnutrition from radiotherapy is twofold:

Table 21.5 Nutritional consequences of radical resection of alimentary tract organs

	Nutritional consequences
Tongue or pharynx	Need for enteral feeding (due to dysphagia)
Thoracic esophagus	Gastric stasis (due to vagotomy)
	Malabsorption of fats (due to vagotomy)
Stomach	Dumping syndrome, anemia, malabsorption of fats, iron, calcium, and vitamins
Duodenum	Biliary-pancreatic deficiency
Jejunum (up to 120 cm)	Reduced absorption of glucose, fats, protein, folic acid, vitamin B_{12}, etc.
Ileum (60 cm) or ileocecal valve	Malabsorption of vitamin B_{12}, biliary salts, and fats
Small intestine (75%)	Malabsorption of fats, glucose, protein, folic acid, vitamin B_{12}, etc., diarrhea
Jejunum and ileum	Complete malabsorption
Colon (subtotal or total resection)	Water and electrolyte loss
Pancreas	Malabsorption and diabetes
Liver	Transient hypoalbuminemia

Table 21.6 Nutritional complications associated with radiotherapy

Region irradiated	Early effects	Late effects
Head and neck	Odynophagia	Ulceration
	Xerostomia (dry mouth)	Xerostomia
	Mucositis	Dental caries
	Anorexia	Osteoradionecrosis
	Dysosmia	Trismus
	Hypogeusia (reduced ability to taste)	Hypogeusia
Thorax	Dysphagia	Fibrosis
		Stenosis
		Fistula
Abdomen and pelvis	Anorexia	Ulceration
	Nausea	Malabsorption
	Vomiting	Diarrhea
	Diarrhea	Chronic enteritis
	Acute enteritis	Chronic colitis
	Acute colitis	

direct hypophagia in patients receiving radiotherapy to regions of the head and neck and chest, and hypophagia associated with malabsorption in patients receiving radiotherapy to the abdomen.

The minimum tolerated dose for other regions (i.e. the dose that may cause severe complications within five years of completion of radiotherapy using the standard high-energy therapeutic modality fractioned into 10 Gy a week, with five sessions a week) varies from 35 to 50 Gy, depending on the organs and tissue of the region (Table 21.7). Head and neck irradiation interferes with nutrition because it causes a rapid exponential loss in the sense of taste. After 3–4 weeks, patients begin to suffer from an affected taste sensation due to lesion of the microvilli of the gustatory cells or their surfaces. This condition returns to normal 2–4 months after the end of treatment.

Table 21.7 Radiation tolerance of the parts of the gastrointestinal tract

Organ	TD 5/5 (rads)	TD 50/5 (rads)
Stomach	4500	5000
Small intestine	4500	6000
Colon	4500	6500
Rectum	5500	8000

TD 5/5 = total dose of radiation which will give rise to a 5% increase in significant complications in five years.
TD 50/5 = total dose of radiation which will give rise to a 50% incidence of significant complications in five years.

Another change caused by head and neck irradiation is the decrease in salivation that occurs in the first 3–4 days of therapy, causing nausea and dysphagia and facilitating the onset of caries. Erythema, mucositis, and oropharyngeal ulceration with odynophagia may develop during the second or third week.

Radiotherapy to the chest may lead to dysphagia when the field of irradiation includes the esophagus; it occurs with fractioned doses of approximately 30 Gy over three weeks and may persist for several weeks after completion of therapy. Radiotherapy to the abdomen and pelvis may cause two different types of nutritional disturbances: those related to decreased food intake due to anorexia, nausea, and vomiting, and those due to chronic X-ray enteropathy.

Negative side effects from chemotherapy occur in several forms (Table 21.8): anorexia due to changes in the sense of taste with perception of a metallic tinge, dysphagia due to ulceration of the mucosa of the lip, tongue, oropharyngeal cavity, and esophagus, decrease in food intake due to nausea and vomiting, as well as constipation or adynamic ileus. The most toxic treatment combination is vinblastine, bleomycin, and cis-platinum (PVB), which is administered for testicular cancers. The combination of chemo- and radiotherapy produces cytotoxicity as a result of their simple additive effect, and as a result of synergism (the final response is greater than the sum of the effects of the single modalities as a result of the use of sensitizing drugs).

The commonest examples of negative effects of combinations of therapy used in cancer treatment are summarized in Box 21.2.

Malabsorption

The malabsorption that occurs in cancer patients may be iatrogenic in origin, or directly related to disease. Recently, in fact, it has been reported that patients with advanced breast cancer exhibit a markedly reduced capacity for active and facilitated absorption of some substrates. However, it should be noted that intestinal enzyme deficiency and significant biochemical changes in the intestinal mucosa (with consequent malabsorption of protein) appear very early under conditions of fasting and hypoalbuminemia, even in the absence of morphological changes. For this reason, it is difficult to determine whether there is an actual 'neoplastic en-

Table 21.8 Negative side effects from chemotherapy

Drug	Severity and duration
Chemotherapeutic drugs commonly associated with severe nausea and vomiting	
Nitrogen mustard (mustine hydrochloride; mechlorethamine hydrochloride USP)	Occurs in virtually all patients
	May be severe, but usually subsides within 24 h
Chloroethyl nitrosoureas	Variable, but may be severe
Streptozotocin (streptozocin)	Occurs in nearly all patients
	Tolerance improves with each successive dose given on a 5-day schedule
Cis-platinum (cisplatin)	May be very severe
	Tolerance improves with intravenous hydration and continuous 5-day infusion
	Nausea may persist for several days
Imidazole carboxamide (DTIC; dacarbazine)	Occurs in virtually all patients
	Tolerance improves with each successive dose given on a 5-day schedule
Chemotherapeutic drugs commonly associated with mucositis	
Methotrexate	May be quite severe with prolonged infusions or if renal function is compromised
	Severity is enhanced by irradiation
	May be prevented with administration of adequate citrovorum rescue factor (folinic acid; leucovorin)
5-Fluorouracil (fluorouracil USP)	Severity increase with higher doses, frequency of cycles, and arterial infusions
Actinomycin D (dactinomycin USP)	Very common; may prevent oral alimentation
	Severity enhanced by irradiation
Adriamycin (doxorubicin)	May be severe and ulcerative
	Increased in presence of liver disease
	Severity enhanced by irradiation
Bleomycin	May be severe and ulcerating
Vinblastine	Frequently ulcerative

- Antitumor antibiotics (adriamycin, actinomycin D, bleomycin) are generally more toxic when administered to patients undergoing radiotherapy
- The incidence and severity of oesophagitis from irradiation increase with the use of actinomycin D, vinblastine, hydroxyurea, procarbazine, and the combination of cyclophosphamide, vincristine, and actinomycin D
- Adriamycin and daunomycin are sensitizing agents which, when combined with radiotherapy, may cause esophageal stenosis
- Fluorouracil, actinomycin D, and adriamycin may enhance damage from irradiation in other regions of the digestive tract
- Actinomycin D and adriamycin are responsible for the so-called 'recall reaction,' in which there is a reactivation of the latent effects of irradiation during medical therapy. In this case, severe irritation of the gastrointestinal mucosa may recur periodically

Box 21.3 Incidences when malabsorption is directly related to the tumor

- The pancreas is involved and there is obstruction of the biliary-pancreatic ducts
- There are lesions in the small intestine from leukemic foci or lymphoma or solid tumors that may directly infiltrate the wall, obstruct lymphatic flow or affect the mucosa and villi
- With protein-losing syndromes, present in patients with lymphoma or gastric carcinoma
- If the digestive tract is the target organ of strong pharmacological substances secreted by certain tumors (e.g. apudomas), such as trophic hormones, steroids, hormonal polypeptides with low molecular weight, quinines, and prostaglandins
- When alterations in the villi and their function are observed in patients with tumors whose origin is extra-gastrointestinal

teropathy,' or if malabsorption is attributable to simple malnutrition and to what degree.

As far as postoperative malabsorption is concerned (Table 21.5), pancreatectomy may cause digestive enzyme deficiency with loss through the stool of fats and proteins as well as a considerable quantity of vitamins and minerals. Radiotherapy to the small and large intestine may cause immediate and late damage, since the epithelium of the small intestine is second only to bone marrow in radiosensitivity. Damage from irradiation, which appears in 70–80% of patients who receive abdomino-pelvic radiotherapy, is clinically expressed as malabsorption of glucose, fat, electrolytes, and, in part, proteins (due to peptidase deficiency). Morphological lesions consistent with flattening of the villi and reduction in mitosis have been demonstrated in asymptomatic patients after a dose of 20 Gy over three weeks or 33 Gy over four weeks. Spontaneous recovery usually occurs within two weeks of completion of radiotherapy. One-third of patients who have had acute enteritis subsequently develop late enteritis.

More recently, the adoption of special measures to dislodge small bowel from the pelvis (Trendelenburg position, use of belly board, maintenance of a full bladder during radiotherapy) has decreased the frequency of severe radiation enteropathy.

Treatment with growth-inhibiting compounds (thioguanine, methotrexate, fluorouracil, vinca alkaloids, hydroxyurea, daunomycin, and alkylating agents) may also cause malabsorption. Folic acid antagonists may cause changes in the intestinal mucosa which are similar to those of sprue, with a reduction in epithelial cell mitosis and absorption of xylose and other nutrients. The administration of fluorouracil leads to a dipeptidase deficiency, and a single intravenous administration of methotrexate (2–5 mg/kg) is followed by inhibition of cell mitosis of the jejunal mucosa as well as other cellular changes. A number of drugs may interfere with normal utilization or elimination of nutrients and may precipitate the onset of (sub) clinical deficiency (Table 21.9). Malabsorption which is directly related to the tumor may be present in a series of circumstances, as summarized in Box 21.3.

Section II: Nutritional support in cancer

21.4 Effect of nutritional support on nutritional status

There is a relationship between weight loss and poor quality of life, and high morbidity and mortality rates have been demonstrated in malnourished cancer pa-tients in both medical and surgical patients. Malnourished or weight-losing patients with breast or testis cancer or Hodgkin's disease have a poorer response to chemotherapy than weight-stable patients. In studies involving the pediatric population nutritional status has been correlated with survival time in lymphoma

Table 21.9 Drug-induced nutrient deficiencies

Drug	Nutrient(s) affected
Aminoglycoside	Magnesium, zinc
Ammonium chloride	Vitamin C
Antacid	Phosphorus, phosphates
Aspirin	Vitamin C
Cholestyramine	Triglycerides, fat-soluble vitamins
Coumadin	Vitamin K
Diphenylhydantoin	Niacin
Diuretics	Sodium, potassium, magnesium, zinc
Doxorubicin and vidarabine	Carnitine
Estrogen and progesterone compounds	Folic acid, vitamin B_6
Hydralazine	Vitamin B_6
Isoniazid	Vitamin B_6, niacin
Laxatives	Sodium, potassium, magnesium
Penicillamine	Vitamin B_6
Phenobarbital and phenytoin	Vitamin C, vitamin D
Phenothiazines	Vitamin B_2
Platinum	Magnesium, zinc
Steroids	Vitamin A, potassium
Tetracycline	Vitamin C
Tricyclic antidepressants	Vitamin B_2

(and histiocytosis) and solid tumors, the greatest impact being most evident in patients with limited tumor spread. The effect of nutritional status on the response to chemotherapy is especially evident in patients with solid tumors, both children and adults. It has been reported that nutritional status is likely to have an impact on response when the response rate to chemotherapy is in the 40–80% range.

Serum albumin level appears to be an excellent predictor of survival. Two studies in Hodgkin's disease and lung cancer reported a 10- and 1.7-fold increase in risk of mortality depending on whether the level of serum albumin was higher or lower than 3.4 g/dl.

The rationale for using artificial nutrition (parenteral or enteral) in cancer patients is primarily based on the assumption that although the final outcome of cancer patients mainly reflects the prognosis of the primary tumor, concomitant malnutrition can affect survival by increasing the complications of the oncologic therapy, reducing tolerance to these treatments and, in some cases, decreasing both the length and the quality of survival.

This approach tends to correlate cancer cachexia with undernutrition, a concept which is only partially true, since, as we have already seen, reduced intake only partially accounts for the onset and progression of cachexia. This is a pivotal aspect of nutritional support: in fact, since hypophagia 'alone' does not account

for the onset and progression of cachexia, the effects of parenteral and enteral nutrition are expected to be more limited than in conditions of simple undernutrition; however, if parenteral or enteral nutrition were totally inefficient in reversing malnutrition or in preventing the progressive deterioration of the nutritional status, there would be no rationale for feeding malnourished cancer patients either in current clinical practice or in randomized trials.

The effects of parenteral and enteral nutrition on nutritional status have been reviewed in previous publications and are summarized in Tables 21.10 and 21.11. The beneficial effects of parenteral nutrition are more evident when compared in controlled studies with a standard oral diet (Table 21.12). It is noteworthy that there is a nutritional benefit even when a vigorous nutritional support is being administered to patients undergoing an oncologic therapy (Table 21.13). Special interest has been focused on the effects of parenteral and enteral nutrition on body cell mass, the component of body compartment which contains the oxygen-exchanging, potassium-rich, glucose-oxidizing, work-performing tissue, and on the protein component of the body which represents the 'functional compartment' par excellence.

Studies evaluating whole body potassium (WBK) have generally had better results than those evaluating total body nitrogen (TBN). There are probably several

Table 21.10 Effects of TPN on the nutritional status of cancer patients

Variable	Response
Body weight	Always increases (Burt, 1982; Bozzetti, 1987; Fan, 1989; Gray, 1990)
Body fat	Usually increases (Evans, 1985; Ota, 1985a)
Muscle mass	
Anthropometry	No change or increase (Bozzetti, 1987; Evans, 1985; Ota, 1985a)
Urinary creatinine or 3-CH$_3$-histidine	No change or decrease (Bozzetti, 1987; Burt, 1983b; Bennegard, 1983)
Lean body mass	
Nitrogen balance	Always positive (Bozzetti, 1987; Fan, 1989; Burt, 1983b; Bennegard, 1983; James, 1985; Moghissi, 1977)
Total body nitrogen	No change or increase (James, 1985; Shike, 1984; Cohn, 1982)
Whole body K	Increase or no change (Bennegard, 1983; James, 1985; Cohn, 1982)
Serum protein	
Total protein albumin	No change (Braga, 1983; Muller, 1982)
Transferrin	Usually no change (Bozzetti, 1987; Gray, 1990; Evans, 1985; Ota, 1985; Burt, 1983; Rasmussen, 1985; Ota, 1984, 1985)
Prealbumin	Usually no change (Bozzetti, 1987; Ota, 1985a; Burt, 1983; Rasmussen, 1985; Ota, 1985; Ota, 1984)
Retinol-binding protein	No change or increase (Ota, 1985; Bennegard, 1983; Ota, 1985a; Ota, 1984; Ota, 1986)
Cholinesterase and ceruloplasmin	Usually increase or no change (Bozzetti, 1987; Ota, 1985a; Ota, 1985; Ota, 1984; Ota, 1986)
Immune humoral response	No change (Bozzetti, 1987; Rasmussen, 1985)
IgA; C$_3$, C$_4$	No change (Rasmussen, 1985; Ota, 1985b)
IgG, IgM, IgA	No change or sometimes increase (Rasmussen, 1985; Ota, 1985b)
Non-specific cellular response	
Neutrophils, total lymphocytes, B, T lymphocytes, helper T, suppressor T, chemotaxis	No change (Bozzetti 1985; Rasmussen 1985; Ota 1985b)
Phagocytosis, killing index, natural killer	No change or increase (Evans 1985; Ota 1985b; Ota 1985b)

Adapted from Bozzetti (1989).
Full list of these references available from www.nutritiontexts.com.

explanations for the discrepancy between the response of WBK and that of TBN, aside from the intrinsic error of the two techniques, since neutron activation measures all protein nitrogen (cellular protein + extracellular collagen) equally without differentiating the site or the metabolic activity of the nitrogen measured. In fact, the intracellular potassium concentration is also influenced by the state of cellular hydration, by glycogen stores, and by the level of insulin and catecholamines; and its depletion may be independent of the loss of body protein. In addition, the K/N ratio changes in different tissues of the body (3 mol of K/kg of N in muscle, to about 1.3 mol/kg in the rest of the lean body mass, to 1 mol/kg in adipose tissue).

The low nitrogen accretion with parenteral or enteral nutrition should come as no surprise. Studies on body composition during weight recovery suggest that the initial percentage of body fat is the most important determinant variable in energy partitioning: the higher it is, the lower the proportion of energy mobilized as protein will be, and hence the greater the propensity

the body has to mobilize fat during semi-starvation and to deposit it subsequently during re-feeding. Consequently, different results may simply reflect different types of tissue depletion and renewal in response to the nutritional support administered.

A number of studies have examined specific protein kinetic response to parenteral nutrition in malnourished cancer patients. Whole body protein turnover has been shown to increase with parenteral nutrition but whole body protein synthesis has been reported both to increase or to decrease. Whole body protein catabolism has been reported to decrease in cancer patients on parenteral nutrition. Few studies have investigated the two components of protein kinetics, namely the muscle compartment and the extra-muscle compartment, and have reported an increase in whole body protein synthesis and in the fractional synthetic rate of protein in muscle, with no change in whole body protein catabolism. In severely malnourished patients with gastric cancer, whole body protein synthesis and catabolism does not significantly change from 'before'

Table 21.11 Effects of enteral nutrition on the nutritional status of cancer patients

Variable	Response
Body weight	Usually increase, sometimes no change (Burt, 1982; Burt, 1983b; Bennegard, 1983; James, 1985; Braga, 1983; Lim, 1981; Balzola, 1984; Daly, 1984; Cristallo, 1984; Ravera, 1986)
Body fat	Increase or no change (Bennegard, 1983; James, 1985; Braga, 1983; Cristallo, 1984; Ravera, 1986)
Muscle mass	
Anthropometry	No change; sometimes increase (Braga, 1983; Daly, 1984; Cristallo, 1984; Ravera, 1986)
Urinary creatinine or 3-CH$_3$-histidine	No change (Burt, 1983b; Bennegard, 1983; Ravera, 1986)
3-CH$_3$-histidine efflux from the leg	Decrease (Lundholm, 1982)
Tyrosine, AA and BCAA efflux from the leg	No change (Bennegard, 1984)
Lean body mass	
Nitrogen balance	Usually positive or equilibrium (Burt, 1982; Bennegard, 1983; Ravera, 1986; Haffeejee, 1979)
Total body nitrogen	No change (James, 1985)
Whole body K	Increase or no change (Burt, 1982; Bennegard, 1983; James, 1985)
Serum protein	
Total protein albumin	No change or increase (Burt, 1983b; Ravera, 1986; Palmo, 1984)
TIBC, CHE, TBPA	Usually no change; sometimes increase or decrease (Burt, 1983; Bennegard, 1983; Braga, 1983; Daly, 1984; Cristallo, 1984; Ravera, 1986; Palmo, 1984)
Ceruloplasmin	No change or increase (Burt, 1983b; Bennegard, 1983; Braga, 1983; Cristallo, 1984; Ravera, 1986)
Immune humoral response	No change
IgG, IgA, IgM, CH$_{50}$	No change (Haffejee, 1979)
C$_3$-C$_4$, C$_3$PA	Increase (Braga, 1983; Haffejee, 1979)
Non-specific cellular response	Increase or no change (Braga, 1983; Ravera, 1986; Haffejee, 1979)

TIBC, total iron-binding capacity; CHE, cholinesterase; TBPA, thyroxin-binding prealbumin.
Adapted from Bozzetti (1989).
Full list of these references available from www.nutritiontexts.com.

Table 21.12 Nutritional effects of TPN versus a standard oral diet

Variable	TPN	Oral diet
Weight	↑ or =	= or ↓
N balance	positive	negative
Total body K	=	=
Urinary 3-methylhistidine	↓	=
Total protein	= or ↑	= or ↓
Albumin	= or ↓	= or ↓
Transferrin	↑ or =	= or ↓ ↑
CHE, RBP	↑	↓
TBPA	=	=
Ceruloplasmin, fibrinogen, IgA	=	=
IgG, IgM, C$_3$A	↑	=

CHE, cholinesterase; RBP, retinol-binding protein; TBPA, thyroxin-binding prealbumin.
Adapted from Bozzetti (1989).

Table 21.13 Effects of total parenteral and enteral nutrition in cancer patients receiving chemotherapy or radiotherapy

Variable	Type of nutrition	Response
Body weight	TPN	Increase or no change
	EN	Increase or no change
Body fat	TPN	Increase
Muscular mass	TPN	Increase
Lean body mass		
Nitrogen balance	TPN	Positive
Total body nitrogen	TPN	No change
Serum protein		
Total protein	TPN	No change
Albumin	TPN	No change
Transferrin	TPN	No change
Retinol-binding protein	TPN	No change
Immune humoral response		
IgA, IgM	TPN	Increase

TPN, total parenteral nutrition; EN, enteral nutrition.
Adapted from Bozzetti (1989).

to 'during' parenteral nutrition, even while the net balance moved from negative to positive. In contrast, the skeletal muscle protein synthesis as well as the protein synthesis rate significantly increased, converting the net balance to a positive value.

Generally it has been shown that parenteral nutrition does not increase the serum level of proteins, albumin transferrin, cholinesterase, or ceruloplasmin.

As regards parenteral nutrition and immunological response, some studies have reported an increase of lymphocyte blastogenesis and production of the helper T lymphocyte lymphokine IL-2 after seven days of a parenteral nutrition regimen, but also a significant impairment of basal natural killer and IL-2-activated natural killer activity. In contrast, it has recently been found that a 10-day course of parenteral nutrition was able to restore to normal a depressed basal or interleukin- or interferon-stimulated natural killer activity in cachectic cancer patients.

Taken as a whole, the data show that parenteral and enteral nutrition are usually able to prevent a further deterioration of the nutritional state and may sometimes improve some metabolic indices. These results are probably dependent on the length of the nutritional support, the biological aggressiveness of the tumor, and the efficacy of the available oncologic therapy. It must be emphasized that even while the nutritional benefit often seems to be limited to maintaining a 'status quo,' it does so in patients who would be condemned to a progressive chronic 'auto-cannibalism' without a nutritional support. However, the nutritional response of cancer patients is always more sluggish and limited than that of undernourished non-cancer patients (Table 21.14).

A study looking at a 10-day course of parenteral nutrition including 29 kcal non-protein/kg per day + 1.6 g amino acid/kg per day significantly decreased protein breakdown (by 50% and 59%) and protein synthesis (by 21% and 33%) in cancer and non-cancer patients, respectively, while it increased protein turnover (by 15%) in cancer patients only. The utilization efficiency of infused amino acid for synthesis of body protein was 39% in both cancer and non-cancer patients. Table 21.15 reports data comparing parenteral and enteral nutrition; and Table 21.16 summarizes the effects of parenteral nutrition and enteral nutrition on protein turnover. It is noteworthy that both techniques are able to improve some nutritional indices, such as body weight, fat mass, nitrogen balance, and whole body potassium. Thyroxin-binding prealbumin

Table 21.14 Response to total parenteral and enteral nutrition in cancer versus non-cancer patients

	TPN		EN	
Variable	Cancer	Non-cancer	Cancer	Non-cancer
Weight	↑	↑↑	↑	↑ or ↑↑
Arm circumference				
Triceps skinfold	↑	↑	= or ↑	↑
Arm muscle area	↑	↑↑	↑	↑
Creatinine-height index	↑	↑↑	↑	↑
N balance	+	+	+	+
Total body K	–	–	↑	↑
Albumin	↑	↑↑	↑	↑
Prealbumin	=	=	=	=
Retinol-binding protein	=	=	–	–
Balance of:				
Na	+	+	–	+
K	+	+	–	+
Cl	+	+	–	+
Mg	+	++	–	+
P	+	+	+	+
Ca	=	=	+	+

TPN, total parenteral nutrition; EN, enteral nutrition.
Adapted from Bozzetti (1989).

Table 21.15 Effects of total parenteral and enteral nutrition on nutritional variables

	Response	
Variable	TPN	EN
Weight	↑	↑
Body fat	↑	↑
Muscle mass[a]	=	=
Lean body mass		
N balance	+	+
Total body K	↑	↑ (=)
Total body N	= ↑	=?
Serum proteins		
Total protein	=	=
Albumin	=	= ↓
TIBC, CHE	=	= ↑
Ceruloplasmin	=	=
TBPA	↑ or =	= or ↑
RBP	↑	–
Protein flux,	↑ or =	=
Synthesis, catabolism	=	=
Immune humoral response		
IgG, IgA, IgM	=	=
C_3, C_4	=	↑
C_3PA	–	↑
CH_{50}	–	=
Immune cellular response		
Neutrophils	=	–
Lymphocytes (total/subpopulations)	=	↑ or =
Chemotaxis/phagocytosis	=	–

[a]3-Methylhistidine, amino acid efflux, anthropometry, creatinine-height index.
TPN, total parenteral nutrition; EN, enteral nutrition; TIBC, total iron-binding capacity; CHE, cholinesterase; TBPA, thyroxin-binding prealbumin; RBP, retinol-binding protein.
Adapted from Bozzetti (1989).

Author	Tumor	Regimen per day		Synthesis (g/kg)		Catabolism (g/kg)	
		kcal/kg	AA/kg	Pre	Post	Pre	Post
Burt (1982)	Esophagus*	38	1.68	2.2	2.7	2.8	2.4
	Esophagus*	44	0.87	2.4	2.3	2.9	2.3
Dresler (1987)	UGI	BEE x 1.2	C/N = 200	2.0	1.8	2.3	1.1
Jeevanandam (1988)	GI	29	1.6	2.1	1.3	2.6	1.3
Hochwald (1997)	GI	25	1.4	–	0.68[a]	–	0.37

Table 21.16 Effects of total parenteral and enteral nutrition on daily protein turnover in cancer patients

*Statistically significant.
[a]μmol leucine/kg/min.
UGI, upper gastrointestinal; BEE, basal energy expenditure; C/N, kcal/nitrogen.
Adapted from Bozzetti (1989).
Full list of references cited are available from www.nutritiontexts.com.

and retinol-binding protein levels increase only with parenteral nutrition, while some immune response indices (complement factors and lymphocyte number) improve only with enteral nutrition. Total body nitrogen shows a small gain only with parenteral nutrition.

The results of three randomized studies comparing parenteral and enteral nutrition were partially conflicting, but only parenteral nutrition showed some significant advantages with regard to weight gain, nitrogen balance, maintenance of serum albumin levels, and some mineral balances (potassium, magnesium, phosphate, sodium, and chloride). However, differences were marginal, and the slight advantage of parenteral nutrition does not support its being used indiscriminately in malnourished cancer patients with a working gastrointestinal tract. In considering the use of parenteral nutrition, some related complications should be considered.

Parenteral nutrition-related complications

Seven studies have demonstrated an increased complication rate in patients receiving parenteral nutrition (catheter and non-catheter sepsis, other infections, febrile episodes, venous thrombosis, and fluid overload). Seven other trials did not demonstrate any difference in complications, while four others did not investigate complications. A recent analysis of the prospective trials of parenteral nutrition and cancer evaluated the potential role played by intravenous lipids in contributing to infectious complications. It was found that the risk of infection in chemotherapy patients receiving parenteral nutrition increased when intravenous fat emulsion was included in the therapy, increasing 2.3-fold when intravenous fat was used intermittently

and 6.3-fold when intravenous fat was used daily. No increase in infectious complications was found when intravenous fat was not used. Although there is no clear explanation for this, it has been postulated that intravenous fat emulsions, which are high in n-6 fatty acids, may result in impaired immune function.

21.5 Effects of nutritional support on clinical outcome

Effects of nutritional support in cancer patients undergoing surgery

The rationale for perioperatively treating malnourished cancer patients with parenteral nutrition or enteral nutrition is mainly based on the following assumptions: Malnourished cancer patients are at higher risk for postoperative complications (especially infections) and cancer malnutrition can be reversed through the use of a nutritional support and consequently the surgical risk can be reduced. However, the value of these statements is limited, since malnutrition is not the only (and also perhaps not the most important, except in extreme cases) cause of surgical complications. Cancer malnutrition can probably be controlled by parenteral or enteral nutrition but this is less easy and it takes more time than in non-cancer patients. Moreover, the length of the preoperative hospital stay has been correlated with increased surgical infection rates. Finally, we do not know whether the parameters of nutritional assessment we use to define a malnourished patient (weight loss, low serum albumin, lymphocyte number, etc.) are the same ones which are pathogenetically involved in the defective defense of the host against the microorganisms, and consequently whether we should aim at normalizing them with parenteral or enteral nutrition before operating on the patient.

Furthermore, it is a common experience that the more severe the malnutrition, the more advanced the stage of the tumor so that the probability of performing an explorative surgery which abates the benefit of artificial nutrition is magnified in severely malnourished patients.

Because of all these intrinsic difficulties, the results of randomized clinical trials have been disparate; only by pooling all these trials together as has been done in meta-analyses is it possible to find a statistically significant advantage in terms of reduction of the complication rate in patients receiving parenteral nutrition, while the reduction in mortality is dubious. The discrepancy in the results obtained by these randomized studies involving parenteral nutrition in the pre- and postoperative periods may be related to the different lengths of preoperative feeding, but mainly to the preoperative nutritional status. It appears in fact that the few studies including patients with at least 10% weight loss were successful in reducing postoperative morbidity and (sometimes) mortality, whereas in normal or less malnourished patients, a benefit was achieved in 50% of the randomized, controlled trials.

Preoperative and postoperative nutrition support

Two studies have compared two ways of preoperatively administering a random nutritional support to patients with cancer of the esophagus or head/neck, demonstrating a marginal advantage for parenteral nutrition as regards body weight and nitrogen balance with no difference in morbidity and mortality. Financial constraints as well as the need to limit the use of enteral or parenteral nutrition to the crucial period of hospitalization have supported the concept of the administration of artificial nutrition in the postoperative period. Whether enteral nutrition is better than parenteral nutrition is matter of controversy. In humans, in fact, it has been found that parenteral nutrition is associated with an exaggerated acute phase and metabolic response after injury or endotoxin challenge, effects that are blunted by enteral nutrition. Early postoperative enteral nutrition in upper gastrointestinal cancer patients undergoing curative resection results in an improvement in protein kinetics, net balance, and amino acid flux across peripheral tissue compared with intravenous feeding.

A recent multicenter randomized clinical trial carried out by the Italian Society of Parenteral and Enteral Nutrition on 317 malnourished patients undergoing surgery for gastrointestinal cancer comparing early postoperative enteral versus parenteral nutrition at regimens similar in energy and nitrogen content has shown that enteral nutrition significantly decreases prevalence of minor and major complications and length of postoperative stay.

Bone marrow transplantation (BMT) is widely used in patients with malignancies since the procedure is often associated with post-transplant diarrhea and weight loss, protein-losing enteropathy, hypoalbuminemia, and biochemical zinc deficiency. The subject of BMT is covered in detail in Chapter 14.

Postoperative immunonutrition

Starting from the concept that a major cause of postoperative infection is the decrease in immune response due to surgical trauma, anesthesia, perioperative care, and the disease itself, irrespective of the nutritional status of the patients, it was felt rational to enrich the usual standard diet with some substrates capable of producing beneficial immune-enhancing and metabolic effects. These substrates include glutamine, arginine, *n*-3 PUFAs, and nucleotides.

The main biological effects of glutamine and arginine in humans are reported in Tables 21.17 and 21.18. Administration of nucleotides to postoperative patients is reported to prevent a decrease in number of lymphocytes as well as in their cytotoxic activity. Administration of *n*-3 PUFAs has been shown to increase the blood monocyte production of IL-1α, IL-1β, and TNF. The main randomized clinical trials in cancer patients (usually non-malnourished) fed with fish oil and structured medium-chain TAGs (MCT) or with intravenous glutamine or with Impact® (an enteral formula enriched in *n*-3 PUFAs, nucleotides, and arginine) are reported in Tables 21.19 and 21.20.

Seven out of 11 randomized controlled trials reported a clinical advantage and all of them a metabolic benefit, thus suggesting that nutrition-unrelated immune depression and consequent clinical complications are favorably affected by nutrition with immune nutrients. The benefit appears to be magnified if enteral support starts six days preoperatively.

Table 21.17 Biological effects of glutamine in humans

	References
Immunity improved	Morlion, 1998; SINPE, 1996; Pastores, 1994; O'Riordain, 1994; Ogle, 1994
No benefit in lymphocyte function	Schilling, 1996
↓ Serum concentration of TNF receptors	Griffiths, 1997
Does not attenuate endotoxin-induced symptoms or proinflammatory cytokine release	Calder, 1994
Muscular glutamine concentration maintained	Braxton, 1995; Stehle, 1989; Hammarqvist, 1989
Muscular glutamine concentration not influenced	Blomqvist, 1995; Ziegler, 1993
Nitrogen balance improved	Morlion, 1998; Braxton, 1995; Karner, 1989; Fürst, 1990
↑ plasma concentration of arginine	Griffiths, 1997
↓ excretion of 3-methylhistidine	Fürst, 1990; Ziegler, 1992
Protein synthesis increased	Stehle, 1989; Schloerb, 1993; Barua, 1992
Stimulates cell proliferation in the gut	Petersson, 1994
Attenuates villous atrophy and mucosal permeability	Scheppach, 1994
Trauma-related intestinal atrophy avoided	Van der Hulst, 1993
Attenuates extracellular fluid expansion	Petersson, 1994; Tremel, 1994

Adapted from Bozzetti (1999).

Table 21.18 Biological effects of arginine in humans

	References
Enhances T lymphocyte response	Scheltinga, 1991; Daly, 1988; Barbul, 1990
Stimulates wound healing	Daly, 1988; Barbul, 1990
Increases plasma insulin and growth hormone	Kirk, 1993
Necessary for synthesis of nitric oxide	Merimee, 1965
No advantage in nitrogen balance	Scheltinga, 1991

Adapted from Bozzetti (1999).
Full list of references cited are available from www.nutritiontexts.com.

Table 21.19 Randomized controlled trials in postoperative patients with fish oil and structured MCT or with intravenous glutamine

Author	Study (No. of patients)	Postoperative start (Duration)	Regimen kcal/kg/day	Results	Comments
Kenler (1996)	FOSMCT vs. O (50)	24 h (× 10 days)	12 vs. 11	FOSMCT: fewer patients with >1 infection	No focus on clinical outcome
Swails (1997)	FOSMCT vs. O (20)	48 h (× 7 days)	111 vs. 14	No difference in infections	High β error
Morlion (1998)	GLU vs. STPN (28)	× 5 po days	29	GLU shorter LOS	Criteria for discharging patients are missing
Petersson (1994)	GLU vs. STPN (17)	× 3 po days	32	No difference on subjective fatigue	

O, Osmolite®; FOSMCT, fish oil and structured MCT; GLU, glutamine; po, postoperative; STPN, standard total parenteral nutrition; LOS, length of postoperative stay.
Adapted from Bozzetti (1999).
Full list of references cited are available from www.nutritiontexts.com.

Effects on outcome in oncologic patients

To date, 19 randomized controlled trials in adults explored the effects of parenteral nutrition as an adjunct to chemotherapy on survival, remission and compli-cations. An important meta-analysis of the American Gastroenterological Association is summarized in Table 21.21. However, the results of these meta-analyses have been severely criticized because of the many flaws contained in the trials. The criticism mainly con-

Table 21.20 Randomized controlled trials in postoperative patients with IMPACT®

Author	Study (No.of patients)	Postoperative start (Duration)	Regimen kcal/kg/day	Results
Daly (1992)	I vs. O (85)	24 h (× 7 days)	I: 20 kcal, 0.2 g N O: 16 kcal, 0.1 g N	I: less infections/complications, shorter LSO
Daly (1995)	I vs. T (60)	24 h (× 7 days)	I: 15 kcal, 0.2 g N T: 16 kcal, 0.1 g N	I: less infections, shorter LSO
Senkal (1997)	I vs. SEN (154)	24 h (× 5 days)	~16 kcal	I: less infections, after 5th po day or with >5 liters, lower cost
Gianotti (1997)	I vs. SEN vs. IV (260)	6 h (× 7 days)	18 kcal	I: vs. S EN vs. TPN, lower LOS
Heslin (1997)	I vs. IV (195)	24 h (× 7 days)	15 vs. 5 kcal	No difference in complications, mortality, LOS
Schilling (1996)	I vs. SEN vs. IV (41)	As early as possible (× 8–10 days)	~14 vs. 14 vs. 34 kcal[a]	No difference in infections and LOS

O, Osmolite®; T, Traumacal®; SEN, standard enteral nutrition; IV, crystalloid; I, impact; LOS, length postoperative stay; po, postoperative.
[a]Median value.
Adapted from Bozzetti (1999).
Full list of references cited are available from www.nutritiontexts.com.

cerns two aspects, the first regarding the statistical and methodological aspects of the studies and the second regarding some practical issues in the selection of the patients and the administration of parenteral nutrition. It is important to point out that although formal sample size calculations for performing meta-analyses do not exist, if this were a single trial, there would be only a 50% chance of detecting and labeling as statistically significant at the 0.05 level a benefit of 10–20% over a baseline of 85% and 50%, respectively (i.e. the expected advantage in three-month survival and in the response rate, respectively) due to the small number of enrolled patients (190 for each outcome, or 15–20 per arm and per study). Furthermore, the quality of the various studies was generally poor, with a score of 0.53 in a scale ranging from 0 to 1.0; and only 46% of the studies met the quality criteria of the reporting of the randomized trials.

The most crucial point, however, was that since the rationale for using parenteral nutrition was the poor tolerance and poor compliance of malnourished patients receiving chemotherapy, one would have expected only severely malnourished patients to be randomized for parenteral nutrition or no parenteral nutrition. Instead, in 20% of the patients nutritional status was not assessed at all, in 16% it was good, and only half of the remaining patients were malnourished. In some studies a 5% weight loss or serum albumin level less than 3.6 g/dl were sufficient to consider the patients suitable for randomization. Patients with gastrointestinal cancer, a group at high risk for developing malnutrition during therapy, were involved in only one or two studies.

The technical quality of the parenteral nutrition regimen was also sometimes inadequate (1500 kcal + 0.2 g amino acids/kg only during the 8 h of chemotherapy), or excessive, more than 50 kcal/kg per day and po-

Table 21.21 Meta-analysis of randomized clinical trial of patients given TPN during chemotherapy.

Outcome	Absolute risk difference %	Confidence intervals %	Number of studies (patients) included
Mortality	0	−5, +5	19 (1050)
Total complication rate	+40	+14, +66	8 (333)
Infectious complcation rate	+16	+8, +23	8 (823)
Tumor response	−7	−12, −1	15 (910)
Bone marrow toxicity	+22	−10, +54	3 (134)
Gastrointestinal toxicity	+1	−9, +11	6 (310)

Adapted from AGA technical review on parental nutrition (*Gastroenterology*, 2001; 121: 970–1001).
Full list of references cited are available from www.nutritiontexts.com.

tentially toxic because of carbon dioxide retention, especially in patients with cancer of the lung. It is therefore difficult to accept the point which the randomized controlled trials were supposed to establish: that parenteral nutrition does not play a beneficial role in malnourished cancer patients undergoing chemotherapy.

Effects on performance status and quality of life

Several studies have examined the effect of nutritional support on performance status and quality of life. Beneficial parameters looked at include:

- a decreased number of medications needed for symptom control,
- decreased radiation enteritis,
- minimizing reduction in white blood count,
- decreased duration of chemotherapeutic-induced nausea and vomiting,
- improved compliance to chemotherapy, and
- fewer treatment delays.

Negative reports of nutrition support in cancer include poorer tolerance to therapy in patients receiving parenteral nutrition, manifested by severe stomatitis, prolonged hospitalization, decreased hemoglobin and white count, and increased frequency of bowel movements.

Home parenteral nutrition and enteral nutrition

There is some controversy as to the indications for artificial nutrition (parenteral nutrition in particular) in cancer patients. The high cost of parenteral nutrition, coupled with the limited life expectancy of these patients, has led some countries or institutions to consider cancer as a relative contraindication for providing such support. In particular, the awareness that cancer patients die 'despite' home parenteral nutrition, whereas patients with benign diseases survive 'thanks' to home parenteral nutrition, argues against the use of home parenteral nutrition in patients with malignancy. Despite this fact, cancer patients account for a high percentage (sometimes even the majority) of subjects receiving home parenteral nutrition.

The proportion of patients with cancer reported on registers of home parenteral feeding in various coun-

Table 21.22 Proportion of patients with cancer reported on registers of home parenteral feeding in various countries

Italy	57%
Japan	55%
USA	46%
Netherlands	60%
Spain	39%
Belgium	23%
Denmark	8%
United Kingdom	5%

tries are shown in Table 21.22. As regards survival, 50% of cancer patients survived six months and 12–13% survived two years by the American registry. A similar percentage of patients (13–18%) in the American and European registries were completely rehabilitated, and another 27% were partially socially rehabilitated. The hospital readmission rate per year was 3.5. Longer survival was associated with treatable neoplasms such as lymphoma and leukemia as well as good performance status at the beginning of parenteral nutrition. The recent experience of the Italian Society of Parenteral and Enteral Nutrition reported a mean survival of four months (range 1–14) with one-third surviving more than three months.

Patients with a Karnofsky performance status >50 at the start of parenteral nutrition had a longer survival. Quality of life parameters remained stable until 2–3 months before death. The conclusions of these studies were that home parenteral nutrition may benefit a limited percentage of patients who may survive longer than time allotted by a condition of starvation and depletion. Provided that these patients survive longer than three months, there is some evidence that quality of life remains stable for some months and acceptable for the patients. Cancer patients, most of whom were affected by gastrointestinal tract tumors, also account for the majority (40%) of patients receiving home enteral nutrition in the American study.

Nutritional regimen

There is no definite consensus on the optimal calorie and protein requirements of the cancer patient. The minimal daily regimen in the literature which improved lean body mass and visceral proteins has ranged from 35 to 55 kcal/kg and from 1.2 to 2 g amino acid/kg for parenteral nutrition and 35 kcal/kg and 1.3 g amino

The comb
following:

- Tumor gr
  tinal can
  cancer stu
- Tumor gr
  tion studi
  tion studi

The overall
has provide
tein synthes
also respon
indirect ma
tein synthes
contrast, m
cancer cells
cleic acids v
phase, are n
is a determ
21.24 clearl
ered – type
or type of 1
– there are c
that increas
when the ar
and feeding

21.8 Per

Several dif
plored to be

Table 21.25

Drug

Megestrol acet

Medroxyproge

Cyproheptadin
Ondanestrone
Dronabinol

Branched chai
Corticosteroid
Anabolic stero
Insulin

Growth horme

---

acid/kg for enteral nutrition. The enteral regimen able to improve some immune responses has included 42 kcal/kg and 2.3 g amino acid/kg.

The calorie requirement of cancer patients has been evaluated in different ways. Using calorimetry it was shown that an energy intake of 30 kcal/kg (approximately 1.4 times the calculated REE) is required to provide a respiratory quotient of 1.0 in non-malnourished cancer patients. However, in malnourished cancer patients, a parenteral nutrition corresponding to 200% of the non-protein energy resting expenditure (49 kcal/kg) and 2.0 g amino acid/kg was necessary to stimulate whole body protein synthesis, an almost identical regimen to the one reported as being able to promote weight gain in cancer patients. Recently a study reported that a parenteral nutrition regimen providing 40 kcal/kg per day (50% glucose and 50% lipid) and protein (1.7 g/kg per day) virtually abolished the net protein catabolism. Current opinion holds that most malnourished cancer patients require a daily regimen of about 35–40 kcal/kg plus 2 g or more amino acid/kg. However, patients receiving home parenteral nutrition usually have widespread abdominal malignancy with involvement of the peritoneum. They often will not tolerate a standard regimen and may require alterations in volume, sodium, glucose, and fat content of solutions.

21.6 Oral nutritional supplementation

The use of oral nutrition supplements (ONS) looks very attractive in many cancer patients in whom anorexia is not extremely severe, the gut is working, and the oral route for introducing nutrients is available. These patients represent the majority of those requiring nutritional support or dietary counseling. In many of them the nutritional problems will be automatically solved as soon as their disease is cured or cytotoxic or radiation therapy ends. In some of them, however, requiring a continuous oncological therapy or harboring a progressive disease, nutritional problems will be magnified throughout the rest of their life.

Many patients are treated with ONS because their nutritional status or food intake are not so severely compromised as to warrant a more aggressive approach such as total enteral or parenteral nutrition. Sometimes such approaches are not accepted by the patients themselves or cannot be adopted for practical

---

reasons. The impossibility of distinguishing in many series of the literature the proper indications for using ONS makes it very difficult to interpret the results and gives a discrepancy between the wide use of ONS and the little scientific evidence of a true benefit.

The results of studies looking at ONS may be summarized as follows:

(1) Only one randomized controlled trial out of nine showed a significantly greater gain in weight in supplemented than control patients after 10–31 days of treatment. The total energy intake ranged between 1500 and 2000 kcal/day.
(2) None of three randomized controlled trials which used arm anthropometry showed a significant improvement with ONS.
(3) Only two studies out of five showed an increased in total energy intake with ONS: patients were supplemented for three months with a prescription of ONS ranging between 500 kcal and an energy supplementation equal to 1.7–1.99 times the basal energy expenditure.
(4) ONS generally did not produce functional benefits, but this may be partly because few studies systematically addressed these outcome measures.

No significant data exist with regard to the role of timing of oral nutritional supplementation, its effect on body functions, the effect of stopping ONS palatability, and comparison with enteral tube feeding. Only one study compared immune nutrition with standard nutrition without drawing any particularly significant conclusion.

On the basis of the current knowledge, it is therefore obvious that prescription of ONS to anorectic and hypophagic patients relies more on the need of the clinician to normalize a physiologic function of the body, the intake of an adequate quantity of food, than on 'evidence-based' demonstration of a beneficial effect on the patients. Clinicians, however, should consider the intrinsic difficulty of getting scientific results from controlled studies like these ones.

21.7 Effects of nutritional support on tumor growth

It has been widely demonstrated in tumor-bearing animals that the intravenous administration of parenteral nutrition and especially amino acids can

lead to
mitotic
tumor
unchar
that so
unifor
recruit
phase (

It m
studies
tion re
after o
cell po
only 2
gradua
in 24–

This
tumor
at the
tional

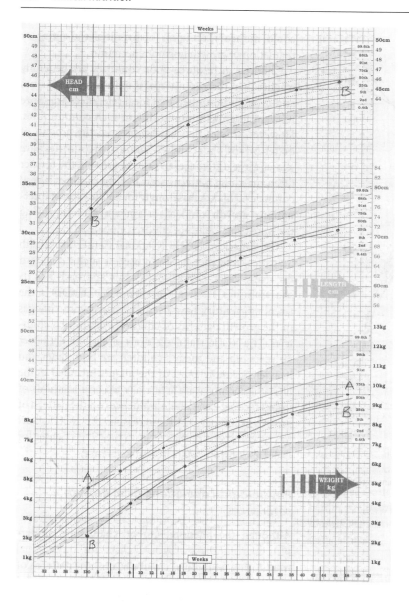

Figure 22.7 'Catch-up' and 'catch-down' in infancy. Growth curves are plotted for two babies. Baby A, the infant of a diabetic mother, has a birth weight above the 97th centile. Excessive weight gain *in utero* was the result of maternal, hence fetal, hyperglycemia and hyperinsulinism. After birth she 'catches down' towards her genetically determined size. Baby B was born at term with birth weight <0.4 centile and head circumference at the 9th centile. This indicates 'head sparing' and is typical of late intrauterine growth retardation (IUGR). After birth the baby crosses several centiles upwards, a pattern indicative of 'catch-up' to genetically determined size following release from intrauterine constraint.

as to seek out his or her genetic potential by exhibiting catch-up growth. Conversely an infant overnourished *in utero*, such as the infant of a diabetic mother, may exhibit catch-down growth. These processes are usually completed by the end of the first year of life but in extreme cases may continue into the second year. It is sometimes important to distinguish clinically between catch-down growth of an unusually heavy baby (e.g. the infant of a diabetic mother) and failure-to-thrive. It is therefore essential to know fully the parental measurements and perinatal history when interpreting growth patterns in infancy.

Puberty

The age at onset of puberty varies greatly between individuals. For example, although pubic hair in girls appears at an average age of 11.9 years, the 2nd and 98th centiles for this stage are five years apart at 14.4 and 9.4 years respectively. Because the 50th centile line on the growth chart reflects the growth trajectory of a child entering puberty at the average age, one exhibiting late puberty may show an apparent downward crossing of centile lines at this age, with later apparent catch-up as puberty occurs (Figure 22.8). The converse may also occur in early puberty: a child

The combined findings from these studies are the following:

- Tumor growth increased in three of five gastrointestinal cancer studies and in three of five head/neck cancer studies.
- Tumor growth increased in one in five enteral nutrition studies and in five out of seven parenteral nutrition studies.

The overall impression is that none of these studies has provided a definitive conclusion. Studies on protein synthesis not only gave conflicting results, but they also respond to the question of tumor growth in an indirect manner since they measure the tumor protein synthesis, but ignore the protein breakdown. In contrast, methods which evaluate the kinetics of the cancer cells with the use of marked precursors of nucleic acids which are incorporated in the DNA at the S phase, are more convincing, since the growth fraction is a determinate of tumor growth. Tables 21.23 and 21.24 clearly show that whatever the variable considered – type of tumor (gastrointestinal or head/neck) or type of nutrition (parenteral nutrition or enteral) – there are conflicting results. However, it is impressive that increased tumor growth was reported, especially when the amount of calories and protein was excessive and feeding given parenterally.

21.8 Perspectives on the future

Several different approaches have been recently explored to better meet the requirements of the host or to feed patients while avoiding an excessive tumor growth stimulation. These are likely to be areas of continued interest in the future.

- The use of antianorexigenic substances or anticachectic drugs
- The modulation of nutrients
- Glutamine supplementation
- *n*-3 PUFA supplementation
- Metabolic manipulation.

Antianorexigenic substances or anticachectic drugs

Drugs used in the management of anorexia and cachexia are shown in Table 21.25.

Medroxyprogesterone acetate (MAP)
There is wide experience with MAP for treating hormone-sensitive breast and endometrial carcinomas. Since its introduction into clinical practice in 1983, it has been reported that MAP at high doses (>500 mg/day) has anabolic effects. A double-blind, placebo-controlled trial further demonstrated that MAP at 100 mg orally three times a day increased appetite in cachectic patients.

Megestrol acetate
Megestrol acetate is available as tablets and a suspension. The precise weight gain mechanism of megestrol is unknown; however, it does increase appetite and non-fluid weight gain, due to adipose tissue rather than fat-free mass. In addition, megestrol produces an-

Table 21.25 Drugs used in the management of anorexia and cachexia

Drug	
Megestrol acetate	Precise weight gain mechanism unknown. Dose response has been demonstrated. Probably does not improve survival. Significant side effects
Medroxyprogesterone acetate (MAP)	High doses (>500 mg) has anabolic effects. Widely used in hormone-sensitive breast and endometrial carcinomas
Cyproheptadine hydrochloride	Works as a serotonin antagonist. Some studies show limited effects
Ondanestrone	Serotonin receptor antagonist and antinausea agent for some patients receiving chemo- or radiotherapy
Dronabinol	Evidence on the use of cannabinoids is scanty. Some studies show increased caloric intake and weight gain, but neuropsychological side effects
Branched chain amino acids	BCAAs may slow down entry of tryptophan (precursor of serotonin) into the brain
Corticosteroids	Ability to stimulate appetite short lived and side effects numerous
Anabolic steroids	Only one trial to date – showing no effects.
Insulin	Reported that added to TPN insulin leads to an improved skeletal muscle protein synthesis and whole protein net balance compared to TPN alone
Growth hormone (GH)	May have an effect in moderately malnourished cancer patients

tigonadotropic effects and could stimulate adipocyte differentiation. Lower circulating levels of IL-1α, IL-1β, and TNFα, were detected following treatment with megesterol acetate.

The effects of and dose response to megestrol administration have been investigated in several randomized, double-blinded, placebo-controlled studies. A dose of 240 mg/day was associated with an increase in appetite along with a moderate increase in weight. A dose of 480 mg/day increased both appetite and subjective energy level. At a dose of 800 mg, it was reported that patients also had less nausea and emesis due to chemotherapy, but 13% of them suffered from edema. Patients with advanced hormone-insensitive malignant lesions using 1600 mg/day were reported to experience weight gain, increased appetite and food intake, and had increased prealbumin levels.

Several randomized trials have evaluated different dosages of megestrol and have demonstrated that 800 mg/day caused an improvement in appetite as compared with the other dosages. There was, however, a certain risk of thromboembolic events with the dosage; in addition, 26% of the male patients reported impotence. In a recent randomized study of patients with hormone refractory cancer it was concluded that dosages >480 mg/day were probably of no value in the majority of patients, and suggested two weeks of therapy before altering the dosage to meet the needs of the patients. The same benefits were observed in a pediatric population. At a dose of 10 mg/kg/day there was a significant increase in appetite, calorie intake, and performance status score, often requiring a decrease in the dosage.

Recently, it has been confirmed in a double-blind randomized controlled trial that megestrol has beneficial effects on appetite and body weight but the study failed to demonstrate any advantage in survival and quality of life. Potential side effects of megestrol acetate administration include impotence in sexually active males and vaginal spotting or bleeding in females. Individual reports of reversible suppression of the pituitary–adrenal axis, hepatic toxicity, diabetes mellitus, and withdrawal response have been published.

Cyproheptadine hydrochloride

Cyproheptadine is available as tablets and syrup. A common dose is 8 mg three times a day. The proposed weight gain mechanism of cyproheptadine is serotonin antagonism. A randomized double-blind trial in cancer patients with anorexia or cachexia failed to prevent weight loss compared with the placebo group. Patients receiving cyproheptadine, however, had less nausea, less energy and more sedation and dizziness compared with placebo patients.

Ondanestrone

Ondanestrone, a serotonin receptor antagonist and an antinausea agent for patients receiving chemotherapy or radiation therapy, has been investigated in malnourished patients who were not receiving chemotherapy. Ondanestrone at 8 mg twice a day failed to correct weight loss or to reverse laboratory parameters of protein malnutrition but improved the ability of patients to enjoy food.

Dronabinol

The literature reporting on the use of cannabinoids in the treatment of cancer cachexia is scanty. It would seem that some benefit in appetite and mood is obtained by an administration of 5 mg/day, with about two-thirds of patients reporting that their appetites were stimulated. There is increased calorie intake and weight gain with 2.5 mg three times daily 1 h after meals, but neuropsychological effects are not uncommon, including nausea and slurred speech.

Branched-chain amino acids (BCAAs)

The use of BCAAs has been proposed recently based on the postulate that increased hypothalamic serotinergic activity could play a role in the development of anorexia. BCAAs might slow down the entry of the precursor of serotonin (tryptophan) into the brain by competing for the same transport system across the blood–brain barrier. Encouraging results have been reported in a pilot study where anorexic patients received oral supplementation of BCAAs.

Corticosteroids

The mechanism underlying the ability of corticosteroids to increase the appetite is unknown, but it may be related to the euphoria produced by these agents. The literature includes at least four randomized, double-blind, placebo-controlled trials with steroids. Despite the fact that these agents were effective in stimulating the appetite of patients, none of these studies documented a significant weight gain. Dexamethasone administered both 0.75 or 1.5 mg four times daily produced a significant increase in appetite after four weeks of therapy in patients with advanced gastrointestinal cancer who were not being submitted to chemotherapy. Methylprednisolone (16 mg) taken orally twice daily increased appetite, food intake, and performance status as well as reducing pain and analgesic consumption in terminal cancer patients. However, this effect was short term, and all nutritional indices returned to baseline after 20 days.

Another study was performed in terminal cancer patients using methylprednisolone at a dose of 125 mg intravenous daily for 56 days. This led to a significant increase in baseline appetite entry during the second week. Other benefits include decreased nausea, vomiting, and anxiety and improved alertness along with a sense of well-being. The effect on appetite was, however, quite transient. Moreover, there was an increase in gastrointestinal and cardiovascular side effects.

Yet another study involving the oral administration of 5 mg prednisolone three times daily for two weeks followed by a dosage reduction in the third week resulted in improved appetite and a sense of well-being compared to the placebo group. The practical conclusions that can be drawn from these studies are that the ability of steroids to stimulate the appetite is short lived, and that the administration of these drugs may entail long-term complications such as cataract formation, weakness, delirium, diabetes, osteoporosis, and immunosuppression.

Anabolic steroids

There is only one randomized controlled trial evaluating the effect of nandrolone decanoate in lung cancer patients with weight loss and receiving chemotherapy. These patients were administered 200 mg of the drug by intramuscular injection every week for four weeks, but continued to lose weight. However, it proved to improve appetite and sense of well-being.

Oxandrolone

Oxandrolone is a chemically unique synthetic derivative of testosterone and is the only oral anabolic agent approved by the US Food and Drug Administration (FDA) for weight gain following disease-related weight loss. It undergoes minimal hepatic metabolism and its nitrogen-sparing activity starts at 0.6 mg/day and progressively increases until 20 mg/day. It stimulates appetite and promotes muscle anabolism through both anabolic (androgen receptors) and anticatabolic (glucocorticoid receptors) pathways. In patients undergoing allogenic bone marrow or stem cell recipients, oxandrolone, 10 mg taken twice daily for 120 days, led to a gain in body cell mass and improved hand grip strength.

Insulin

Administration of insulin has resulted in a decreased whole body protein breakdown rate and in an appropriate response of muscle protein synthesis. Insulin (1 mU/kg body weight per minute for four days) added to total parenteral nutrition resulted in improved skeletal muscle protein synthesis and whole body protein net balance compared with parenteral nutrition alone.

Growth hormone

There is some concern regarding the use of growth hormone because of the possible stimulation of tumor growth, despite the fact that experimental data have not shown tumor progression. One clinical study reported an increase in whole body protein synthesis greater than the stimulation of whole body protein breakdown, with no change in muscle protein turnover. It has been shown that in moderately malnourished cancer patients growth hormone at 0.2 mg/kg per day was able to improve the nitrogen balance and the grip strength, whereas there was no effect in patients at <90% of ideal body weight.

Metabolic inhibitors and anticytokine therapy

The enzyme that catalyzes the conversion of oxaloacetate to phosphoenolpyruvate is phosphoenolpyruvate-carboxykinase (PEPCK). Hydrazine sulfate is a noncompetitive inhibitor of PEPCK which inhibits *in vitro* gluconeogenesis in animal systems. Some controlled studies have demonstrated an improved tolerance to glucose and weight stabilization with the administration of hydrazine sulfate, while little benefit has been reported in clinical trials aimed at decreasing tumor size. It would seem that while this agent has a limited efficacy alone, it would be opportune to test it in association with modulated diets.

Pentoxifylline

The ability of pentoxifylline to decrease TNF messenger RNA levels (an effect probably mediated by inhibition of the cAMP phosphodiesterase activity) has been tested in cancer patients with contrasting results. Pentoxifylline has been reported to decrease TNF secretion and to increase appetite and promote weight gain. However, a randomized controlled trial failed to report any benefit deriving from its administration.

Thalidomide

There is little information about the potential of thalidomide, a drug capable of lowering the plasma level of TNFα in animals as well as in patients with cancer cachexia. Recently, a study reported on 37 patients treated with 100 mg of thalidomide per day for at least 10 days. The effects on appetite, energy intake, and well-being were significantly better in comparison with an historical group of patients treated with megestrol acetate (480 mg/day). These results warrant further investigation.

Melatonin

Melatonin, the pineal hormone that regulates the circadian rhythm, has recently been investigated for the treatment of cancer cachexia. The proposed explanation for its use in cancer cachexia is that cancer patients have disrupted circadian rhythms, which in turn stimulate the release of TNFα. In fact, patients receiving a daily 20 mg oral dose of melatonin in the evening for three months had lower TNFα serum levels and less weight loss compared with the control group.

Other anticachectic agents

Recently it has been reported that simple therapy with anti-inflammatory agents such as ibuprofen may prolong survival in undernourished patients with metastatic solid tumors. Ibuprofen leads to a reduction in acute phase protein activity and a control of the resting metabolic expenditure in patients with pancreatic cancer.

Modulation of nutrients

Further formulations will surely investigate the effects of the incorporation of new substrates such as *n*-3 fatty acids, MCTs, nucleotides, arginine, and glutamine in nutritional regimens. The safety and efficacy of these nutrients are being tested in many experimental conditions and future trials will undoubtedly include patients with cancer. Present experience is more limited and is mainly concerned with the amino acid content and the calorie component of the diet. It has been shown that a 50% BCAA-enriched parenteral nutrition formula (energy at 1.3 × basal energy expendi-

ture) and 1.2 g protein/kg per day has a significant effect on whole body protein synthesis, leucine balance, and incorporation of ^{14}C leucine into plasma albumin as compared with a parenteral nutrition solution enriched with only 19% BCAA. It has also been suggested that the BCAA-enriched solution could be less efficient than a standard solution at increasing tumor protein synthesis.

As regards the quality of the energy source, a few studies have compared two different parenteral nutrition regimens, one based on glucose and amino acids and the other on glucose, fat, and amino acids. Data are summarized in Table 21.26 and show either no difference or only a marginal advantage for glucose-based parenteral nutrition. Similarly, a few authors have compared a total or 'near total' glucose regimen to a total or 'near total' fat regimen. It has been demonstrated that the infusion of glucose (23 kcal/kg per day) or fat (31 kcal/kg per day) resulted in a significant suppression of the net protein catabolism (approximately 15%) in patients with lower gastrointestinal cancer, but was ineffective in those with upper gastrointestinal cancer. Glucose infusion resulted in a suppression of endogenous glucose production (at least 55%), while lipid infusion was associated with a minor suppression (9%). Lipid infusion did not decrease the glucose production.

Only one study has compared the metabolic effect of two enteral isonitrogenous (1.5 g protein/kg per day), isocaloric (4.4 kcal/kg per day) diets containing different qualities of energy, one 31% as fat and the other 70% as MCT plus arginine D-3-hydroxybutyrate. There was no significant alteration in host N balance, whole body protein synthesis, degradation, or turnover rates.

Table 21.26 Effects of glucose (G) and glucose lipid (GL) TPN on nutritional status

Category	G	GL
Body weight	↑ usually or = ↑	↑ usually or =
Albumin	=	=
TBPA, RBP	↑ or =	=
Transferrin	↑ or =	↑ or =
Total protein, fibrinogen, IgA, C_4	=	=
IgG	↑	=
IgM, C_3A	↑	↑

TBPA, thyroxin-binding prealbumin; RBP, retinol-binding protein.

Glutamine supplementation

There is some debate regarding the role of glutamine-supplemented diets in the cancer patient, since the potential benefits in protecting the gut from the enterotoxic effects of chemotherapy and radiation therapy might be counteracted by the stimulation of tumor cell metabolism. Experimental work in tumor models has shown that glutamine-supplemented parenteral nutrition can maintain higher intestinal levels of gluthathione to promote the jejunal villous height in rats treated with 5-fluorouracil, and to decrease bacterial translocation compared with standard parenteral nutrition formulas. Providing a glutamine-supplemented enteral diet to tumor-bearing rats increased the small bowel mucosal content of DNA and resulted in a significant reduction in the severity of methotrexate-induced enterocolitis, as reflected by improved morphometric parameters, as well as in the incidence of positive cultures in the spleen, and in morbidity and mortality associated with chemotherapy.

A substantial body of experimental evidence indicates that glutamine is the major respiratory fuel cell in some experimental tumors, for example in hepatomas and fibrosarcomas, where the rate of glutamine uptake was quantified, leading to the concept that the tumor behaves as a sort of 'glutamine trap'.

In 1935 it was demonstrated that the proliferation of cultured HeLa cells (malignant cervical cells) is greatest when glutamine concentrations are at least 1 mmol/l. This *in vitro* requirement may reflect the continuous demand for glutamine in the absence of the normal *in vivo* supply (0.6–0.9 mmol/l). Failure to provide glutamine in the growth medium of cultured malignant cells retards cell division and usually results in cell death. In contrast, *in vivo* studies using tumor-bearing rats have shown that glutamine-supplemented enteral or parenteral nutrition did not apparently stimulate tumor growth even though the ratio of euploid to diploid cells in the tumor mass increased by 20% in animals receiving glutamine intravenously. No data are available on humans, and it is important to keep in mind that due to the discrepancy between tumor weight/host weight ratio and cell kinetics in experimental versus human tumors, it is quite difficult to extrapolate laboratory findings to the clinical setting.

Data on human cancer is scanty. Some authors have reported than human hepatoma cells consume glutamine at a rate five- to ten-fold faster than do normal hepatocytes, and that patients with leukemia exhibit an extremely high rate of glutamine consumption. *In vivo* human data show a considerable range in the exchange rate of glutamine in gastrointestinal cancer with the most common finding being a slightly negative balance. The clinical effects of glutamine supplementation in cancer patients receiving bone marrow transplantation and/or chemotherapy are summarized in Table 21.27. A possible explanation for the discrepancy between the experimental literature and clinical results is the fact that changes in circulating glutamine concentration occur when tumor size accounts for at least 10% of the body weight. At this point there is a 20% drop in the muscle glutamine concentration, with an accelerated glutamine efflux from the hindquarter, a drop in gut glutamine extraction, and a consequent increase in bacterial translocation, suggesting a defect in the gut mucosal barrier. Usually at this stage the animal begins to show visible signs of cachexia, and appears unwell. However, in clinical practice the majority of patients reported in the literature and receiving glutamine were not severely depleted, and tumor weight almost never accounted for as high a percentage of the host body weight in humans as it does in experimental tumors. It is therefore possible that antineoplastic chemotherapy intestinal toxicity occurs by way of a mechanism that is completely independent from that mediated by the glutamine intracellular concentration that occurs during nutritional depletion.

n-3 Polyunsaturated fatty acids

Eicosapentaenoic acid (EPA) is an essential polyunsaturated fatty acid of the *n*-3 class found in relatively large quantities in fish oil. It is a precursor in prostanoid synthesis and leads to less inflammatory and prothrombotic prostaglandins, leukotrienes, and thromboxanes than those derived from arachidonic acid. Studies on *n*-3 PUFAs, especially EPA (C 20:5) and DHA (C 22:6), indicate that these fatty acids may prevent the occurrence of cachexia and metastatic

Table 21.27 Effects of glutamine supplementation on mucositis and diarrhea in cancer patients receiving BMT and/or CT

	References
No effect	
Mucositis in BMT: IV L-GLN, 30–40 g/day	Ziegler *et al.*, 1992; Schloerb and Amare, 1993
Mucositis/diarrhea in BMT: oral L-GLN, 16 g/day	Jebb *et al.*, 1995
Mucositis/diarrhea in BMT: oral L-GLN, 30 g/day ± IV L-GLN	Schloerb and Skikne, 1999
Mucositis/diarrhea/oral food intake in BMT: oral L-GLN, 30 g/day	Coghlin-Dickson *et al.*, 2000
Mucositis in acute leukaemia chemotherapy: IV ALA-GLN, 26 g/day	Van Zaanen *et al.*, 1994
Mucositis with 5-FU-based chemotherapy: oral L-GLN 8 g/day	Okuno *et al.*, 1999
Mucositis with 5-FU-based chemotherapy: oral L-GLN 16 g/day	Jebb *et al.*, 1994
Diarrhea in breast cancer + doxifluridine: oral L-GLN, 30 g/day	Bozzetti *et al.*, 1997
Beneficial effect	
Mucositis in autologous BMT: oral L-GLN, 4 g/m² per day	Anderson at al., 1998a
Mucositis in autologous MBT for breast cancer: oral L-GLN, 24 g/day	Cockerham *et al.*, 2000
Diarrhea after high-dose combined chemotherapy for leukemia: oral L-GLN, 18 g/day	Muscaritoli *et al.*, 1997
Diarrhea and need for loperamide therapy after 5-FU therapy for colorectal cancer: oral L-GLN, 18 g/day	Daniele *et al.*, 2001

GLN, glutamine; IV, intravenous; BMT, bone marrow transplantation; CT, chemotherapy.
Modified from Ziegler (2001).
Full list of references cited are available from www.nutritiontexts.com.

disease in experimental tumor models. Although the mechanism has not yet been fully elucidated, EPA might inhibit cell proliferation and induce its apoptosis. Cytotoxicity may be related to lipid peroxidation and production of superoxide radicals. Furthermore, the beneficial metabolic effects of *n*-3 PUFAs may be attributed to the inhibition of LMF-related lypolysis through the block of cAMP activity in adipocytes.

In clinical practice, the efficacy of dietary supplementation with fish oil capsules (1 g each) containing EPA and DHA acids has been demonstrated in patients with advanced pancreatic carcinoma. In fact, EPA and fish oil lowered the levels of proinflammatory cytokines in patients with pancreatic cancer and, despite weight loss prior to entry into the study, after three months of fish oil supplementation (2–6 g EPA per day), median weight gain of 0.3 kg/month ($p < 0.002$) and significant reduction in acute phase protein production were obtained.

In a recent paper, 60 patients with solid tumors were randomized to receive dietary supplementation with either fish oil (18 g of *n*-3 PUFA) or placebo until death. Despite no effect on body weight, the *n*-3 PUFA group had a significantly prolonged survival.

Metabolic manipulation

The hypothesis of feeding the host without stimulating tumor growth through the use of a selective nutrition has been extensively investigated in animals, but clinical applications have been very few, and mainly based on diets which were selectively deficient of some amino acids. Experimental data are extremely controversial: some studies have shown that PUFAs may be capable of promoting tumor growth by directly stimulating mitosis. Others have suggested that tumors may not actually deplete host lipid stores to support their own growth since fat utilization by the tumor is poor due to the lack of key enzymes for NEFA and ketone body degradation. In human trials, dietary supplementation with *n*-3 fatty acids has been shown to inhibit tumor genesis. There is, however, some evidence that the energy metabolism of *in vivo* sarcoma and carcinoma in humans relies predominantly on glucose, with fat-derived calories making no appreciable contribution. The association of lipid-based parenteral nutrition with hydrazine sulfate, a gluconeogenic-blocking agent, aims at selectively starving the tumor by interrupting the cycle of tumor energy gain/host energy loss at the enzymatic level of phosphoenolpyruvate carboxykinase (Figure 21.2).

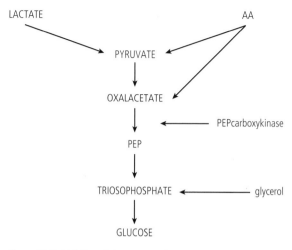

Figure 21.2 Inhibition of gluconeogenesis.

References and further reading

Bozzetti F. Effects of artificial nutrition on the nutritional status of cancer patients. *JPEN J Paren Enteral Nutr* 1989; 13: 406–420.

Bozzetti F. Nutritional support in adult cancer patients. *Clin Nutr* 1992; 11: 167–179.

Bozzetti F. Lessons learned from studies on immune nutrition in post-operative patients. *Clin Nutr* 1999; 18: 193–196.

Bozzetti F. Nutrition support in patients with Cancer. In: *Artificial Nutrition Support in Clinical Practice* (J Payne-James, G Grimble, D Silk, eds). London: Greenwich Medical Media, 2001.

Bozzetti F, Gavazzi C, Cozzaglio L, Costa A, Spinelli P, Viola G. Total parenteral nutrition and tumour growth in malnourished patients with gastric cancer. *Tumori* 1999; 85: 163–166.

Klein S, Simes J, Blackburn GL. Total parenteral nutrition and cancer clinical trials. *Cancer* 1986; 58: 1378–1386.

McGeer AJ, Detsky AS, O'Rourke K. Parenteral nutrition in cancer patients undergoing chemotherapy: a meta-analysis. *Nutrition* 1990; 6: 233–240.

Ziegler TR. Glutamine supplementation in cancer patients receiving bone marrow transplantation and high dose chemotherapy. *J Nutr* 2001; 131: 2578S–2584S.

22
Pediatric Nutrition

Anthony F Williams

Key messages

- A child varies enormously both in maturity and in size, from the 500-g 23-week gestation neonate to the fully-grown adult.
- The challenge of optimal childhood nutrition is to match supply with demands throughout this period of age, so that full genetic potential can be realized.
- Worldwide, about 11–12 million children die each year before reaching the age of five. Malnutrition is considered to be a sole or contributory cause in about 60%.
- Childhood growth not only involves increase in body size but changes in body proportions, the relative sizes of organ systems, and chemical composition.

- Nutrition has an important role to play in neurological, gastrointestinal, renal, and metabolic maturation.
- Breastfeeding is associated with better health outcomes for mother and baby, even in industrialized countries.
- Failure-to-thrive among young children in industrialized countries is most commonly the result of chronic energy deficiency arising from inappropriate care practices, rather than underlying physical disease or food shortage.
- A range of dietary products and delivery devices is now available for specialized enteral and parenteral nutritional support of sick children of all ages and sizes.

22.1 Introduction

'Pediatrics' is the treatment of disease during growth and development. As a clinical discipline it is inextricably linked to 'child health' – the promotion and maintenance of health in children. The child or 'pediatric patient' varies enormously both in maturity and in size, from the 500-g 23-week gestation neonate to the fully-grown adult. The challenge of optimal childhood nutrition is to match supply with demands throughout this period of age, so that full genetic potential can be realized. Failure to do so compromises the child's health and chance of survival. It also strongly influences health in adult life.

Why are children nutritionally vulnerable?

Worldwide, about 11–12 million children die each year before reaching the age of five. Malnutrition is considered to be a sole or contributory cause in about 60%. The particular vulnerability of children can be explained by considering influences which act on nutrient demand and supply.

Demands

Growth imposes high metabolic demands throughout childhood, particularly during infancy (the first year of life) and adolescence. Growth is not merely an increase in size. As children grow their body proportions alter, reflecting maturation in body composition and changes in the partitioning of nutrients between organ systems. These events are developmentally programmed so that the effects of supply failure depend to a large extent upon the age of the child. For example, severe energy restriction in early childhood, when the normal pace of growth is rapid and the brain is still developing, may never be recoverable. The end result is 'stunting' with associated impairment of cognitive development.

Supply

Failure of nutrient supply in children may be attributable many causes. In the case of babies born too early immaturity of the absorptive, metabolic, and excretory systems may constrain supply. In older children illness (acute and chronic, somatic, or psychological) may both increase demands and deleteriously affect supply. However, probably the most important factor is simply the availability of food. This is a key distinction between supply failure in children and adults. Adults can usually find the food they need, whereas young children (those with the highest demands) need others to find it for them. Where children are concerned, food shortage is not confined to resource-poor countries; it occurs even in industrialized nations as the result of parenting failure, educational deficiencies, and socioeconomic deprivation.

Imbalance of supply and demand

Children are also more disadvantaged than adults when supply does not meet demand. The smaller the child, the smaller are nutrient stores, and the shorter the period they will last. Additionally, immaturity of the metabolic and excretory systems, coupled with the relatively high demands of essential organs (such as the brain), constrain the capacity for reductive adaptation. The reasons why children are nutritionally vulnerable are summarized in Box 22.1.

These points will be revisited in more detail at later points in the chapter.

Box 22.1 Vulnerability of children

High demands
Demands are related to:
- The rate of growth
- Amount of metabolically active tissue (e.g. brain) per unit of body mass
- Occurrence of disease

Supply limitations
Supply may be limited by:
- Immaturity of the absorptive, metabolic, and excretory systems
- Developmental stage (ability to forage and eat)
- Neurological impairment
- Psychological disorder
- Social and educational disadvantage

Body composition
Nutrient stores are related to:
- Absolute body size
- Tissue composition (protein, fat, and water)

Box 22.2 How nutritional science is applied in pediatrics and child health

Promotion of child health
- Primary prevention, e.g. breastfeeding, vitamin supplementation
- Secondary prevention, e.g. screening for iron deficiency or phenylketonuria

Primary treatment of disease
- e.g. exclusion diets (celiac disease, allergy), therapeutic diets (inborn errors)

Nutritional support
- e.g. feeding the extremely low birth weight (<1000 g) baby, treatment of inflammatory bowel disease

---

Applications of nutritional science in pediatrics and child health

People practising in pediatrics and child health apply nutritional principles daily. Box 22.2 lists some examples relevant to practice in both industrialized and resource-poor countries. Advances in clinical nutrition have had a major impact on child survival globally – for example well-controlled trials have shown that vitamin A supplementation in resource-poor countries can reduce mortality amongst preschool children by about 30%. In industrialized countries improved techniques of nutritional support have greatly improved the survival of sick children, such as those born extremely early and those who develop chronic disease or intestinal failure.

Long-term relevance of pediatric nutrition

Optimizing nutrition in early life is increasingly seen to have relevance to long-term health. Although many of the mechanisms still require clarification, epidemiologic data clearly show that patterns of growth in fetal life and infancy are correlated with later risk of cardiovascular disease and the metabolic syndrome. Although effects seem most marked amongst individuals whose early growth was severely restricted it is important to realize that there is in fact a gradation of risk across the normal range of body size and shape. Thus the potential later health dividends of providing optimal early nutrition could be considerable at population level.

Figure 22.1 shows conceptually how early life interventions could integrate with later (adult and old-age)

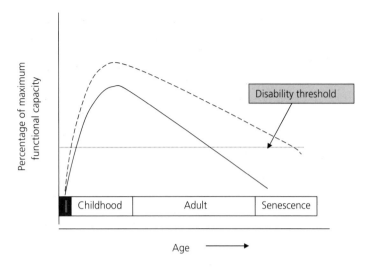

Figure 22.1 Model for promoting lifelong health through optimizing early nutrition. Maximum functional capacity is achieved as the result of tissue growth and maturation during fetal life (black area) and childhood. Functional capacity then declines during adult life at a rate determined by health, lifestyle, and environmental factors, eventually crossing a "disability threshold". The time taken to reach this point is partly determined by the height of the initial peak around adolescence. Reproduced with permission from Stein and Moritz (1999).

interventions to improve health outlook with aging. If functional capacity is maximized in the early years the individual has a greater reserve from which decline begins in adult life. Such an approach acts synergistically with interventions in later life aimed at slowing the rate of decline. The effect of both is to prolong the period elapsing before functional capacity crosses a 'disability threshold.' One example of such an effect might be bone health. Bone mass in later years might theoretically be optimized by attainment of peak bone mass during childhood and adolescent growth, coupled with measures (such as optimal nutrition and lifestyle) to slow decline in adult life.

22.2 Growth

Growth, physical and mental development are the processes which distinguish children from adults. Physical growth involves an increase in both the size and complexity of body structure, occurring under genetic and endocrine regulation. The pattern of growth has a characteristic tempo which is disturbed if nutrient supply is inadequate or disease impairs nutrient uptake and utilization. Therefore growth monitoring is a key clinical tool in pediatrics and child health.

The process of growth has a number of corollaries for nutrient demands. First, depending on the child's age, it is 'expensive.' For example, in early infancy when growth is most rapid it may consume half the energy intake. Secondly, because the dominance and rela-

tive size of organ systems change substantially during growth, the partitioning of nutrients also changes, affecting to some extent the balance of nutrient requirements.

Measuring growth: growth references and charts

The normal pattern of growth can be defined in the form of a growth reference compiled by measuring normal healthy children. One approach to constructing a growth reference is to measure children of differing ages at the same time (cross-sectional sampling). Another is to follow a cohort of children as they grow (longitudinal sampling). The data obtained may be reproduced graphically in the form of growth charts or be transformed into the properties of a normal distribution as z-scores (i.e. the number of standard deviations from the mean). The former are most commonly used for day-to-day clinical monitoring of individual children, whereas the latter are most widely used for handling population data. Weight, height (or length), and occipito-frontal circumference (OFC; head circumference) are the most widely used parameters clinically, though references exist for others too, such as skinfold thickness, mid-arm circumference, knee–heel and foot length. Cross-sectional charts may not adequately depict substantial interindividual variations in normal growth patterns, particularly during infancy and at adolescence. This observation has clinical implications and is further discussed later.

Distance and velocity charts

Reference data may be displayed either in terms of absolute attainment (i.e. distance traveled) for age or the speed of growth at a particular age (Figure 22.2). Clinical monitoring is most commonly performed using charts of the former type, interindividual variation being depicted in the form of centile lines. Charts commonly used in UK practice today are compiled from over 25 000 cross-sectional weight and height measurements of white English, Welsh, and Scottish children sampled in seven separate studies conducted 1978–1990. This is known as the UK 1990 growth reference (Figure 22.3). The chart used in clinical practice actually uses nine lines, rather than the seven shown in the figure. These represent the 0.4th, 2nd, 9th, 25th, 50th, 75th, 91st, 98th, and 99.6th centiles, each band being spaced two-thirds of a standard deviation above or below the next. Thus it is easy to calculate how many standard deviations a child's height (or weight) is above or below the mean (Figure 22.4).

A key assumption in using growth charts for clinical monitoring is that an individual child's growth trajectory parallels a centile line on the chart: a phenomenon known as 'channeling' or canalization. With a few physiological exceptions, deviation from such a course signifies under- or overnutrition, or the presence of an underlying disease process modifying nutrient assimilation, demands, or losses.

Growth data depicted in velocity/age format are now less commonly used clinically. They have a specialist use in investigation and monitoring in endocrine/growth clinics but the need for extremely accurate measurements limits their clinical value, as the error in any difference estimate is double that of the individual measurements used. Nevertheless, for the purpose of considering nutrient demands a useful insight into the overall pattern of growth can be obtained by examining a velocity chart. In fact the pattern can be resolved mathematically into three overlapping curves: the infant, child and pubertal phases (Figure 22.5). This is known as the ICP model of infant growth and reflects changes in the dominant influences of growth with age:

- Infant growth is primarily nutrient/insulin led, an extension of the fetal pattern.
- Childhood growth is predominantly growth hormone led.
- Pubertal growth is primarily driven by the influence of sex steroids on growth hormone secretion.

The increase in velocity at puberty is called the pubertal growth spurt. This occurs at a substantially younger age in girls, first because they enter puberty earlier than boys and, secondly because the growth spurt occurs at an earlier stage and is beginning to subside by menarche (Figure 22.6). This adaptation helps

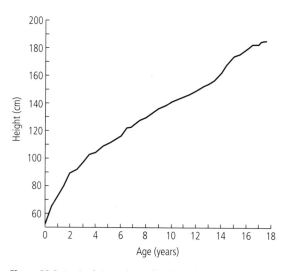
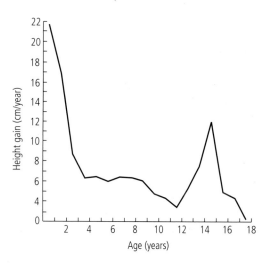

Figure 22.2 Attained size and growth velocity plots. Philippe de Montbeillard, an eighteenth-century French aristocrat, made serial measurements of his son's height throughout childhood. These are plotted in two ways: the left-hand plot shows height attained and the right-hand one the velocity of growth at any particular age. Reproduced with permission from Tanner (1989).

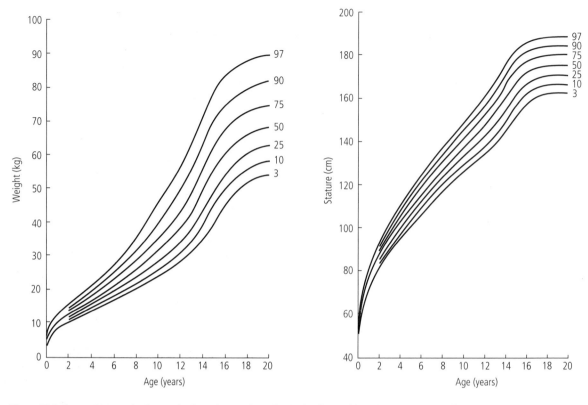

Figure 22.3 The UK 1990 growth reference. The charts show weight and height data for British boys. These were compiled from cross-sectional measurements of over 25 000 white children made between 1978 and 1990. Reproduced with permission from Freeman *et al.* (1990).

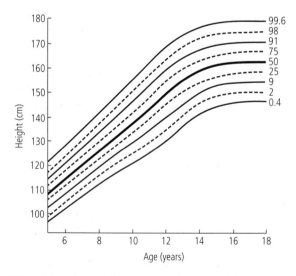

Figure 22.4 A 'nine-centile' growth chart, showing centile bands spaced at intervals of two-thirds of a standard deviation (i.e. *z*-score 0.66). This presentation is now most commonly used in UK clinical practice. Data shown here are for British girls aged 5–18 included in the UK 1990 growth reference. Reproduced from Cole (1994) with permission of the BMJ Publishing Group.

to ensure both that the child's growth is completed before pregnancy occurs and that fetal nutritional demands are anticipated by the deposition of maternal body stores.

Optimal growth: the place of international standards

Growth references are *descriptive*: they merely describe the growth pattern of the sample selected. Yet they are often used clinically in a *prescriptive* sense, for example as a standard or yardstick against which to judge whether a child's size at some age is normal or abnormal, or to evaluate the growth of groups of children. If they are used in this way it is clearly important that they reflect a pattern associated with optimal social, functional, and health outcomes. Growth is affected by a numerous factors, including poverty, ethnic background, and emotional wellbeing. It is possible that these may adversely affect growth by mechanisms apart from a reduction in nutrient supply. For example higher centers

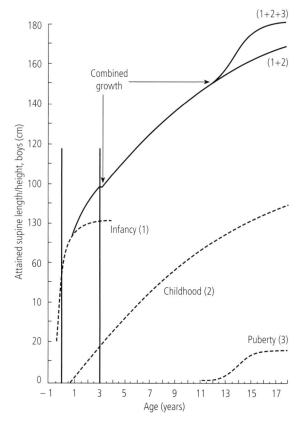

Figure 22.5 The Karlberg 'ICP' model of human growth. The chart shows three dotted lines which represent the infancy (1), childhood (2), and puberty (3) curves. These summate to form the 'combined growth' curve (solid line). From Kelnar *et al.* (1998).

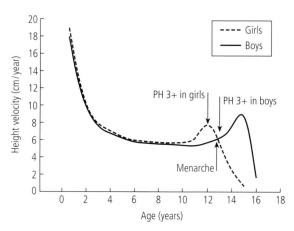

Figure 22.6 Differences in timing of the pubertal growth spurt. Height velocity curves for boys and girls are overlapped. Comparable stages of puberty (pubic hair rating 3) are indicated by the arrows. The growth spurt is clearly an earlier pubertal event in girls than boys.

could, in theory, act upon the hypothalamo-pituitary regulation of growth hormone secretion.

Children in resource-poor countries are generally smaller than their counterparts in industrialized ones and it might be argued that local references are more relevant to growth monitoring in such communities. However, studies that have compared the growth of better-off and poor children *within* such countries have shown large differences in rates of growth, the former often matching patterns seen in richer industrialized countries. This argues strongly for application of international growth standards as a measure for improving the nutritional status of children globally.

The American NCHS (National Center for Health Statistics) reference has been used as such a standard for many years. Unfortunately this approach has its shortcomings. First, important secular changes in the twentieth century have been associated with changes in the growth patterns of children even in rich countries. The NCHS standards draw on growth data over 50 years old and today's children are both taller and heavier. Secondly, most of the infants included in the NCHS reference were artificially fed and methods of infant feeding exert major influences on the pattern of growth in infancy. For these reasons the NCHS chart has recently been revised to form the CDC (Center for Disease Control) 2000 Growth Reference.

Physiological deviations from growth references

Although the phenomenon of 'channeling' underpins the clinical use of growth charts for longitudinal monitoring, individual children can show patterns of growth which deviate from the centile lines for valid physiological reasons. This tendency to cross up or down centile line channels is particularly marked at two stages of life: infancy and puberty.

Infancy

As charts are compiled from cross-sectional data there is a tendency for babies at the extremes of the birth weight range to show regression towards the mean during the early months, crossing centiles up or down (Figure 22.7). At a given gestational age birth size is principally affected by placental function (nutrient supply) and maternal, rather than paternal, size. An infant constrained by intrauterine environment will, if optimally nourished after birth, grow in such a way

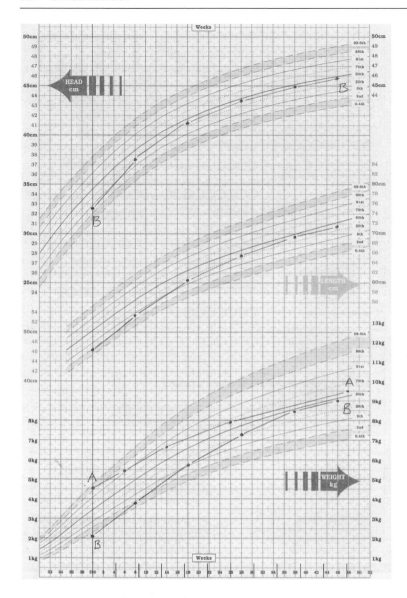

Figure 22.7 'Catch-up' and 'catch-down' in infancy. Growth curves are plotted for two babies. Baby A, the infant of a diabetic mother, has a birth weight above the 97th centile. Excessive weight gain *in utero* was the result of maternal, hence fetal, hyperglycemia and hyperinsulinism. After birth she 'catches down' towards her genetically determined size. Baby B was born at term with birth weight <0.4 centile and head circumference at the 9th centile. This indicates 'head sparing' and is typical of late intrauterine growth retardation (IUGR). After birth the baby crosses several centiles upwards, a pattern indicative of 'catch-up' to genetically determined size following release from intrauterine constraint.

as to seek out his or her genetic potential by exhibiting catch-up growth. Conversely an infant overnourished *in utero*, such as the infant of a diabetic mother, may exhibit catch-down growth. These processes are usually completed by the end of the first year of life but in extreme cases may continue into the second year. It is sometimes important to distinguish clinically between catch-down growth of an unusually heavy baby (e.g. the infant of a diabetic mother) and failure-to-thrive. It is therefore essential to know fully the parental measurements and perinatal history when interpreting growth patterns in infancy.

Puberty

The age at onset of puberty varies greatly between individuals. For example, although pubic hair in girls appears at an average age of 11.9 years, the 2nd and 98th centiles for this stage are five years apart at 14.4 and 9.4 years respectively. Because the 50th centile line on the growth chart reflects the growth trajectory of a child entering puberty at the average age, one exhibiting late puberty may show an apparent downward crossing of centile lines at this age, with later apparent catch-up as puberty occurs (Figure 22.8). The converse may also occur in early puberty: a child

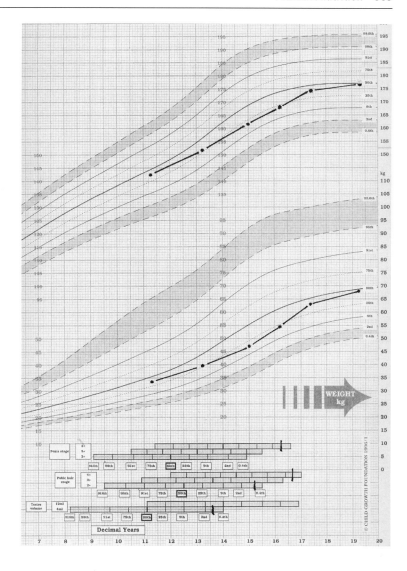

Figure 22.8 Late puberty. This boy has developed signs of puberty at late age. Pubic hair stage 4 was not reached until 16½ years (<2nd centile; average age at PH 4 would be 14½). Because his pubertal growth spurt is delayed there is the apparent effect of crossing down one centile space for both weight and height. This is because the cross-sectional chart best reflects the growth trajectory of boys entering puberty at average age.

may show apparent early upward and later downward centile crossing. (Earlier Tanner–Whitehouse growth charts (based on data collected in the 1960s) made some allowance for this by showing as a shaded area the age at which variations attributable to puberty might occur.) Interpretation may be further confounded by the observation that taller, heavier children tend to develop puberty earlier than ones who are shorter and lighter, whereas those with chronic disease may show later puberty. This adaptation may help them catch-up to their genetically determined final height despite long-term disease-associated undernutrition.

Body composition and growth

Childhood growth not only involves increase in body size but changes in body proportions, the relative sizes of organ systems, and chemical composition. These changes have implications for:

- the nature and amount of body nutrient stores,
- the partitioning of nutrients between organ systems, and
- the potential for nutrient restriction to have lifelong effects.

Sexual differences in body composition become apparent after puberty but not before.

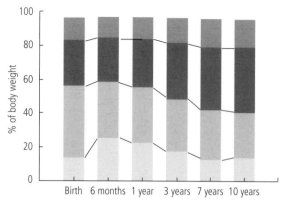

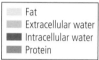

Figure 22.9 Change in the relative size of body compartments with age. Drawn using data from Fomon *et al.* (1982). Reproduced with permission by the *American Journal of Clinical Nutrition* © Am J Clin Nutr. American Society for Clinical Nutrition.

Table 22.1 Percentage of body weight accounted for by various tissues and organs at various stages of human development

	24-week fetus	Full-term newborn	Adult
Muscle	25	25	40
Bone	22	18	14
Heart	0.6	0.5	0.4
Lungs	3.3	1.5	1.4
Liver	4	5	2
Kidneys	0.7	1	0.5
Brain	13	12	2.0

From Widdowson (1981).

Organ systems and nutrient partitioning

Table 22.1 illustrates the relative contribution of various organ systems to body weight in the infant and adult. A notable difference is the relative size of the brain, which is growing at peak velocity around term and completes most of its growth in the first two years of life. These changes have major effects on the contribution brain metabolism makes to resting energy expenditure (Figure 22.10). As glucose is the principal

Nutrient stores

Changes in the amount and distribution of body fat reserves exemplify the implications of growth for nutrient stores. Figure 22.9 shows how the body mass is distributed between fat, protein, and water as the child grows to ten years. The extracellular fluid compartment is relatively large at birth but quickly decreases in size, a process which largely accounts for the normal weight loss of newborn infants in the first week of life. In the first six months of life body weight more than doubles and proportion of fat increases from about 14% to 25%. Thus the average fat mass of a six-month-old baby is about four-fold greater than that of a normal newborn – some 2 kg as opposed to 500 g. This need to deposit large amounts of fat (9 kcal/g) partly explains why growth is so energetically demanding at this stage of development, consuming up to 50% of the baby's energy intake.

The connotations for surviving a period of starvation are equally important, and even more dramatic if the extremely preterm baby is considered. The fat compartment of a 500-g 25-week gestation baby represents only 2–3% of body weight – about 10–15 g or 90–130 kcal. Provision of nutritional support is therefore a matter of urgency in such a patient.

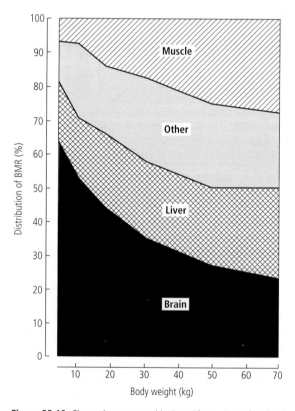

Figure 22.10 Change in energy partitioning with age. Reproduced with permission from Holliday (1971).

brain fuel it also explains why glucose requirements change so greatly with age. In the adult hepatic gluconeogenesis can be suppressed by an intravenous infusion of 1–2 mg glucose/kg body weight per min. However the term newborn needs 3–5 mg/kg body weight per min and the preterm, growth-retarded newborn (with a relatively much larger brain) some 6–8 mg/kg body weight per min. If glucose requirements were expressed instead per 100 g of brain weight a different picture would emerge: requirements are similar across the age spectrum.

This example clearly shows how changes in body composition associated with growth affect nutrient partitioning between organ systems and hence nutrient requirements if expressed on a per unit body weight basis.

Nutrient restriction and critical growth periods

Figure 22.11 shows the stages in childhood at which various organ systems are undergoing most rapid growth. It is particularly important to note that brain growth is virtually completed in the early years of childhood. Prolonged and severe nutrient restriction at this age may be associated with lifelong functional deficit.

Chronic early life undernutrition results in stunting (linear growth restriction) which is extremely common in resource-poor countries, as many as one-third to one-half of all children being affected. At two years of age, in such settings, a height more than 2 standard deviations below the mean on WHO charts (z-score −2.0) seems to be associated with a later IQ deficit of around 10 points. The extent to which this reflects deprivation of nutrients, as opposed to the effects of numerous confounders (e.g. poverty and low birth weight) is uncertain. Mechanisms exist to spare brain nutrition in the presence of nutrient shortages. For example, the newborn who has suffered intrauterine growth retardation as the result of placental failure has a small body with thin limbs and a large head because blood flow and nutrients are diverted away from the somatic organs to the brain. To a lesser extent brain sparing, with similar changes in body proportions, is also evident in malnourished young children

Sexual differences in body composition

In early life the body composition of boys and girls is closely comparable, yet important differences arise at puberty, as shown in the Figure 22.12. In girls fat rep-

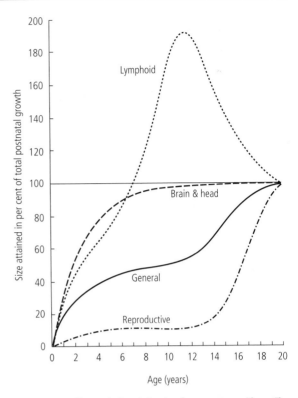

Figure 22.11 Changes in the relative size of organ systems with age. The graph shows age at which organs attain a given percentage of their size at age 20 (100%). Note that 90% of brain growth is completed in the first three years, and that the relative size of the lymphoid organ in childhood significantly exceeds that of the adult. Reproduced with permission from Tanner (1989).

resents a much higher proportion of pubertal weight gain than in boys, who deposit more lean body tissue. These differences reflect the dominance of androgenic steroids in boys, but also serve to ensure that girls have more adequate energy reserves to meet the later demands of pregnancy and lactation.

Key points on growth and body composition are summarized in Box 22.3.

22.3 The impact of development on nutrition

'Children are not just small adults' – they are growing and exhibit developmental changes which better equip them to meet metabolic demands. For example developmental changes in the gastrointestinal system enhance the efficiency of nutrient absorption, while

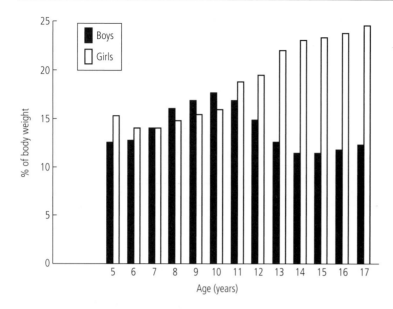

Figure 22.12 Differences between boys and girls in development of the fat compartment. The bars represent fat as a percentage of body weight. Difference between sexes becomes significant only after puberty. From Widdowson (1981).

Box 22.3 Growth

- A growth reference can be compiled from cross-sectional or longitudinal data
- Growth references can be represented graphically (centile charts) or statistically (z-scores)
- Cross-sectional charts can conceal normal variation in growth patterns during infancy and at puberty
- Growth is a sensitive measure of health, nutrient supply, and socioeconomic status. These influences are much stronger than ethnic background
- The pattern of growth can be resolved into infant, child, and pubertal phases (the Karlberg ICP model). These reflect differing endocrine influences
- Body composition and the relative sizes of organ systems change as growth proceeds. The timing of a nutritional insult therefore determines the outcome
- Sex differences in body composition appear at puberty
- The growth spurt occurs early in female puberty, but late in male puberty

---

those in the liver and kidney progressively increase the child's ability to adapt to over- or undersupply of nutrients. Perhaps the most important of all is the child's neurological maturation, which facilitates transition from total dependence during infancy to the independent adult, capable of seeking out and selecting a food supply. This section examines some of the major nutritional changes that occur as the child develops.

Neurological maturation

Infancy, the first 12-months of life, is a particularly rapid period of developmental change during which the typical term infant will treble in weight and move from total dependence on milk to the acceptance of a mixed diet compatible with the family's culture. This process of nutritional diversification is gradual and the pace of change needs particularly to respect the timing of normal psychomotor and mental developmental changes, often referred to as 'developmental milestones'. Those particularly relevant to the development of eating behaviour are shown in Table 22.2. Note that these are approximations only and there can be substantial normal variation between individual children.

When considering the table it may be useful to know that pediatricians generally think about developmental milestones in four groups (or 'fields'):

- gross motor function and maintenance of posture,
- fine motor function (manipulation) and vision,
- speech and hearing, and
- psychological and social.

Successful feeding requires convergence in all fields. The child must be able to sit comfortably, hold the head erect and be able to turn (gross motor), have coordinated oropharyngeal movements in order to swallow (speech), be able to locate food with the hand and transfer it to the mouth (vision and fine motor),

Table 22.2 Developmental 'milestones of neurological maturation relevant to feeding

Milestone	Age achieved
Sucking and swallowing	From about 34 weeks of gestation
	Reflex sucking disappears about 4 months.
Rooting reflex	Present at term. Disappears about 4 months
Co-ordinated acceptance of a spoon	About 6 months
Puts hands to mouth	About 5–6 months
Sits unsupported	About 7 months
Transfers objects from hand to hand	About 8 months
Pincer grip	About 10 months
Full rotary chewing movements	1–2 years
Holds spoon or cup to feed	12–18 months
Feeds self (but messily)	18 months–2 years

and interact with a carer (psychological). As a result, children with cerebral palsy (a disorder of posture and movement caused by a non-progressive lesion of the developing brain in which muscles become stiff or 'spastic', making coordinated movements hard to achieve) often have major feeding problems and fail-to-thrive because of their difficulty with muscular control, despite normal intellectual ability and intact special sensation. They need help with body positioning and careful attention to the texture and consistency of foods offered in order to learn to eat.

Thinking about the development of complementary feeding skills in this way emphasizes a number of other points too:

- The child needs to be 'developmentally ready': there is no point in offering solids before the child is able to take food from a spoon. Indeed, to do so may result in force-feeding and negatively affect eating behaviour.
- The introduction of complementary feeding at appropriate times may also help to stimulate development by promoting the coordinated use of muscle groups. For example, encouraging the introduction of solids from about six months probably helps to 'train' muscles which will later be important for speech. Sucking from the breast or bottle teat requires the tongue to move only in a sagittal plane, whereas forming solids into a bolus requires the gradual attainment of rotary tongue movements necessary for speech. Anecdotally there is a frequent association between early feeding problems and speech delay, though whether one is a consequence of the other, or both reflect the underlying delay in neurological maturation is not clear.

The impact of neurological development on nutrition is summarized in Box 22.4.

> **Box 22.4** Impact of neurological development on nutrition
>
> - Children mature neurologically in a well-defined sequence marked by 'milestones'
> - The development of feeding requires integration of milestones in all fields: gross motor, fine motor, speech and psychosocial
> - Appropriate timing and progression of complementary feeding must recognize this process

Gastrointestinal maturation

The gut is anatomically mature by about 24 weeks of gestation and there is transit of fluid through the upper intestine from early in the second trimester of pregnancy. Fetal swallowing can be observed on ultrasonography, and obstruction related to congenital anomalies (e.g. esophageal or duodenal atresia) results in accumulation of excessive amniotic fluid (polyhydramnios). Swallowed water is absorbed in the small intestine and excreted through the fetal kidneys; thus there is turnover of the water compartment of the amniotic fluid. There is no net transit through the large intestine which accumulates meconium, a sticky dark green material. Meconium is usually excreted within 24 h of birth (excretion during labor may be an indication of fetal stress resulting from hypoxia and ischemia). Delayed excretion of meconium is often an indication of lower intestinal obstruction or dysmotility, such as Hirschsprung's disease.

Animal studies have shown that feeding is the important trophic stimulus to further postnatal development of the gut. Milk feeding results in both a hypertrophy (increase in cell size) and a hyperplasia (increase in cell number) of the small intestine. Homologous milk (i.e. that of the animal's own species) appears more effective than artificial milks in this respect. This probably reflects the presence of peptide growth factors, such as epidermal growth factor and lactoferrin, in the colostrum. In this way the newborn's capacity for mucosal absorption increases rapidly after birth in response to enteral feeding. Early feeding also stimulates the release of 'gut hormones' including cholecystokinin, motilin, and enteroglucagon, which respectively help to stimulate bile flow, intestinal transit, and the integration of liver metabolism with feeding.

Despite the observation that about half the infant's energy intake is provided by fat, the pancreas is relatively small at birth, and secretion of pancreatic lipase reduced. This apparent paradox is explained by the existence of other effectors of luminal fat digestion. One compensating factor is the initiation of fat digestion in stomach, at acid pH, through the release of lingual lipase during sucking. Another is the presence in breastmilk of a lipase active at duodenal pH and stimulated by bile salts. The presence of the latter is one reason that breastmilk lipids are more effectively absorbed than those in formula or other milks.

When infants are born prematurely fat digestion is even less well developed than at term. The initiation of enteral feeding is further hampered by the absence of effectively coordinated propulsion due to maturational delay in the propagation of a migrating motor complex. The latter appears at a gestation of about 34 weeks, concomitant with the presence of effectively coordinated sucking and swallowing. It is known, however, that the initiation of feeding can effectively 'call forward' the maturation of motility patterns. Enteral feeding in even very preterm infants (from about 24–26 weeks gestation) is usually therefore commenced in small quantities as soon as possible after delivery, increasing gradually in volume, in order to effect this change.

Another important aspect of gut maturation is the evolution of immune protection during infancy. Gut infection is a leading cause of death in infants and young children. Moreover mechanisms must develop which allow the infant to recognize harmful antigens yet become tolerant to foods. A number of factors are important in this respect:

- The provision of specific passive secretory immunity (secretory immunoglobulin A) through the enteromammary axis of breastfeeding.
- The presence of non-specific immune factors in breastmilk (e.g. lysozyme, lactoferrin, the lactoperoxidase system).
- The promotion of a large bowel flora dominated by bifidobacteria, rather than coliform organisms. This is partly attributable to the prebiotic effect of non-absorbable oligosaccharides in breastmilk, in which they constitute about 10% of the carbohydrate content.

Although the last has long been cited as important in protecting the gut from infection, the nature of large bowel flora may also be important in the determination of systemic immune tolerance through regulating the relative balance of T helper/suppressor activity (see Chapter 7).

The role of gastrointestinal maturation on nutrition is shown in Box 22.5.

Box 22.5 Gastrointestinal maturation

- Enteral feeding is an important stimulus to early gut maturation
- Pancreatic fat digestion is relatively immature at birth, though the actions of lingual lipase and a lipase in breastmilk help to compensate for this
- Breastmilk particularly helps to promote gut development and is important in protecting the gut from infection
- The nature of the large bowel flora (especially the presence of lactobacilli) is influenced by feeding and probably influences the development of systemic immune tolerance

---

Renal maturation

At birth both glomerular filtration rate (GFR) and renal tubular concentrating capacity are reduced. This limits the amount of solute that can be cleared from the blood, and increases the demand for free water needed to eliminate dietary excess in a relatively dilute urine. The term renal solute load (RSL) is used to describe the amount of absorbed dietary solute surplus to growth demands that must be eliminated through the kidneys. Stressors such as fever or diarrhea may further compromise excretory capacity by increasing insensible and stool water losses, reducing water availability for urine. Retention of solute then leads to hyperosmolar dehydration.

Carbohydrate and fat do not contribute to renal solute load because they are entirely eliminated through non-renal routes (oxidation to CO_2 and water). The principal components of RSL are sodium (Na), potassium (K), chloride (Cl), and absorbed phosphorus (P_a), together with the amount of urea formed by oxidation of protein excess to growth demands. These form the potential renal solute load (PRSL). However the actual RSL depends not only on the composition of the feed, but on the baby's rate of growth (influencing the rate of solute retention) and non-renal water losses. In the absence of diarrhea the latter can be ignored so that RSL can be calculated as:

Estimated RSL =
PRSL − (0.9 × weight gain in g/day) mosmol/l

PRSL can in turn be expressed by the formula:

PRSL = N/28 + Na + Cl + K + P_a mosmol/l

In both formulas elemental composition is expressed in mmol/l. The factor 0.9 in the first equation is an estimate which allows for the disposal of solute through growth (0.9 mmol for each gram of weight gained). This observation re-emphasizes R.A. McCance's dictum that growth constitutes the infant's 'third kidney,' and explains the paradox by which infants tolerate protein intakes that would be proportionally far too high for an adult with similarly low GFR resulting from kidney disease (see Chapter 13). The divisor of 28 in the second equation, applied to the total fraction of nitrogenous solute (N/mg), assumes that the modal number of nitrogen atoms per molecule of urinary nitrogenous solute is 2, i.e. that it is urea.

A final complication is that the amount of water consumed is partly determined by the energy density of a feed: infants consuming an energy-dense feed will take a lower volume, hence less water. Thus, whereas the calculations above show PRSL in terms of mosmol/l, it is more logical to express it as mosmol/100 kcal. Table 22.3 shows the PRSLs of various feed types calculated in both ways. On both theoretical and epidemiologic grounds (risk of hypernatremic dehydration) it can be shown that feeds with a PRSL <27 mosmol/100 kcal are safe, whereas those >38 mosmol/100 kcal are associated with increased risk of developing hyperosmolar dehydration. For regulatory purposes limits of 30–35 mosmol/100 kcal have been proposed for infant formulas.

The role of renal maturation in nutrition is shown in Box 22.6.

> **Box 22.6** Renal maturation
>
> - Young infants, especially those born preterm, have both reduced glomerular filtration rate (GFR) and tubular concentrating capacity (TCC)
> - The amount of dietary solute in excess of the need for growth is known as the renal solute load (RSL)
> - Low GFR, particularly in the very preterm baby, reduces clearance of RSL through the kidneys, contributing to uremia
> - Impaired tubular concentrating capacity requires that the infant is given sufficient water to eliminate RSL or the plasma will become hyperosmolar
> - The potential renal solute load (PRSL) of a feed is normally greater than the RSL because growth consumes solute, effectively acting as a 'third kidney'

Metabolic maturation

At birth the normal newborn must switch rapidly from continuous transplacental nutrient supply to a pattern of intermittent enteral feeding. Initially, during the onset of stage II (postpartum) lactogenesis,

Table 22.3 Calculation of potential renal solute load (PRSL) for various milks

Type of milk feed	Protein (g/l)	Na (mmol/l)	Cl (mmol/l)	K (mmol/l)	P_a (mmol/l)	Urea (mosm/l)	Σ elecs (mosm/l)	mosm/l	mosm per 100 kcal
Human milk	10	7	11	13	5	57	36	93	14
Milk-based formula	15	8	12	18	11	86	49	135	20
Whole cow's milk	33	21	30	39	30	188	120	308	46

Reprinted from Fomon and Ziegler (1999) with permission from Elsevier.

the amount of energy delivered by breastmilk is small. Typically volumes of only 50–100 ml may be taken on the first day of life, rising to 600–800 ml by the end of the first week. In keeping with the need to meet high obligatory metabolic demands (at this stage cerebral metabolism accounts for over half of the resting energy expenditure, see Figure 22.10), in the face of such low intake counter-regulatory mechanisms are well developed. With the cessation of transplacental glucose supply there is a surge in glucagon secretion, resulting in glycogenolysis. About 1% of the newborn's body weight is glycogen, which forms an important short-term energy reserve. The glucagon surge also promotes gluconeogenesis: glycerol (from fat stores), alanine (from muscle), lactate, and pyruvate acting as substrates.

Adrenaline secretion is also important in opposing the action of insulin, which dominates the fetal metabolic milieu. It stimulates lipolysis in fat stores, and protein breakdown in muscle (releasing alanine to fuel gluconeogenesis) during the early hours of life. Growth hormone and cortisol also play important roles: indeed children with growth hormone or cortisol deficiency may present with significant neonatal hypoglycemia. This switch from carbohydrate to fat metabolism is evident as:

- a fall in respiratory quotient from 1.0 in the first hour to 0.8–0.85 by about 8–12 h of age, and
- the appearance of significant ketonemia at 24–48 h of age ('suckling ketogenesis').

In contrast, some pathways important for the metabolism of protein are less mature in the young infant, particularly if preterm. The ability to synthesize urea following deamination of amino acids is reduced, as is capacity to interconvert certain essential amino acids. This particularly increases metabolic requirements for cysteine and taurine (less easily synthesized from methionine), and for tyrosine (normally synthesized from phenylalanine).

These apparent metabolic deficiencies possibly reflect the observation that the young infant is strongly anabolic and in health has little need to dispose of excessive amino acid. Indeed the young infant's metabolic milieu is characterized more by the need to conserve nitrogen in the interests of protein economy. Thus the intake of nitrogen from breastmilk is relatively low but the infant is able to maintain nitrogen balance by virtue of:

- the high quality of breastmilk protein (conventionally used as the reference for calculating the amino acid scores of alternative proteins – such as cow's milk or soya – used in infant formulas) and
- the existence of mechanisms for colonic salvage. Almost a quarter of the nitrogen in breastmilk is 'non-protein nitrogen' (much of it urea), and there is good evidence that the infant can incorporate this into body protein. (The observation of a high level of non-protein nitrogen has caused some to observe that it is not appropriate to express the protein content of breastmilk by applying the conventional factor of 6.38 to nitrogen measured using the Kjeldahl technique. A factor of 5.18 probably reflects more closely the nutritional protein content.)

The role of metabolic maturation in nutrition is shown in Box 22.7.

> **Box 22.7** Metabolic maturation
>
> - Counter-regulatory mechanisms are well developed in the term newborn
> - They are instrumental in effecting the change from continuous transplacental delivery of nutrients to intermittent enteral feeding controlled by appetite
> - High metabolic demands and immaturity of some metabolic steps mean that a greater number of amino acids is essential or conditionally essential for the young infant
> - The protein quality of breastmilk is high
> - High protein quality and the existence of mechanisms promoting nitrogen economy in the baby explains why the nutritional protein content of breastmilk seems relatively low

22.4 Infant feeding

Previous sections have shown that infancy is a period of particular nutritional vulnerability: the potential rate of growth is rapid, body stores are small, and functional immaturity constrains adaptation to both over- and undersupply. Feeding during infancy therefore warrants close attention.

Breastfeeding

The establishment of successful breastfeeding is crucial to the general health of mother and baby in all environments (see chapters 15, 16, and 18 in the *Public Health Nutrition* textbook in this series). In summary, the principal health gains associated with breastfeeding are reduced vulnerability to gastrointestinal and respiratory (including ear) infections and suppression of ovulation, leading to a reduction in demands on family resources. Long-term gains may also include an advantage in the child's cognitive development and a reduction in the mother's risk of premenopausal breast cancer. Although these factors were once considered less relevant to industrialized countries, cohort studies in the United Kingdom have clearly shown that breastfed babies suffer fewer gastrointestinal and respiratory infections and are significantly less likely to be admitted to hospital.

Key points about breastfeeding are listed in Box 22.8.

Composition of breastmilk

Nutritionally, breastmilk alone is viewed as the reference diet of infants younger than six months of age. Table 22.4 summarizes its composition and compares it with that of a typical infant formula and unmodified cow's milk. There is pronounced interindividual variability in the composition of breastmilk. This is attributable to a number of factors including the gestational age of the baby, the postnatal age of the baby, the volume produced, and the time of the day. Even within

> **Box 22.8** Breastfeeding
>
> - Breastfeeding is associated with better health outcomes for mother and baby, even in industrialized countries
> - Data on the consumption and composition of breastmilk constitute a dietary reference for young infants
> - The production of breastmilk is controlled by infant demand: unrestricted access to the breast and effective feeding technique are both important to success
> - There are technical problems in measuring precisely both the amount of milk the infant consumes and its composition

a single mother–baby pair the fat concentration rises significantly during a feed.

The nitrogen moiety of breastmilk is particularly complex for a number of reasons. First, many of the proteins serve 'non-nutritional' biological functions, such as specific and non-specific immune protection of the gut and mucosal surfaces. For example about 10% of the protein is secretory immunoglobulin A (IgA) which is not absorbed. Secondly, about a quarter of the nitrogenous compounds exist as the so-called 'non-protein nitrogen' fraction, which comprises free amino acids, urea, and other small peptides. There is

Table 22.4 Summary of the composition of human milk, infant formula, and cow's milk

	Constituent	Human milk	Infant formula	Cow's milk
Protein nitrogen	Total protein (g/l)	8.9[a]	18	31
	Secretory IgA (g/l)	0.5–1	0	trace
	Lactoferrin (g/l)	1	0	trace
	Lysozyme (g/l)	0.05–0.25	0	trace
Non-protein nitrogen	(% of total N)	25	0	5
Carbohydrate	Lactose (g/l)	65	25 (minimum)	45
	Oligosaccharides (g/l)	12	0	1
	Other (e.g. glucose polymer) (g/l)		Up to 10 g in total as: lactose, maltose sucrose, glucose syrup, starch, or maltodextrins	
Fat	Total (g/l)	40 (very variable – see text)	35	40
Energy	kcal/l	600–>800	600–750	600–800
Minerals	Na (mmol/l)	7	12	20
	K (mmol/l)	15	20	39
	Ca (mmol/l)	9	10	30
	Mg (mmo /l)	1	3	5
	P (mmol/l)	5	14	30
	Ca:P ratio (by weight)	2:1	0.5:1 to 2:1	1.3:1
	Fe (mmol/l)	0.014	0.125	0.01

Data for composition of infant formula are taken from *The Infant Formula and Follow-on Formula Regulations, 1995* (Statutory Instrument 1995 No. 77), taking the mid-point of the legally permissible range unless otherwise stated. Data for composition of cow's milk and human milk are taken from Williams (1991).
[a]See note in the text about the uncertainty surrounding the true (nutritional) protein content of human milk.

evidence that much of this can be salvaged in the colon. For these reasons the true, nutritionally available, protein content of breastmilk is not easily measurable and cannot be simply expressed as a fraction of the total nitrogen content.

The economic utilization of the nitrogenous compounds in breastmilk to match the demands of growth helps to prevent the accumulation of urea, which would otherwise need to be eliminated through the kidneys. This, together with the low macroelement content, minimizes the PRSL of breastmilk to the extent that the breastfed baby need not be offered additional free water to facilitate renal solute clearance. Thus breastmilk is entirely sufficient as both a food and a drink for the first six months of life.

Establishment of breastfeeding

The endocrine control of lactation ensures that breastmilk supply matches demands made by the infant sucking. In practical terms the key requirements for successful establishment of breastfeeding at birth are:

- unrestricted access to the breast when the infant is hungry, and
- effective milk removal by the infant.

Many clinical problems with breastfeeding, for example breast pain, cracked and sore nipples, mastitis, early dehydration, and poor weight gain, result from errors of breastfeeding technique which hamper the second of these requirements. In order for the baby to remove milk from the breast effectively he or she must be properly positioned (or held correctly by the mother) and attached at the breast (i.e. take sufficient breast tissue into the mouth, not just the nipple). An account of the skills required to assess and correct such problems is beyond the scope of this text, but early referral to a professional skilled in breastfeeding management is essential should such problems develop.

Consumption of breastmilk

The volume of breastmilk consumed by a breastfeeding baby has been measured in a number of ways. The oldest is 'test-weighing' – measuring the difference in the baby's (or occasionally the mother's) weight before and after a feed. Although improvements in the accuracy of scales have reduced the errors inherent in weighing a moving baby, there remains considerable variation in the volume of milk consumed from day to day. The procedure is also intrusive and may alter the

mother and baby's feeding pattern, making measurements of limited value. For these reasons test-weighing is no longer used for clinical purposes, the best measurement of breastfeeding adequacy being the baby's growth rate. Measurements of the breastmilk intake of 'free living' breastfed babies have been made using isotopic dilution techniques, administering either ^2H_2O or $^2H_2{}^{18}O$ to the baby or mother and baby. These suggest that breastfed babies consume some 400–800 ml/day of breast milk.

The composition of the milk which the baby consumes is also difficult to measure, because it changes during the feed. A number of solutions to this problem have been tried:

- *Expressing the entire content of the breasts at a feed.* An objection to this is that the baby may not remove all milk from the breast, but choose to leave some behind. Because the fat concentration rises progressively as the breast empties the expressed sample may overestimate the energy content of milk consumed.
- *Expressing samples before and after a feed.* This technique has been widely used, but the assumption that changes in concentration follow a linear trend during a feed may not be valid.
- *Doubly-labeled water ($^2H_2{}^{18}O$) technique.* As the ^{18}O exchanges with both the CO_2 and ^2H-labeled water pools, differences in the rate of elimination can be used to calculate both energy expenditure and milk intake, allowing energy intake to be inferred (see chapter 2 in *Introduction to Human Nutrition* in this series).

Formula feeding

Unmodified animal milks (for example cow's milk) are unsuitable for young infants for several reasons:

- protein and mineral content impose too high an RSL,
- micronutrient content (e.g. iron, folic acid, vitamin D, vitamin A) is inadequate, and
- fat and protein are relatively indigestible.

When a mother chooses not to breastfeed, therefore, the infant should be fed an infant formula. According to UK (*The Infant Formula and Follow-on Formula Regulations, 1995* define the terms 'infant formula' and 'follow-on formula,' setting out legally permissible minimum and maximum nutrient concentrations) and European law this label defines a commercial product which provides the nutritional requirements of infants in good health for the first 4–6 months of life, as set out in legally enforceable compositional requirements.

Infant formula is based on a cow's milk or soy protein source, the amount and type of protein (whey : casein ratio) being adjusted to match better the baby's metabolic needs. The carbohydrate moiety of infant formula is usually supplied by lactose and other permissible carbohydrates (Table 22.4) in amounts intended to approximate those of breastmilk (about 70 g/l). Vegetable oil blends usually provide the fat: these are substituted for cow's milk fat because it is less digestible, having a higher saturated fatty acid content. The mineral content of infant formulas is also adjusted. Notably the sodium content is reduced and the ratio of calcium : phosphorus increased. Finally infant formulas are fully supplemented with trace minerals and vitamins.

In order to avoid the complications associated with use of animal milks the non-breastfed infant should receive infant formula for at least the first 12 months of life – alone for the first 4–6 months and later as part of a progressively diversified weaning diet (see 'complementary feeding' below). Infants over six months are, however, sometimes given a follow-on formula. The composition of 'follow-on formulas' is legally defined in UK and European law but, unlike infant formulas, they are not required to meet the infant's whole nutritional requirements. Like infant formulas, they are micronutrient enriched and promoted principally for their value in preventing iron deficiency. Although there is good evidence that they are superior to whole cow's milk in this respect they have not been shown to be any better than infant formula, which remains a suitable choice at this age for the non-breastfed infant.

All powdered infant formulas need careful reconstitution:

- All utensils must be sterilized.
- Water must be boiled and of appropriate electrolyte composition. It should be tap water drawn from the mains supply (not through an ion exchange softener) or a bottled water of similar composition. The main concern here is the sodium concentration: EU regulations set a maximum [Na] of 200 mg/l at the tap.

- Level measures in the correct measuring scoop (usually supplied with the tin) must be used.
- Powder should be added to the measured amount amount of water, not vice versa, or the feed may be hazardously overconcentrated.

The amount of formula infants consume averages about 150 ml/kg per day at 2–3 months of age. However this is merely a guideline and, as with breastfeeding, there is large interindividual variation. For example in a well-known study of a group of three-month-old American infants consumption varied from 120 to over 220 ml/kg per day.

Key points on infant formula are summarized in Box 22.9.

Box 22.9 Infant formula

- An infant formula is based on modified cow's milk or soya protein
- It is designed to provide the nutritional requirements of healthy, full-term infants for the first 4–6 months of life
- Extensive modification of cow's milk reduces potential renal solute load, enhances protein quality, alters macronutrient balance, and adjusts Ca : P ratio
- Infant formula is enriched with trace minerals and vitamins
- Powdered infant formulas must be reconstituted carefully, according to the manufacturer's instructions
- The amount of formula consumed averages about 150 ml/kg per day at 3 months of age, but varies greatly between babies

---

Complementary feeding

Complementary feeding is the introduction of foods other than breastmilk or infant formula into the infant's diet. The term is now generally considered preferable to 'weaning' which misleadingly implied a role in the cessation of breastfeeding. In fact the primary role of complementary feeding is rather to increase dietary diversity, not to reduce breastmilk intake. Complementary foods themselves are sometimes also referred to in the literature as beikost (USA) or solids (UK).

Although complementary feeding is generally thought of as a mechanism for increasing the nutrient density of the diet, it serves a number of other developmental functions too (see section on neurological maturation). There has been much controversy over the optimum time at which to introduce foods other than breastmilk into the infant's diet. Introducing them too early will undesirably increase renal solute load, increase the risk of infection, compromise the maintenance of lactational amenorrhea, and possibly expose the infant too early to dietary antigens such as gluten (see Chapter 7). Leaving complementary feeding too late may, on the other hand, impair growth because the nutrient density of a liquid diet is relatively low. Moreover, the concentrations of some important micronutrients in breastmilk, particularly zinc, declines with the length of lactation.

Historically a number of different philosophical approaches have been applied to defining the appropriate age for introducing complementary foods:

- *Factorial calculation* of the intake required to support 'optimal growth.' If the expected rate of growth is known it is possible to calculate what energy intake is required after making allowance for losses and maintenance expenditure. Although this approach seems intuitively sensible, considerable problems arise in agreeing what is meant by 'optimal growth' and it is now acknowledged that many growth references (such as NCHS) do not accurately describe the early growth pattern of breastfed infants. The use of such charts was one factor which led to the overestimation of the energy and protein requirements of growing breastfed infants. Others were underestimation of breastmilk intake and miscalculation of the nutrient content of breastmilk. Better estimation of these quantities subsequently led to a postponement of the recommended age for complementary feeding from 'about 3 months' to '4–6 months.' More recently recommendations have been further revised to 'about 6 months' on the basis of evidence discussed below.
- *Consideration of developmental and biological factors.* An alternative way of considering the problem is to ask by what age infants are developmentally prepared to receive foods other than breastmilk. Maturation of neurological, gastrointestinal, renal, and immune function can be taken into account and considered together with available data on the morbidity associated with complementary feeding at particular ages. On this basis the World Health Organization (WHO) review concluded that exclusive breastfeeding can be continued with benefit for 'about the first six months' in healthy infants of appropriate birth weight, though alternative strategies may need to be considered for at-risk groups such as those of low birth weight.
- *Controlled studies of interventions.* A limited amount of information is available from small controlled

trials conducted in a less-developed country setting. Commercially prepared complementary foods were introduced at four or six months and the effects on growth and breastmilk intake studied. Introduction at four months did not confer a detectable growth advantage although it was associated with a reduced breastmilk intake. Clearly such studies are difficult to perform and a particular problem with the controlled work described was differential dropout from the study groups, which could have biased the findings.

Taking all this evidence together there seems no good reason to suppose that introduction of complementary foods earlier than six months benefits the majority of breastfed infants. Diversification of the diet in infancy is a gradual process which needs to be conducted at a pace compatible with the infant's development. Initially foods need to be pureed and are offered from a spoon 2–3 times a day after breastfeeds. As they are accepted the amount offered can be increased and the consistency allowed to change. Home-prepared foods must be puréed at this stage and salt, sugar, and strong spices must not be added. Once liquids are well accepted solid foods which will dissolve in the mouth (e.g. banana, toast) offer a useful stage in the transition to finely, then coarsely, chopped and ultimately lumpier foods which require chewing or which the infant can hold. The eventual aim should be that by one year of age the infant is having three main meals a day, plus snacks and 3–4 breastfeeds to supply the fluid portion.

Key points on growth and complementary feeding are listed in Box 22.10.

Effect of feeding on infant growth

Breastfed and bottlefed infants show different patterns

Box 22.10 Growth and complementary feeding

- The timing of complementary feeding should reflect the pace of the individual baby's development
- Controlled studies suggest that introducing complementary foods at four months (as opposed to six months) does not lead to faster growth but is associated with compensatory reduction in breastmilk intake
- Breast- and bottlefed babies show different patterns of growth in the first year of life, breastfed babies being lighter at a year of age
- There is no evidence that these growth differences are due to shortage of breastmilk
- The mechanisms which explain these growth differences and their long-term significance are currently unclear

of growth in early life. Figure 22.13 illustrates this. Breastfed infants gain weight particularly rapidly in the first two months, but velocity then slows relative to the NCHS norms (see previous section on growth). This trend was once believed to signify 'growth faltering' as a consequence of inadequate breastmilk supply but more recent work has shown that it occurs amongst breastfed infants in all societies, and that weight gain is not influenced by introduction of solids at four or at six months. Bottlefed infants, on the other hand, show sustained weight gain above NCHS norms throughout the first year of life. The reasons for these differences are currently unclear, though they may represent the effect of different protein intakes on the release of insulin and insulin-like growth factors. Whatever the mechanism, there is current speculation that they influence metabolic programming and explain the predisposition of bottlefed babies to be fatter than breastfed ones in later childhood.

It is important to note the breastfed baby's growth pattern when giving clinical advice so that an initial tendency to veer upwards on the growth chart, followed by a tendency to cross downwards is not attributed to feeding problems. Rather it is a problem with currently available charts. (Note, however, that the average magnitude of this effect is unlikely to result in the crossing of more than 1 centile line when plotted on a UK 1990 growth reference chart.) For this reason the WHO is compiling a new growth reference, based on

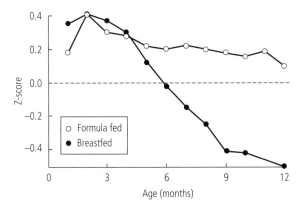

Figure 22.13 Differences in weight gain between breastfed and bottlefed infants. The curves show weight as variation (in fractions of a *z*-score) from the 50th centile of NCHS reference. Thus breastfed babies, on average, quickly rise 0.4 standard deviations above the 50th centile then fall 0.4 standard deviations below by the end of the first year of life. Adapted from Dewey *et al.* (1995, 1993).

the growth of infants in various countries exclusively breastfed for the first 4–6 months.

Dietary supplements in infancy

Vitamin K
All babies should receive vitamin K at birth, in order to prevent hemorrhagic disease of the newborn (HDN), a rare but potentially fatal bleeding disorder. 'Classical' HDN occurs in approximately 1/10 000 unsupplemented infants during the first week of life. It usually presents as apparently innocuous bleeding from, for example, the umbilicus, scalp, or gut. If unheeded such 'warnings' may be followed by major internal (e.g. intracranial) hemorrhage with significant morbidity and mortality. More rarely HDN can present later on in the early months of life. Unfortunately this 'late' form often presents only after severe bleeding has already occurred. Consequently it is associated with high risk of death or lifelong disability. Breastfed babies are at greater risk than bottlefed babies because infant formula is supplemented with vitamin K. Babies who are preterm, delivered instrumentally, or have liver disease are also more commonly affected, as are those whose mothers are taking certain drugs, notably anticonvulsants.

Vitamin K can be given orally or intramuscularly. The intramuscular route is associated with lowest risk of both early and late HDN (about 1 per million births) and is therefore the route of choice for all those in high-risk groups (see above). It is, however, unpopular with some parents because a case–control study some ten years ago suggested an association between childhood leukemia and intramuscular, but not oral, administration. Fortunately subsequent work has not substantiated this. If chosen, oral dosing should be repeated, at least at the end of the first week and then monthly whilst exclusively breastfeeding. A number of oral dosing regimens are in use though their relative safety and efficacy has not yet been determined.

The fat-soluble form of vitamin K, phytomenadione, is currently used for neonatal administration. Early reports of the induction of hemolytic jaundice by vitamin K were associated with the water-soluble analogue acetomenaphthone, which is no longer used.

Vitamin drops
Supplementary vitamins A, C, and D (in the form of

'children's vitamin drops') are advised for all children under two years of age in the UK. In the case of breast-fed babies they should be started from about six months of age, but they may be deferred until one year of age in babies fed infant formula (which is fortified). Vitamin D is probably the most important component of the drops, particularly among high-risk ethnic groups in whom clinical rickets is still seen. In a UK national study some 20–30% of toddlers from Asian backgrounds had low (<25 nmol/l) plasma concentrations of 25-hydroxy vitamin D, about a half of whom had levels typically associated with rickets. UK recommendations therefore suggest that vitamin drops are started much earlier in these groups, from about 2–3 months of age.

Special circumstances

Some groups of infants have particular nutritional needs, including preterm and low birth weight infants (i.e. those born before 37 completed weeks of gestation or weighing <2.5 kg at birth). These reflect low nutrient stores, high growth potential, and the need to catch-up on, for example, bone mineralization. These infants should receive a multivitamin supplement soon after birth, normally until at least two years of age.

Low birth weight (LBW) infants are particularly vulnerable to iron deficiency in later infancy or early in the second year of life. This so-called late anemia of prematurity arises because expansion of the blood volume with growth exhausts iron reserves present at birth. These are limited because most (about 75%) of the body iron is in the form of hemoglobin and preterm babies have both a slightly lower hemoglobin concentration and low blood volume (about 80 ml/kg of body weight). Iron supplements are usually prescribed for LBW infants from about one month of age and continued until complementary feeding is well established. Iron is not started earlier because it favors colonization of the gut with coliform organisms.

Key points relating to dietary supplements are summarized in Box 22.11.

22.5 Preschool children

Children between one and five years of age remain at significant risk of undernutrition. They are still growing rapidly but have not fully developed independent feeding skills: in the earlier years of this era they remain totally dependent on an adult.

Box 22.11 Dietary supplements

- Infancy is a period of rapid tissue deposition: reference nutrient intakes for certain vitamins at this age are high and may not be met by diet
- Vitamin supplements are therefore recommended as a safety net to catch vulnerable individuals in the population
- All newborn babies should be given vitamin K to prevent hemorrhagic disease of the newborn
- Breastfed babies should receive supplements of vitamins A, C, and D from about six months until at least two years of age
- Formula-fed babies should receive them from about one year
- Vulnerable groups (e.g. dark skinned) may benefit from commencing vitamin D from about two months onwards
- Low birth weight infants are at greater risk of iron deficiency and should receive iron supplements with multivitamins for at least the first six months

---

Common dietary problems of young children

By about a year of age a child should be established on a pattern of three meals per day plus snacks and breastfeeds. Even at this stage breastmilk (or formula/cow's milk) will be providing about a quarter of the energy and about a third of protein requirements. In situations where food is short, sustained breastfeeding into the second year therefore acts as an important nutritional safety net; indeed cessation of breastfeeding associated with the arrival of another baby at this stage can be a factor that precipitates malnutrition. Globally, continued insufficiency of food into the second year of life is a prime cause of chronic energy deficiency, manifesting as 'stunting' or restricted linear growth. This failure to achieve growth potential as a consequence of chronic food shortage in early life remains the commonest manifestation of nutritional deficiency today (see earlier section on growth).

In industrialized countries nutritional problems of a different sort arise and commonly present to primary care services. Growth may falter ('failure-to-thrive') because of problems with the establishment of an appropriate eating pattern even where there is an abundance of food in the household. Parents may, for example, offer excessive amounts of milk or fruit juice, often because solids are refused. In these circumstances it is advisable to limit milk intake to <600 ml/day, and continue to offer three meals. Uneaten food should merely be removed and no more offered until the next mealtime. The temptation to coax or force young children into eating should always be resisted as it is usually counterproductive and negatively reinforces eating behavior.

Sometimes growth failure may occur even in the presence of normal meal patterns because the energy density of the diet is inadequate. Parents may be relatively affluent and deliberately offer foods which they perceive as 'healthy,' for example high in fiber and low in fat. This has been labeled 'muesli malnutrition'. Its occurrence emphasizes that energy needs at this stage are still relatively high and that fat plays a role in providing a diet of sufficient energy density. The transition from the young infant's milk diet in which 50% of energy is provided by fat to an adult-appropriate target of <35% must occur gradually over the first five years. To facilitate this full-fat milk should be used until the age of two, when it may be replaced by semi-skimmed. Skimmed milk and low-fat spreads are unsuitable dietary items for under-fives.

Excessive consumption of fruit juice or squash is also common in toddlers. Recent evidence suggests that the 'squash syndrome' can be associated with growth failure (short, fat children) and that the drinks replace the intake of more nutritious food. This suggests that the overall dietary intake does not allow children to reach their genetic potential in height, but leads to a deposition of excess energy. Consumption of squash may even be so high as to cause diarrhea and provoke suspicion of malabsorption. Frequent loose stools, often containing undigested vegetable material, are generally a very common problem in this age group but almost always innocuous and associated with normal growth. This presentation is described as 'toddler diarrhea'. It is probably related to an immature pattern of small bowel motility and can sometimes be ameliorated by increasing dietary fat intake to enhance ileal braking.

Preschool children are also vulnerable to micronutrient deficiencies, notably of vitamin A, iron, vitamin D, and zinc. These are particularly common in resource-poor countries and multifactorial in origin. Low birth weight (hence low stores) and chronic low intake are compounded by both increased urinary losses during recurrent acute infection and chronic gastrointestinal losses caused by parasite infestation (such as hookworm). Children in industrialized countries are not however immune to micronutrient deficiency. Iron deficiency, hypovitaminosis D, and even frank rickets are often seen, particularly amongst children from South Asian and Afro-Caribbean backgrounds.

Behavioral eating problems in young children

Eating problems are very common among toddlers, and cause much concern to parents. Some degree of faddism and food refusal can however be construed as a normal phase of toddler development, provided it does not persist or lead to overt signs of nutrient deficiency (such as failure-to-thrive, see Section 22.7 on undernutrition).

Sometimes more persistent eating problems are encountered. These include such things as severely selective eating (e.g. jam sandwiches, chocolate biscuits) and eating food of inappropriate texture (e.g. the child will take only liquids or puréed food and spits out lumps). Another prevalent problem in children who have required nutritional support as the result of illness in early in life is difficulty withdrawing tube feeding and establishing an eating pattern.

Problems such as these almost never have a basis in organic disease but develop out of a complex variety of etiologic factors including:

- early aversive experience of eating, e.g. vomiting or choking on particular foods, force-feeding during weaning or use of inappropriate complementary foods,
- abnormal developmental experiences, and
- conflict with parents.

These may be reinforced by neglect, abuse, parental disagreement, and lack of support. The primary management of such problems is behavioral. A multidisciplinary team approach is most successful, coordinating the skills of psychologist, dietitian, health visitor, and, if necessary, a speech and language therapist to assist with the assessment of swallowing. The nutritional aim is ultimately to provide normal food in sufficient quantities, not to resort to supplements or other nutritional interventions as a means of increasing intake. Indeed to do so may actually be counter-productive and 'medicalize' the problem. Solving it can take time and persistence. Thus it may be necessary to accept suboptimal intake in the short term in the interests of long-term gain associated with establishing normal dietary patterns.

Key nutritional points on young children are listed in Box 22.12.

> **Box 22.12** Young children
>
> - Young children are still growing relatively quickly and have high nutrient requirements
> - Successful transition to a varied diet and the establishment of eating patterns can be demanding on parenting skills
> - Behavioral eating problems are common in this age group and require multidisciplinary management. Coaxing or force-feeding must always be avoided
> - Globally children are at high risk of chronic energy deficiency (causing stunting) and several specific micronutrient deficiencies

22.6 Schoolchildren and adolescents

Children of this age can eat independently of a carer, and by completion of adolescence are capable of providing for themselves – indeed capable of reproducing and caring for their offspring. The emergence of independence is associated with nutritional problems of a different sort: children are learning to make choices of their own and this has many implications. They are a population susceptible to marketing and peer-group influences which will impact on both patterns of diet and activity. For the health educator nutritional education at this age has at least the potential to influence habits for life. Many of the overt problems which present to health services during this era of development are related to the behavioral extremes of lifestyle choice, for example childhood overweight, obesity, and adolescent eating disorders.

National data collected in the UK show that in addition to these conditions the diet and activity patterns of schoolchildren and adolescents are cause for concern. Low consumption of vegetables and fruit and increasing reliance on snack and 'fast' food eaten outside the home are associated with low intakes of many micronutrients. Reduced activity levels, particularly amongst adolescent girls, can be expected to impact unfavorably in several areas: they may partially explain the increasing prevalence of fatness and obesity, and can be expected to affect adversely the attainment of peak bone mass (see Chapter 18).

Eating disorders

Although a number of disordered eating presentations have been described in this age group, anorexia nervosa and bulimia nervosa are the most frequently encountered, the former being commonest (see Chapter 6). These syndromes share many features, particularly overconcern with body weight and shape, but are distinguished by the pattern of intake. In bulimia food is consumed (often in large quantities – 'bingeing') and then eliminated through vomiting or purgation, whereas food refusal and preoccupation with exercise predominate in anorexia. Children from higher socio-economic groups are more frequently affected: often they are high achievers with perfectionist or frankly obsessive traits but they lack self-esteem. Their overwhelming ambition is to be thin. Family psychodynamics are often complex and the presentation is believed to indicate the child's attempt for autonomy and self-control in some area of life. It is also argued that the illness represents an attempt to regress from puberty, but this has been questioned on the grounds that it may present before indications of puberty appear.

The prevalence of eating disorders amongst adolescents and young adults appears to be increasing in western countries, where it has always been more common than in the developing world. Psychosocial and media pressures stigmatizing obesity and associating thinness with success have probably contributed to this trend.

The classical form of anorexia described in young adults differs in an important respect from that encountered in children. When anorexia nervosa presents during (or sometimes before) puberty it will significantly delay progression of endocrine development and the pubertal growth spurt (see Section 22.2 on growth). In most cases recovery is accompanied by resumption of progress through puberty with full attainment of final height, breast development, and commencement of menstruation. However in some severe, chronic cases puberty is arrested with prolonged delay in appearance of menses and ultimately a deficit in final height. It is also worth remembering that although classical (postmenarchal) anorexia affects almost exclusively women, boys are occasionally affected both before and during puberty.

The presentation of anorexia in young girls may be quite insidious. Preoccupation with exercise, calorie counting, and static weight (or loss of small amounts) may at first be viewed as normal. Overt refusal of food becomes apparent only later, often after the child has resorted to other strategies such as hiding food, exercising in secret, or abusing laxatives. Detection at an early stage may be compatible with management in the community but later admission to hospital may become necessary. Criteria for inpatient management include:

- weight <80% of expected weight-for-height,
- dehydration, hyperkalemia, and peripheral circulatory failure,
- persistent vomiting (sometimes hematemesis), and
- evidence of complicating psychiatric features (usually depression).

The management of children with anorexia nervosa is difficult and the disease has a significant mortality over the long term, variously estimated at between 2% and 10%. It is essential that a multidisciplinary approach is followed, coordinated by the psychiatric team with input from a pediatric dietitian, and pediatrician. The general principles of nutritional management are as follows:

- Parents are made responsible for the child's eating as the key to resuming health. Initially this can cause resentment and objection on the part of the child, but this can sometimes be traded against freedom to choose in other aspects of lifestyle.
- A target weight range needs to be agreed with the child and parents (usually in the range 90–100% of expected weight-for-height).
- Once electrolyte deficiencies and hydration state have been corrected, refeeding is instituted (see Section 22.7 on undernutrition). Competing needs to replete tissue with the child's sensitivities to eating large amounts of food will need to be balanced. Attempting immediate hyperalimentation will be counterproductive, and it is better to increase amounts of normal food more gradually. Although children can participate if they wish by discussing the daily menu it is important not to hand over control at this early stage. A multivitamin supplement is usually given, although clinical micronutrient deficiency is not so common as might perhaps be expected given the degree of weight loss present.
- Sometimes (in the face of severe weight loss, dehydration, or persistent refusal to eat) it may prove necessary to embark on enteral nutritional support or parenteral therapy. If so, it can be made clear that the amount of support will be reduced as more oral diet is accepted.

Clearly these steps must be instituted hand-in-hand with psychotherapeutic measures addressing the child's underlying problems, her relationships with family and friends, and her continuing education (bearing in mind that absence from her school may be prolonged).

Key nutritional points on schoolchildren and adolescents are listed in Box 22.13.

> **Box 22.13** Schoolchildren and adolescents
>
> - At this stage children are developing, and learning to assert, their independence. Many nutritional problems arise from this
> - Children of this age are vulnerable to media and peer-group influences
> - Eating disorders – bulimia and anorexia – are common in young girls, and can occur before puberty
> - They may also occur in boys, but are much less common
> - The management of eating disorders is complex and demands a multidisciplinary approach in consultation with both the child and the family
> - Correction of undernutrition and re-establishment of normal eating patterns cannot be achieved quickly

22.7 Undernutrition in children

Causes of undernutrition

Childhood undernutrition has many origins: psychological disturbance, socioeconomic deprivation, and underlying illness. All may act in concert and the treatment of undernutrition therefore involves more than the mere provision of nutrients. For example, interventions may be needed at societal level to increase food supply, at family level to improve parenting skills, and with the child to treat associated problems such as infection.

Nutritional assessment (see also Chapter 2)

A child's nutritional status is assessed by taking a history, performing a physical examination (including anthropometry) and, sometimes, performing special investigations.

Key points on nutritional assessment in children are shown in Box 22.14.

History
The history should be taken from the parent, carer, or close relative and must be thorough because nutritional status at the time of consultation reflects what has happened since conception. For example a school-age child may be small because of severe fetal growth

Box 22.14 Nutritional assessment in children

- History, examination, and special investigations provide complementary information
- The history must encompass details of the child's previous life, including the pregnancy
- The examination must include anthropometry and assessment of growth
- Growth measurements provide information about body composition and body function (adequacy of growth)

retardation, critical illness, or malnutrition in early life from which catch-up has been incomplete, leading to stunting.

Questions asked may include:

- *Pregnancy and birth.* Was the pregnancy uncomplicated or was fetal growth slow? What was the gestation at birth and the birth weight? Were there neonatal illnesses (which might have led to early postnatal growth failure)?
- *Infant feeding.* Was the child breastfed or formula-fed? When was the child first given foods other than milk and what where they (specifically, when were gluten-containing foods started)? Did the child thrive in infancy? If not, when were there first concerns? Was there vomiting or diarrhea in infancy? Were dietary supplements (such as iron or vitamins) given?
- *Developmental history.* Enquiry should be made into 'milestones' to ensure that developmental delay or motor disability have not caused feeding difficulty.
- *Current dietary history.* Recent intake of food and fluids. If breastfeeding: has there been any change in feeding pattern, and has the mother experienced any problems such as pain or mastitis? If formula feeding: what is being given, how exactly is the mother making up the feeds, and how much is consumed? For older children enquiries should be made about change of appetite, meal patterns, behavior disturbance, and food refusal. Is the child considered to be intolerant of particular foods, and why?
- *Family history.* How tall and heavy are the parents and siblings? Is there any family history of food intolerance or gastrointestinal problems?
- *Social history.* Who is/are the child's primary carer(s) throughout the day; what are the family's dietary habits?

- *Illness.* Ask particularly about diarrhea and vomiting, features of malabsorption, chronic disease, recurrent and recent acute infections.

Clinical examination

- Weight and height should be measured, recorded, and plotted on a growth chart. Head (occipito-frontal) circumference is also measured routinely in infancy and other measurements such as mid-arm circumference, triceps, and subscapular skinfolds may be made as appropriate. Previous measurements are usually easily obtainable from sources such as the parent-held child health record (a multi-disciplinary record of the child's medical care which parents in the UK are encouraged to bring to all consultations).
- Note the child's affect: malnourished children are withdrawn and miserable; 'frozen watchfulness' may signify neglect.
- Assess the child's development. Infants and toddlers who show developmental delay may fail to thrive because of difficulty communicating their needs, or problems with handling, chewing, and swallowing food.
- Look for signs of micronutrient deficiency such as pallor (iron deficiency), dermatoses, cheilosis (B vitamin deficiencies), xerophthalmia (vitamin A deficiency), acrodermatitis (zinc deficiency), goiter (iodine deficiency).
- In older children note the pubertal stage attained: chronically undernourished children or those with growth failure attributable to chronic disease often undergo late puberty and allowance may be needed for this, particularly where cross-sectional growth references are being applied.
- Conduct a full systemic examination, looking especially for signs such as muscle wasting, abdominal distension, heart murmurs (sometimes due to high cardiac output in anemia).

Anthropometric measurements can provide two kinds of information: body proportions (BMI or weight-for-height; Figure 22.14) and body function (adequacy of growth – if a series of measurements is available).

Special investigations

In circumstances where special investigations are feasible those chosen will clearly depend on the findings of

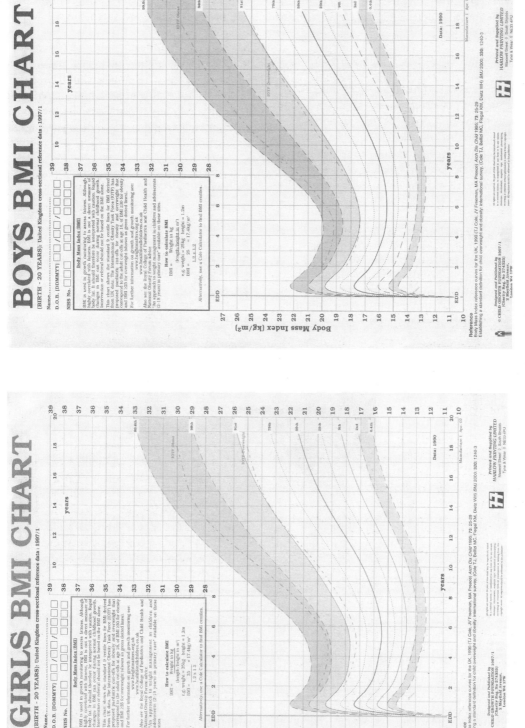

Figure 22.14 Body mass index (BMI) charts. These charts are drawn from the UK 1990 reference. Note the earlier 'adiposity rebound' (upward inflection preceding puberty) amongst the heavier children. Reproduced from Cole *et al.* (1995) with permission of the BMJ Publishing Group.

history and examination. The possibilities are numerous but they can help in assessment of status by providing information in complementary ways (see Chapter 2). Examples include:

- Assessment of nutrient balance (e.g. microscopy of stool for fat globules in infants failing to thrive, urinary sodium concentration in preterm infants).
- Assessment of body composition (e.g. hemoglobin and serum ferritin as measures of iron stores; X-ray of wrist for features of rickets).
- Assessment of metabolic and physiological function (e.g. plasma alkaline phosphatase as a measure of bone turnover; X-ray of wrist to assess bone age).

Screening for malnutrition

Opportunistic weighing of babies and young children is common in primary care, for example when immunizations are given during the first six months. Nevertheless, for reasons previously stated, the interpretation of weight measurements at this age can be difficult: catch-up and catch-down growth associated with 'regression to the mean' during the first year (see Section 22.2 on growth) mean that a proportion of normal babies cross weight-centile lines on the growth chart. In the case of the UK 1990 growth reference, up to 5% of children under two cross two centile spaces down, and about 1% three centile spaces. It follows that, where serial measurements are available, any baby who has crossed two centile spaces, particularly in less than a year, needs close assessment (see section on failure-to-thrive).

A good deal of thought has been given to the problem of correcting mathematically for the phenomenon of regression to the mean and thereby separating more objectively babies who are merely 'catching-down' from those who are failing to thrive. These include calculation of the 'thrive index' and the use of 'thrive lines' (available as a transparent overlay for the growth chart). These do, however, have practical problems and it may be better to view all children crossing centile channels downwards as warranting close observation and further assessment. Recommendations about centile crossing are complex, vary with age, and initial centile position. There are no internationally agreed cut-off points for application throughout childhood, although tentative suggestions have been made for

certain age ranges. The direction of change, and likely future changes are also important considerations.

Where only single measurements are available, any child who measures <0.4th centile for weight or length on the chart requires early medical assessment: only 4 in 1000 normal children can be expected to be so small, so the chance that an abnormality is present is quite high. A baby weighing <9th centile should be weighed again after an interval of at least two weeks, and repeatedly until it is established that the growth trajectory is satisfactory.

Failure-to-thrive

'Failure-to thrive' (FTT) is a term used to describe slow weight gain in the infant and young child. It is not in itself a diagnosis, but implies that growth (usually in weight) is faltering pathologically and does not merely reflect simple interindividual variations in patterns of growth.

Key points on failure-to-thrive are listed in Box 22.15.

Box 22.15 Failure-to-thrive

- Failure-to-thrive (FTT) is a term used to describe inadequate growth (most commonly weight gain) in the early years of life
- FTT is evident as downward crossing of two or more centile spaces on a growth chart
- FTT needs to be distinguished from other causes of centile crossing, such as 'catch-down' growth
- FTT can be caused by underlying illness but is most commonly due to low intake of nutrients, particularly energy
- Low intake can arise through physical illness, but is most commonly a reflection of parenting difficulty
- Sometimes FTT is a consequence of neglect or abuse
- The management of FTT requires a coordinated multidisciplinary approach to increasing the intake of normal food. Prescription of dietary supplements is not the solution

---

The underlying cause of FTT is chronic energy insufficiency. This may result from many causes, simply classified as:

- inadequate intake (e.g. a breastfeeding problem, inadequate parenting, frank neglect, or abuse),
- excessive losses (e.g. vomiting and regurgitation, diarrhea and malabsorption, high resting energy expenditure in acute infection, or chronic disease), and
- abnormal nutrient partitioning.

Note that these factors usually operate in combination, rather than independently. For example children with infection will become anorexic, may vomit and often show increased urinary losses of trace minerals and vitamins. Resting energy expenditure may be increased in the presence of fever and tachycardia, and nutrient demands of the immune system increased. Following infection there will be increased nutrient (particularly energy) requirements to meet the demands of 'catch-up' growth (see also Section 22.8 on nutrition as treatment).

It is important to recognize that growth faltering in an industrialized country is usually 'non-organic' in origin (see Figure 22.15). Low food (particularly energy) intake may result from some combination of the following:

- developmental abnormality,
- oral-motor dysfunction,
- abnormal mealtime interactions with a carer,
- feeding insufficient amounts, either as the result of parental perceptions or poor appetite in the child, and

- sometimes frank neglect, physical or emotional abuse.

The management of these problems demands a multi-disciplinary approach, directed at identifying and rectifying the eating problem – rather than resort to special formulas or food. The first step is direct observation at mealtimes, preferably in the child's home environment. Video-recording can assist later review or facilitate sharing of information with other professionals. Problems may then be addressed in a coordinated fashion by appropriate disciplines. For example, a dietitian may be able to make simple recommendations about food choices to increase the nutrient density of meals. A physiotherapist or occupational therapist might advise on improving the child's positioning at mealtimes and a speech and language therapist may be able to identify disordered oral-motor function. These aspects are particularly suitable if there is coexisting developmental delay or neuromuscular disability.

In summary, failure-to-thrive amongst young children in industrialized countries is most commonly the

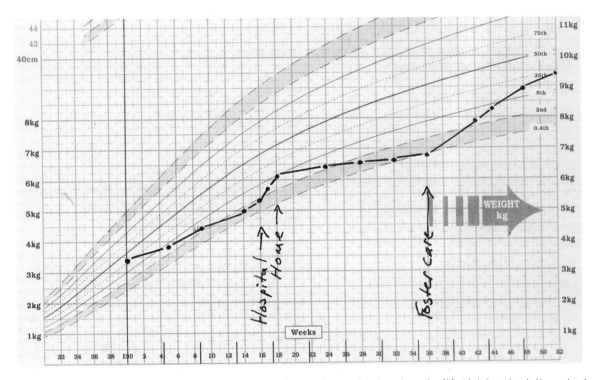

Figure 22.15 Failure-to-thrive. The baby's weight has crossed three centile spaces downwards in the early months of life. Admission to hospital is associated with rapid weight gain followed by a further period of growth faltering. Rapid catch-up then occurs in foster care. This pattern of growth is typical of parental neglect.

result of chronic energy deficiency arising from inappropriate care practices, rather than underlying physical disease or food shortage. The treatment is predominantly behavioral and directed at rectifying the deficit in intake of normal food. Mere prescription of food supplements or nutrient-enriched formulas is neither an appropriate nor sustainable solution in the majority of instances. Such measures should be reserved for the infant with disturbed energy balance as the result of underlying chronic illness (for example of the cardiac or respiratory system) requiring nutritional support.

Severe malnutrition

Severe undernutrition in children is life threatening. Injudicious treatment is itself dangerous and can increase mortality further. Most severe primary undernutrition occurs in resource-poor countries, though it can occur in industrialized countries too – for example as the result of anorexia in teenagers. It may also develop as the result of severe underlying disease. Whatever the cause, and wherever severe undernutrition occurs, some common principles apply to its assessment and treatment. In particular it is important that the metabolic perturbations which are associated with chronic energy deficiency are corrected at an appropriately gradual pace to prevent refeeding syndrome (see Chapter 8).

Diagnosis

Classically, two patterns of malnutrition were recognized in young children. These were known as kwashiorkor (edematous malnutrition, most commonly in the young child) and marasmus (severe wasting, usually in infancy). Recently a more unifying treatment approach has been adopted though weight measurements must always be interpreted carefully for two important reasons:

- Presence of edema ('pitting' elicited by applying digital pressure over feet and ankles) will cause the child's true body weight to be overestimated.
- Absence of edema may mean the child's low weight is due to chronic energy insufficiency (or 'stunting') rather than recent weight loss (or 'wasting'). Thus weight must be interpreted along with a measurement of length (or height if over two years of age).

Assessment of wasting and stunting

A 'stunted' child is below his or her appropriate height-for-age, whereas a 'wasted' child is under the appropriate weight-for-height. Severity of stunting can be calculated from the child's height as a percentage of the median (50th percentile) height for one of that age. Similarly the degree of wasting can be expressed by calculating the child's weight as a percentage of the weight which would be appropriate for a child of that height and age. The latter can be estimated by first plotting the child's height against age on a growth chart to establish the percentile line on which it falls. The weight associated with the corresponding percentile for age is then read off the weight chart (Figure 22.16). An alternative method, less prone to errors of reading and interpolation, is simply to read the percentage weight-for-height from tables. Weight-for-height <70% equates with a standard deviation score of −3 SD and is classified as severe wasting. Likewise a height-for-age <85% represents an SD score of −3 SD, viewed as severe stunting. Weight-for-height of 70–79% (−2 to −3 SD) and height-for-age of 85–89% (−2 to −3 SD) represent moderate malnutrition.

Treatment

A child who presents with clinical features of malnutrition has survived low food intake for a very variable period. As a result adaptive changes in metabolism and body composition will have occurred. For example the intracellular compartment will be more depleted than the extracellular, resulting particularly in deficiency of intracellular cations such as potassium and magnesium. The extracellular compartment may even be expanded to the extent that edema is present. This may coexist with a contracted blood volume, causing secretion of antidiuretic hormone (ADH) leading to water retention and hyponatremia despite a normal or increased total body sodium content. It is worth noting that these changes are the converse of those observed in the child with acute diarrhea. As a result, one of the greatest dangers in treating malnourished children is to refeed too quickly. Administering excessive amounts of fluid and/or high-energy feeds will shift fluid between the intra- and extracellular fluid compartments which can dangerously derange plasma electrolyte concentrations and sometimes kill the child. Management is therefore considered to have three phases:

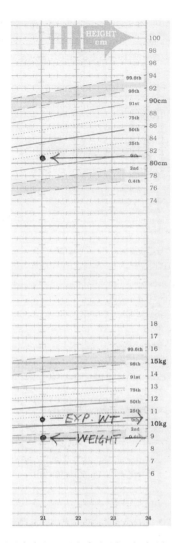

Figure 22.16 Calculating weight-for-height. The height is plotted and centile position noted (25th). The expected weight is then established by interpolating from the weight centile appropriate for the height, in this case 25th centile, 10.5 kg. The actual weight is then expressed as a percentage of this, in this case 86%.

- resuscitation,
- stabilization and tissue repair (the first few days), and
- tissue repletion and rehabilitation (subsequent weeks to months).

Resuscitation, stabilization, and repair
The key priorities are:

- to diagnose and treat underlying infection, for example respiratory infection, gastrointestinal infection, malaria, measles, or HIV-related illness (Note, however, that physical signs such as fever may be absent in severe malnutrition. 'Blind' broad-spectrum antibiotics are usually therefore given initially to all severely malnourished children),
- to reverse hypoglycemia and hypothermia (often signs of infection),
- to begin the correction of fluid and electrolyte imbalance, and
- to start correction of micronutrient deficiencies (which are universally present in severe protein–energy malnutrition) by administration of a multivitamin preparation with folic acid, zinc, and copper.

Small, frequent (e.g. 2-hourly) oral or nasogastric feeds are given, restricting the amount to about 100 ml/kg per day if the child is edematous. Otherwise up to 130 ml/kg per day of specially formulated milk- or cereal-based feed, low in osmolality and lactose content (e.g. 'F75 starter formula') are given. This provides about 100 kcal/kg per day of energy and 1–1.5 g/kg per day of protein, which can be supplemented by breastfeeds.

Children who are both dehydrated (for example as the result of diarrhea) and malnourished should be treated differently. They can be fed a solution called 'ReSoMal' which contains less sodium and more potassium and magnesium than standard oral rehydration solution. It is given orally in small amounts frequently. Intravenous therapy is reserved for shocked children, i.e. those who are hypotensive with evidence of impaired peripheral circulation. These aspects are discussed further in the next section.

Repletion and rehabilitation
After about a week the child's appetite begins to return. The aim of treatment now is to replete stores and promote catch-up growth. Energy intake is gradually increased to achieve growth rates exceeding about 10 g/kg per day. This can be achieved by using high-energy formula (about 100 kcal/100 ml) and gradually increasing the amount offered. Breastfeeds should be offered after the high-energy formula to ensure that high-energy intake is maintained. Iron can now be given with the micronutrient supplement (it is usually deferred initially because of its possible effect on Gram-negative infection; see also section on dietary supplements).

Rehabilitating the child involves much more than feeding. Play and environmental stimulation have been shown to accelerate catch-up growth and be associated with improved longer term cognitive outcomes. Parents may need re-education about feeding and teaching about food preparation for their child. Sometimes abnormal behavior such as 'frozen watchfulness,' rumination or head-banging, possibly signifying frank neglect, need more careful assessment. This is also an opportunity to bring the child's immunization status up to date and to diagnose and treat any chronic underlying problems such as anemia, parasitic infestation, or tuberculosis.

Key points on severe malnutrition are summarized in Box 22.16.

Box 22.16 Severe malnutrition

- Careful note should be taken of body proportions, to establish whether a child's low weight is attributable to wasting or stunting
- Management comprises the resuscitation, repair, and repletion stages

During the resuscitation and repair phase:
- Fluid and electrolyte balance need careful assessment – they influence the choice of initial feed
- They must be closely monitored throughout treatment.
- Underlying infection and micronutrient deficiencies must be quickly treated
- Hypoglycemia and hypothermia must be addressed quickly

During the repletion stage:
- Sufficient food is needed to promote catch-up growth
- Play and stimulation are important
- Carers will need re-education about feeding, and about other aspects of their child's health care

---

Micronutrient deficiencies

Deficiencies of trace minerals (particularly iron and zinc) and vitamins (particularly vitamin A and D) are very common in young children. They occur in both industrialized and resource-poor countries. Many others are seen in specific circumstances. These include iodine deficiency, selenium deficiency, scurvy, and B vitamin deficiency.

The underlying causes of micronutrient deficiency reflect the general vulnerabilities of children and are:

- low body stores (for example as the result of low birth weight),

- low intake as the result of improper feeding practices, and
- increased losses, for example during acute intercurrent infection.

Some deficiencies (especially selenium and iodine) are important because they occur endemically in particular geographical areas where the mineral is lacking in the earth's crust. The effects of these are particularly important in infants and young children because they impair thyroid function, which will impact adversely on development of the brain during its critical growth period, causing cretinism.

Iron deficiency

Dietary iron deficiency is the commonest cause of a microcytic, hypochromic anemia in young children. Important differential diagnoses to consider at this age are hemoglobinopathies (usually beta-thalassemia) and causes of malabsorption (particularly celiac disease). Blood loss is unusual at this age in industrialized countries, though occult losses associated with hookworm and parasitic infestations are very important globally.

Concern about the effects of iron deficiency in young children relate not so much to the physiological effects of anemia as to the possible consequences for cognitive function and development. Iron deficiency is associated with a delay in the acquisition of cognitive skills which appears to be reversible on treatment. This concern, though still controversial, has been the principal justification for programs aimed at the prevention, detection, and treatment of deficiency.

It has been claimed that between 10% and 20% of inner-city toddlers in the United Kingdom are iron deficient, though one of the problems associated with determining the exact prevalence is definition. Although the WHO defines iron deficiency as a hemoglobin concentration <11 g/dl many 'iron-deficient' toddlers may have a hemoglobin concentration only just below this diagnostic threshold. Consequently if children are tested repeatedly, substantial numbers of individuals move between iron-sufficient and iron-deficient categories. These natural fluctuations in hemoglobin concentration present considerable barriers to the introduction of effective screening programs.

Other parameters of iron status are susceptible to similar criticisms; for example serum ferritin concentration rises in the presence of acute infection.

Factors associated with iron deficiency are: low birth weight, early introduction of whole cow's milk, vegetarian weaning, use of tea as a drink, South Asian ethnic background, and low socioeconomic status. Medicinal supplements are a useful preventive strategy for some high-risk groups (e.g. low birth weight infants), though some concern has been expressed about the possible detrimental effects of supplements on weight gain among children who are iron-replete. It has been suggested that this may reflect reduced availability of zinc, which competes with iron and copper for absorption.

Some large controlled studies conducted amongst non-breastfed infants have shown that continuing the use of iron-fortified infant formulas rather than cow's milk for the first 12–18 months of life is associated with reduced incidence of anemia and, probably, some developmental advantage. Other simple measures include the use of a vitamin C source (such as fruit juice or vitamin drops), avoidance of tea, and introduction of red meat into the weaning diet. Unfortunately, at least in the UK, controlled studies have shown little benefit associated with the provision of parental education programs designed to prevent the condition.

Vitamin D deficiency

Vitamin D deficiency is common in parts of North Africa, the Middle East, and Pakistan. It is also prevalent in ethnic minority communities living at northerly latitudes, including the UK. In the UK a reference nutrient intake (RNI) for vitamin D intake is set for infants and young children, pregnant and lactating women. This cannot be achieved by diet, making the consumption of supplements important among these groups. Children from Afro-Caribbean and South Asian backgrounds are most commonly affected in the UK. Important etiologic factors are season (winter and spring), prolonged (>six months) exclusive breastfeeding, and cultural factors (e.g. purdah and concealing clothing).

Clinical presentations of vitamin D deficiency in childhood include hypocalcemic tetany in young infants and nutritional rickets. The latter is usually detected radiologically when the child presents with, for example, coexisting iron deficiency anemia and growth faltering. Frank clinical signs are now rarely seen in the UK but may include swelling of epiphyses, beading of the ribs (the 'rickety rosary'), bossing of the frontal bones, and softening of the cranium ('crani-

otabes'). Closure of the fontanelles and appearance of teeth may be delayed. Hypotonia may also hold back gross motor development (see section on neurological maturation).

Severe rickets in early life may also affect adult health: for example, linear growth and bone mineralization may be suboptimal, and bony deformity of the lower skeleton may result. In the latter context pelvic deformity in girls may cause later problems in childbirth.

An X-ray of the wrist is the quickest and most helpful diagnostic test (Figure 22.17). The radiological signs include a general reduction in bone density, loss of metaphyseal density with 'cupping', and a frayed appearance to the edges of the bone. These reflect increased bone turnover at the growth plate resulting from secondary hyperparathyroidism. These changes are not, however, diagnostic of vitamin D deficiency and can sometimes be caused by rarer inherited diseases (e.g. familial hypophosphatemic rickets, in which there is excessive tubular loss of phosphate, or vitamin D-resistant rickets, in which there is either inability to synthesize 1,25-dihydroxy vitamin D or insensitivity of the receptor) or chronic renal failure. Rickets may also be due (particularly in parts of Africa) to very low

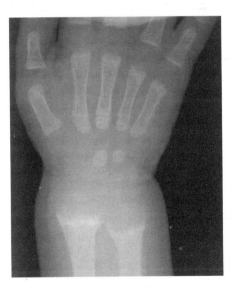

Figure 22.17 Rickets. This is the wrist X-ray of a nine-month old baby of Asian ethnic origin. The baby was still exclusively breastfed. Neither the mother nor the baby had received vitamin D supplements. Characteristic 'cupping' of the radial metaphysis can be seen, together with a 'frayed' appearance of the bone edges. These changes are the consequence of bone reabsorption caused by secondary hyperparathyroidism.

calcium intake rather than vitamin D deficiency. For this reason it is useful if possible to confirm vitamin D status by measuring the serum concentration of 25-hydroxy vitamin D: a level below 25 nmol/l is indicative of inadequate vitamin D status.

To treat nutritional rickets a large dose of vitamin D (about 1000–5000 IU/day) is usually given for the first 4–6 weeks with the aim of repleting stores. During treatment plasma calcium and phosphorus concentrations must be monitored to ensure toxicity is avoided. Gradually the plasma alkaline phosphatase concentration will return to the normal range. Thereafter the RNI (about 400 IU or 10 µg) should be given as a daily supplement to continue healing and prevent recurrence.

Vitamin A deficiency

Vitamin A deficiency remains globally the most important and cheaply preventable cause of early blindness. It is endemic in many parts of the world, particularly Africa, South-East Asia, and South Asia and considered a public health problem when the prevalence of night blindness exceeds 1% or >0.05% of individuals show corneal scarring. Randomized trials in such areas have demonstrated that significant reduction in childhood mortality and infectious morbidity can be achieved by supplementation.

Factors causing vitamin A deficiency include:

- low intake of fat and fat-soluble vitamins,
- curtailment of breastfeeding,
- poverty, and
- increased losses in, for example, acute infections – particularly measles and diarrhea.

Deficiency can be documented by measuring serum retinol concentration (<0.35 µmol/l) or by detection of changes in corneal impression cytology. However, these tests are rarely practicable for clinical purposes in countries where deficiency is endemic. In such circumstances oral vitamin A therapy should be given to all children presenting with diarrheal diseases, malnutrition, measles, and acute respiratory infections. If deficiency is identified in a child it is advisable to treat siblings and the mother as well (particularly if breastfeeding). Dietary education should also be given: foods rich in vitamin A include red palm oil, carrots, oily fish and liver, and green leaves.

Zinc deficiency

Foods high in protein, such as meat and fish, are rich sources of dietary zinc. Human milk contains zinc in a highly bioavailable form though the zinc content of human milk falls several-fold over the first six months of lactation. Iron and copper compete with zinc for gastrointestinal absorption, one reason multinutrient supplements may be preferred to use of single nutrients in populations at risk of micronutrient deficiency. Globally, diarrheal disease is an important precipitant of zinc deficiency. There is also a rare disorder of gastrointestinal zinc absorption known as acrodermatitis enteropathica, in which infants fail to thrive and develop the classical skin rash of zinc deficiency.

Clinical zinc deficiency is characterized by slowing of growth, particularly affecting the lean tissue compartment. Edema is often present, and the plasma concentration of alkaline phosphatase (a zinc metalloenzyme) characteristically falls. Eventually the characteristic rash appears as a severe desquamative eruption affecting the hands, feet, peri-oral and peri-anal areas (Plate 7). In view of its peripheral distribution (probably reflecting the areas of highest cell turnover) this is described as an acrodermatitis. Initiation of zinc repletion (as oral zinc sulfate) leads to rapid healing, within a week.

Subclinical zinc deficiency is extremely common in resource-poor countries and is associated with both stunting and impaired immunity. Supplementation in such circumstances has been associated with improved growth and reduced infectious morbidity, particularly from pneumonia and diarrhea. Zinc deficiency is occasionally seen also in industrialized countries, usually among sick children. Children on parenteral nutrition may be at risk because some commercial trace mineral solutions are relatively low in zinc concentration. Those with severe, prolonged diarrhea are also vulnerable. Late (after about 3–4 months of age) zinc deficiency occasionally occurs in human milk-fed extremely low-birth-weight (<1000 g) preterm infants: this reflects the combined effects of low stores at birth, rapid somatic growth, and extended duration of lactation with associated fall in zinc supply.

Iodine deficiency

Iodine deficiency is important in children because globally it is a major cause of disability through impairment of thyroxine synthesis. It is endemic in some parts of the world, particularly remote mountainous areas. Deficiency encompasses a spectrum of problems from mild cognitive impairment to cretinism in which bone age is delayed, growth impaired, and neurological deficit sometimes severe (incorporating deafness, cerebral palsy, and severe learning difficulty). Treatment after clinical presentation is associated with universally poor prognosis: even early recognition will be associated with some deficit. In view of this much effort has been directed at population-scale prevention in affected communities. Strategies employed include food fortification (table salt is the commonest vehicle employed) and medicinal supplementation of pregnant women (using a single oral dose). The latter is important both because much brain development occurs before birth, and because goiter (thyroid swelling) in an affected fetus may give rise to problems in labor if neck extension causes face presentation.

Other vitamin deficiencies

A number of B vitamin deficiencies may occur in areas where severe malnutrition is common. These include:

- thiamine deficiency, resulting in beri beri (cardiac failure, peripheral neuropathy, and encephalopathy),
- nicotinic acid deficiency, resulting in pellagra (diarrhea and photo-dermatosis), and
- riboflavin deficiency, associated with cheilosis and anemia.

The common coexistence of these deficiencies with severe malnutrition re-emphasizes the importance of early micronutrient supplementation in treatment.

Vitamin B_{12} deficiency is much less common in children than in, for example, the elderly, but can occur rarely in breastfed infants of vegan mothers and some vegan children. It is also sometimes seen in children who have undergone resection of the terminal ileum, usually as a consequence of necrotizing enterocolitis in the neonatal period. In such circumstances deficiency may take many years to present clinically – perhaps until puberty. This reflects the adequacy of stores in the face of low turnover rates, until stressed by the additional metabolic demands of the pubertal growth spurt.

Folic acid deficiency results in megaloblastic anemia. It is uncommon as an isolated dietary deficiency in children and usually signifies the presence of malabsorption, commonly celiac disease.

Vitamin C deficiency in children is now rare in the absence of severe malnutrition and causes scurvy. Historically it is of interest because it became endemic in the latter part of the nineteenth century when artificial feeds were introduced. Subsequently this was found to be due to inactivation of vitamin C by heat treatment. The scorbutic child typically presents with bruising, bleeding, and bone tenderness – sometimes sufficiently marked as to cause a pseudoparesis. X-rays show severe subperiosteal hemorrhage with calcification and loss of trabecular bone mineral. The subperiosteal swellings may cause obvious swelling of the limbs and anterior ends of the ribs.

Vitamin K deficiency has been covered in a previous section.

Finally, vitamin E deficiency may occur in children with inherited disorders causing severe fat malabsorption – such as abetalipoproteinemia and cystic fibrosis. It eventually manifests as a demyelinating disorder of the spinocerebellar tracts, by which stage changes are not reversible. This observation emphasizes the importance of vitamin E supplementation in such children. Rarely it may also cause hemolytic anemia in preterm infants.

Other trace mineral deficiencies

Copper deficiency is rare but has been described in babies of extremely low birth weight. It causes anemia and severe osteopenia, sometimes giving rise to fractures.

Selenium deficiency is also rare but has been observed in a few children on long-term parenteral nutrition. As it is associated with the development of a cardiomyopathy (cf. 'Keshan disease') it should be considered in any such child developing signs of heart failure.

22.8 Nutrition as treatment

Nutritional support for the sick child

Technical advances in the provision of techniques of nutritional support have greatly increased prospects of survival for sick children. Some of the most striking advances have been in the field of neonatal medicine: indeed it is of interest to note that the earliest applications of parenteral nutrition in human patients were amongst newborn infants undergoing bowel surgery.

General principles

There is one important conceptual difference between pediatric and adult medical practice in the aims of providing nutritional support. While in both there will

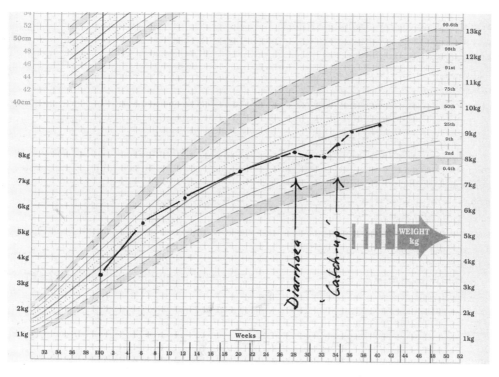

Figure 22.18 Weight loss and catch-up. An episode of protracted diarrhea causes significant weight loss over a month. On treatment weight gain is extremely rapid. This process of catch-up after illness is associated with very high nutritional requirements.

have been tissue depletion of variable extent by presentation (depending on balance and the size of body stores), the child will additionally have undergone a period of suboptimal growth. Thus nutritional support must provide for:

- maintenance demands (as in the adult),
- tissue repletion (as in the adult), *plus*
- growth, *and*
- catch-up growth (Figure 22.18).

Consequently nutrient demands are much greater than those of a healthy child of similar age and size. Moreover they must be delivered within the constraints imposed by immature homeostatic systems, and complicating morbidity.

Aside from this consideration, the general principles of nutritional support in adults (see Chapter 8) also apply to sick children.

- The gut should be used when it is functioning.
- Potential intake of normal food should be maximized before resorting to commercial supplements or specialist feeds.

- Careful attention to hygiene should be observed both when handling enteral feeds and managing parenteral lines.
- A multidisciplinary team approach to management should be followed, both in hospital and the community.
- Clear guidelines and care pathways must be in place to support children and parents managing nutritional support in the community.
- Nutritional support should be organized in such a way as to minimize disruption to the child's daily life (particularly schooling). In order to accomplish this in the case of children receiving long-term nutritional support it may be necessary to make a formal statement of Special Educational Needs to the local education authority (in the UK) and consider application for benefits such as Disability Living Allowance or Attendance Allowance (UK).
- Growth, fluid balance, and plasma biochemistry must be closely monitored because normal homeostatic controls (especially thirst and hunger) may be overridden when nutritional support is provided.

Routes of access for enteral nutritional support

The most commonly employed at all ages is nasogastric tube feeding. Polyvinyl chloride (PVC) tubes are most commonly used, particularly in young infants. If long-term tube feeding is considered silicon rubber or polyurethane tubes are softer and can be left in place for weeks. These need a guidewire to stiffen them sufficiently for introduction, but parents and adolescent children can be taught the technique. This allows them, for example, to use them for overnight feeding and remove them for school. In very young infants, especially if preterm, nasogastric tubes increase upper airway impedance and hence the work of breathing (young infants are obligate nose-breathers). Tubes passed by the orogastric route are therefore preferable in the presence of respiratory distress.

Each time a gastric tube is passed its position should be checked by aspirating and testing for an acid reaction with indicator paper. If there is doubt, tube position should be confirmed by X-ray. This precaution is necessary to exclude accidental intubation of a bronchus, something which can happen particularly with young preterm infants, unconscious children, or those with neuromuscular disability who have a weak gag reflex.

Naso- or orojejunal tubes were once used quite commonly as an alternative to gastric tubes, particularly in preterm infants. These are weighted to facilitate passage through the pylorus, but a degree of skill is needed (sometimes it helps to stiffen the tube in a freezer first). It is also difficult to aspirate the tube and an X–ray is usually needed to confirm its position. Another, more theoretical, disadvantage is that this method of feeding seems less 'physiological' than gastric feeding. For example, the neurenteric peptide responses to feeding gastrically and jejunally are different, and feeds must be given by continuous infusion rather than by bolus as the jejunum will not tolerate such large volumes as the stomach. This may impair fat digestion. For all these reasons jejunal feeding has declined in popularity, though it can still be particularly useful in babies who have severe gastroesophageal reflux or who are receiving continuous positive airways pressure (CPAP) applied to the oropharynx.

Where long-term access to the gut is required gastrostomy has become an increasingly popular procedure. Classically this was performed as a surgical procedure, an inflatable balloon being used to fix the catheter. Most gastrostomies are now, however, inserted endoscopically (percutaneous endoscopic gastrostomy (PEG)) and retained by a flat disk (or 'button'). This can be simply closed off or opened (e.g. for overnight tube feeding) which aids concealment and makes it popular with older children. A considerable disadvantage of gastrostomy is that it tends to exacerbate any gastroesophageal reflux present, so any vomiting may worsen. Occasionally this may be so marked as to necessitate surgical fundoplication of the stomach. Gastrostomy is particularly common in the management of children with severe neuromuscular disability, for example those with cerebral palsy.

Types of enteral feed

Breastmilk (or infant formula if the mother is not breastfeeding) is used for the majority of young infants. This may be given in volumes of up to 180–200 ml/kg body weight per day, the caloric density approximating 0.7 kcal/ml. Preferably the mother's own breastmilk is used. If her baby is unable to feed at the breast the mother will need support and help to express and store her milk. She can either express manually or use a hand-, battery-, or electric-powered pump. Whatever her preference she will need to do this at least 6–8 times per day to maintain her supply. When a mother's own milk is not available milk from a donor may be used. If so it is vital to follow available guidelines about donor deferral (declining high-risk donors), serological testing (for HIV, HTLV, hepatitis, and other infections), processing (including pasteurization), and microbiological testing in order to prevent transmission of infection. It is not usually necessary to microbiologically test or process a mother's own milk so long as simple hygiene instructions in relation to cleaning pumps and bottles are followed.

If there is a need to increase energy intake further, or to reduce the fluid volume administered (for example because of cardiac or renal disease) several options are available.

- High-fat breastmilk can be obtained by showing the mother how to separate hindmilk (richer in fat) when she expresses.
- Commercial supplements can be used to increase energy density to as much as 1 kcal/ml. These include glucose polymer powder, Calogen (a long-chain triglyceride emulsion), or Duocal (a combined fat/carbohydrate supplement).

160 mmol/l the risk of death or disability is particularly high. Rehydration in such cases must aim to correct the electrolyte derangement more slowly, over at least 24–48 h.

Fluid replacement

WHO rehydration schedules for children with diarrhea envisage three scenarios, based on the degree of dehydration at presentation (Table 22.6).

Children presenting with signs of severe dehydration need urgent replacement of water and electrolytes or they will die (Table 22.6, schedule C). This should be given intravenously, initially as 0.9% saline or Ringer's lactate solution. It is dangerous to give a hypotonic fluids such as 5% glucose or 4% glucose with 0.18% saline as they will precipitate a rapid fall in plasma sodium concentration with attendant risk of cerebral edema (particularly if the child is hypernatremic at presentation). WHO recommends the following infusion rates for a child with severe dehydration:

- Child under one year: 30 ml/kg over first hour, followed by 70 ml/kg over the next 5 h (equating to a total of 75 ml/kg body weight over the first 4 h).
- Child over one year: 30 ml/kg in the first 30 min, and 70 ml/kg over the next 2½ h.

These amounts occasionally need to be repeated if the child remains unconscious with continuing high stool losses, but in most cases there is immediate improvement and the child recovers consciousness sufficiently to drink. It is important at this stage to offer additional oral rehydration solution (ORS) to replace the ongoing losses: roughly 1 ml of ORS will be needed for each ml (or g) of loose stool. Breastfeeding may then be resumed and ORS given by mouth, aiming to provide about 5 ml/kg per h.

Table 22.7 Comparison of ReSoMal and WHO oral rehydration solutions

	ORS (mmol/l)	ReSoMal (mmol/l)
Sodium	75	45
Potassium	20	40
Magnesium	0	3
Glucose	75	55
Sucrose	0	69

If a child has features of severe malnutrition ReSoMal should be used instead of ORS. The composition of these two fluids is compared in Table 22.7. They differ in important respects, particularly sodium and potassium concentration. This reflects the fact that the child with malnutrition often has a surplus of extracellular fluid and hence excessive total body sodium balance (even if hyponatremic) but is deficient in the intracellular electrolytes potassium and magnesium. The child with diarrhea, on the other hand, has lost principally extracellular fluid and is acutely depleted in sodium.

Remember that children with malnutrition may quickly become edematous (looking puffy in the face and eyelids) during rehydration. If this occurs additional ORS should be stopped but normal feeding continued. Once fluid balance is stabilized ORS can be recommended if losses continue.

Feeding

Breastfeeding should not be interrupted and the child allowed to feed on demand. Infants under six months who are not breastfed are given 100–200 ml of boiled water in addition to ORS during the rehydration period. Formula and other foods are reintroduced when rehydration has been completed, usually after about

Table 22.6 Summary of WHO guidelines for managing diarrhea

Dehydration	Rehydration	Plan
None	Not needed, but extra fluid as demanded	'Schedule A': home treatment with extra fluid as ORS, water, or food-based fluid. Continue feeding
Some (mild or moderate)	Oral rehydration with measured amounts of ORS, depending on age and weight	'Schedule B', rehydrate with ORS over 4 hours. Continue breastfeeding. If not breastfed re-feed within 4 h. Continue to replace losses with extra ORS
Severe	Intravenous rehydration with isotonic fluid	'Schedule C', rehydrate over 4–6 h. Give ORS as soon as child can drink. Continue to replace losses and feed as soon as possible

From World Health Organization.

4 h. The old practice of using half-strength diluted milk and waiting for the diarrhea to settle before 're-grading' is no longer endorsed: it led to significant reduction in nutrient intake without any improvement in the rate of recovery.

Persistent diarrhea

In resource-poor countries between 5 and 20% of acute diarrheal episodes become prolonged. If diarrhea continues for more than 14 days it is defined as 'persistent diarrhea.' This is commonly associated with growth faltering, compromised immunity (especially if associated with HIV infection), and micronutrient deficiency (especially of zinc and vitamin A). It often leads to death. The causes may be persisting infection or mucosal injury which has caused intolerance to food constituents (usually lactose or cow's milk proteins).

The important aspects of initial management are the following:

- Correction of water and electrolyte imbalance, usually orally with ORS. Although children may not be severely dehydrated they may be hypokalemic and weak as a result.
- Detection and treatment of underlying systemic infections, parasitic infection (amebiasis or giardiasis), or dysentery.
- Micronutrient supplementation and continued/frequent breastfeeding on demand.

If these are unsuccessful and the mother is not breastfeeding, a modified diet may be needed to reduce or eliminate lactose intake. A formula based on hydrolyzed cow's milk protein and sucrose (or glucose polymer) may be used when available. Sometimes it is necessary to use a modular feed based on ground chicken. An inexpensive lactose-free diet can also be made from egg (or ground chicken meat), rice, glucose, and vegetable oil.

Key points on the management of childhood diarrhea are listed in Box 22.18.

The chronically ill child: general remarks

A range of dietary products and delivery devices are now available for specialized enteral and parenteral nutritional support of sick children of all ages and sizes. Equally, improvements in pediatric treatment now mean that, with the exception of conditions caused by intolerance and allergy to food constituents

---

Box 22.18 Diarrhea

- Acute and chronic diarrhoeal disease is a major cause of death, especially in children under two
- Most of these episodes could be prevented by exclusive breastfeeding, followed by prolonged breastfeeding as part of a more varied diet
- The main cause of death amongst children with diarrhea is mismanagement of fluid replacement – too little, or too much too quickly
- In uncomplicated diarrheal disease the need is mainly to replace sodium and water as principally the extracellular fluid compartment is depleted
- The amount, rate, and route of salt and water replacement is determined by clinical assessment of the extent of dehydration
- Breastfeeding should continue, supplemented with oral rehydration solution (ORS)
- Children with diarrheal disease superimposed on malnutrition must be managed differently to reduce the risk of acute extracellular fluid overload and to replace intracellular electrolytes
- Persistent diarrhea requires further investigation and further dietary management to prevent continued growth faltering

---

such as celiac disease, dietary restriction is not used to control symptoms. For example, children with cystic fibrosis were once advised to follow strict low-fat diets to control steatorrhea. The resulting chronic energy deficiency led to severe stunting now rarely seen. The availability of modern pancreatic enzyme supplements, coupled with the use of high-energy diets and supplementation (if necessary by overnight tube or gastrostomy feeding) has meant that children survive longer and in most cases achieve weight and height in the normal range for age (see Chapter 23). Children with renal disease and heart disease similarly are no longer advised to follow severely restrictive diets.

It is not possible here to provide details of the nutritional management of the many chronic disorders affecting children. The general constraints which disease in various systems places upon nutrient assimilation, metabolism, and the excretion of waste products are covered in other sections of this chapter and elsewhere in the book.

Exclusion diets

Exclusion diets should not be given to children without good clinical justification. There are a number of reasons for this:

- The nutrient demands of growing children are high and the restrictive nature of exclusion diets poses a risk of specific nutritional deficiencies.

- The diet may be unpalatable, and lead to energy deficiency.
- The normal development of eating patterns can be disturbed because meals are not shared with family and friends.

If an exclusion diet is prescribed it must be supervised by a pediatric dietitian. Unfortunately parents of young children may unjustifiably attribute causally a number of symptoms to particular foods and may introduce informal dietary restrictions. Symptoms related to food can be categorized in the following way:

- *Food aversion* – the child has a psychological objection to particular foods. Such symptoms can be distinguished from true intolerance if the food components are given in blinded circumstances.
- *Food intolerance* – there is a reproducible reaction to the food, even if the child and parents are blinded to its presence in the diet. Food intolerances are not always 'allergic' in origin and may be due to a number of causes:
  - abnormal absorption (e.g. milk causing diarrhea in lactase deficiency),
  - abnormality of metabolism (e.g. fruits causing vomiting and hypoglycemia in fructose intolerance),
  - presence of toxins or pharmacologically active compounds in food (e.g. histamine releasing sarcotoxins in some fish, caffeine in drinks), or
  - immune reactions to food ('food allergy'). These may be of the immediate or delayed hypersensitivity type.

The types of diet used to manage food intolerances in children are:

- *Simple exclusion* of a food to which the child is reproducibly sensitive. Usually, but not always, the reaction is immediate making the causal link clear. Examples include peanuts and milk. Very careful counseling is needed as even trace amounts present in commercially prepared foods can have significant consequences. One of the most widely used therapeutic exclusion diets in pediatrics is the gluten-free diet employed in celiac disease. The principles of managing this condition are covered in Chapter 10.
- *Empirical diets.* Some diets have been shown to be effective in clinical trials for ill-understood reasons. Examples include milk and egg avoidance for eczema, additive avoidance in hyperactivity.

- *'Oligoantigenic' (few antigens) diets.* These very restrictive diets use only a few foods and are generally used only for diagnostic purposes over short periods. New foods can be added one at a time in order to identify troublesome items.
- *'Hypoallergenic diets'.* These involve using specialized enteral feeds. They are usually bland and unpalatable, hence may often be given by tube. They have, however, been used particularly successfully to induce remission in Crohn's disease among children. This is a great advantage because the alternative therapeutic option, corticosteroids, has an number of undesirable side effects – particularly growth suppression.

Food intolerance – suspected or proven – is an increasingly common problem in pediatric practice and a number of hypotheses have been raised to explain this trend. These issues, and further aspects of management, are covered in Chapter 7.

Inborn errors of metabolism

Genetically determined abnormalities have been recognized in virtually every metabolic pathway. Indeed understanding these 'experiments of nature' has provided considerable insight into the phenotypic significance of particular enzyme steps. This is because a single gene deletion gives rise to a single enzyme deficiency, the great majority following an autosomal recessive pattern of inheritance. Individually they are rare, but collectively they are quite common affecting up to 1 in 1500–2000 children in the UK, for example. Incidence varies considerably from country to country, reflecting variation in the gene frequency; for example phenylketonuria (the commonest of the inherited disorders of amino acid metabolism) affects about 1 in 10 000 children in the UK but about 1 in 5000 children in Ireland.

Some inborn errors are not treatable (e.g. respiratory chain disorders) and may cause death very soon after birth. Others (e.g. phenylketonuria, type I glutaric aciduria, medium chain acyl CoA dehydrogenase deficiency) are associated with metabolic decompensation, death, or severe neurological handicap which is preventable if detected sufficiently early. All newborn infants in the UK have for many years received the so-called 'Guthrie test' which screens for phenylketonuria (PKU) by measuring blood phenylalanine. This is usually done around the end of the first week of life once milk feeding has become established.

Historically it has not been cost-effective to screen for other metabolic diseases but the development of new techniques (tandem mass spectrometry) has made it practically feasible to test for multiple disorders on a single small sample. The resulting world-wide escalation of multidisease screening programs is increasing very substantially the number of children requiring specialist nutritional management. The more common amino and organic acid metabolism disorders are summarized in Table 22.8, selected disorders of carbohydrate metabolism managed by diet are summarized in Table 22.9, and some selected disorders of lipid metabolism managed by diet are summarized in Table 22.10.

Key points about inborn errors of metabolism are shown in Box 22.19.

For most inborn errors diet remains the mainstay of management despite the promise of technological advances. There are a few exceptions: for example enzyme replacement has proven effective in some (e.g.

Table 22.8 The more commonly occurring disorders of amino and organic acid metabolism managed by diet

Metabolic disorder	Metabolic defect	Aim of dietary treatment
Phenylketonuria	Phenylalanine hydroxylase deficiency (or, rarely, a defect in recycling of biopterin a cofactor for the enzyme)	Restriction of dietary phenylalanine
Maple syrup urine disease	Branched chain 2-ketoacid dehydrogenase complex deficiency	Leucine restriction Thiamine supplementation (thiamine responsive form; 2 ketoacid dehydrogenase cofactor)
Homocysteinuria	Cystathionine beta synthase deficiency	Methionine restriction. Pyridoxine supplementation (cystathionine beta synthase cofactor)
Tyrosinemia (types I and II)	Deficiency of fumarylacetoacetate hydrolase (type I) or tyrosine aminotransferase (type II)	Low phenylalanine, low tyrosine diet
Urea cycle disorders	Many, e.g. carbamoyl phosphate synthetase deficiency, ornithine carbamoyl transferase deficiency	Protein restriction; use of sodium benzoate or phenylbutyrate to facilitate alternative N-excretion pathways; arginine supplementation (to replace intermediate compounds not formed)
Propionic acidemia; methylmalonic acidemia (MMA)	Deficiency of propionyl carboxylase or methylmalonic acid mutase respectively. In MMA sometimes deficiency of the enzyme cofactor adenosylcobalamin	Protein restriction. Avoid fasting (to limit oxidation of fat and protein). Possible benefit from vitamin B_{12} in MMA and from use of antibiotics (metronidazole) to suppress synthesis of propionic acid by colonic flora
Isovaleric acidemia	Deficiency of isovaleryl co-A dehydrogenase.	Protein restriction. Supplementation with carnitine and glycine (to conjugate isovaleric acid and enhance urinary excretion)

Table 22.9 Selected disorders of carbohydrate metabolism managed by diet

Metabolic disorder	Metabolic defect	Aim of dietary treatment
Glycogen storage diseases (GSD) (types I, III)	Glucose-6-phosphatase deficiency (type I); amylo-1,6-glucosidase (debranching enzyme) deficiency (type III). Other steps also affected	Avoidance of hypoglycemia by frequent (or continuous) feeding of glucose polymer/cornstarch to meet glucose oxidation requirments
Galactosemia	Classically deficiency of galactose-1-phosphate uridyl transferase	Avoidance of lactose from milk and covert sources (such as medicines)
Galactokinase deficiency	Galactokinase	As galactosemia
Hereditary fructose intolerance	Deficiency of fructose-1-phosphate aldolase	Avoidance of fructose (together with sucrose and sorbitol)
Congenital disorders of glycosylation (CDG)	Several types: deficiencies of the glycosyltransferases and other enzymes which glycate proteins	Varies, e.g. use of mannose in CDG type Ib (phosphomannose isomerase deficiency) to circumvent the production of mannose from fructose
Fructose 1,6-biphosphatase deficiency	Fructose 1,6-biphosphatase deficiency; ineffective gluconeogenesis leading to fasting hypoglycemia	Diet low in fructose; otherwise similar approach to GSD using frequent feeding and glucose polymer/uncooked cornstarch supplements. Avoid alcohol (which also impairs gluconeogenesis)

Table 22.10 Selected disorders of lipid metabolism managed by diet

Metabolic disorder	Metabolic defect	Aim of dietary treatment
Disorders of beta-oxidation	Medium and long-chain acyl CoA dehydrogenase deficiency (MCAD; LCAD); 3-hydroxyacyl-CoA dehydrogenase deficiencies; multiple acyl CoA dehydrogenase deficiencies	High-carbohydrate diet and avoidance of fasting. The patient does not have normal ketogenesis and will become hypoglycemic. Fatty acids and accumulated CoA derivatives are also toxic in LCAD. Thus diet aims to minimize long-chain fat intake
Abetalipoproteinemia	Inability to make apolipoprotein B, therefore absence of chylomicra, LDL, and VLDL in the blood. Results in severe fat malabsorption with failure to thrive, acanthocytosis of red cells, ataxia, and retinopathy	Reduce long-chain triglyceride intake and supply energy as medium-chain triglyceride and carbohydrate
Hyperlipoproteinemias	Many types. Commonest is type IIA resulting in high LDL concentrations and hypercholesterolemia	Reduce fat intake to 30% of energy, increase intake of non-starch polysaccharide; drugs (statins and bile salt chelators such as cholestyramine to reduce fat absorption)

Box 22.19 Inborn errors of metabolism

- Inborn errors are individually rare, but collectively affect up to 1 in 500 children
- The prevalence of inborn errors is likely to increase as more are identified by new screening technology
- The only treatment for most is dietary modification
- As they are single-gene disorders affecting single enzyme steps these 'experiments of nature' have taught us much about normal metabolism
- Dietary treatment may entail:
  - reducing the supply of precursors whilst ensuring sufficiency of other nutrients
  - use of supraphysiological doses of vitamin cofactors to increase activity of vitamin dependent enzymes ('vitamin dependency')
- High-energy feeding during illness reduces catabolism of fat and protein stores, thus minimizing the unwanted release of precursors from body tissues

Gaucher's disease, Fabry's disease) and gene replacement in others (e.g. urea cycle disorders, adenosine deaminase deficiency) at least in the short term. The general principles of dietary management are:

- to restrict the intake of precursor metabolites in order to prevent accumulation of the precursors themselves or their metabolites,
- to augment the activity of defective metabolic pathways (Sometimes this can be accomplished by using a supraphysiological dose of the relevant vitamin cofactor. This situation is known as 'vitamin dependency' not to be confused with deficiency), an example of which is the use of vitamin B_6 in pyridoxine dependent seizures,

- to provide sufficient intake of other nutrients (especially energy, trace minerals, and vitamins) to meet the demands of maintenance and growth, and
- to restrict the extent of catabolism during any intercurrent illness, preventing metabolic stress due to release of precursors form body stores.

Phenylketonuria

As phenylketonuria (PKU) is one of the commonest inherited metabolic disorders it is illustrative to understand some general principles of management. Classical PKU occurs when there is an absence of phenylalanine hydroxylase (Figure 22.19) or the enzyme is present in extremely low quantities. Without treatment blood phenylalanine concentrations may exceed 1 mmol/l, a level sufficient to cause cerebral damage resulting in severe learning difficulty, seizures, and microcephaly. There is often a striking absence of skin, eye, and hair pigmentation because of the inability to convert phenylalanine to tyrosine, which is a precursor of the skin pigment melanin. Rarely PKU is caused not by a defect in the protein structure of phenylalanine hydroxylase itself but by an abnormality in the pathway which reduces and recycles biopterin, the enzyme cofactor (Figure 22.19). Such patients need supplementation with folate and other compounds, in addition to dietary phenylalanine restriction.

The cornerstone of management in classical PKU is restriction of phenylalanine intake, titrating this against blood phenylalanine concentrations. In young infants this can be accomplished by using a low phenylalanine formula alone or in combination with breastmilk. As breastmilk has a much lower phenylalanine

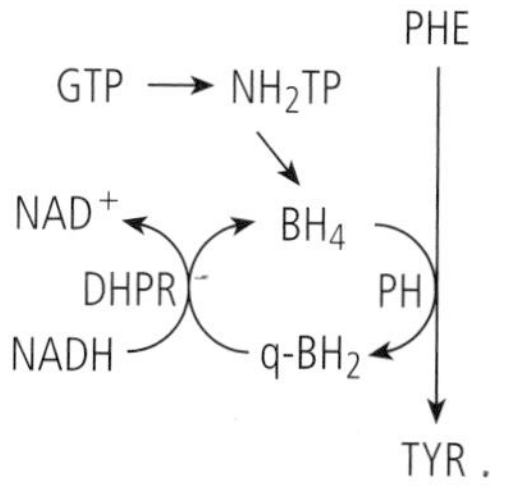

$$GTP \longrightarrow NH_2TP$$

$$NAD^+ \quad BH_4$$

$$DHPR \quad PH$$

$$NADH \quad q\text{-}BH_2$$

$$PHE$$

$$TYR.$$

Figure 22.19 Phenylketonuria. 'Classical' phenylketonuria is caused by reduced activity in the phenlalanine hydroxyase (PH) pathway. Thus phenylalanine (PHE) cannot be converted to tyrosine (TYR). Rarely, there is instead a deficiency in the associated pathway responsible for synthesizing and regenerating reduced (tetrahydro-) biopterin (BH_4), the enzyme cofactor. DHPR, dihydropteridin reductase; q-BH_2, quinoid dihydrobioptein; GTP, guanosine triphosphate; NH_2TP, dihydroneopterin triphosphate. From McLaren *et al.* (1991).

concentration than cow's milk (or infant formulas) partial breastfeeding is fortunately possible in most cases. Management becomes more challenging with the introduction of complementary foods. Only very limited quantities of 'natural' dietary protein can be allowed, and staple protein sources such as meat, fish, cheese, and soya protein must be avoided completely. Those lower in protein content (such as cereals, rice, and vegetables) become the principal 'normal' components of the diet and are offered in 'exchanges' (i.e. measured portions) containing 50 mg phenylalanine. In recent years dietary goals have become much stricter and, whereas once fruit and vegetables with low phenylalanine content were offered freely, even these are now incorporated in the 'exchange' scheme.

Such a diet might control phenylalanine intake but is grossly insufficient in total dietary protein (and hence other essential amino acids), not to mention trace minerals and vitamins. Potential dietary deficiency of protein is prevented by prescribing phenylalanine-free amino acid mixtures as substitutes for natural dietary protein. A range is available, the exact choice depending on age (which affects essential amino acid requirement). Most are complete in vitamin and essential mineral content, though these can be provided separately. Analogous products depleted in amino acids other than phenylalanine are used to treat other inherited amino- and organic acidemias. All are listed in the 'Borderline substances' section (Appendix 7) of the British National Formulary, together with a range of prescribable prepared foods such as low protein breads, pasta, confectionery bars, etc.

Clearly the diet of a child with PKU is very different to that of his or her peers. This can lead to substantial behavioral problems among children of all ages. Young children may ingest normal foods accidentally whereas older ones, particularly adolescents, may rebel. The need to eat such a restrictive diet is potentially a considerable social handicap as meals outside the home present difficulties. Food refusal can also be a major management problem.

Setting such behavioral issues aside, blood phenylalanine levels may also fluctuate for valid physiological reasons. Fasting, infection, energy, or essential amino acid deficiency and other stresses (e.g. surgery) may enhance endogenous protein breakdown, liberating phenylalanine from body protein and significantly increasing blood levels. Such effects can be minimized by maintaining a high energy intake through provision of high-carbohydrate drinks or even parenteral supplementation. On the other hand growth spurts (e.g. at puberty or during catch-up after infections) may increase physiological demands and depress blood levels. Again similar considerations apply to the management of other amino- and organic acidemias.

Children with PKU have always remained on their diet throughout childhood, though traditionally the diet was relaxed in adolescence and abandoned in adult life because the completion of central nervous system development was believed to eliminate the need for strict dietary control. Views on this have changed for a number of reasons:

- In the case of girls the relative unpalatability of the diet always led to problems with regaining dietary control prior to conception and throughout pregnancy. In order to achieve a normal fetal outcome metabolic control in such circumstances must be even tighter than in young infants. This is hard to achieve once a taste for 'normal' foods has been acquired.
- Neuropsychological studies have demonstrated superior cognitive function in well-controlled adult patients.
- Recent neuroimaging (MRI) studies have demonstrated white matter lesions in the long tracts of adults of both sexes who had relaxed their diets.
- Paraplegia, sometimes irreversible, has developed in young adults who have stopped their diet.

Most now recommend diet for life. In recent years it has been recognized that maintaining diet is associated both with improved cognitive performance in early adult life and reduced risk of the neurological abnormalities associated with white matter changes on brain MRI scans.

Other inborn errors of metabolism

It is not possible here to give a detailed description of the management of other inborn errors of metabolism. This is a highly specialized, technically and clinically demanding subject. Tables 22.8, 22.9, and 22.10 give a glimpse of the variety of problems that may be encountered and the general principles of nutritional management.

22.9 Overweight in children: fatness and 'obesity'

Defining 'obesity' in childhood

Body mass index (BMI) changes throughout childhood so it is impossible to follow the approach familiar in adult practice of defining overweight and obesity in terms of simple arithmetical values. Recently BMI centile charts have entered clinical use (Figure 22.14). They are based on the body proportions of children forming the UK 1990 growth reference. It would, of course, be simple to follow the usual principles associated with the use of growth charts (see Section 22.2 on growth) and define the condition in terms of a particular centile, such as the 99.6th. Unfortunately there are problems associated with this too:

- First, it is now well established that BMI in children continues to undergo rapid secular change. Thus the proportion of children labeled as 'obese' on current charts would rise in successive years.
- Secondly, the long-term implications of any particular BMI are much less clear for children than for adults. In other words cut-offs cannot clearly be defined in terms of clinical risk. One solution (recommended by the International Task Force on Obesity) has been to impose on the BMI chart lines which correspond to the likely attainment of an adult BMI of 25 or 30. These lines now appear on the UK 1990 nine-centile charts and are indicated in Figure 22.20. The lack of clear data on clinical risk and childhood BMI centile has persuaded some that the term 'fatness' is preferable to 'obesity' at this stage of life.
- Thirdly, the charts are cross-sectional and children may change their relative position on the chart as they grow older. This raises the question of how children 'track' along particular centiles as they grow (see below). While there is a high year-on-year correlation between the centile position of any single individual, it is considerably lower over longer periods. Thus there is little relationship between fatness in adult life and infant BMI, but a much stronger relationship with BMI after puberty.

In addition to the child's position on the centile chart at any one time, other indicators that the child is at high risk of adult obesity include:

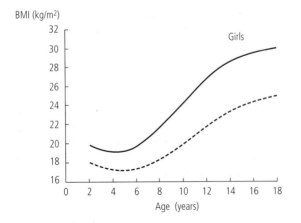
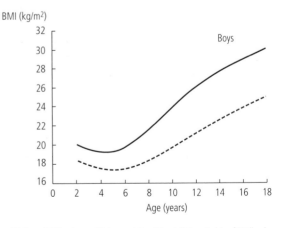

Figure 22.20 BMI 'risk' lines extrapolated into childhood. These lines indicate the childhood BMI values which correlate with adult thresholds of 25 (broken line) and 30 (solid line). Reproduced from Cole *et al.* (2000) with permission of the BMJ Publishing Group.

- one or two overweight or obese parents, or
- early 'adiposity rebound', i.e. the normal upwards inflection of the BMI curve associated with puberty begins relatively early (see charts: the curve is inflected earlier in the upper centiles than the lower; Figure 22.20).

Complications of 'obesity' in childhood

Although much attention has been focused on the possible consequences of childhood fat mass for adult health, being overweight increases the risk of certain conditions presenting in childhood. A list is given in Box 22.20.

Box 22.20 Complications of 'obesity' in childhood

- Orthopedic (slipped femoral epiphysis; Blount's disease)
- Sleep apnea/hypoventilation
- Hyperlipidemia
- Non-insulin-dependent diabetes mellitus (NIDDM)
- Pseudotumor cerebri
- Hypertension

Currently there is particular concern about the increasing prevalence of non-insulin-dependent diabetes mellitus (NIDDM) among children. This seems especially a problem amongst those of South Asian ethnic origin.

Less common causes of 'obesity' in childhood

Most fat children have 'simple' obesity arising from energy imbalance. However, a few uncommon causes exist and are shown in Box 22.21. A useful general pointer to the presence of an underlying endocrine disorder is the presence of associated short stature or recent growth failure, in addition of course to physical signs specific for each condition.

The presence of learning disability, dysmorphic features, or precocious/late puberty are also of concern and should prompt referral to a pediatrician. Most 'simple' obesity in children is, however, best managed by a primary care multidisciplinary team in the community.

Treating 'obesity' in children

Treatment is unlikely to succeed unless:

- the child and the family want to change,

Box 22.21 Less common 'medical' causes of obesity in children

- Genetic
- Prader–Willi syndrome
- Rarer syndromes
- Endocrine
- Hypothyroidism
- Cushing's syndrome
- Growth hormone deficiency
- Iatrogenic
- Glucocorticoid therapy
- Poorly controlled diabetes mellitus (insulin excess)
- Illnesses associated with immobility (decreased energy expenditure)
- Spina bifida
- Muscular dystrophy

- the goals set are realistic and acceptable to the child and family, and
- the solution is sustainable.

The goals may include maintenance of weight or just slowing of weight gain so that height and weight centiles converge with growth. It is usually inappropriate to aim for weight loss though if obesity is severe or complications (for example diabetes) are present it may be necessary. Even then weight loss should be gradual – no more than 500 g per month. Rapid weight loss and strict diets are rarely appropriate for young children. Avoidance of severe energy restriction is especially important in young children and during the pubertal growth spurt, since it may lead to restriction of final height attainment.

Treatment should address the following areas:

Food and eating patterns
- Establish a regular meal pattern, avoiding 'grazing' and snacks.
- Use low-calorie drinks, spreads, and foods, to conserve as far as possible the apparent amount on the plate.
- Substitute complex carbohydrate in the form of whole grains, vegetables, and fruits for products containing fat and refined sugars such as confectionery (these foods also have the advantage of taking more time to eat!).

Lifestyle changes
- Introduce sustainable changes in moderate activity – such as outdoor rather than sedentary pastimes.

- Increase the activity component in daily life (e.g. walking to school, using stairs).

Psychosocial adjustment

Obese children may have low self-esteem and are frequently bullied. Dealing with these aspects may necessitate referral of the family for specialist psychological counseling.

Preventing obesity

The causes of the secular trend towards increasing BMI and fatness are many but particularly include:

- A reduction in physical activity associated with increased dependence on motorized transport and indulgence in sedentary pastimes. One study in the United States, for example, showed a statistically significant correlation between BMI and the number of hours children spent watching television!
- An increase in the consumption of snack and convenience foods, high in refined carbohydrate and fat content. Media and peer pressure reinforce this behavior.

The solutions are therefore complex and lie not just in the hands of individual parents and children but government and the commercial sector. Community initiatives facilitating the enhancement of exercise opportunities for children may be particularly important.

Key nutritional points on obesity in children are listed in Box 22.22.

22.10 Perspectives on the future

This chapter has described both normal and abnormal patterns of child growth and development, and touched upon the scope of nutrition as it is currently applied to the prevention and treatment of disease during childhood. Currently our understanding of the interactions between the environment, nutrients, and genes is increasing very rapidly, and this will offer new therapeutic horizons.

Within the childhood era better understanding of the relationships between nutrition, host defense, and inflammation could enable us to make further inroads

---

Box 22.22 Obesity

- Defining 'obesity' in children is difficult because:

  - adiposity changes normally with age
  - there is considerable continuing secular change in body mass
  - there are no clear disease-risk thresholds

- Body mass index (BMI) charts can be used to adjust for age and sex effects
- Obesity is associated with complications in childhood, particularly insulin resistance
- Although most children have simple obesity some, particularly short, fat children, have underlying disease
- The treatment of obesity in children demands:

  - motivation of the child and family
  - a whole family approach to change in eating patterns
  - a whole family approach to change in lifestyle (activity level)

- The aim of treatment should generally be reduced rate of gain, rather than weight loss
- Excessively strict dieting may restrict height gain and should be avoided, particularly during the adolescent growth spurt

---

into early child mortality – a stage of life at which malnutrition and communicable diseases account for over 80% of deaths and a similar proportion of morbidity.

We will also be able to take a much longer view and turn attention to stemming the epidemic of non-communicable diseases – such as cardiovascular disease, diabetes, and cancer accounting for the burden of ill-health in later life. In other words we shall become more concerned with fine-tuning patterns of childhood growth and metabolic development in order to maximize lifelong metabolic fitness, thus optimizing functional capacity not just throughout childhood but into the adult years. This will require:

- Specialists in clinical nutrition who can take more of a life cycle view of human growth and development, transcending boundaries of disease-based specialities such as obstetrics, pediatrics, adult diabetology.
- Development of methods that can be used in a clinical context to measure: the (a) growth of separate body tissues and compartments, (b) the metabolic relationships between those compartments, and (c) the factors that control partitioning of nutrients between them.
- The identification of key stages in the life cycle for nutritional interventions.

- The development of interventions that are cost-effective, recognizing that the greatest burden of such disease and the accompanying disability will be borne by resource-poor countries.

References and further reading

Campbell AGM, McIntosh N (eds) *Forfar & Arneil's Textbook of Pediatrics.* New York: Churchill Livingstone, 1998.

Cole TJ. Do growth chart centiles need a face lift? *BMJ* 1994; 308: 641–642.

Cole TJ, Freeman JV, Preece MA. Body mass index reference curves for the UK, 1990. *Arch Dis Child* 1995; 73: 25–29.

Cole TJ, Bellizzi MC, Flegal KM, Dietz WH. Establishing a standard definition for child overweight and obesity worldwide: international survey. *BMJ* 2000; 320: 1240–1243.

Committee on Medical Aspects of Food and Nutrition Policy. *Scientific Review of the Welfare Food Scheme. Reports on Health and Social Subjects* 51. London: The Stationery Office, 2002. *Rep Health Soc Subj (Lond)*; 2002: 51: i–xxi, 1–147.

Department of Child Health and Adolescent Development. *Management of the Child with a Serious Infection or Severe Malnutrition.* Geneva: World Health Organization, 2000.

Dewey KG, Heinig MJ, Nommsen LA, Peerson JM, Lonnerdal B. Breast-fed infants are leaner than formula-fed infants at 1y of age: the DARLING study. *Am J Clin Nutr* 1993; 57: 140–145.

Dewey KG, Peerson JM, Brown KH *et al.* Growth of breast-fed infants deviates from current reference data: A pooled analysis of US, Canadian and European data sets. *Pediatrics* 1995; 96, 495–503.

Edmunds L, Waters E, Elliott EJ. Evidence based management of childhood obesity. *BMJ* 2001; 323: 916–919.

Fomon SJ, Ziegler EE. Renal solute load and potential renal solute load in infancy. *J Pediatr* 1999; 134: 11–14.

Fomon SJ, Haschke F, Ziegler EE, Nelson SE. Body composition of reference children from birth to age 10 years. *Am J Clin Nutr* 1982; 35: 1169–1175.

Freeman JV, Cole TJ, Chinn S, Jones PRM, White EM, Preece MA. Cross sectional stature and weight reference curves for the UK, 1990. *Arch Dis Child* 1995; 73: 17–24.

Holliday MA. Metabolic rate and organ size during growth from infancy to maturity and during late gestation and early infancy. *Pediatrics* 1971; 47: 169–179.

Kramer MS, Kakuma R. *The Optimal Duration of Exclusive Breastfeeding: a systematic review.* Geneva: World Health Organization, 2002.

McLaren DS, Burman D, Belton NR, Williams AF. (eds). *Textbook of Pediatric Nutrition*, 3rd edn. Edinburgh, Churchill Livingstone, 1991.

Michaelsen KF, Weaver L, Branca F, Robertson A. *Feeding and Nutrition of Infants and Young Children.* WHO Regional Publications, European Series, 87. Copenhagen: World Health Organization, 2000.

Scottish Intercollegiate Guidelines Network (SIGN). Management of obesity in children and young people. A national clinical guideline. 2003; No. 69.

Shaw V, Lawson M. *Clinical Paediatric Dietetics.* Oxford: Blackwell, 1994.

Stein C, Moritz I. *A Life Course Perspective of Maintaining Independence in Older Age*, pp. 1–20. Geneva: World Health Organization, 1999.

Tanner JM. *Foetus into Man: Physical growth from conception to maturity*, 2nd edn. Ware: Castlemead, 1989.

Widdowson EM. Changes in body composition during growth. In: Chapter 17 in *Scientific Foundations of Paediatrics*, Davis JA, Dobbing J (eds). Second edition. Heinemann, London, 1981.

Williams AF. Lactation and infant feeding. In: *Textbook of Paediatric Nutrition*, 3rd edn (DS McLaren, D Burman, NR Belton, AF Williams, eds). Edinburgh: Churchill Livingstone, 1991: 26–27.

Wright CM. Identification and management of failure to thrive: a community perspective. *Arch Dis Child* 2000; 82: 5–9.

23
Cystic Fibrosis

Olive Tully and Julie Dowsett

Key messages

- Cystic fibrosis is the most common life-shortening genetic disorder among white populations, with approximately 1 in 25 people being carriers for the condition.
- Cystic fibrosis patients are at an increased nutritional risk and malnutrition has been shown to have a negative effect on prognosis.
- The etiology of malnutrition is complex and arises as a result of the energy imbalance resulting from a combination of decreased energy intake, increased energy needs, and increased energy losses.

- Early nutritional management should be instituted from diagnosis in an attempt to minimize nutritional complications and maximize quality of life and survival.
- Many other features of cystic fibrosis may require specific nutritional intervention including diabetes, liver disease, and osteoporosis. A qualified dietitian experienced in the area of cystic fibrosis should give specialized nutritional counseling.

23.1 Introduction

Cystic fibrosis is the most common life-shortening genetic disorder among white people. It can impact on nutritional status in a number of ways to produce a negative energy balance and the ensuing malnutrition negatively impacts on quality of life and survival. Early identification and treatment of malnutrition has played a significant role in the increased survival in cystic fibrosis seen in the last four decades (Figure 23.1). Factors contributing to this improved survival are summarized in Box 23.1. Despite recent advances in nutrition management strategies, malnutrition continues to be a significant clinical issue for many cystic fibrosis patients at some time in their lives. This chapter will outline the main clinical features of cystic fibrosis and summarize their nutritional management.

23.2 Definition and pathology

Cystic fibrosis is a genetic disorder caused by the mutation of a single gene that encodes for the cystic fibrosis transmembrane regulator protein (CFTR). It is inherited in a Mendelian recessive manner, i.e. both parents of a child with cystic fibrosis carry at least one abnormal gene, as illustrated in Figure 23.2. The incidence of cystic fibrosis is 1 in 2500 in white people, with 1 in 25 being carriers. Table 23.1 shows the estimated frequency of cystic fibrosis at birth in different populations. Since the cystic fibrosis gene was first identified in 1989, over 1000 CFTR mutations have been reported.

The CFTR protein regulates the passage of chloride through the cell wall of secretory epithelia. The dysfunction of this protein results in altered fluid composition of epithelial secretions. The resultant dehydrated and sticky secretions lead to a dysfunction of many organ systems throughout the body. The transport of sodium, and more importantly chloride, is central to

Box 23.1 Factors contributing to an improved survival in cystic fibrosis

- Improved nutritional status
- Improved antibiotic treatment
- Early diagnosis
- Better physiotherapy techniques
- Treatment in specialist centers

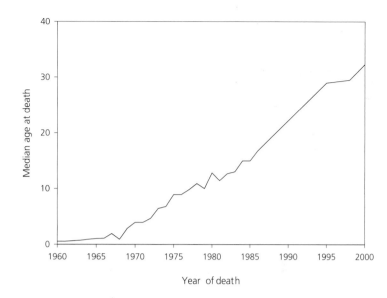

Figure 23.1 Expected survival for cystic fibrosis patients.

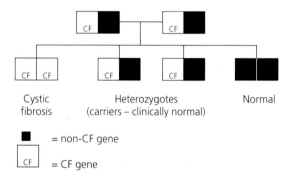

Figure 23.2 Mode of inheritance of cystic fibrosis – a Mendelian inherited recessive characteristic.

Table 23.1 Estimated frequency of cystic fibrosis at birth in different populations

National group	Birth incidence
UK	1/2500
USA (white)	1/3500
USA (African American)	1/14 000
USA (Asian)	1/25 500
Sweden	1/7700
The Netherlands	1/3600
Ireland	1/1500
Finland	1/25 000
Israel	1/3300
Japan	1/323 000
Faroe Islands	1/1800

the basic defect in cystic fibrosis. Diagnosis of cystic fibrosis is generally made on the basis of an elevated sweat sodium concentration.

23.3 Clinical features of cystic fibrosis

Clinically, cystic fibrosis is characterized by chronic lung disease, pancreatic insufficiency, and excessive losses of sweat electrolytes. The wide range of CFTR mutations are responsible, in some part, for the wide variety and severity of clinical manifestations of the disease.

The clinical features of cystic fibrosis can be broadly divided into respiratory and gastrointestinal manifestations, both of which have an effect on nutritional status and survival. As early as the 1980s a positive correlation was shown between nutritional status and survival. While progressive lung disease puts extra nutritional demands on patients with cystic fibrosis and can ultimately lead to nutritional failure, it also limits their ability to achieve these increased requirements.

There are many other clinical features of cystic fibrosis, including diabetes, liver disease, and osteoporosis, that will all have influences on a patient's nutritional needs. These are discussed later in the chapter.

The clinical features of cystic fibrosis are summarized in Box 23.2.

Box 23.2 The main clinical features of gastrointestinal and respiratory disorders related to cystic fibrosis

Gastrointestinal features of cystic fibrosis
- Gastroesophageal reflux
- Regurgitation
- Pancreatitis
- Pancreatic insufficiency
- Maldigestion
- Malabsorption
- Distal intestinal obstruction syndrome (DIOS)
- Cholelithiasis
- Cirrhosis
- Portal hypertension
- Splenomegaly
- Fibrosing colonopathy
- Rectal prolapse

Respiratory features of cystic fibrosis
- Bronchiectasis
- Bronchitis
- Pneumonia
- Atelectasis
- Pneumothorax
- Hemoptysis
- Sinus disease

Table 23.2 Nutritional consequences of respiratory disease in cystic fibrosis

Respiratory disease	Nutritional complication
Bronchitis	Increased energy requirements
Excessive coughing	Increased energy expenditure
	Risk of regurgitation
Pneumonia	Increased energy requirements
	Nutrient loss through sputum
	Poor appetite
Hemoptysis	Anemia
Sinusitis	Altered taste and smell

Table 23.2 summarizes the nutritional consequences of respiratory disease in cystic fibrosis.

Gastrointestinal features

Pancreatic insufficiency

The major gastrointestinal features of cystic fibrosis are as a result of malabsorption due to pancreatic insufficiency and a reduction in the production of digestive enzymes and bicarbonate. Pancreatic insufficiency results from cell atrophy due to the obstruction of pancreatic ducts by thickened secretions. The production of pancreatic secretions, including enzymes and bicarbonate, is reduced when more than 97% of the normal structure of the pancreas is lost. It is estimated that at least 85% of the cystic fibrosis population have some level of pancreatic insufficiency (PI) resulting in the malabsorption of macro- and micronutrients. Fat malabsorption (steatorrhea) leads to foul-smelling bulky stools, flatulence, and abdominal bloating and discomfort. As fat is the most calorie-dense nutrient this contributes to poor weight gain and has a negative impact on nutritional status. Fat malabsorption will also give rise to fat-soluble vitamin deficiencies (see Section 23.7 on vitamin supplementation).

A number of tests are available to assess pancreatic function, both direct and indirect, but there is no single 'ideal' test. Direct tests measuring pancreatic fluids are very useful and highly specific but their invasive nature precludes them from routine clinical use. Indirect tests including 72-h fecal fats are the most common but difficult in the clinical setting. Recently an enzyme-linked immunosorbent assay (ELISA) assay for the detection of the pancreatic enzyme elastase 1 in stool has begun to be used. This test is a sensitive and specific marker of exocrine pancreatic function and can be carried out in

Respiratory features of cystic fibrosis

The lungs of people with cystic fibrosis may be normal at birth but thereafter may rapidly develop pathological changes due to infection and chronic inflammation. Bacterial, viral, and fungal infections are all seen in cystic fibrosis with the most commonly isolated bacteria being *Pseudomonas aeruginosa*, *Staphylococcus aureus*, and *Haemophilus influenzae*.

Chronic pulmonary inflammation superimposed with periods of acute respiratory infection lead to an increased energy requirement, which may be difficult to achieve with the associated poor appetite and breathlessness. This can often be corrected in the short term, but if respiratory exacerbations become more frequent, nutritional status can deteriorate rapidly. Repeated coughing can cause vomiting, and large meals can exacerbate shortness of breath. Severe or prolonged coughing of blood (hemoptysis) may result in low iron stores and even iron deficiency anemia. Sinus disease, which is present in many cystic fibrosis patients, can have a negative impact on nutritional status as it may cause altered taste and smell sensations, leading to a decrease in overall dietary intake (see chapter 9 in the *Nutrition and Metabolism* textbook in this series).

the clinical setting. There may be logistical problems in measuring stool elastase in some patients.

Exocrine pancreatic dysfunction is treated with supplemental oral pancreatic enzyme replacement therapy (PERT). Due to the progressive nature of pancreatic disease in cystic fibrosis, patients who were originally pancreatic sufficient may, as they get older, develop pancreatic insufficiency and require enzyme supplementation.

PERT comes in the form of capsules, which must be taken with all meals, snacks, and drinks containing fat and or protein. Foods containing sugar only do not require enzymes for digestion. The active form of the enzyme is protected from the acid medium of the stomach by a pH-sensitive coating, which is activated in the more alkaline pH environment of the duodenum. Due to the reduced production of bicarbonate by the pancreas and the resulting lower pH in the duodenum of patients with cystic fibrosis, the enteric coating of the enzyme may fail to dissolve, in which case the enzyme will not become activated at the absorptive surface. Increasing the duodenal pH by taking proton pump inhibitors may improve enzymatic action.

Distal intestinal obstruction syndrome

Distal intestinal obstruction syndrome (DIOS) is a condition unique to cystic fibrosis that occurs when undigested food in combination with thick intestinal secretions causes partial or complete obstruction of the small bowel. Inadequate PERT, dietary changes, and dehydration appear to be the main precipitating factors in DIOS. Clinically the patient presents with abdominal cramps, pain, and distension. Partial obstruction can lead to complete obstruction with increasing severity of symptoms. DIOS is treated by using either large volumes of oral laxatives or enemas to clear the obstruction. All patients presenting with DIOS should have careful assessment of their diet and enzyme compliance and doses adjusted where necessary to maximize absorption.

Cystic fibrosis-related liver disease

The incidence of cystic fibrosis-related liver disease varies from 2% to 25% and is probably related to genetic mutation. Hepatic manifestations vary through all stages of liver disease from bile sludging, through stone formation to decompensated liver disease with portal hypertension, ascites, and cirrhosis. The early stage of cholestatic liver disease, demonstrated by an elevated serum alkaline phosphatase and gamma glutamyl-transferase, can be reversed by treatment with ursodeoxycholic acid. Organomegaly due to hepatomegaly, which may be accompanied by splenomegaly, can impact on a patient's ability to consume large volumes of food. This resultant 'small stomach syndrome' will have a negative effect on dietary intake and nutritional status. Liver disease is also a risk factor for vitamin K deficiency.

The primary cellular abnormality in cystic fibrosis affects the cells of bile ductules, with consequent reduced bile production and altered bile acid composition. Dehydrated secretions in the gallbladder can lead to bile sludging. Stone formation is probably related to large fecal losses of bile acids and a reduced bile acid pool, which causes the bile to become supersaturated with cholesterol and form stones.

The presence of esophageal varices should not be a contraindication to nasogastric feeding with fine-bore tubes. However, the presence of gastric varices is usually a contraindication to the placement of percutaneous gastrostomy tubes which may be needed for nutrition support.

Gastroesophageal reflux

Gastroesophageal reflux is common in cystic fibrosis. The exact cause of this is unknown. It may be related to increased abdominal–thoracic pressure caused by coughing and physiotherapy. H_2 antagonists or proton pump inhibitors are used in its treatment. Excessive early morning coughing can lead to regurgitation of gastric contents if patients have had overnight tube feeding. This problem can be overcome by postpyloric feeding methods.

Pancreatitis

The etiology of acute or chronic pancreatitis in cystic fibrosis is not fully clear but the viscous secretions from the pancreas may play a role in its development. It is more commonly seen in adults than in children. Recurrent pancreatitis in pancreatic sufficient patients can eventually lead to pancreatic insufficiency.

Fibrosing colonopathy

Fibrosing colonopathy is characterized pathologically by dense submucosal fibrosis, which leads to a narrowing and shortening of the colon. Associations have been seen between high-dose pancreatic enzyme intake and colonic strictures. More recently there have been suggestions that it is the substance methacrylic acid, used to coat certain brands of enzyme preparations, that causes this fibrosis of the colonic wall.

23.4 Malnutrition in cystic fibrosis

The etiology of malnutrition is threefold. A combination of decreased dietary intake, increased energy requirements, and increased energy losses gives rise to a negative energy balance. The majority of patients are capable of balancing these factors, but in those who do not, protein–energy malnutrition may develop. Malnutrition is defined as a weight-for-height value below 90% in children and a body mass index (BMI) below 19 kg/m² in adults.

Decreased dietary intake

People with cystic fibrosis are now recommended to consume a diet high in energy with no fat restriction. Prior to the development of enteric-coated enzymes in the mid-1980s, patients with cystic fibrosis were advised to follow a low-fat diet in an attempt to minimize steatorrhea. Because of this, some older patients

may continue to avoid eating foods high in fat. Some patients mistakenly follow dietary advice given to the general public. Many factors including repeated respiratory tract infections, gastrointestinal complications, drug side effects, reduced sensations of taste and smell, and social factors can all contribute to a reduced oral intake.

Increased energy requirements

Energy requirements are increased during periods of infection due to catabolism and fever and continue to increase with advanced pulmonary disease. As lung function deteriorates, energy requirements increase and appetite decreases. Total energy expenditure may be increased in some individuals, but a reduction in energy intake is by far the most important cause of a negative energy balance during acute exacerbations of respiratory infections.

Increased energy losses

The factors contributing to a negative energy balance in cystic fibrosis are summarized in Figure 23.3.

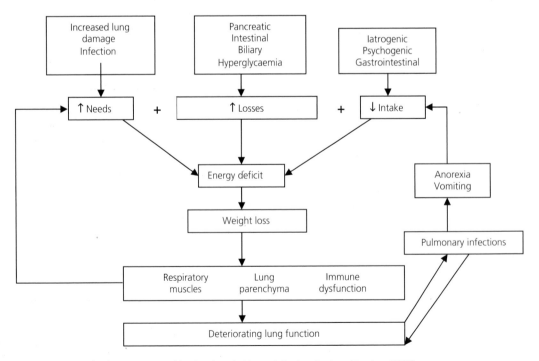

Figure 23.3 The etiology of malnutrition in cystic fibrosis. Adapted with permission from Durie and Pencharz (1989).

Malabsorption remains the most common reason for increased energy losses. Even with maximal PERT it has been estimated that up to 10% of ingested energy will be malabsorbed. Reduction of bile acid secretion can cause maldigestion as lipids fail to be emulsified in the lumen of the duodenum. Poorly controlled diabetes can lead to a negative energy balance due to glycosuria. Energy losses through sputum have been shown to be as high as 274 kcal daily. This energy loss could be significant in a patient whose overall nutritional intake is already compromised.

23.5 Other nutritional considerations in cystic fibrosis

As people with cystic fibrosis are living longer, the incidence of numerous other clinical complications is increasing. Many of these have either minor or major implications to nutritional status.

Cystic fibrosis-related diabetes

As the prognosis for patients with cystic fibrosis improves, the incidence of glucose intolerance and cystic fibrosis-related diabetes (CFRD) is becoming increasingly common. It is estimated that up to 50% of cystic fibrosis patients over 30 years of age will have some degree of impaired glucose tolerance. Many post-transplant patients are at high risk of developing CFRD secondary to steroid use. While CFRD shares features of both type 1 and type 2 diabetes, it is a clinically distinct entity. The primary cause of CFRD is insulin deficiency but other factors unique to cystic fibrosis can also affect glucose metabolism. These are summarized in Box 23.3. The diagnostic criteria for CFRD is similar to those of type 1 and type 2 diabetes. Random outpatient glucose measurements are useful for early diagnosis of CFRD. Fasting and 2-h postprandial blood sugar levels should be routinely measured to screen for impaired

---

Box 23.3 Factors affecting glucose metabolism

- Malnutrition
- Chronic and acute infection
- Glucagon deficiency
- Malabsorption
- Abnormal intestinal transit time
- Liver disease

Box 23.4 Diagnostic criteria for the diagnosis of cystic fibrosis-related diabetes

- 2-h postprandial glucose level >11.0 mmol/l during 75 g oral glucose tolerance test
- Fasting plasma glucose >7.0 mmol/l on two or more occasions
- Fasting plasma glucose >7.0 mmol/l and random glucose level >11.1 mmol/l
- Random glucose level >11.1 mmol/l on two or more occasions

---

glucose tolerance and CFRD. Box 23.4 summarizes the diagnostic criteria for CFRD. Glucose intolerance and CFRD may be intermittent, only occurring during times of infection or steroid use.

As the patient population ages it is likely that more micro- and macrovascular complications of CFRD will be seen. The nutritional management of CFRD should concentrate on optimizing nutritional status. Some dietary modification may be necessary to control blood sugars, including reducing intake of refined carbohydrate foods, especially sugar-containing drinks and those with a high glycemic index. Dietary advice given to patients with CFRD differs significantly from the advice given to non-cystic fibrosis diabetics (Box 23.5).

The medical management of choice in this group of patients is nearly always insulin therapy. Using new very short-acting insulin allows for greater dietary flexibility.

Cystic fibrosis-related osteoporosis

Recently there have been numerous reports of low bone density and osteoporosis in cystic fibrosis. Mean bone mineral density of patients with cystic fibrosis is one or more standard deviations below that expected for age and sex. There is a growing consensus

---

Box 23.5 Dietary advice given to patients with CFRD compared with type 1/type 2 diabetes

- High energy intake advised – calorie restriction is never advised to control blood sugars
- High fat intake is recommended to provide extra calories since macrovascular disease is not a concern
- Protein restriction is not recommended because of the potential for malnutrition
- Salt restriction is never advised
- Flexible meal plans are necessary to allow for periods of infection and poor intake

that osteopenia is widely prevalent in cystic fibrosis, although its cause is debated. Box 23.6 lists the possible causes of cystic fibrosis bone disease. Optimizing nutritional status is crucial in the prevention of osteopenia and osteoporosis. Daily supplementation with 400–2000 IU vitamin D is recommended to maintain normal levels of the vitamin. Keeping vitamin D levels in the higher end of the normal range is advisable to ensure optimal bone health. Vitamin K is also involved in bone metabolism given its role in osteocalcin production. Good compliance with pancreatic supplements is vital to maximize the absorption of the macro- and micronutrients necessary for achieving and maintaining bone health. Where possible, steroid use should be minimized and only used to treat respiratory disease when absolutely necessary due to the clear associations between steroid use and low bone density.

Eating disorders in cystic fibrosis

Atypical eating patterns have been reported amongst cystic fibrosis patients of differing age groups, particularly young children and adolescent females. Early identification of abnormal eating patterns and nutritional counseling are essential to reduce the further risk of malnutrition in this group.

Fertility issues in cystic fibrosis

Almost all males with cystic fibrosis are infertile as a result of the congenital bilateral absence of the vas deferens. Semen analysis is useful to identify the small percentage of males who may be fertile. Fertility in males is more likely with specific genotypes.

Fertility in females is usually normal as they have anatomically normal reproductive tracts. There are many reports of successful pregnancies in cystic fibrosis women, the first case being described in 1960. Women considering pregnancy should be advised of the potential risk to their own health as a result of the pregnancy as in some cases there may be a decline in lung function. Prepregnancy counseling should be encouraged and this should include carrier screening for the partner. Folic acid should be supplemented for the non-CF population. The most important determinant for a good outcome for mother and infant is minimal pulmonary disease and good nutritional status prepregnancy. Ideally in the preconception period every effort should be made to maximize respiratory and nutritional status. Regular monitoring with the cystic fibrosis and obstetric teams is crucial during the pregnancy, including regular monitoring of blood sugar levels in all individuals. Preconceptually women should be advised to reach their ideal body weight as there is evidence to show that women with a body weight closest to ideal had the least chance of delivering prematurely and had the highest chance of a normal delivery. In women with severe respiratory disease and malnutrition, outcome is poor for both mother and child. For women who are not gaining sufficient weight during pregnancy, supplementary nutrition as oral supplements or enteral feeding should be considered.

Lung transplantation in cystic fibrosis

Progressive lung disease continues to be the leading cause of morbidity and mortality in the cystic fibrosis population. Now bilateral lung transplantation offers a new hope for cystic fibrosis patients with end-stage pulmonary disease. Adequate nutritional status pretransplantation is an important factor in minimizing postoperative complications. Cystic fibrosis patients awaiting transplantation will frequently have impaired nutritional status as a result of their severe respiratory disease. Nutritional support of these patients both before and after transplantation may improve their survival and quality of life. In recent times patients who are unable to achieve and maintain an acceptable nutritional status pretransplant are encouraged to have gastrostomy tubes inserted to provide nocturnal nutritional support. Postoperatively patients will be prescribed steroids so care must be taken to monitor and treat blood glucose levels.

In general, transplantation is associated with an improvement in nutritional status. However, despite the improved lung function, patients will still have the gastrointestinal features of cystic fibrosis.

23.6 Nutritional management

The correlation between suboptimal nutritional status and the severity of lung disease has long been recognized. Good nutritional status is associated with improved prognosis and, for this reason, the goal of nutritional management in cystic fibrosis is to achieve and maintain ideal body weight for height by maximizing nutritional intake, minimizing malabsorption and maldigestion, monitoring vitamin intakes and serum levels, and adapting eating patterns in the advent of other complicating factors.

Box 23.7 summarizes the main goals of nutrition therapy.

Assessment of nutritional status

Body composition and anthropometry
Studies of body composition in cystic fibrosis patients have shown deficits in total body mass, lean body mass, and body fat. Generally cystic fibrosis patients weigh less than age- and sex-matched controls. Other anthropometric measurements including mid-arm circumference are not used routinely in cystic fibrosis. The reliability and reproducibility of these anthropometric measurements tends to be poor in cystic fibrosis and thus they are rarely used.

Total body potassium (TBK) measurements have been used to assess body composition in cystic fibrosis patients. Using TBK as an indicator of nutritional status has identified larger numbers of nutritionally compromised patients. There is also decreased bone mineral density in patients with cystic fibrosis as a result of many contributing factors, as discussed above in the section on osteoporosis.

The most frequently measured anthropometric measurements are weight and height. These should be plotted on a percentile chart for patients <19 years (see Chapter 22). Weight is expressed as a percentage of the ideal weight for height in adults. Table 23.3 summarizes the categories of weight for height classifications

Table 23.3 Categories of malnutrition

Percentage of ideal body weight	Category
90–110	Acceptable
85–89	Underweight (early malnutrition)
80–84	Mild malnutrition
75–79	Moderate malnutrition
<75	Severe malnutrition

Ramsey BW, Farrell PM, Pencharz P. (1992).

as used in the 1992 Nutrition Consensus Document. BMI is used in cystic fibrosis to express nutritional status. The goal in cystic fibrosis is to have BMI values of 20–25, which is the acceptable range for the normal population.

Assessing energy requirements
Until recently, it was thought that the energy requirements of cystic fibrosis patients were greater than those of their age- and sex-matched peers. More recently it has been suggested that despite an increased resting energy expenditure (REE) in people with cystic fibrosis total daily expenditure is not elevated due to reduced activity levels within this group. Increased energy and protein intakes should be encouraged during periods when patients are not acutely unwell to allow for repletion of fat and lean body mass. In practice energy requirements should be determined by assessing total energy expenditure. There are many ways of assessing nutritional requirements (see Box 23.8).

After calculating basal metabolic rate (BMR), additions are then made for degree of stress and mobility. Note that this calculation of energy requirements does not consider energy losses through malabsorption, sputum, and hyperglycemia.

Dietary assessment
All patients with cystic fibrosis should have an annual detailed dietary assessment by an experienced dietitian

to assess nutritional adequacy. It is important to ensure that patients are meeting their requirements of all nutrients. Computerized dietary analysis programs can be useful in this regard.

PERT should be maximized in an attempt to optimize the digestion and absorption of macro- and micronutrients. The correct number of pancreatic enzymes for a patient is the amount that results in normal bowel function in both consistency and frequency of defecation.

Nutritional support in cystic fibrosis

Diet and nutritional supplements
Cystic fibrosis patients are usually advised to consume a high-protein, high-calorie diet. Emphasis should be put on the importance of meeting nutritional requirements and preventing deterioration in nutritional status. Frequent meals and snacks should be encouraged, with specific and individual advice given regarding enzyme supplementation. As with other patients requiring nutritional support, if diet or fortified food is not successful in meeting energy needs, sip or tube feeding may be required (see Chapter 8).

Enteral nutrition
Where diet and nutritional supplements fail to achieve or maintain optimal nutritional status, supplementary enteral nutrition should be considered. When weight falls below 85% ideal body weight (IBW) or a BMI = 19 kg/m^2, patients should be advised to consider nocturnal gastrostomy feeding. A sustained weight gain and a slowing decline in respiratory function has been associated with supplemental feeding. Gastrostomy tubes can be passed surgically, endoscopically, or under fluoroscopic guidance and are generally well tolerated with infrequent complications.

The types of tubes used vary between cystic fibrosis centers but over the last decade the low-profile 'button' devices have become popular as they are cosmetically more acceptable for this patient group. Postpyloric feeding by adapting gastrostomy tubes with a jejunal extension usually solves the problems of gastroesophageal reflux, delayed gastric emptying, and early morning regurgitation associated with coughing.

Whole protein polymeric feeds can be used successfully in some patients; in older patients with reduced pancreatic function semi-elemental formulas can be used. These specific formulas contain medium-chain triglyceride (MCT) fat and protein in the form of peptides and amino acids, thus requiring fewer pancreatic enzymes for digestion. Enzymes are usually given in divided doses at the beginning and end of the feeding period. In some cases elemental feeds will be used where other formulas are poorly tolerated. The type of feed to be used must be assessed on an individual basis by the dietitian as the optimum feed will depend on many factors including degree of pancreatic function, and individual patient tolerance. Feeds are usually administered overnight in an attempt to maximize oral intake during the day. For patients with impaired glucose tolerance or cystic fibrosis-related diabetes, blood sugar levels should be monitored carefully as extra insulin may be required to control blood glucose levels.

Pancreatic enzyme replacement therapy (PERT)
All people with cystic fibrosis probably have some level of pancreatic dysfunction but the requirements of PERT are variable and must be assessed individually. The recommended daily dose of pancreatic enzymes is less than 2500 units of lipase per kilogram body weight per meal (10 000 units/kg per day). Higher doses should be used with caution, and only if quantitative measures demonstrate substantially improved absorption.

23.7 Vitamin supplementation in cystic fibrosis

Subclinical and frank clinical deficiencies of several vitamins have been reported in cystic fibrosis. Fat-soluble vitamin deficiency is common as a direct result of pancreatic insufficiency and dietary fat malabsorption. With the use of pancreatic enzyme replacement therapy and routine vitamin supplementation, clinical problems arising from deficiencies of vitamins have become rare. However, cystic fibrosis patients are at risk from developing clinical or subclinical vitamin deficiencies if:

- the diagnosis of cystic fibrosis is made late,
- patients have had previous small bowel resection,
- there is poor compliance with vitamin supplements or enzymes, or
- liver disease is present.

Factors other than the malabsorption of fat may play a role in the development of specific vitamin deficien-

Table 23.4 Current recommendations for vitamin doses

Vitamin	Recommended dose
Vitamin A	4000–10 000 IU daily
Vitamin D	400–800 IU daily
Vitamin E	100–400 IU daily
Vitamin K	No consensus
Water-soluble vitamins	200% RDA

RDA, recommended dietary allowance.

cies. The most recent Nutrition Consensus Statement made specific recommendations for vitamin supplementation (Table 23.4). More detailed information about the role of vitamins is found in chapter 8 of the *Introduction to Human Nutrition* in this series.

Vitamin E

Vitamin E is a highly effective antioxidant. Alpha-tocopherol is the most bioactive form of vitamin E and is the form most frequently measured in cystic fibrosis. The absorption of vitamin E is dependent on the ability to absorb fat from the small intestine, and due to its high lipophilic nature vitamin E deficiency correlates closely with degree of malabsorption. The subsequent transport of the vitamin within the body and its uptake appears largely to follow the paths available to other relatively non-polar lipids such as triacylglycerols and cholesterol.

Functions of vitamin E

In humans chronic deficiency of vitamin E results in progressive neurological degeneration. This neurological decline has been recognized in patients with cystic fibrosis not receiving supplementation. Vitamin E may also be important in controlling the progression of lung disease in cystic fibrosis. A proportion of the lung injury that occurs is thought to be due to the host inflammatory response, in particular the release of free radicals and proteolytic enzymes from neutrophils. The antioxidant properties of alpha-tocopherol are thought to protect tissues from damage by free radicals and stabilize cell membranes. However, there are as yet no long-term studies of vitamin E supplementation in cystic fibrosis that have been able to show a beneficial effect on the lung. Correction of vitamin E deficiency has also been associated with a significant rise in hemoglobin levels. This effect is most likely to be due to

increased erythrocyte survival time once vitamin E deficiency is corrected, since vitamin E deficiency is a recognized cause of hemolytic anemia in low-birth-weight infants.

Supplementation of vitamin E

The recommended daily dosage of vitamin E is 100–400 IU daily. Where possible, this should be given in the more efficiently absorbed form of a water-miscible preparation. The supplements should be taken at mealtimes with pancreatic enzymes – again to aid absorption. It is important to remember that standard multivitamin preparations will not provide sufficient amounts of vitamin E for a cystic fibrosis patient.

Vitamin A and beta-carotene

Vitamin A consists of retinoids and carotenoids. One of the first signs of vitamin A deficiency is night blindness and there have been several reports of this in cystic fibrosis. Deficiency of vitamin A is again largely due to pancreatic insufficiency and malabsorption. Vitamin A and carotenoids tend to aggregate with lipids into globules, which then pass into the small intestine. The upper intestine is the main site of lipid hydrolysis. Patients with cystic fibrosis have been shown to have low serum levels of retinol but normal or even elevated liver levels of the vitamin indicating a failure in the mobilization or transportation of the hepatic stores to other tissues by retinol-binding protein (RBP). People with cystic fibrosis often have low levels of RBP which may be due to an abnormality in its production in the liver, zinc deficiency, or protein–energy malnutrition. Fecal loses of retinol may also have an effect on serum levels of vitamin A. There may be a specific defect in the handling of retinol by the gastrointestinal tract in cystic fibrosis, which may be unrelated to the digestion and absorption of dietary fat.

Vitamin A levels must be monitored carefully in cystic fibrosis patients who become pregnant as high levels have been shown to be damaging to the developing fetus.

Beta-carotene is one of the carotinoids present in plasma and is a precursor of vitamin A. It is effective as an antioxidant at lower oxygen saturation states than vitamin E. Routine supplementation with beta-carotene could diminish lipid peroxidation and improve essential fatty acid status.

Functions of vitamin A

Whilst clinical problems directly attributable to vitamin A deficiency are relatively uncommon in cystic fibrosis the effects of subclinical deficiency on the progression of lung disease are not known. Animals made deficient in vitamin A commonly die of respiratory and genito-urinary infections before xerophthalmia becomes established. In animal models, carotenoids have been shown to boost the immune response. The method of their action is unclear. Studies need to be performed in cystic fibrosis to assess the long-term effects of vitamin A deficiency on lung disease.

Vitamin A supplementation

The recommended dose of vitamin A is 4000–10 000 IU daily. It should be given daily in the form of a water-soluble preparation if possible. Vitamin A deficiency also correlates with malabsorption and low levels may indicate poor compliance with both pancreatic enzymes and vitamin supplements. In view of the toxicity of vitamin A, a daily dosage greater than 20 000 IU should not be given if RBP is low.

Vitamin D

Much interest has been generated recently regarding vitamin D deficiency and cystic fibrosis because of the increased prevalence of low bone density and osteoporosis among cystic fibrosis populations. A variety of factors may lead to this deficiency state, including fat malabsorption leading to malabsorption of vitamin D, inadequate calcium intakes, underexposure to sunlight, and, in rare cases, defects of metabolism due to liver disease.

Recently many studies have demonstrated low levels of vitamin D despite daily supplementation with between 400–800 IU vitamin D. Recent evidence suggests that vitamin D levels should be maintained towards the upper level of the normal range to ensure optimal bone health.

Supplementation of vitamin D

The current recommendations for vitamin D supplementation in cystic fibrosis are 400–800 IU daily. As many patients display suboptimal levels at this dose serum levels should be monitored and supplements adjusted accordingly. It has been recently suggested that a dose of 400–2000 IU/day may be required to keep levels within the normal range.

Vitamin K

There is currently no consensus on routine vitamin K supplementation. Protein induced in vitamin K absence (PIVKA II) is probably the most useful marker of vitamin K deficiency in cystic fibrosis. Using PIVKA II levels, vitamin K deficiency has been shown to be present in more than three-quarters of cystic fibrosis patients with pancreatic insufficiency. It would seem prudent to prescribe vitamin K supplements to all patients with any of the following risk factors:

- Pancreatic insufficiency
- Severe liver disease
- Extensive small bowel resection
- Chronic broad-spectrum antibiotic use
- Hemoptysis.

Given the role of vitamin K in the formation of osteocalcin, subclinical deficiency may play a role in osteopenia and osteoporosis in cystic fibrosis patients.

Monitoring of fat-soluble vitamins

Fat-soluble vitamins should be checked regularly, especially vitamins A, D, and E. These levels should be checked annually if stable and more frequently if abnormal. Vitamin doses may need to be altered depending on serum levels. When the blood is taken it should be covered with foil to protect the sample from degradation by sunlight. Serum levels of vitamins should be monitored in those patients with pancreatic sufficiency, as low levels may highlight the transition from pancreatic sufficiency to insufficiency that can occur in older cystic fibrosis patients.

Water-soluble vitamins

Low levels of water-soluble vitamins have been reported in this population but are rare. Recent recommendations state that if the patient has a well-balanced diet, routine supplementation of water-soluble vitamins should not be required.

23.8 Mineral status in cystic fibrosis

The minerals most likely to be deficient in cystic fibrosis are iron, zinc, and selenium.

Iron

Iron deficiency has been reported in up to one-third of patients with cystic fibrosis. There are many possible causes of iron deficiency in cystic fibrosis including:

- Chronic inflammation
- Dietary deficiency
- Gastrointestinal or pulmonary blood loss
- Malabsorption.

Cystic fibrosis patients should have routine iron studies to assess iron stores. Routine supplementation with oral iron is not advised but should be considered in deficient patients.

Zinc

In normal situations, zinc absorption from the diet is in the region of 25–30%. This is affected by host factors including diarrhea, mucosal defects, and nutritional status. In cystic fibrosis, zinc absorption may be compromised due to steatorrhea. Zinc status in cystic fibrosis is thought to worsen as the severity of disease increases. Zinc supplementation should be considered where there is growth retardation and severe steatorrhea.

Selenium

There is no current consensus on selenium supplementation. Where selenium deficiency as been reported, some authors suggest that it may be the result of a maternal malabsorptive syndrome or of an abnormality of selenium transfer. The deficiency can occur either prenatally or postnatally and particularly in the preschool rapid growth years. Selenium, being a precursor of the antioxidant enzyme glutathione peroxidase, may have an important role in lung health. Selenium levels may also fall with increasing age in cystic fibrosis. Selenium deficiency is rare, but two disorders of selenium deficiency are known: Keshan disease (China and East Asia affected) and Kashin–Bech disease, which are both due to environmental factors (lack of selenium in soil).

23.9 Perspectives on the future

In recent years new treatments have evolved which may significantly affect the course of cystic fibrosis. These new treatments include gene therapy, correction of the abnormality in airway epithelial cell ion transport, and the use of newly developed anti-inflammatory/antimicrobial agents.

Gene therapy

The identification of the cystic fibrosis transmembrane regulator protein (CFTR) has created the potential for gene therapy. The fundamental idea is to administer a normal version of the cystic fibrosis gene or protein so as to restore normal cellular function and therefore prevent and treat the disease. For gene therapy to work successfully an efficient therapeutic gene that can transfer easily to the correct cells *in vivo* must be developed. Despite much early positive work in gene therapy this has not yet been achieved.

Ion transport therapy

Pharmacological products that correct the abnormal cellular transport of chloride are being tested both *in vitro* and *in vivo*. They can work by either improving the function of CFTR, activating alternate chloride channels and therefore enhancing chloride transport and by reducing the increased transport of sodium in the airways. Some promising results have been achieved but as yet there are not enough data to allow these agents to be used in routine use.

Anti-inflammatory agents

The inflammatory response in cystic fibrosis is so excessive that it can produce a cycle of immune hyperresponsiveness which can ultimately cause further tissue damage which favors more bacterial growth. Counteracting this inflammatory damage has become as area of major interest. These include steroid treatment, α_1-antitrypsin, and the use of non-steroidal anti-inflammatory medications. Current research favors using non-steroidal anti-inflammatory drugs in order to minimize the damaging side effects of steroids, such as diabetes and osteoporosis.

While these new treatments have the potential to significantly improve prognosis and quality of life in cystic fibrosis, they are not currently in routine use. Until these therapies are widely available for routine clinical use, the focus must remain on the more conventional treatment options, which are currently improving the prognosis of cystic fibrosis patients. Within this routine nutritional assessment, counseling, and support have an essential role to play.

References and further reading

Dowsett J. An overview of nutritional issues for the adult with cystic fibrosis. *Nutrition* 2000; 16: 566–570.

Durie PR, Pencharz PB. A rational approach to the nutritional care of patients with cystic fibrosis. *J R Soc Med* 1989; 82(Suppl 16): 11–20.

Moran A, Hardin D, Rodman D *et al.* Diagnosis, screening and management of cystic fibrosis related diabetes mellitus. A consensus conference report. *Diabetes Res Clin Pract* 1999; 45: 61–73.

Pencharz PB, Durie PR. Pathogenesis of malnutrition in cystic fibrosis, and its treatment. *Clin Nutr* 2000; 19: 387–394.

Ramsey BW, Farrell PM, Pencharz P. Nutritional assessment and management of cystic fibrosis: a consensus report. *Am J Clin Nutr* 1992; 55: 108–16.

Sinaasappel M, Stern M, Littlewood J *et al.* Nutrition in patients with cystic fibrosis: a European Consensus. *J Cyst Fibros* 2002; 1: 51–75.

24
Water and Electrolytes

Meritxell Girvent, Guzmán Franch, and Antonio Sitges-Serra

Key messages

- Water represents the most abundant component of the human body, accounting for up to 60–70% of its weight.
- Total body water (TBW) is contained in two main compartments: the intracellular (ICW) and the extracellular water (ECW).
- The ICW is the site of all the metabolic processes of the body and the ECW provides a constant external environment in which the cells function. It is through the ECW that all exchanges of water and solutes between the cells and the external environment occur.
- Thirst is a behavioral response to losses of body fluid. Together with reflex endocrine and neural responses, thirst

is responsible for maintaining the homeostasis of body fluids, and more specifically for the regulation of the ECW.
- In certain pathological conditions water accumulates in a so-called 'third space' causing profound alterations in hemodynamics, endocrine responses regulating water and sodium, and in the distribution of plasma proteins.
- Starvation, severe trauma, and sepsis as well as several disease processes can cause alterations in the sizes of the body water compartments and in exchangeable ions and may acutely alter the volume and composition of the ICW.

24.1 Introduction

Since the days of the Ancient Greeks, it has been recognized that the biosphere is composed of four basic elements: earth, wind, fire, and water. These elements were thought to combine or segregate according to forces of attraction and repulsion. Central to our understanding of human nutrition is the knowledge that the four constituent elements of life are still relevant, although three of them are currently known under names quite different from those given to them by the Ancient Greeks. 'Earth' contains most of the nutritional substrates including vitamins and trace elements. 'Winds' are the respiratory gases required supporting cell life or produced as by-products of metabolic processes occurring within the cell. 'Fire' is the energy resulting from substrate. Water is the only element that is still called by its original name.

This chapter will review some basic aspects of water and electrolyte metabolism relevant to several major areas of clinical nutrition such as body composition, undernutrition, nutrition assessment, and refeeding.

24.2 Water, electrolytes, and body composition

Life emerged on our planet a billion of years ago from a 'cosmic broth' which probably contained concentrations of sodium and other electrolytes similar to those of the extracellular fluid of mammals. In fact, the independent life of mammals was made possible only after a very long evolutionary process led to the internalization of this original sea. Claude Bernard, a renowned French physiologist, coined the term '*milieu intérieur*' to refer to this internalization of the *milieu extérieur*, the sea of life.

As a result of this process, water represents the most abundant component of the human body, accounting for up to 60–70% of its weight. The proportion of total body water (TBW) is lower in women, in the obese, and in the elderly, due to a higher content of body fat. Conversely, TBW may account for over 75% of the body weight in infants and in excessively lean individuals because of their low levels of depot fat.

Through the evolutionary process, mammals have developed a very sophisticated and efficient system to preserve water and sodium, allowing them to survive in a dry environment. Thus, from a general point of view, water- and sodium-retaining mechanisms are much more developed and powerful than those designed for water and electrolyte excretion. This is particularly true for sodium excretion. This concept of relative inefficiency or weakness of sodium excretion mechanisms will appear repeatedly in this chapter, since many disease processes, and particularly those related to undernutrition and stress, are very often associated with an increase of the extracellular pools of water and sodium.

24.3 Body water distribution

Body water is contained in two main compartments: the intracellular (ICW) and the extracellular water (ECW). The ICW is the site of all the metabolic processes of the body and contains approximately two-thirds of the TBW (40% of the body weight). The ECW (20% of the body weight) provides a constant external environment in which the cells function. It is through the ECW that all exchanges of water and solutes between the cells and the external environment occur.

The ECW is itself subdivided into several compartments, the largest of which are the interstitial-lymph water and the plasma water, separated from each other by the capillary wall. There are also three further small ECW compartments: connective tissues such as cartilage and tendons, the bone matrix, and the epithelial secretions also known as transcellular water (digestive tract, sweat, cerebrospinal, pleural, synovial, and intraocular fluids). For practical purposes, we shall consider that the ECW is subdivided into just two components: the plasma water, which accounts for one-quarter of the ECW, and the interstitial water compartment, roughly accounting for three-quarters of the ECW (Figure 24.1).

In certain pathological conditions water accumulates in a so-called 'third space' causing profound alterations in hemodynamics, endocrine responses regulating water and sodium, and in the distribution of plasma proteins. This 'third space' is not constant from the anatomical point of view and can be located in the retroperitoneum (e.g. in acute pancreatitis), in the abdominal cavity (e.g. ascitis or within the bowel lumen), or as generalized edema in the subcutaneous tissue.

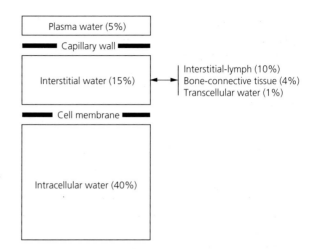

Figure 24.1 The body water compartments. Figures are percentages of body weight in the average individual.

24.4 Body electrolyte content: distribution and exchangeable fractions

The concentrations of the major cations and anions found in the ECW and ICW are summarized in Table 24.1. Na^+ is the major cation found in the ECW, and Cl^- and HCO_3^- are the major anions. The ionic compositions of the two subcompartments of the ECW (interstitial and plasma water) are almost identical since they are separated by the capillary wall which is freely permeable to small ions. The most significant difference between interstitial and plasma water is that the latter contains significantly more protein. Since pro-

Table 24.1 Concentrations of major cations and anions in the ECW and ICW

	ECW	ICW
Anions (mEq/l)		
Cl^-	105	60
HCO_3^-	25	50
$H_2PO_4^{2-}$	2	50
Proteins	14	50
Other[a]	6	80
Cations (mEq/l)		
Na^+	145	12
K^+	4	150
Ca^{2+}	5	0.001
pH	7.4	7.1

ECW, extracellular water; ICW, intracellular water.
[a]Largely represents organic phosphates such as ATP.

teins constitute a fraction of the plasma anions, their presence in plasma affects the distribution of cations and anions across the capillary wall (Gibbs–Donnan effect). This effect is rather small and so, for practical purposes, the ionic composition of the interstitial fluid and plasma can be considered identical.

In contrast to ECW, the concentration of Na^+ in the ICW is low, and K^+ is the predominant cation of this compartment. This uneven distribution of Na^+ and K^+ across the cell membrane is maintained by the enzyme Na^+/K^+ ATPase, which continuously pumps Na^+ out of the cell in exchange for K^+. The anion composition of the ICW also differs notably from that of the ECW. Concentrations of Cl^- and HCO_3^- are lower than those of the ECW. Other major ICW anions are phosphates, organic anions, and proteins.

The exchangeable fraction of a given electrolyte is the percentage of total body content for that particular ion that can easily move between the ECW and ICW compartments, and between the ECW compartment and the external environment. It is the exchangeable fraction that permits adjustments of the ion concentration in a given body fluid. The non-exchangeable fraction is that percentage of the total body ion that is combined with other substances (i.e. bone or collagen) and so will not diffuse between compartments.

Total body sodium averages 60 mEq/kg weight in the normal adult, and is mostly distributed across the ECW with only 3% found in the cells. Some 70% of the total body sodium is readily exchangeable (Na_e).

The average normal adult has a total body potassium of 53 mEq/kg weight, with an exchangeable fraction (K_e) of 92%, which is mostly distributed within the cells. Only 2–3% of exchangeable body potassium is located outside the cells and this is the reason why measurements of plasma potassium concentrations do not appropriately reflect the total body potassium pool. Nevertheless, this small extracellular potassium pool is extremely important for the acid–base balance and for the transmission of electrical impulses along nerves and cell membranes.

24.5 Intracellular water and the body cell mass concept

Potassium within the cells reaches a concentration of 150–165 mEq/l. Phosphate is also an important intracellular anion salt. Body pools of these two ions are related to the total body protein, and closely follow changes of the total body protein pool. In catabolic conditions, protein is lost from the cells and so are potassium and phosphate. In contrast, during anabolism, protein accrual is paralleled by positive potassium and phosphate balances. The quantitative physiological relationship between potassium and nitrogen is approximately 3 mEq K/g N. Accordingly, the interrelationship between free or exchangeable potassium, nitrogen, and cellular mass is used in body composition analysis to calculate the so-called body cell mass (BCM), the metabolically active, oxygen-consuming compartment of the organism. Thus:

$$BCM\ (g) = K_e\ (mEq) \times 8.33$$

In addition, in conditions of stable hydration of the body cell mass, it is assumed that:

$$K_e\ (mEq) = 150\ (ICW\ in\ liters) + 60$$

The relationship between exchangeable potassium and body protein may change in pathological conditions. Potassium depletion and repletion during catabolism and refeeding may be more rapid than changes in body protein. This finding may explain the early positive clinical response to nutritional repletion in malnourished individuals even prior to any measurable change of the body protein.

Extracellular water

The intravascular or plasma water volume is of critical importance in maintaining appropriate organ perfusion, transporting oxygen and nutrients to cells, and in facilitating communication between organs and tissues through transfer of humoral mediators such as hormones, cytokines, and neurotransmitters. Accordingly, the 'nutritional' relevance of ECW is substantial. Severe circulatory and/or respiratory distress results in impaired tissue perfusion and oxygen supply, which makes uptake and oxidation of substrates by cells impossible. There is an intimate relationship between cardiorespiratory homeostasis and alteration of energy consumption and substrate oxidation. These have been very well delineated by the Buffalo group and their work is an important reference in the area (Siegel JH et al., 1979). In view of the critical importance of the intravascular volume for survival, it is not surprising that the volume, composition, and osmolality of this subcompartment of the ECW remains tightly controlled by cardiac, renal, vascular, and endocrine responses (see below).

The interstitial space

The interstitial water acts as a buffer for changes occurring in the plasma volume. In contrast to the systemic regulatory mechanisms controlling the ECW, the regulation of the interstitial volume is largely local, governed by Starling's law (Figure 24.2), which regulates fluid exchange across the different capillary beds. Briefly, Starling's law postulates that the net fluid exchange across a capillary bed is the final result of opposing forces: the hydrostatic capillary and the oncotic (protein-related) interstitial pressures tend to draw water out of the capillary while the hydrostatic interstitial and the plasma oncotic pressures tend to retain fluid within the capillary.

Increased vascular hydrostatic pressure, decreased plasma oncotic pressure (Figure 24.3), or increased

(a) Hydrostatic pressure

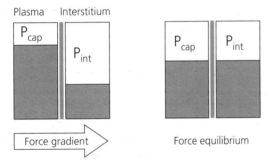

(b) Oncotic (colloidosmotic) pressure

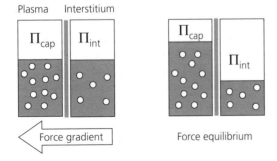

Figure 24.2 Diagrammatic model showing the effect of hydrostatic and oncotic pressure gradients on fluid movements across the capillary wall. P, hydrostatic pressure; π, oncotic pressure; cap, capillary; int, interstitial.

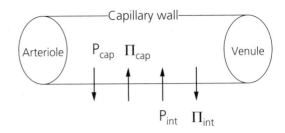

Net filtration = Lp S (Δ hydraulic pressure - Δ oncotic pressure)
= Lp S [(P_{cap} - P_{int}) - σ (Π_{cap} - Π_{int})]

Figure 24.3 Different hydrostatic and oncotic pressure forces involved in fluid movement across the capillary wall. The equation that calculates the net filtration force represents Starling's law. P, hydrostatic pressure; π, oncotic pressure; cap, capillary; int, interstitial; Lp, porosity of the capillary wall; S, surface area available for filtration; Δ gradient; σ reflection coefficient of proteins across the capillary wall.

permeability of the capillaries all facilitate water flowing out of the vessels towards the interstitium and from there, via the lymphatic system, back to the circulation. Lymph drainage of the interstitium is of paramount importance to prevent edema formation. If, however, a shift of water towards the interstitium exceeds the lymphatic drainage (which can increase up to 30 times) then edema ensues. This occurs typically in circumstances of aggressive fluid therapy for resuscitation (trauma or sepsis), heart failure, or a combination of both. In the more chronic situation, extreme hypoalbuminemia (serum albumin <25 g/l) is associated with a low colloidosmotic capillary pressure, allowing more water to flow out of the capillaries and causing interstitial edema.

Distribution of macromolecules within the ECW

Plasma proteins do not move freely across the capillary wall. There is, however, a constant transcapillary flux of proteins, depending on their molecular weight and electric charge. There are also different degrees of impermeability to plasma proteins in the different capillary beds, a physiological phenomenon reflected in Starling's law by the capillary reflection coefficient (σ) (Figure 24.3). For example, the hepatic sinusoidal capillaries are permeable to plasma proteins while the pulmonary capillary bed is almost totally impermeable to them. In the case of albumin (the most important plasma protein in terms both of concentration and volume of transfer across the capillary membrane) the physiological transcapillary flux may amount to 150 g/day, which means half of its total body mass. Overall, 60% of the total albumin pool is situated in the interstitial space while the remaining 40% is in the intravascular compartment. These proportions may change, however, when alterations of the interstitial matrix occur.

The normal interstitium is composed of a hyaluronan glycosaminglycan gel matrix embedded in collagen fibers. Experimental evidence shows that the physical space occupied by this interstitial matrix is partially excluded for macromolecules and plasma proteins. Nevertheless, the available space for macromolecules may rapidly change when variations in the interstitial gel matrix hydration occur: the more hydrated the interstitial matrix, the more available space there is for protein distribution. Hence, the movement of proteins across the capillary wall may be consistently affected by both changes in the hydration of the interstitium and/or changes of the hydrostatic capillary pressure forcing water and a protein equivalent to move out of the vascular bed (convective protein transport). These mechanisms explain why a substantial decrease in the albumin plasma concentration occurs after a rapid increase of the ECW volume (Figure 24.4).

Fluid shifts between ECW and ICW compartments

Water moves freely across cell membranes. Except for brief periods of time, ECW and ICW are in osmotic equilibrium. Hence, a measurement of plasma os-

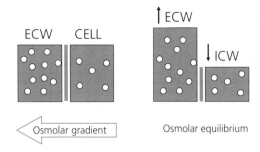

Figure 24.5 Diagrammatic model showing the effect of the osmotic pressure gradient on water movement across the cell membrane.

molarity provides a measure of both ECW and ICW osmolarity. On the other hand the movement of ions across cell membranes depends on the presence of specific transporters that maintain constant intracellular ion concentrations. For the sake of simplification, it can be assumed that there is no appreciable shift of ions across the cell membrane. Thus, it can then be assumed that equilibration between ECW and ICW osmolarity occurs only by a movement of water, and not by movement of osmotically active solutes. These water shifts occur only when the ECW osmolarity is altered (Figure 24.5).

24.6 Regulation of body water compartments

The volume and the osmolarity of the body water are very tightly controlled by systemic regulatory mechanisms through two major physiological actions:

(1) the regulation of water and electrolyte balance (equilibrium between the intake and output of water and electrolytes), and
(2) the regulation of the body water distribution.

Both major physiological mechanisms aim at the same target: regulating within narrow limits both the osmolarity of body fluids and the extracellular fluid volume that is effectively perfusing the tissues (effective circulating volume).

Control of body fluid osmolarity

Body fluid osmolarity is maintained through a tight control of water balance in the range of 285–295 mosmol/l. Normally, thirst (see below) is the

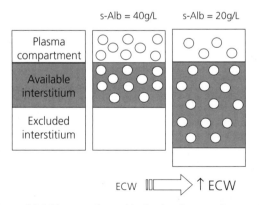

Figure 24.4 Diagrammatic model showing how an increase in extracellular water (e.g. after acute saline infusion) induces a distribution related decrease in serum albumin. The excluded interstitium represents the glycosaminglycan and collagen interstitial gel matrix. Dots represent arbitrary units of albumin mass. S-alb, serum albumin; ECW, extracellular water. Adapted from Franch-Arcas *et al.* (1998).

major signal to increase water intake. On the other hand, the kidneys are responsible for adjusting the water balance by diluting or concentrating the urine. Vasopressin (antidiuretic hormone or ADH) is the major endocrine mediator between changes in plasma osmolarity and the appropriate renal response.

A decrease in blood volume or arterial pressure also stimulates ADH secretion. The receptors activated are the baroreceptors located in both the low- (atria and pulmonary vessels) and high-pressure (aortic arch and carotid sinus) sides of the circulatory system. Signals from these receptors, activated by an increased blood volume or arterial pressure, inhibit ADH secretion. This effect is less sensitive than that of osmoreceptors. Thus, a decrease of 5–10% in blood volume or arterial pressure is required to stimulate ADH secretion.

Control of the effective circulating volume

Salts of sodium are the major solutes of the ECW, and in normal circumstances sodium balance closely regulates the fraction of the ECW that is effectively perfusing the body tissues, the so-called effective circulating volume. Alterations of the osmolarity due to changes in sodium balance are rapidly counteracted by changes on ADH secretion and thirst that maintain body fluid osmolarity. Hence, fluctuations that occur physiologically in sodium intake do not to disturb the ECW osmolarity since this is rapidly compensated by an increase or decrease of body water balance mediated by ADH and the thirst mechanism. Thus, in the steady state, addition of sodium to the ECW is equivalent to adding an isotonic solution and increasing the ECW

volume. Conversely, a negative sodium balance results in a decrease of the ECW volume.

Under normal conditions, the kidneys also share responsibility for keeping the ECW volume constant by adjusting the excretion of sodium through the activation of the renin secretion at the juxtaglomerular apparatus. Baroreceptors (volume-sensing system) present in the circulatory system detect changes in blood volume and pressure (afferent signal). In order to counteract the changes of effective circulating volume by corresponding modifications of the sodium balance, the afferent signal stimulates or inhibits the sympathetic nervous system, the renin–angiotensin–aldosterone system, and the secretion of atrial natriuretic peptide. Table 24.2 gives a summary of these efferent signals and their effects on renal sodium excretion.

Thirst regulation and water balance

Thirst is a behavioral response to losses of body fluid. Together with reflex endocrine and neural responses to these losses, thirst is of the utmost importance for maintaining the homeostasis of body fluids, and more specifically for the regulation of the ECW. From a behavioral and psychological point of view, thirst can be defined as a strong motivation to seek, to obtain, and to consume water in response to deficits in body water. Thirst is stimulated mainly through changes in plasma osmolality and in plasma volume.

Thirst stimulated by plasma osmolarity and sodium concentration.

Animal experiments have been of crucial importance in investigating the mechanisms integrating the com-

		Table 24.2 Efferent signals as a response to changes in blood volume/pressure, and their actions on renal sodium excretion
Renal sympathetic nerves ($\uparrow$ activity = $\downarrow$ Na$^+$ excretion)	$\downarrow$ Glomerular filtration rate $\uparrow$ Renin secretion $\uparrow$ Proximal and distal nephron sodium reabsorption $\uparrow$ Angiotensin II levels $\uparrow$ proximal nephron Na$^+$ reabsortion	
Renin–angiotensin-aldosterone ($\uparrow$ secretion = $\downarrow$ Na$^+$ excretion)	$\uparrow$ Aldosterone levels $\uparrow$ distal nephron Na$^+$ reabsorption $\uparrow$ Angiotensin II levels $\uparrow$ ADH secretion $\uparrow$ Glomerular filtration rate	
Atrial natriuretic peptide ($\uparrow$ secretion = $\uparrow$ Na$^+$ excretion)	$\downarrow$ Renin secretion $\downarrow$ Aldosterone secretion $\downarrow$ Distal nephron Na$^+$ reabsorption $\downarrow$ ADH secretion and action on distal nephron	

ADH, antidiuretic hormone.

plex neuroendocrine and psychological response to water deficiency. Thirst and motivation to seek and drink water are stimulated when an increase in the ECW (plasma compartment) osmolarity is detected by the hypothalamic osmoreceptors. Small changes of the extracellular fluid osmolarity (as small as 1%) are sensed by specialized cells located in the subfornical organ and organum vasculosum of the lamina terminalis of the hypothalamus (osmoreceptors). These cells respond only to solutes that are effective osmoles. Hence, urea or glucose, which are able to freely move across the cell membrane, are ineffective osmoles and do not affect the function of osmoreceptors.

The osmoreceptors send signals to the nearby neuroendocrine cells located within the supraoptic and paraventricular nuclei of the hypothalamus that synthesize ADH. ADH is then released to the bloodstream from the posterior lobe of the pituitary gland. This small peptide hormone acts on the collecting tubules of the nephron, increasing their permeability to water. When plasma ADH levels are low, the collecting tubule are relatively impermeable to water and a large volume of diluted urine is excreted, but when plasma ADH levels are elevated, the urine is concentrated and its volume reduced.

In addition to the role of osmoreceptors in regulating thirst, there seem to exist pathways that regulate water intake other than via plasma osmolarity. In animal experiments, drinking is aborted before plasma osmolarity returns to normal, indicating the presence of signals reaching the brain to terminate drinking. Several studies support the suggestion that gastric water absorption is detected mainly by splanchnic osmosensors that send their signals through the vagus nerve to the area postrema and adjacent nucleus of the solitary tract for an anticipated termination of drinking.

Thirst stimulated by hypovolemia
Thirst is also strongly stimulated by a reduced effective circulatory volume. An endocrine and a neural mechanism mediate this response. Hypovolemia stimulates the juxtaglomerular apparatus, inducing the synthesis and release of renin. Increased plasma renin activity results in a subsequent increase in angiotensin II, the most powerful dypsogenic substance known. Angiotensin II stimulates thirst and, in addition, the secretion of aldosterone from the adrenal cortex. It also acts on the central nervous system promoting ADH secretion. The preferred site of action of angiotensin II to

stimulate drinking appears to be the subfornical organ, in the hypothalamus, which, in addition, is connected to the endocrine cells in the supraoptic and paraventricular responsible for ADH secretion. The subfornical organ also has efferent connections to the autonomous nervous system nuclei located in the brainstem. Finally, it also seems to have a behavioral influence through its connections with the anterior region of the third ventricle.

As previously discussed, hypovolemia is also detected by the baroreceptors the stimulation of which results in parasympathetic signals reaching the solitary tract nucleus from which efferent pathways reach the paraventricular nuclei enhancing the secretion of ADH.

24.7 Metabolic links: glucose, water, and sodium

Transport of glucose across the intestinal epithelium and the proximal renal tubules is closely linked to a parallel transport of sodium and water. The first hint of the antinatriuretic effect of glucose derived from physiological information gained during studies carried out during the World War II in pursuit of the minimal liferaft ration. The basic aims of this work were to determine both the minimal water requirement in the state of fasting and whether this minimum requirement changed according to the quantity and quality of food intake. The studies showed that glucose intake has a sodium-sparing effect by diminishing the renal excretion of this cation. Briefly, it was found that the administration of 100 g of glucose per day induced a sparing effect on sodium balance that even surpassed the effect of a daily intake of 4.5 g of sodium chloride. When sodium and glucose were given together, this sodium-sparing effect was potentiated (Figure 24.6).

These studies set up the basis for our current standards of intravenous fluid therapy during short periods of fasting. Other authors later confirmed the sodium sparing effect of glucose.

24.8 Body water compartments in chronic starvation

Starvation, severe trauma, and sepsis are linked to alterations in the sizes of the body water compartments

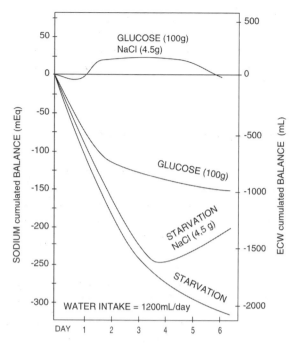

Figure 24.6 The effect of salt and glucose intakes on water and sodium balance in fasting normal volunteers. Adapted from Gamble (1946).

and in the concentrations of exchangeable ions, particularly Na_e. Basically, severe disease is associated with an expansion of the ECW and a corresponding increase in the Na_e pool. In fact, in the early 1980s, Shizgal's group went so far as to suggest that a $Na_e/K_e > 1.22$ was diagnostic of malnutrition.

Prolonged reduced intake of protein and energy results in subtle alterations of water and electrolyte metabolism. The best-known phases of these changes are the early diuretic and natriuretic phases, the relative expansion of the ECW as depletion progresses, and the final phase of a kwashiorkor or kwashiorkor-like picture dominated by an absolute expansion of the ECW, edema (famine edema), and hypoalbuminemia.

Starvation: early diuretic and natriuretic phase and late relative ECW expansion

Shortly after a drastic reduction of food intake occurs, there is an early diuretic and natriuretic renal response, probably mediated by the low insulin plasma concentrations. Excretion of sodium salts of ketones during early ketonuria has also been implicated in sodium losses. Some degree of ECW depletion may occur during this phase. This diuretic and natriuretic renal re-

sponse is, however, short-lived and may not be present if fasting is not complete. In fact, from the nutritional point of view, it seems not to be particularly relevant since partial starvation is far more common than complete fasting both in the clinical setting and in countries where a shortage of food is widespread.

Prolonged partial starvation results in a complex and only partially understood renal response characterized by sodium retention or, at least, by an abnormal renal handling of sodium and a tendency towards positive sodium balance. In fact, despite severe weight and body cell mass loss occurring after prolonged reduction of food intake, the ECW compartment does not diminish. In their classical studies, Keys and his co-workers found that in semi-starving volunteers the volume of the ECW, assessed by the distribution space of thiocyanate, remained constant despite a severe (around 30%) body weight loss. Thus, it is now well established that protein–energy malnutrition results in an ECW expansion that is relative or absolute to the weight of the patient.

Famine edema versus marasmus

Chronic undernutrition results in 'dry' cachexia (marasmus) or in 'wet' cachexia (kwashiorkor). In both cases, a severe depletion (25–35%) of protein and fat stores are present, but they differ from each other on water and sodium metabolism. Marasmus is characterized by maintenance of normal extracellular fluid volume, which is only expanded in relationship to body weight, and normal or normal–low serum albumin concentrations, i.e. anorexia nervosa or depletion due to swallowing disorders. Conversely, by mechanisms not completely understood, some individuals with protein–energy malnutrition develop dependent edema and severe hypoalbuminemia (serum albumin <25 g/l). In these cases, the ECW expansion is absolute; this is well above the normal ECW volume for a given weight and body size.

Observations made in concentration camps during the early 1940s drew attention to the fact that malnutrition edema was only seen in subjects with a combination of low protein with normal–high carbohydrate intakes. In further observations made with prisoners of war it was also noted that edema developed when sodium intake was increased. It has been suggested that elevated plasma insulin can be found in kwashiorkor at variance with the low plasma insulin concentrations observed in marasmus. This would favor the current hypothesis that carbohydrate intake may be essential for the development of absolute ECW expansion through sodium retention, possibly mediated by normal plasma insulin concentrations.

Chronic anemia may also facilitate water and sodium retention. Several endocrine and hemodynamic parameters have been investigated in patients with severe anemia (mean hematocrit of 13%), including retention of sodium and water, reduction of renal blood flow, and glomerular filtration rate associated with a high cardiac output and a low systemic vascular resistance and blood pressure. It has been suggested that the low concentration of hemoglobin causes an inhibition of basal endothelium-derived relaxing factor activity, leading to generalized vasodilatation. The consequent low blood pressure may be the stimulus for neurohormonal activation and salt and water retention.

Finally, a kwashiorkor-like picture can result when patients with marasmus suffer from an acute disease process such as trauma or infection. In these cases, the association of fluid infusion and the antidiuretic drive of stress lead to further sodium retention and absolute ECW expansion, resulting in edema and distributional hypoalbuminemia.

24.9 Impact of acute pathological conditions on the ICW

Several disease processes may acutely alter the volume and composition of the ICW through two major mechanisms: altered osmolarity of the ECW and cell membrane dysfunction. While the first falls largely in a non-nutrition area, the second has important implications for clinical nutrition.

In protein–energy malnutrition as well as in certain acute conditions (trauma, sepsis, major surgery), cells become energy deficient, the energy-consuming membrane ATPase activity is reduced, and water, sodium, and chloride tend to accumulate within the cell, causing a spurious potassium-poor ICW expansion. On the other hand, there may exist a healthy 'cell swelling' promoted by anabolic agents which determine the increase in the ICW compartment associated with an anabolic process leading to protein synthesis.

The ICW volume decreases when the osmolarity of the ECW increases, thus bringing water out of the cells. These circumstances are most often found in conditions associated with pure water loss or deficit, a phenomenon likely to occur in enteral nutrition if substrates are not administered together with the appropriate volume of water.

24.10 Body water in acute illness

Shock, severe sepsis, polytrauma, and burns are associated with profound translocation of body fluids. ECW expansion is the hallmark of acute disease and is usually the result of a multifactorial process involving the physiologic response to disease (sepsis and trauma), the underlying nutritional status, and the infusion of intravenous fluids and nutrients.

Briefly, the mechanisms that have been implicated to explain the expansion of the ECW in acute illness are:

- Activation of water and sodium retaining mechanisms by hypovolemia and pain
- Increased capillary permeability and 'albumin leak' to the interstitium
- Aggressive fluid therapy during resuscitation
- Excessive administration of water and sodium during the flow phase
- Reduction of effective plasma volume
- High-glucose low-protein diets.

Some of these will be discussed below.

The antidiuretic drive, volume expansion, and hypoalbuminemia in acute injury

The pioneering work of Moore in the sixties (Moore FD, 1965) demonstrated the antidiuretic renal response observed after hemorrhage, surgery, and trauma. While some of this response may be due to inappropriate resuscitation, there is no doubt that activation of the sympathetic and renin–angiotensin–aldosterone systems do occur in acute illness, particularly in severe sepsis and hypovolemia, and clinically they translate into oliguria and positive water and sodium balance. Reduction of effective plasma volume due to massive shift of fluid and albumin to the interstitium may also contribute to a reduction of the glomerular filtration rate, oliguria, and further activation of sodium-retaining mechanisms.

Absolute extracellular water expansion

While chronic malnutrition results in an ECW expansion, which is relative to the actual weight, in critically ill patients the expansion of the ECW occurs in absolute terms. If, under normal conditions, the ECW represents 20% of the body weight, in acute injury this compartment may increase to up 50% of the body weight. After resuscitation from hypovolemic shock, studies have found a 55% increase of the ECW, mainly affecting the interstitial compartment, associated with a significant decrease in the plasma oncotic pressure. Increase of the ECW, assessed by the muscle biopsy technique, has also been proved after elective colon resection.

The expansion of the ECW has several undesirable consequences. Interstitial edema may be detrimental to the lungs, impairing gas exchange and, possibly, predisposing to lung infection. Hypervolemia may precipitate heart failure in susceptible individuals. Edema may also impair wound healing. The pharmacokinetics of many drugs (antibiotics, dopamine, antiarrythmics) may be altered due to the considerable increase of their distribution space. All these may account for the fact that ECW expansion closely correlates with clinical outcome. When the normal ECW is doubled, that is increased up to 40% of total body weight, the risk of death approaches 80%. In summary, ECW expansion and edema may interfere with normal physiologic processes such as gas exchange in the lungs, wound healing, cardiac function, pharmacokinetics of drugs, oxygen delivery to tissues, and soft tissue defenses against infection.

The risk of extracellular fluid overexpansion is higher in those patients with a physiologically reduced ECW, namely, thin adults (40–45 kg), very obese short people, and the old frail patient. In these cases, the volume of the extracellular compartment can be as low as 6–8 liters; thus, a rapid infusion of just 2.5 liters of saline represents a 25–40% increase of this compartment.

Low serum albumin concentrations

Hypoalbuminemia is a complex multifactorial phenomenon associated with a poor outcome in many clinical conditions. In acute injury and in some chronic conditions, the transcapillary escape rate of albumin, as measured by plasma disappearance of labeled albumin, is increased up to fourfold. The mechanisms underlying this albumin shift to the interstitium are not completely understood at present. Two major hypotheses have been advanced (Figure 24.7): increased available space in the interstitial compartment due to matrix degradation, and increased capillary permeability to macromolecules.

Degradation of interstitial matrix occurs because hyaluronan, an essential component of the glycosaminoglycan, is washed out from the interstitial space. This can occur by a simple clearing mechanism related to increased interstitial hydrostatic pressure due to overhydration, or may be induced by mediators or sepsis products, as has been experimentally demonstrated in a sheep model of *E. coli* sepsis. On the other hand, it has been postulated that in acute injury inflammatory mediators such as tumor necrosis factor (TNF) may increase the permeability of the endothelial capillary lining. A recent study suggests that both hypotheses may be complementary since TNF was found to interfere with the synthesis of glycosaminoglycans by endothelial cells.

In this clinical context, hypoalbuminemia is a symptom, or an epiphenomenon, of disease and is not related to any primary nutritional derangement. For that reason, therapeutic efforts should be directed towards treatment of the underlying illness rather than focusing on the management of a low plasma albumin concentration. There seems to be no role for exogenous human albumin administration either in resuscitation protocols or in the more specific setting of nutrition support. In fact, exogenous albumin may worsen the situation by increasing the interstitial colloid osmotic pressure, thus facilitating the immobilization of water in the extravascular space.

In addition, aggressive nutrition either by the enteral or parenteral route may not be an ideal approach to 'manage' the hypoalbuminemia of the severely ill patient, who may not tolerate substrates given via the gastrointestinal tract or may show biochemical signs of poor plasma substrate clearance such as hyperglycemia and hypertriglyceridemia. When possible, usually after the underlying process has improved, diuretics may be given to promote a negative water and sodium balance, which will be paralleled by an increase in the serum albumin concentration. At this 'non-stressed' stage, some authors have recommended low doses of human albumin to mobilize fluid excess and facilitate diuresis.

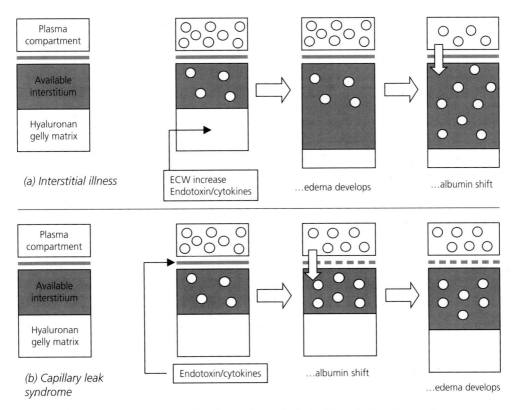

(a) Interstitial illness

Plasma compartment

Available interstitium

Hyaluronan gelly matrix

ECW increase Endotoxin/cytokines

...edema develops

...albumin shift

(b) Capillary leak syndrome

Plasma compartment

Available interstitium

Hyaluronan gelly matrix

Endotoxin/cytokines

...albumin shift

...edema develops

Figure 24.7 Schematic representation of the two major hypotheses explaining distributional hypoalbuminemia in acute illness.

24.11 Water and electrolyte metabolism during refeeding

Refeeding of the malnourished non-stressed patient should lead to progressive increase of the depleted fat and protein stores, improved muscular strength, diuresis of any ECW excess, and restoration of subjective wellbeing. This is commonly followed by a phase of postinjury weight gain during which the protein and energy intakes surpass the daily requirements, possibly due to behavioral changes. In severely depleted individuals, however, aggressive refeeding either by the enteral or parenteral route may lead to complications through two major metabolic responses: acute intracellular cation shift and water and sodium intolerance.

Early works on refeeding reported inappropriate physiological responses consisting mainly of disturbances affecting the ECW and the cardiovascular system: hemodilution, congestive heart failure, hypertension, edema, and excessive weight gain. After the siege of Stalingrad during World War II, refeeding of the population led to an epidemic of hypertension and congestive heart failure. In different clinical settings, cardiac decompensation was reported when aggressive glucose-based total parenteral nutrition (TPN) was given to undernourished patients and in other works an increase of the blood volume and hemodilution during oral refeeding of malnourished children has been reported. Briefly, water and electrolyte metabolism appears to be an important determinant of an appropriate response to refeeding in undernourished individuals.

The anabolic response. Intracellular cation shift

Chronic protein–energy depletion is associated with a reduction in body cell mass. Not only are cytoplasm and intracellular protein lost during malnutrition but also potassium and other intracellular ions such as phosphate and magnesium. In addition, the intracellular concentration of potassium is reduced in depleted individuals, probably because of a diminished activity of the Na/K ATP-dependent pump. Thus, during refeeding, two anabolic phenomena occur: a positive nitrogen balance with an increase of the body cell mass and a correction of the reduced intracellular potassium concentration. Both result in increased demands of potassium and may lead to hypokalemia if potassium salts are not administered in adequate amounts. The requirements of phosphate and magnesium are also increased in this period.

Both hypokalemia and hypophosphatemia have been noted to occur rapidly if aggressive hypercaloric glucose-based parenteral nutrition is administered to cachectic patients. Hyperinsulinemia facilitates the uptake of nutrients and electrolytes into cells and this may result in life-threatening dyselectrolytemia, rhabdomyolisis (rupture of muscle fibers with myoglobinuria), and seizures.

The refeeding syndrome: water and sodium retention and hypoalbuminemia

Soon after the introduction of parenteral nutrition, it became evident that undernourished patients refed by the intravenous route tended to gain weight rapidly and showed signs of ECW overexpansion. In carefully conducted balance studies, it has been shown that between 35% and 50% of the weight gain observed shortly after refeeding was accounted for by extracellular fluid. Withdrawal of sodium from the TPN formula stops weight gain and induces negative sodium, weight, and extracellular fluid balances. Similarly, rapid expansion of intracardiac volume may occur early after starting oral plus parenteral refeeding of malnourished individuals, some of whom developed signs and symptoms of congestive heart failure. These authors administered refeeding regimens with a very high content of glucose (350–850 g/day) and achieved a mean weight increase of 6 kg in 20–35 days.

This inappropriate ECW response to parenteral nutrition in depleted non-stressed patients and its clinical consequences have been well characterized. Some patients being refed preoperatively with TPN showed an expansion of the ECW, which was linked to an increase of postoperative complications. This may help to explain previous reports on hemodilution following refeeding and also a subsequent report indicating that 60% of esophageal cancer patients receiving preoperative parenteral nutrition showed a dilutional response characterized by increasing weight and decreasing serum albumin concentrations. In the subgroup of pa-

tients with an inappropriate response, death related to respiratory problems may occur.

Administration of high glucose and sodium loads during TPN can now be definitely implicated as a cause of ECW expansion. Early TPN studies demonstrated a rapid expansion of the ECW in patients receiving inappropriately high quantities of glucose, water, and sodium. Body composition studies have shown that glucose-based parenteral nutrition regimens result in more water retention and fat gain than those including fat as a source of 60% of the non-protein calories.

To help elucidate the role of parenteral nutrition formulas in inducing ECW expansion, the response to refeeding with low sodium/low water TPN regimens has been investigated. In a series of experimental studies, malnourished rabbits with a weight loss of at least 15% were refed using all-in-one TPN mixtures with different fat/glucose calorie ratios, and sodium and water intakes. Animals refed with high-glucose regimens and larger sodium loads exhibited a more positive weight balance largely due to ECW expansion secondary to diminished natriuresis. Furthermore, rabbits receiving high-glucose regimens had higher urinary metanephrine excretion, pointing towards an increased sympathetic activity as a result of the high glucose intake (Figure 24.8).

In the clinical setting a glucose and salt-restricted TPN formula has also proved superior in terms of

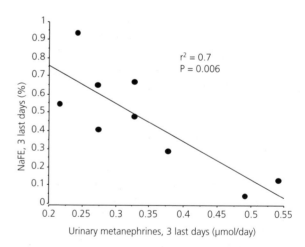

Figure 24.8 Correlation beween urinary metanephrine excretion and sodium fractional excretion in malnourished rabbits receiving glucose-based TPN. This response could not be observed in animals receiving a lipid-based TPN. Reproduced from Domingo et al. (1994) with permission from Elsevier.

Table 24.3 Metabolic response to TPN in severely depleted gastrointestinal cancer patients refed with two different formulas

	Glucose-Na group (n = 19)	Lipid group (n = 22)	P-value
Serum albumin (g/l)	31.7 ± 4.1	35.3 ± 3.8	0.008
Δ Serum albumin (g/l)	−0.7 ± 2.8	2.3 ± 3.5	0.006
Δ Weight (kg)	0.8 ± 0.9	−1.5 ± 1.1	0.0001
Daily diuresis (ml)	1,230 ± 310	959 ± 245	0.003
Water balance (10 days)	478 ± 1134	−1091 ± 1256	0.001
Na balance (mEq/day)	40 ± 3	−27 ± 18	0.0001
Urea (mg/dl)	41 ± 12	61 ± 34	0.02

From Gil *et al.* (1997) with permission from Elsevier.

physiological response and avoiding ECW expansion. Patients given larger doses of glucose and sodium exhibit a linear relationship between water and weight balances (Figure 24.9) and show positive sodium and water balances, weight gain, and decreased serum albumin concentration levels. On the other hand, when sodium and glucose are restricted the opposite response is observed (Table 24.3). Respiratory complications are predominantly observed in patients showing fluid retention and lowering of serum albumin concentrations.

Other authors have found a clear-cut relationship between weight decrease and increases in serum albumin concentrations when refeeding malnourished edematous patients with low sodium and volume diets to facilitate a negative water and sodium balance.

These concepts may also apply to patients with ongoing infection receiving TPN. Experimental data have shown that the septic animal with an intra-abdominal abscess is also susceptible to further expansion of the ECW by high-volume and high-glucose parenteral nutrition and that, in sepsis, ECW expansion is favored by the hypoalbuminemia already present at the start of intravenous feeding.

It is interesting to note that the three human studies investigating water and sodium metabolism during preoperative TPN have shown that only 50–60% of patients refed with large glucose loads did in fact exhibit an inappropriate response characterized by weight increase and decreasing serum albumin concentrations. This has also been observed in animal studies. The reasons for this are unclear. A hypothesis can be put forward implicating genetic differences in the ability to handle glucose loads and, specifically, differences in the ability of glucose to retain sodium via an increase in plasma insulin and/or catecholamines.

24.12 Implications of water and sodium metabolism in nutrition therapy for specific clinical conditions

Congestive heart failure and cirrhosis

Sodium retention is a hallmark of congestive heart failure and advanced liver cirrhosis. A unifying hypothesis for these and maybe other edematous states has been put forward by Schrier (Schrier RW *et al.*, 2001), emphasizing the role of arterial underfilling as the initial pathophysiological phenomenon. This phenomenon consists of reduced effective blood flow in the arterial system despite relative or absolute expansion of the ECW. Arterial underfilling would be caused by poor cardiac contractility and/or arteriolar vasodilation. The renal consequences of arterial underfilling have been well summarized in a recent review on congestive heart failure. Arterial underfilling leads to:

(1) reduction in renal blood flow produced by the almost simultaneous operation of alpha- and beta-catecholamines, antidiuretic hormone, the endothelins, and angiotensin II;
(2) activation of the tubuloglomerular feedback system enhancing intrarenal angiotensin II release;
(3) activation of apical sodium channels of principal cells in the cortical collecting tubule by aldosterone and by ADH; and
(4) resistance of the inner medullary collecting ducts to the action of atrial natriuretic peptide.

In the presence of edema and overt heart failure sodium should be eliminated or severely reduced from feeding formulas, either enteral or parenteral. As has already been mentioned, ECW expansion – and even edema and heart failure – may occur during aggressive refeeding of the severely undernourished patients given too much glucose, sodium, and water. Thus, refeeding should be done cautiously using, when possible, the enteral route.

Obstructive jaundice

Extrahepatic cholestasis is linked to profound alterations of appetite and thirst. Animals subjected to bile duct ligation immediately become anorectic and develop negative energy, water, and sodium balances. The consequences of these behavioral changes can be observed in humans with obstructive jaundice, who often show malnutrition and water depletion.

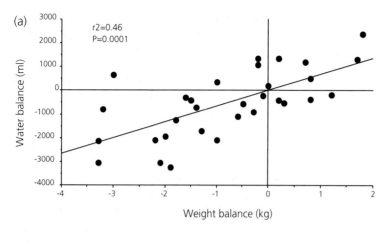

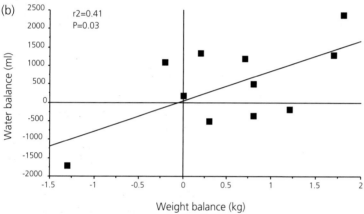

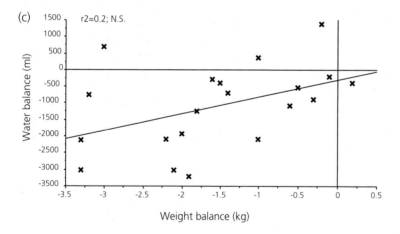

Figure 24.9 Correlations between weight balance and water balance in severely malnourished patients receiving preoperative TPN for 10 days. (A) The whole population study; (B) correlation found in patients receiving high-glucose/high-Na TPN contrasting with (C) the lack of correlation in patients receiving a lipid-based low-Na formula. Reproduced from Gil MJ et al. (1997) with permission from Elsevier.

Anorexia and malnutrition in obstructive jaundice

Two-thirds of the patients with obstructive jaundice present a significant reduction of food intake when prospectively investigated with a controlled diet. Although the cause of anorexia in this condition is not well established, a good correlation between raised plasma concentrations of cholecystokinin and reduced spontaneous food intake has been observed. Cholecystokinin has been implicated in the physiology of satiety and has both a central anorectic action and a

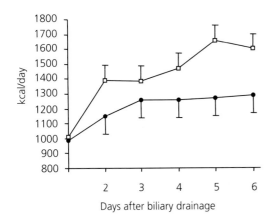

Figure 24.10 Improvement of food intake (kcal/day) after internal biliary drainage. ANOVA test: Open squares, benign obstruction: $P < 0.01$; Black dots, malignant tumors: $P < 0.05$. Data are expressed as mean ± SD. Reproduced from Padillo *et al.* (2001) with permission from the American College of Surgeons.

gastric motility inhibitory effect. The absence of bile salts in the duodenal lumen in obstructive jaundice may be an important stimulus for cholecystokinin secretion in this condition.

Roughly half of the patients with obstructive jaundice are malnourished (33% prevalence in patients with benign obstructions and 57% in those malignant disease). The patient's age, duration of jaundice, liver function tests, and cholecystokinin levels all correlate with impaired nutrition status. Biliary drainage significantly increases spontaneous food intake (Figure 24.10).

In addition, patients with advanced obstructive jaundice often show hypoalbuminemia of a multifactorial origin, possibly involving chronic reduction of food intake, cytokine activation, and liver failure. Hypoalbuminemia has been demonstrated to increase surgical risk in patients with obstructive jaundice.

Loss of thirst and water depletion in obstructive jaundice

Hypodipsia is a very early finding after common bile duct ligation in the experimental animal. Increased atrial natriuretic peptide and nitric oxide have been postulated as possible humoral mediators of hypodipsia because they both have a central antidipsogenic activity. This reduced water intake is not associated with a predictable decrease in urinary output. Conversely,

urinary losses of water and sodium appear to be inappropriately high with respect to water and sodium intakes, which leads to a negative fluid balance.

Although data on the drinking behavior of humans with bile duct obstruction are lacking, several studies have reported water depletion in this setting, suggesting that at the time of diagnosis some of the patients are water-depleted. One study detected increased plasma levels of renin in up to one-quarter of patients newly diagnosed with obstructive jaundice. Loss of ECW has been found in patients with obstructive jaundice by means of both tracer dilution techniques and bioimpedance analysis. ECW depletion involves the plasma volume in advanced cases and this would help to explain the tendency of patients with obstructive jaundice to renal failure when challenged by a severe infection, bleeding, or nephrotoxic agents.

Stroke and dysphagia

Inadequate water intake is a hallmark of patients with cerebrovascular accidents who suffer from swallowing difficulties. In a recent study, patients with a newly diagnosed acute stroke and dysphagia had a water intake that amounted to only 60% of the daily requirements. The authors concluded that hospital staff must ensure adequate fluid intakes in patients at risk of dehydration, which should include both an adequate prescription and provision of supplementary fluids. Prethickened drinks improve oral fluid intake in patients with dysphagic acute stroke on non-specialist wards.

In this group of patients, and more broadly speaking in the elderly with acute disease, dehydration due to poor water intake may go unnoticed due to a diminished threshold for thirst and cognitive impairment. The aging process alters important physiological control systems associated with thirst. Recent evidence suggests that older men and women:

- have a higher baseline osmolality and thus a higher osmotic operating point for thirst sensation (with little or no change in sensitivity), and
- exhibit diminished thirst and satiety in response to the unloading (hypovolemia) and loading (hypervolemia) of baroreceptors.

Attention to hydration then becomes an essential part of clinical management in the elderly. In addition, since some of these patients may also be candidates for enteral feeding, attention should be paid to adequate provision of fluids to prevent dehydration due to both hypodipsia and substrate load.

24.13 Perspectives on the future

Our knowledge of fluid and electrolyte balance has increased steadily over the past 50 years, although it is still an area that is often poorly understood. Inappropriate prescribing can cause increased postoperative morbidity and mortality. It remains a vital component of the metabolic care of surgical and critically ill patients with important consequences for gastrointestinal function and hence nutrition. It is also of importance when prescribing enteral or parenteral nutrition, and should be given the same careful consideration as other nutritional and pharmacological needs.

References and further reading

Almond DJ, King RFGJ, Burkinshaw L, Laughland A, McMahon MJ. Influence of energy source upon body composition in patients receiving intravenous nutrition. *JPEN J Parenter Enteral Nutr* 1989; 13: 471–477.

Cochrane Injuries Group Albumin Reviewers. Human albumin administration in critically ill patients: systematic review of randomised controlled trials. *BMJ* 1998; 317: 235–240.

Domingo MI, Lladó L, Guirao X *et al.* Influence of calorie source on the physiological response to parenteral nutrition in malnourished rabbits. *Clin Nutr* 1994; 13: 9–16.

Fleck A, Raines G, Hawker F *et al.* Increased vascular permeability: a major cause of hypoalbuminaemia in disease and injury. *Lancet* 1985; 1: 781–784.

Franch-Arcas G, Sitges-Serra A. Fluid and sodium problems in perioperative feeding: what further studies need to be done? *Curr Opin Clin Nutr Metab Care* 1998; 1: 9–14.

Gamble JL. Physiological information gained from studies on life raft ration. *Harvey Lectures* 1946; 42: 247–273.

Gil MJ, Franch G, Guirao X *et al.* Response of severely malnourished patients to preoperative parenteral nutrition: a randomized clinical trial of water and sodium restriction. *Nutrition* 1997; 13: 26–31.

Hill GL. Body composition research: Implications for the practice of clinical nutrition. *JPEN J Parenter Enteral Nutr* 1992; 16: 197–218.

Klahr S, Davis TA. Changes in renal function with chronic protein-calorie malnutrition. In: *Nutrition and the Kidney* (WE Mitch, S Klahr, eds), pp. 59–79. Boston: Little, Brown and Co., 1988.

Lobo DN, Bjarnason K, Field J, Rowlands BJ, Allison SP. Changes in weight, fluid balance and serum albumin in patients referred for nutritional support. *Clin Nutr* 1999; 18: 197–201.

Mac Fie J, Smith RC, Hill GH. Glucose or fat as a nonprotein energy source? A controlled trial in gastroenterological patients requiring intravenous nutrition. *Gastroenterology* 1981; 80: 103–107.

Moore FD. Energy and the maintenance of the body cell mass. *JPEN J Parenter Enteral Nutr* 1980; 4: 228–260.

Moore FD. The effects of haemorrhage on body composition. *N Engl J Med*, 1965; 273: 567–577.

Padillo FJ, Andicoberry B, Naranjo A, Miño G, Pera C, Sitges-Serra A. Anorexia and the effect of internal biliary drainage on food intake in patients with obstructive jaundice. *J Am Coll Surg* 2001; 192: 584–590

Schrier RW, Gurevich AK, Cadnapaphornchai MA. Pathogenesis and management of sodium and water retention in cardiac failure and cirrhosis. *Semin Nephrol* 2001; 21: 157–172.

Siegel JH, Cerra FB, Coleman B *et al.* Physiological and metabolic correlations in human sepsis. *Surgery* 1979; 86: 163–193.

Sitges-Serra A. Renal failure in obstructive jaundice. In: *Liver and Kidney* (V de Arroyo, P Ginés, P Schrier, J Rodés, eds), pp. 79–98. Oxford: Blackwell, 1999.

Sitges-Serra A (Chairman). ESPEN Symposium: hypoalbuminaemia. *Clin Nutr* 2001: 20: 265–284.

25
Illustrative Cases

Simon P Allison

Key messages

- A simple and rapid screening process, linked to an action plan, is the first step in alerting staff to the possibility that the patient is at nutritional risk.
- A patient who screens at risk may then need a more detailed and expert nutritional assessment, taking into account anthropometry, biochemistry and hematology, clinical picture, and dietary intake.
- The results of the nutritional assessment will determine the level of nutritional support or dietary counseling required and allow a clinical management plan to be developed.

25.1 Introduction

The purpose of this chapter is to give the reader the opportunity to apply the knowledge gained from previous chapters to real clinical situations with all their challenging variety and interest. As in other branches of medicine, accurate diagnosis of nutritional problems, obtained from the full range of history, examination, and investigations, is the key to appropriate and successful treatment. Amidst the host of patients attending clinics, admitted as emergencies, or suffering the consequences of disease and its treatment, a large proportion have problems of nutritional excess, deficiency, or imbalance which affect their long-term health or the outcome of their current disease. A simple and rapid screening process, linked to action plans, is the first step in alerting staff to the possibility that the patient is at nutritional risk. You would be rightly criticized for failing to test urine or blood for glucose and missing the diagnosis of diabetes. The same principle applies to malnutrition.

A patient who screens at risk may then need a more detailed and expert assessment leading to a clinical decision and management plan. This process will be applied to each of the patients described in this chapter, beginning with the screening tool we use for inpatients (Box 25.1) to identify patients with actual or potential protein–energy deficit or excess. This addresses the following questions:

- Where is the patient now? Body mass index (BMI) or some surrogate such as mid-arm circumference (MAC).
- Where has the patient come from? Percentage weight change over the previous 3–6 months.
- Where is the patient going? This depends on change in appetite and food intake as well as disease severity.

In addition, micronutrient deficiencies may be suspected from the history (e.g. alcoholism or restrictive diet), and other factors need to be considered at the extremes of life (e.g. growth velocity and development in children and poor dentition, swallowing problems, or disability in the elderly). For these reasons, illustrative growth charts are included with Case 1 and the mini-nutritional screening tool for the elderly with Case 3.

Further assessment will include not only nutritional requirements but the consequences of undernutrition (e.g. muscle weakness) and of overnutrition (e.g. complications of obesity). A similar format will therefore be applied to each case under the following headings:

- Screening for nutritional risk
- Nutritional assessment in depth of those screened at risk
- List of problems to be addressed
- Clinical decisions
- Nutritional requirements
- Treatment
- Monitoring of progress

Box 25.1 Nutrition screening tool for adults. Reproduced from Schofield (1985) with permission of Nature Publishing Group

Is YOUR patient at nutritional risk?

Q1 a **Height**   Q2 a **Weight**
   □.□□ metres   □□.□ kg
Q1 b □ Estimated or   Q2 b □ Estimated or
     □ Measured   □ Measured

Q3 **Body Mass Index** (BMI) = kg/m^2 □□
   (refer to ready-reckoner)

		Score	
Greater than 20		□	0
18 to 20		□	2
Less than 18		□	3

Q4 **Food intake** – has this
   decreased over the last
   month prior to admission
   or since the last review
   (or is the patient NBM)?

		Score	
	No	□	0
	Yes	□	1
	Not known	□	2

Q5 Has the patient **unintentionally
   lost weight** over the last 3 months
   or since the last review?

		Score	
	No	□	0
Up to ½ stone (3 kg)	A little	□	1
More than ½ stone (3 kg)	A lot	□	2

Q6 **Stress factor/severity of illness**

		Score	
None	None	□	0
Moderate	Moderate	□	1

(Minor or uncomplicated surgery, minor infection, chronic disease, pressure sores, CVA, inflammatory bowel disease, other gastrointestinal disease, cirrhosis, renal failure, COPD, diabetes)

Severe	Severe	□	2

(Multiple injuries, multiple fractures, burns, head injury, multiple deep pressure sores, severe sepsis, malignant disease, severe dysphagia, pancreatitis, post-op complications)

Q7   **TOTAL SCORE** □

Review patient in three days

Q8 Action
   If score 0-2   Repeat screening   □
                    within 7 days
   If score 3-4   Keep food record charts
                    and start supplements
                    if food intake poor   □
   If score ≥ 5   Refer for expert advice   □

- Outcome and prognosis
- Learning points.

Cases are grouped according to problem category.

25.2 Children

Case 1

A healthy eight-year-old boy, on the 50th centile for height and weight, presented to the clinic feeling unwell with diarrhea and abdominal pain after eating. Radiological and laboratory investigations led to a diagnosis of Crohn's disease, necessitating treatment with steroids and later with mesalazine and azathioprine. There were a series of exacerbations and remissions over the years. Between the age of eight and 17 years his growth velocity fell to less than 2 cm per year, so that at the age of 17 he was below the 3rd centile for height and weight, had no sexual development, and a radiological bone age of only 12 years. Inflammatory markers including C-reactive protein (CRP) were raised and the serum albumin was low at 29 g/l.

Screening for nutritional risk

Screening tools for adults are not so useful in the growing child in whom changes in growth rate, development, and bone age are more useful. Nonetheless, at 17 years, with a BMI of 16.5 kg/m^2, slight weight loss of 2% over three months, poor appetite and diminished food intake, and moderately severe disease, he still scored 6 (see Box 25.1). Considering also the data on growth failure, this puts him at high nutritional risk.

Assessment and clinical decisions

The history, examination, laboratory tests, and nutritional data at the age of 17 led to a clear diagnosis of disease-related malnutrition whose main manifestation was delayed growth and development. Previously, his doctors had focused on the treatment of the underlying disease process and had ascribed growth failure largely to this and the treatment with steroids and immunosuppressants. The doctor who saw him for the first time at the age of 17 realized that the effect of his disease on food intake and catabolic rate were the major cause of his growth failure and that this might be corrected by nutritional support.

Problems to be addressed

- Active Crohn's disease causing low food intake and increased catabolic rate
- Anti-anabolic effects of steroids and immunosuppressants
- Undernutrition causing failure of growth and development.

Nutritional requirements

These should be calculated on the basis of his biological age of 12, the repair of nutritional deficit, and the needs for growth and development catch-up. His estimated requirements were 11.0 MJ (2630 kcal) and 65 g protein per day. It was also likely that he needed vitamin and mineral supplements including vitamin D and calcium. Elemental diets (i.e. glucose and amino acids) were shown to have benefit in Crohn's disease, but later studies have suggested that polymeric diets (oligosaccharides, fat, and whole protein) may be just as effective.

Treatment

In view of his anorexia, treatment began using a nasogastric polymeric feed of 4.2 MJ (1000 kcal) and 70 g protein/l, starting slowly at 25 ml/h, building gradually over a week to 100 ml/h for 16 h/day, allowing normal oral intake when desired. Once initial improvement had been obtained after four weeks, the nasogastric feed was discontinued and oral intake was continued using food of high energy and protein density supported by proprietary oral supplements. The management of his underlying Crohn's disease continued in the previous manner.

Monitoring and outcome

Height, weight, growth velocity, and sexual development were used as the main criteria of response to treatment (Figure 25.1a–c). His growth velocity returned rapidly to normal and he regained some lost ground, reaching the 5th centile for height. This illustrates the phenomenon described by Widdowson that with delays in growth through malnutrition, renutrition may restore growth velocity but the patient never reaches an ultimate height commensurate with genetic potential – remember he started at the 50th centile. Over the next two years he entered puberty, his bone age advanced, and his epiphyses closed with cessation of growth by the age of 20.

Learning points

- Failure of growth and development are the main manifestations of malnutrition in children.
- It is not always just the disease and its treatment, but the secondary malnutrition which is responsible for some of the clinical manifestations of illness.
- Serum albumin is low because of inflammation and protein losing enteropathy rather than malnutrition (see later cases).

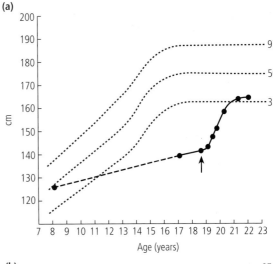

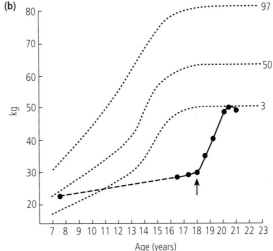

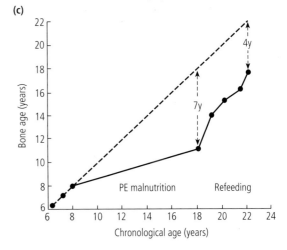

Figure 25.1 Illustrative growth charts for Case 1 showing (a) height, (b) weight, and (c) bone age compared to age.

- Nutritional support where appropriate can be extremely effective and is an important part of management.
- Early diagnosis and treatment of malnutrition is essential if unnecessary loss of growth potential is to be prevented.

25.3 Anorexia of psychological origin and refeeding syndrome

Case 2

A young woman aged 22 had started to lose weight in her mid-teens when anorexia nervosa was diagnosed. She was being followed up, appropriately, by a psychiatrist with a special experience in eating disorders. Her menstruation had ceased at the age of 16 as her BMI fell below 17 kg/m². BMI continued in the range 15–17 kg/m² until six months before admission when her condition worsened. She became very weak and her family and carers feared for her life.

Screening

On admission her height was 1.66 m and weight 29 kg, giving a BMI of 11.0 kg/m². Screening score was estimated at 7 and she was referred for more detailed assessment and for nutritional support.

Nutritional assessment

Life-threatening malnutrition. Life-saving artificial nutritional support indicated.

Problems to be addressed

- Severe anorexia nervosa
- Life-threatening malnutrition.

Clinical decision

She agreed to accept nasogastric feeding. Since in the

UK, legally, anorexia nervosa comes under the Mental Health Act, sectioning the patient and feeding under sedation, without the patient's consent, is not only legal and ethical, but mandatory if the patient's life is deemed to be at risk, since survival below a BMI of 10 kg/m² in women is unusual.

Nutritional requirements

Estimated resting energy expenditure (REE) (calculated by Schofield prediction equation, see Table 25.1) was 3.8 MJ (912 kcal), although with such severe malnutrition it may be 10–15% below this. Assuming 1.5 × REE for weight gain, the target intake should be approximately 6.3 MJ (1500 kcal) and 1.5 g protein/kg or 45 g protein.

Treatment

An oral multivitamin preparation and folate were prescribed. A standard polymeric enteral feed of 4.2 kJ/ml was started at 30 ml/h and increased to 60 ml/h over the next three days. Oral intake was encouraged by day.

Monitoring and progress

After three days of enteral feeding using a standard polymeric feed of 4.2 kJ/ml starting at 50 ml/h and increasing slowly to 80 ml/h, she had gained 2 kg in weight and edema was observed. At the same time, potassium and phosphate levels fell (see Table 25.2) necessitating intravenous supplementation with potassium phosphate.

On day 3 intravenous supplements were started with potassium phosphate. Note the low serum creatinine level reflecting a low muscle mass.

Outcome

After a week she became more active and lively and after three weeks was transferred to the psychiatric unit

Table 25.1 Schofield equations for basal metabolic rate (BMR)

Age (years)	BMR (male)		BMR (female)	
	kcal/day	MJ/day	kcal/day	MJ/day
10–17	17.7 W + 657	0.074 W + 2.754	13.4 W + 692	0.056 W + 2.898
18–29	15.1 W + 692	0.063 W + 2.896	14.8 W + 487	0.062 W + 2.036
30–59	11.5 W + 873	0.048 W + 3.653	8.3 W + 846	0.034 W + 3.538
60–74	11.9 W + 700	0.0499 W + 2.930	9.2 W + 687	0.0386 W + 2.875
75+	8.4 W + 821	0.035 W + 3.434	9.8 W + 624	0.041 W + 2.610

W = weight in kg.
Reproduced with permission from Schofield (1985).

Table 25.2 Biochemical changes with enteral nutrition (Case 2)

	Day 2	Day 3	Day 5	Normal values
Na (mmol/l)	131	132	135–145	
K (mmol/l)	3.6	3.1	4.0	3.5–5.3
Urea (mmol/l)	4.0	2.2	2.0–6.5	
Creatinine (μmol/l)	37	40	50–100	
Glucose (mmol/l)	5.5	6.0	3–5	
PO_4 (mmol/l)	0.31	0.2	0.6	0.7–1.4
Mg (mmol/l)	0.71	0.62	0.7–1.0	
Albumin (g/l)	39	37	39	35–45

for further treatment, having gained 2 kg tissue weight without edema. One of the long-term nutritional concerns was the development of osteoporosis associated with low oestrogen, malnutrition, and low calcium and vitamin D intake.

Learning points

- The refeeding syndrome consists of (a) salt and water gain due to intolerance associated with severe malnutrition (famine edema), (b) a fall in serum levels of potassium, phosphate, and sometimes magnesium due to anabolism of protein and glycogen causing cellular uptake (see also Chapter 24).
- Refeeding of severely malnourished patients should begin slowly for this reason. Diarrhea may also be provoked with too rapid oral or enteral refeeding.
- Careful biochemical monitoring during the initial period of refeeding is important.
- A BMI below 10 kg/m^2 in women or 11 kg/m^2 in men is usually fatal.
- Medico-legally anorexic patients may be fed against their will in some countries, and this should be undertaken if life is at risk.
- Nutrition support only improves the patient's physical condition and does not improve the basic psychiatric disease.
- Serum albumin is often normal in anorexic patients unless there is intercurrent inflammation or dilution with retained fluid.
- Amenorrhea usually occurs below a BMI of 17 kg/m^2. Menstruation usually returns when the BMI rises above this level. With malnutrition the hypothalamic release of luteinizing hormone-releasing factor (LHRH) is reduced and in both sexes gonadotropin and sex hormone levels are reduced.

- Low estrogen levels with malnutrition and low calcium and vitamin D intake predispose to the early development of osteoporosis.

25.4 Malnutrition in the older person

Case 3

A 73-year-old woman and her twin sister both developed thyrotoxicosis and lost weight due to the increased metabolic rate associated with that condition. The thyrotoxicosis was cured and the twin sister regained her normal weight. The patient, however, then developed severe depression and anorexia leading to persistent weight loss. On admission to hospital she was cachectic, weak, and depressed with bruising and edema of the leg. She was severely depressed but a Mini-Mental Score revealed no evidence of dementia. Her temperature was low at 35°C. Her nutritional data are shown in Table 25.3.

Screening

Box 25.2 shows the Toulouse Mini-Nutritional Assessment (MNA) validated for nutritional screening of the elderly, and the scores for this particular patient. In contrast to the nutritional screening tool in Box 25.1, a low rather than high score indicates malnutrition, which in this case was severe.

Nutritional assessment

The screening tool was sufficient in this case to diagnose malnutrition. More detailed assessment showed profound loss of function. Depression not only causes anorexia and weight loss, but more than 15–20% weight

Table 25.3 Nutritional data – Case 3

Height	1.55 m
Weight	
Now	36 kg
Allowing for 3 kg edema	33 kg
Remembered 2 years previously	51 kg
% weight loss	35%
BMI	
Now	13.8
Two years previously	21.3
Serum albumin	41 g/l
Hemoglobin	12.8 g/dl
Lymphocyte count	0.51 (normal 1.5–4.0) × 10^9/l
Creatinine	40 (normal 50–100) μmol/l
Urea	1.5 mmol/l

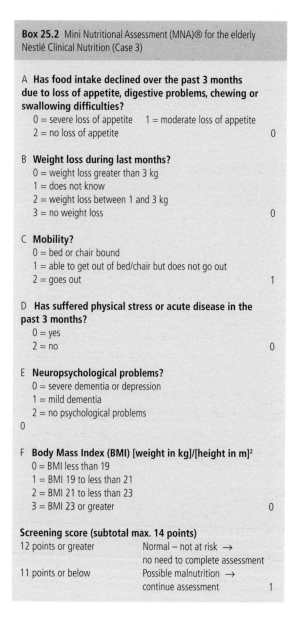

Box 25.2 Mini Nutritional Assessment (MNA)® for the elderly Nestlé Clinical Nutrition (Case 3)

A Has food intake declined over the past 3 months due to loss of appetite, digestive problems, chewing or swallowing difficulties?
0 = severe loss of appetite   1 = moderate loss of appetite
2 = no loss of appetite   0

B Weight loss during last months?
0 = weight loss greater than 3 kg
1 = does not know
2 = weight loss between 1 and 3 kg
3 = no weight loss   0

C Mobility?
0 = bed or chair bound
1 = able to get out of bed/chair but does not go out
2 = goes out   1

D Has suffered physical stress or acute disease in the past 3 months?
0 = yes
2 = no   0

E Neuropsychological problems?
0 = severe dementia or depression
1 = mild dementia
2 = no psychological problems
0

F Body Mass Index (BMI) [weight in kg]/[height in m]²
0 = BMI less than 19
1 = BMI 19 to less than 21
2 = BMI 21 to less than 23
3 = BMI 23 or greater   0

Screening score (subtotal max. 14 points)
12 points or greater   Normal – not at risk →
    no need to complete assessment
11 points or below   Possible malnutrition →
    continue assessment   1

loss can itself cause depression, creating a vicious circle requiring not only antidepressants but nutritional support. The latter was particularly indicated in this case since few women survive a BMI below 10 kg/m², or men below 11 kg/m². Her low temperature and low lymphocyte counts were typical of the failure of thermoregulation and of immunity associated with severe weight loss. She had so-called 'famine edema,' since, with severe weight loss, the extracellular fluid volume as a percentage of body weight increases, and salt and water may be retained in excess.

Despite severe malnutrition, the serum albumin concentration was normal, in the absence of any inflammatory condition. The low blood urea reflected low protein turnover and the low creatinine her diminished muscle mass. Her food intake had been so poor in quantity and quality that multiple micronutrient deficiencies must be presumed. This might account for some of the bruising on her legs. Measurement of vitamin and trace element concentrations in blood are possible in specialized laboratories, but are not routine.

Problems
- Previous thyrotoxicosis and weight loss.
- Severe depression causing anorexia.
- Profound protein–energy malnutrition exacerbating her depression and causing major functional impairment, including failure of the thermogenic response to cold or the febrile response to infection.
- Presumed multiple micronutrient deficiencies.

Clinical decision
Ethical considerations should always inform clinical decisions, particularly at the extremes of life. Ceasing to eat and drink is a feature of dying from whatever cause and terminal dementing illness is no exception. Artificial nutritional support in those circumstances is contraindicated since it exposes the patient to all the risks and confers none of the benefits of the treatment (the ethical principles of beneficence and non-maleficence – see Chapter 9). This patient, however, has two major treatable and reversible conditions – depression and malnutrition. As well as antidepressants, therefore, she requires nasogastric feeding since her anorexia precludes taking sufficient by mouth. The patient's permission was therefore obtained (the ethical principle of autonomy must be observed, except in anorexia nervosa) to pass a fine-bore nasogastric tube whose position was ascertained radiologically.

Nutritional requirements
At 33 kg, her estimated resting metabolic rate was 4.1 MJ (990 kcal) (by Schofield predictive equation see Table 25.1), but with advanced starvation this was reduced by about 10%. Since the aim of treatment is first to avoid refeeding syndrome by too rapid renutrition, secondly to achieve functional improvement in the short term, and thirdly to restore body weight to

normal in the longer term (i.e. over 3–6 months), continuous pump feeding was begun using a polymeric enteral feed of 4.2 kJ/ml at an initial rate of 25 ml/h, increasing to 40 ml/h over three days (i.e. sufficient to meet 1.1 × REE). Tolerance was established and over the next few days the feed was increased to achieve 1.5 × REE. In the second week the nasogastric feed was given at 100 ml/h overnight only, allowing oral intake and activity by day. Continuous enteral feeding may disinhibit the appetite so that increasing voluntary oral intake can be used as a monitor of response to this as well as the antidepressants.

Treatment

By the end of the first week, therefore, she was established on an intake of 5 MJ (1200 kcal) per day and 1.5 g/kg per day of protein. A standard multivitamin preparation plus folate 5 mg/day was sufficient to repair deficiencies and meet her needs. Additional thiamine, potassium, and phosphate were also given. Lofepramine 70 mg daily was prescribed for her depression since this is better tolerated by the elderly than tricyclics or selective seratonin reuptake inhibitors (SSRIs).

Monitoring and outcome

After two weeks of antidepressants and overnight nasogastric feeding, her voluntary oral intake had risen sufficiently to meet her requirements and there was improvement in both mental and physical function. Her edema had resolved with loss of 3 kg in weight, but this was partially offset by a 1-kg gain of real tissue. After the first four days her basal temperature had risen from 35 to 36.5°C. She was then transferred to a convalescent unit and ultimately discharged with gradual and steady weight gain of 0.5 kg per week. Careful observations were made for any complications such as reflux, aspiration of feed, abdominal distension, diarrhea, or tube displacement, but after some initial mild diarrhea 2–3 times daily, responsive to loperamide, there were no further complications.

Learning points

- The syndrome of anorexia of psychological origin is not confined to young women. It may be difficult to treat at any age but in the elderly sometimes responds to antidepressants, addressing precipitating factors such as social isolation, and nutritional support.

- Refeeding should be introduced gradually by the oral and enteral route, with careful observations made for complications such as refeeding syndrome, diarrhea, or aspiration.
- Enteral feeding overnight may help to disinhibit appetite and also allows oral intake and activity by day.

25.5 Bowel disease

Case 4

A 63-year-old patient with active Crohn's disease for five years was admitted with weight loss from 54 to 44 kg over a six-month period. She had developed an enterovaginal and enterovesical fistula and had edema, suggesting a true tissue weight of <42 kg.

Screening

Nutritional screening showed a BMI of 14 kg/m², 20% weight loss, diminished food intake, and active disease, giving a high risk score of 10.

Assessment

Nutritional assessment revealed depression, apathy, and weakness with edema and a serum albumin of 15 g/l, reflecting inflammation and serous losses from infected fistulas.

Problems
- Gastrointestinal failure
- Gross protein–energy malnutrition
- Probable micronutrient and mineral deficiencies
- Fistula and fluid losses
- Active inflammation due to Crohn's disease and infection.

Clinical decision

Due to the intestinal fistulas, this woman clearly needed parenteral nutrition. A tunnelled subclavian line was inserted. Initial objectives of nutritional care should have been:

- Gradual introduction of feeding to avoid metabolic disturbance.
- Correction of fluid, electrolyte, mineral, and micronutrient deficiencies.

- To minimize bowel contents and hence fistula losses, allowing spontaneous healing of the fistula if possible.
- Improved function in the short term.
- To improve her general condition to allow successful medical and surgical management of her underlying condition.
- In the long term to allow regain of lost body tissue.

Nutritional requirements

Her estimated REE was approximately 4.5 MJ (1080 kcal)/day and 1.5 times this figure would be required for weight gain. Her protein needs were 1.5 g/kg or 60 g per day (9–10 g N).

Treatment

Unfortunately she was treated with excessive enthusiasm, being infused parenterally with 12 MJ (2870 kcal) (including 400 g of glucose) and 18 g N per day. Her Crohn's was managed by a combination of medical and surgical treatment.

Monitoring

Within 24 hours she became extremely short of breath. A pulmonary embolus was suspected until the infusion rate was halved and her respirations returned to normal as her feed-induced increase in oxygen consumption and CO_2 production resolved.

Outcome

She ultimately required two months of parenteral nutrition before her fistula closed spontaneously and bowel function returned sufficiently to allow normal oral intake. She was well at discharge after regaining 3 kg in weight. Six months later she weighed 52 kg.

Learning points

- Parenteral nutrition is the management of gastrointestinal failure in the same sense that dialysis is the treatment of renal failure and ventilation is of respiratory failure, i.e. it supports organ function until the underlying cause of the problem is resolved.
- This patient's life expectancy without nutritional support was less than six weeks. Survival is unlikely below a BMI of 10 kg/m² or with weight loss of more than 35%, especially in the presence of active disease. Parenteral nutrition was therefore life-saving.
- Carbohydrate and protein/amino acids cause diet-induced thermogenesis and increased demands for

gas exchange. Glucose should rarely be infused at a rate greater than 0.3 g/kg per h, since above this it merely increases CO_2 production and O_2 consumption without useful effect and may be dangerous in those with respiratory failure or in those with respiratory muscle weakness due to disease or malnutrition. Her initial glucose infusion rate was 0.42 g/kg per h, not to mention the 0.4 g N/kg per day – more than twice her requirements.

Case 5 – Chronic gastrointestinal failure

In a 57-year-old man with a ten-year history of intestinal disease the initial diagnosis was Crohn's disease, but this was changed four years before admission to celiac disease with microscopic colitis and gastritis. He was admitted in the past with extensive obstructing strictures in the duodenum and jejunum and underwent partial jejunal resection and gastrojejunostomy. His diet was gluten-free. He suffered osteoporosis from a combination of previous steroid treatment and malnutrition (with cachexia, sex hormone levels fall). Intake and absorption of calcium and vitamin D was also impaired.

Over four years he took an elemental diet, but intestinal strictures, small bowel bacterial colonization, and protein-losing enteropathy continued to be a problem.

He was first seen in the nutrition clinic with serial measurements of weight, function, tests of mood and muscle strength, and serum biochemistry.

Screening

Height 1.7 m, weight 56 kg, BMI 19.1 kg/m². Percentage weight change in three months was +3 kg, although over one year it was –9.7 kg (score 0). Oral intake with elemental supplements appeared adequate (score 0). Disease was quiescent (score 0).

Assessment

Despite the overall picture suggesting that he might need parenteral nutrition in the long term, his recent weight gain and score of 3, combined with some anxiety as to his capacity to cope with the demands of parenteral feeding, led to a decision to rely on oral intake and to follow him in the clinic, measuring weight, muscle strength, biochemistry, and hematology. Results of his anthropometric and biochemical and hematological measurements are shown in Table 25.4.

Table 25.4 Serial data for Case 5

Date	Wt (kg)	BMI	R Handgrip	Albumin (g/l)	Hb (g/l)
Day 0	56.1	20	31.6		10.3
Day 7	52.6	18.7	33.5	26	9.5
Day 20	51.4	18.3	32.4		
Day 29	51.2	18.2	24	21	10.7
Day 49	48.8	17.4	23	19	
Parenteral nutrition started on Day 59					
Day 79	57.5	20.5	32.4	23	11.0
Day 130	61.2	21.8	32.6	28	12.1

Medication
- Prednisolone 5 mg
- Budesonide CR 9 mg
- Lansoprazole 30 mg
- Ferrous sulfate 200 mg
- Calcichew one daily.

As can be seen from Table 25.4, his condition deteriorated with declining weight, muscle strength, serum albumin, and hemoglobin. Selenium concentration was low at 0.44 mmol/l, but magnesium was normal at 0.77 mmol/l.

Problems
- Chronic gastrointestinal failure, unlikely to improve as a result of any further medical or surgical intervention.
- Worsening malnutrition with weight loss and impaired function, with muscle weakness and fatigue, hypoalbuminemia, anemia, selenium depletion, and osteoporosis.
- Fluid depletion from diarrhea.

Clinical decision
- To start parenteral nutrition to restore and maintain nutritional status, while continuing to allow oral intake at will.
- To admit for two weeks of training by an expert nursing team – the mechanical metabolic, thrombotic, and infectious complications of parenteral nutrition are prohibitive without an expert nutrition team to manage both short and long-term administration.

Nutritional requirements
At 50 kg his REE (by Schofield predictive equation – Table 25.1) was 6.0 MJ (1434 kcal). Diet-induced thermogenesis will increase this by 10% and moderate activity by 40%, suggesting an approximate intake to maintain weight of 1.5 × REE, i.e. 9 MJ (2170 kcal) per day. However, the aim was also to increase his weight over 2–3 months back to more than 60 kg and restore his lean mass, meeting the energy cost of protein synthesis. It was decided to allow an extra 30% of energy over basal to meet this need, giving a total energy intake of 12 MJ (2870 kcal) per day.

To maintain nitrogen balance in a healthy man, a minimum of 0.8 g protein/kg per day are required, providing energy needs are met, i.e. a minimum of 40 g in this case. In addition, however, he had continuing protein-losing enteropathy and a requirement for lean mass restoration, i.e. an intake of at least 1.5 g/kg per day of protein (0.24 g N/kg per day). Micronutrient supplements and extra selenium as Na selenite were also required.

The standard ready-made all-in-one feed nearest to these requirements was one of 2.5 liters containing 14 g N (87.5 g protein) and 10.7 MJ (2560 kcal) (1.5 MJ from protein, 3.8 MJ from fat, and 5.4 MJ from carbohydrate (including the glycerol component of the lipid emulsion)).

Treatment and progress
The parenteral nutrition was given for 14 h overnight, seven nights per week, and supplemented by a modest oral intake. The most dramatic initial change, as always, was a large improvement in mood, energy, and muscle strength, occurring before any weight increase. Part of his initial weight gain was due to restoration of extracellular fluid deficit from diarrhea and some gain in intracellular fluid as glycogen stores were replenished. After two months, the parenteral nutrition was reduced to four nights per week, with a reduced energy (7.9 MJ/1890 kcal)) and nitrogen (11 g) composition. In combination with oral intake, this was sufficient to maintain his weight, function, and quality of life. Despite initial apprehensions, he managed his parenteral nutrition perfectly and had no complications during two years of follow-up.

Learning points
- Function is an even more important criterion of nutritional status than changes in body composition. It correlates well with malnutrition and responds rapidly to refeeding even before gain in tissue mass.

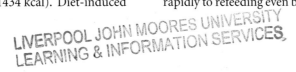

- Home parenteral nutrition is the management of chronic gastrointestinal failure causing malnutrition.
- The parenteral nutrition prescription should take account of likely requirements for tissue regain and maintenance and compensate for fluid, electrolyte, mineral, and micronutrient losses or deficiencies.
- Steroids which are catabolic in respect of bone, connective tissue, and muscle should be kept to the minimum dose necessary.
- Cachexia causes impaired gonadotropin and sex hormone secretion. This with poor nutrient absorption, including Ca and vitamin D, causes osteopenia, which must be treated.
- A parenteral nutrition service requires an expert nutrition team.

Case 6 – Liver disease

A 55-year-old man, height 1.73 m, weight six months previously 52 kg (BMI 17.4 kg/m^2) presented with a current weight of 45 kg (including edema, BMI 15.0 kg/m^2). He had a history of high alcohol intake (more than 1 bottle of whiskey daily) and poor food intake and developed acute confusion, dysuria, and fever 38.5°C. On examination he was jaundiced, with spider nevi, bruising, small testes, ankle edema, liver enlarged 5 cm below the costal margin, no enlargement of the spleen, and distended bladder.

Investigations
- Hemoglobin 13.6 g/dl
- International Normalized Ratio (INR) 1.6
- Mean cell volume (MCV) 121.8 fl = macrocytosis
- Total white cell count 9.25 × 10^9/l
- Erythrocyte sedimentation rate (ESR) 58 mm/1 h
- Blood glucose low at 3.0 mmol
- Blood urea elevated at 8.1 mmol/l
- Sodium 145 mmol/l, potassium 4.4 mmol/l, magnesium 0.59 mmol/l (low), phosphate 1.58 mmol/l
- Liver enzymes elevated. Serum albumin 30 g/l (low). Bilirubin 45 µmol/l (high)
- Urine cloudy and infected

Screening
His nutrition screening scores are 3 for BMI of 15 kg/m^2, 2 for weight loss, 1 for impaired food intake and 2 for disease severity = total score 8.

Assessment and problems
- Alcoholic hepatitis causing liver failure, hypoglycemia, hypoalbuminemia, and hypomagnesemia.
- Urinary retention and infection secondary to prostatic hypertrophy, causing fever, postrenal failure and precipitating hepatic encephalopathy.
- Gross protein–energy malnutrition through anorexia and low intake. Interestingly, one bottle of 40% whiskey (75 cl) containing 300 g alcohol (31.5 kJ/g) provides 9.5 MJ (2270 kcal) energy.
- Impaired immunity secondary to protein–energy malnutrition and liver disease.
- Probably multiple vitamin deficiencies, particularly thiamine, absence of which causes Wernicke's encephalopathy.
- Low prothrombin level secondary to liver disease, requiring vitamin K.

Treatment
- Intravenous antibiotics and urinary catheterization.
- Thiamine 100 mg × 3 daily and oral multivitamin preparation.
- Vitamin K 1 mg.
- Enteral nutrition via nasogastric tube using a standard polymeric diet (as in European Society of Parenteral and Enteral Nutrition guidelines).
- Later, counseling concerning alcohol intake.
- Chlordiazepoxide to cover alcohol withdrawal symptoms.

Nutritional requirements
It takes a 3-liter salt and water overload before edema is manifest, so this man's real weight is a maximum of 42 kg. REE was therefore 5.7 MJ (1360 kcal)/day. Allowing a 10% increase for diet-induced thermogenesis, and a 13% increase per 1°C rise in temperature, this gives a total energy requirement of 7.8 MJ (1860 kcal)/day to maintain zero energy balance. Once his catabolic phase is over, however, he will need another 2 MJ (480 kcal)/day to meet the cost of restoring lost tissue. Cirrhotic patients without infection also have a raised resting energy expenditure at 10% over estimated for weight and height. Although branched-chain amino acid preparations are available for either enteral or parenteral use and can help to reverse encephalopathy, they are unbalanced in their amino acid profile.

Standard polymeric feeds are therefore preferred in most cases of malnutrition secondary to liver disease. Remarkably, increasing protein intake, up to a point, does not usually worsen encephalopathy in most cases. In this case, 0.2 g N/kg per day would be a reasonable starting point, increasing as tolerated up to 0.3 g/kg per day during recovery (52 g protein, increasing to 78 g per day).

Progress

Despite starting a 4.2 kJ/ml (1 kcal/ml) enteral feed at only 30 ml/h increasing to 80 ml/h over five days, his serum magnesium fell from 0.59 to 0.49 mmol/l (0.74–1.0), his serum phosphate from 1.58 to 0.31 (0.8–1.5), and his serum potassium from 5.5 to 2.9 mmol, necessitating intravenous administration of magnesium sulfate and potassium phosphate in dextrose. This refeeding syndrome (see Case 2) is typical of the response to feeding in extremely cachectic individuals and may be fatal if untreated. For a further three weeks, the patient received 9 MJ (2150 kcal) and 12.4 g N/day enterally before beginning oral intake. As this increased, so his enteral feeding was limited to the night hours and then withdrawn. Overnight enteral feeding usually disinhibits appetite. After 45 days of admission, he was discharged weighing 50 kg. He subsequently stayed off alcohol, his liver function returned to normal and his weight gradually rose over six months to over 60 kg.

Learning points

- Liver disease is associated with anorexia, poor food intake, protein–energy malnutrition, increased metabolic rate, and multiple vitamin deficiencies.
- In acute liver failure secondary to alcoholism, give thiamine in therapeutic doses as well as a multivitamin preparation. Vitamin K may be required if INR (International Normalized Ratio – an indicator of clotting ability) is prolonged.
- True weight loss may be marked by edema and/or ascites.
- If oral intake is inadequate, enteral feeding using a standard polymeric feed is the treatment of choice.
- The feed should be introduced slowly and gradually increased to meet targets.
- Electrolytes, phosphate, and magnesium levels should be monitored for refeeding syndrome and any falls in concentration corrected.

25.6 Catabolic illness

Case 7 – Sepsis, anorexia, and the effect of drugs

A man aged 45 years underwent arthroscopy of the knee. A week later he developed pain in the thigh which worsened over two weeks, accompanied by fever and malaise. He then underwent drainage of osteomyelitis of the right femur and received antibiotics for a *Streptococcus milleri* infection. One month later he developed a large abscess of the thigh with fever of 38°C and underwent further drainage, with antibiotics in the form of penicillin and metronidazole. His premorbid weight had been 70 kg and he now weighed 59 kg but with marked edema. He was anorexic and nauseated, managing an energy intake of only 1 MJ (240 kcal)/day despite all attempts at oral intake including supplements.

Screening

Height 1.7 m, weight 59 kg (real weight 54 kg after resolution of edema). Based on 54 kg his BMI was 19 kg/m^2 (score 2). Percentage weight loss was 20% (score 3). Grossly reduced intake (score 2). Disease severity (score 2). Total 9, indicating high nutritional risk.

Assessment

In view of his poor intake with nausea and vomiting, the nutrition team were asked to see him to provide parenteral nutrition. His symptoms, however, appeared disproportionate to his underlying disease, and suspicion fell on the side effects of his drugs. Albumin 29 g/l, hemoglobin 9.7 g, secondary to sepsis.

Problems

- Sepsis and abscess causing increased metabolic rate (+13% per 1°C rise in temperature).
- This combined with decreased intake resulted in 20% weight loss, weakness, and immobility.
- Nauseating effect of metronidazole preventing adequate oral intake.

Clinical decision

- Treat infection by drainage and penicillin.
- Stop metronidazole.
- Observe oral intake.

Nutritional requirements

At least $1.5 \times$ REE for weight gain and 1.5 g protein/kg per day.

Monitoring and outcome

With successful treatment of the infection his fever subsided. After stopping metronidazole all his nausea and anorexia disappeared and his spontaneous oral intake rose to over 10 MJ (2400 kcal) daily. He regained weight rapidly, mobilized, and was discharged three weeks later.

Learning points

- Trauma, infection, and inflammation increase metabolic rate, accelerating weight loss and protein catabolism. Cytokines released by inflammation also depress appetite.
- First treat the underlying catabolic disease to reduce rate of weight loss, e.g. by draining an abscess.
- Drugs have many side effects that can affect nutritional status. Always consider the nutritional effects of medications.
- Use oral feeding where possible.

Case 8 – Burns

A man of 36 years (weight 70 kg, height 1.8 m, BMI 21.6 kg/m^2) and previously fit, suffered burn injury of 50% of his body surface (half being full thickness and half partial). He also suffered smoke inhalation necessitating ventilation in the intensive care unit (ICU) for a period of two weeks. After the initial 24-h resuscitation period, the question of feeding arose.

Screening

Although zero food intake and a disease severity score of 2 gave a total score of 4, this does not reflect the severity of the metabolic problem. Like all measurements, therefore, screening must be interpreted intelligently in the light of the clinical circumstances and a knowledge of the likely natural history of the disease.

Assessment

Although nutritionally normal at the time of injury, his subsequent catabolic illness and inability to eat will necessitate artificial nutritional support, preferably by the oral and enteral route.

Problems

- Prolonged catabolic illness with consequent wasting of lean body mass which can be reduced but not abolished by feeding.
- Prolonged immobility enhancing muscle wasting.
- Sepsis, ventilatory failure, and repeated surgical procedures.
- Additional micronutrient requirements due to excess loss of copper, zinc, and selenium and the need for extra vitamins, e.g. vitamin C.
- Need to design nutrient intake accurately to give maximum benefit without the problems of metabolic overload, e.g. increasing demand for gas exchange, hyperglycemia, increasing risk of infection, etc.
- May need extra amounts of special substrates, e.g. glutamine, ornithine alpha-ketoglutarate.

Nutritional requirements

In the past, such a burn injury would have been associated with a total energy requirement in excess of $1.5 \times$ REE. With modern methods of management – (1) nursing in a thermoneutral environment (normal 28–29°C, burned patients 30–32°C), (2) early debridement and grafting, and (3) better management of infection, pain, and fluid balance – the formerly reported high energy expenditures are no longer seen and it is rarely necessary to give more than $1.3 \times$ estimated REE (see Schofield predictive equation, Table 25.1), which in this case was 9.1 MJ (2175 kcal)/day. Centers with facilities for daily measurement of REE can achieve more accurate energy balance since estimated and measured may differ by 30% or more during critical illness.

Nitrogen intakes in excess of 0.25 g/kg per day ($\times$ 6.25 = 1.56 g protein/kg per day) are converted to urea, increasing osmotic load and not contributing usefully to nitrogen balance. Energy requirements were met from 105 g protein = 1.8 MJ (430 kcal), 250 g glucose = 4.2 MJ (1000 kcal) (well below the 0.3 g/kg per h at which gas exchange is adversely affected) and fat to meet an additional 3.2 MJ (765 kcal). There is also need for extra micronutrients (see above) and benefit is obtained from giving glutamine or ornithine alpha-ketoglutarate to enhance antioxidant and immune function as well as improving nitrogen balance. The role of immune-enhancing cocktails containing arginine, *n*-3 fatty acids, and nucleotides is controversial.

Clinical decision

- To begin feeding after 24 h, by the enteral route if possible, starting at 20 ml/h of a 1.0 kcal/ml standard polymeric feed by the nasogastric route, aspirating every 4 h to test gastric emptying. Nurse patient in a semi-recumbent position (if allowed by the distribution of burn injury) to minimize risk of aspiration.
- To supplement the feed by the parenteral route, if necessary, to meet nutritional targets.
- To give micronutrient supplements.
- To give additional glutamine.

Treatment and clinical course

Clear and realistic goals of evidence-based nutritional support were

- to minimize loss of lean mass,
- to correct or prevent mineral, electrolyte, and micronutrient abnormalities,
- to support muscle (particularly respiratory) function,
- to maintain antioxidant status,
- to support gut and immune function and reduce the risk of invasive infection,
- to avoid metabolic, mechanical or other complications of artificial nutritional support, and
- to optimize healing of wounds and grafts.

Initially, gastric aspirations were high and enteral feeding was not tolerated. After the first week, however, enteral feeding could be introduced and increased to the full target of 9 MJ (2150 kcal) and 105 g of protein. Initially, therefore, parenteral nutrition was begun using a glutamine dipeptide-containing 'all-in-one' solution via a central catheter. Nutritional targets were maintained by this route until the 10th day, when parenteral feeding was tailed off as full enteral feeding became tolerated. His blood glucose rose to 12 mmol/l and therefore a high-dose insulin infusion was begun to maintain normoglycemia (4–7 mmol/l), since insulin used in this way has been shown to improve nitrogen economy, enhance capacity to excrete excess salt and water, reduce infection, and improve survival and outcome in critically ill patients including burns.

Despite these measures, the patient lost 15% of his body weight during his three-week stay in the ICU. On his return to the ward, someone decided to feed more aggressively and doubled his enteral protein intake. After a few days, his blood urea had risen to 30 mmol/l

and he appeared dehydrated. A consultation for 'renal failure' resulted in a realization that the problem was excessive protein intake causing a high urea production rate and an osmotic diuresis. The consequent fluid deficit was also exacerbated by diarrhea. Reducing the enteral feed rate and increasing fluid intake corrected the problem. His subsequent course was uneventful, although nutritional supplements were continued, since insulin resistance and impaired protein synthesis persist for many weeks. As he became more mobile and started to eat, his energy and protein intake could be usefully increased to restore lost tissue.

Learning points

- Burn injury is the most potent cause of catabolic illness, but modern management has reduced the stress stimulus.
- Loss of lean mass can be minimized but not abolished by feeding in catabolic illness. The goals of feeding include preservation of as much lean mass as possible, maintenance of tissue function, reduced complications, and more rapid recovery.
- Feeding should be begun as early as possible, preferably by the enteral route but supplemented parenterally if necessary, to achieve nutritional goals.
- To optimize benefit and minimize risk, avoid the complications of artificial nutrition by using strict protocols and an expert team.
- Nutritional requirements for most burned adult patients are met by supplying 1.3 × estimated REE and 0.25 g N/kg per day. Micronutrient and mineral supplementation is beneficial. The use of substrates, e.g. glutamine or ornithine alpha-ketoglutarate is also helpful.
- During catabolic illness, the former hyperalimentation regimens have been abandoned in favor of a more conservative approach, with higher nutritional intakes during convalescence and rehabilitation when high nutrient loads can be utilized.
- High-dose insulin and maintenance of normoglycemia have metabolic and clinical benefits.

25.7 Dysphagia

When the swallowing mechanism is impaired by neuromuscular disease (e.g. motor neuron disease) or mechanical obstruction (e.g. upper gastrointestinal tract cancer), artificial enteral feeding is indicated. Early assessment and nutritional intervention should be undertaken before significant weight loss occurs. Since gastrointestinal function is usually intact apart from swallowing, enteral feeding via a gastrostomy or jejunostomy is the preferred feeding method, although nasogastric feeding may be employed for short periods.

Case 9 – Motor neuron disease

A 60-year-old woman presented with dysarthria and dysphagia due to bulbar manifestations of motor neuron disease. At first she was able to swallow semi-solids and could maintain her weight. This became an increasing struggle and she began to choke on liquids and solids and was unable to swallow her medication. Her weight had fallen from 55 kg to below 50 kg by the time of her referral by the neurologists to the nutrition unit.

Screening
Height 1.63 m, weight 49 kg, BMI 19 kg/m^2 (score 2). Weight loss >3 kg (score 2). Food intake decreased (score 1). Disease severity (score 2). Total 7.

Assessment and clinical decision
In view of her worsening dysphagia she will clearly die of starvation or aspiration pneumonia without artificial feeding. Since, at this stage, she had well-preserved limb function, she was advised to have a percutaneous endoscopic gastrostomy (PEG) placed to allow self-administration home enteral nutrition and a reasonable quality of life.

Nutritional requirements
Estimated REE (calculated by Schofield, see Table 25.1) was 4.7 MJ (1120 kcal). Since she was mobile and needed weight gain, a target of $1.5 \times$ REE was set at 7 MJ (1670 kcal). Protein requirement was estimated to be 1.5 g/kg initially for weight gain, falling to 1.0 g/kg for maintenance. Care was needed to ensure that the dose of proprietary enteral feed to achieve these targets also contained sufficient micronutrients to meet her requirements.

Treatment
A PEG was inserted without complications and following our strict management protocols. Over the next week she was trained to give herself overnight enteral feeding at between 100 and 125 ml/h. Rates greater than this may induce reflux, especially in the horizontal position, and may increase diet-induced thermogenesis and demand for gas exchange. In the presence of respiratory muscle weakness (as in motor neuron disease), this may induce shortness of breath. Additional bolus feeding was also given by day, with additional water. Care was taken to avoid tube blockage by flushing with water after each period of feeding.

Progress and monitoring
She managed her feeds extremely well for 18 months until muscle weakness developed and a carer had to administer them. Weight was restored to 53 kg and maintained at this until the terminal phase. She died of her condition two years after initial presentation.

Learning points
Home enteral feeding using a gastrostomy or jejunostomy may maintain life of reasonable quality in dysphagic patients. It has been shown to confer benefit in about 25% of patients with motor neuron disease, particularly when bulbar symptoms predominate.

Combine overnight pump with daytime bolus feeding, avoiding rates of administration in excess of 125 ml/h to avoid reflux with aspiration or excessive diet-induced thermogenesis.

Best results are obtained by an expert team using strict protocols and a program of training, hot-line contact, and follow-up for the patient and carers.

25.8 Obesity

Case 10

A 23-year-old man with learning difficulties admitted to hospital with a respiratory infection.

On examination
Morbidly obese (height 1.6 m, weight 180 kg, BMI 62 kg/m^2). Fever 37.8°C. Cough and purulent sputum. Cyanosed. Dependent edema and raised jugular venous pressure, indicating right heart failure.

Investigations
- Hemoglobin 18 g/l
- Pao_2 9 kPa
- Pco_2 7.3 kPa

- HCO_3 32 mmol/l
- Blood glucose 15.0 mmol/l.

These tests may be interpreted as showing a chronic anoxic state (compensatory polycythemia) and chronic CO_2 retention (compensatory increase in HCO_3). The random blood glucose >11.0 mmol (15 mmol) showed that he was already developing type 2 diabetes from insulin resistance caused by obesity.

Screening and assessment
Screening data with BMI of 62 kg/m² showed morbid obesity. (Obesity is defined as BMI >30 kg/m² and morbid obesity >40 kg/m².) History from mother revealed constant eating.

Problems
- Morbid obesity causing impaired ventilation with respiratory failure (Pickwickian syndrome) and secondary pulmonary hypertension and right heart failure.
- Exacerbation of respiratory problems by acute infective bronchitis.
- Huge food intake.

Treatment and progress
Five-day course of antibiotics and physiotherapy for his acute bronchitis.

Long-term food restriction and exercise program. Since he had no independent access to food and his mother was his sole carer, it was possible to ensure dietary compliance, which is not usually the case in morbidly obese patients. Additional measures could include drugs, e.g. sibutramine (appetite suppressant) or orlistat (intestinal lipase inhibitor to cause fat malabsorption). Bariatric surgery is the most successful form of treatment and can be undertaken in suitable cases if all else fails (see Chapter 3).

This patient was able to lose 50 kg in nine months as a result of dietary restriction and exercise under supervision. His blood glucose fell to normal and his respiratory and cardiac failure resolved to the point where his exercise tolerance was virtually normal.

Learning points
- Morbid obesity (BMI >40 kg//m²) is a dangerous condition with many complications including diabetes, hypertension, arterial disease, cardiorespiratory failure, increased cancer risk, and crippling arthritis.
- Obesity of any degree is identified by routine screening allowing appropriate referral and treatment.
- Obesity is difficult to treat by diet alone except in highly motivated patients. The same applies to exercise. Additional drug support is effective. Bariatric surgery used appropriately is the most effective.
- The prevalence of obesity in the UK has increased from 6 to 20% over 20 years and represents a major health problem for the future.

Useful weblinks for core nutrition journals

American Journal of Clinical Nutrition.
www.ajcn.org
British Journal of Nutrition.
www.nutsoc.org.uk/Publications/bjn.htm
Clinical Nutrition.
www.harcourt-international.com/journals/clnu/
European Journal of Clinical Nutrition.
www.nature.com/ejcn/
Journal of Human Nutrition and Dietetics.
www.blackwellpublishing.com/journal
Journal of Nutrition. www.nutrition.org
Journal of Pediatric Gastroenterology and Nutrition.
www.jpgn.org
Journal of the American Dietetic Association.
www2.adajournal.org
Nutrition in Clinical Practice.
www.clinnutr.org/publications/ncpabstracts/ncpabs.htm
Nutrition Research.
www.journals.elsevierhealth.com/periodicals/NTR
Nutrition.
www.journals.elsevierhealth.com/periodicals/nut
Proceedings of the Nutrition Society.
www.nutsoc.org.uk/Publications/bjn.htm
PubMed.
www.ncbi.nlm.nih.gov/entrez/query.fcgi?db=PubMed

References

Schofield WN. Predicting basal metabolic rate, new standards and a review of previous work. *Hum Nutr Clin Nutr* 1985; 39C (Suppl 1): 5–41.

Index